I0072101

Insomnia Treatments: Therapeutic Potential of Orexin Antagonist

Insomnia Treatments: Therapeutic Potential of Orexin Antagonist

Edited by Matthew Woods

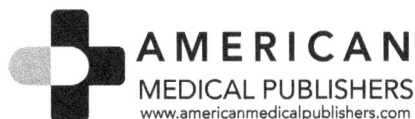

AMERICAN
MEDICAL PUBLISHERS
www.americanmedicalpublishers.com

American Medical Publishers,
41 Flatbush Avenue,
1st Floor, New York,
NY 11217, USA

Visit us on the World Wide Web at:
www.americanmedicalpublishers.com

© American Medical Publishers, 2022

This book contains information obtained from authentic and highly regarded sources. Copyright for all individual chapters remain with the respective authors as indicated. All chapters are published with permission under the Creative Commons Attribution License or equivalent. A wide variety of references are listed. Permission and sources are indicated; for detailed attributions, please refer to the permissions page and list of contributors. Reasonable efforts have been made to publish reliable data and information, but the authors, editors and publisher cannot assume any responsibility for the validity of all materials or the consequences of their use.

ISBN: 978-1-63927-542-7

Trademark Notice: Registered trademark of products or corporate names are used only for explanation and identification without intent to infringe.

Cataloging-in-Publication Data

Insomnia treatments : therapeutic potential of orexin antagonist / edited by Matthew Woods.
    p. cm.
Includes bibliographical references and index.
ISBN 978-1-63927-542-7
1. Insomnia--Treatment. 2. Orexins--Therapeutic use. 3. Sleep disorders.
4. Psychopharmacology. I. Woods, Matthew.
RC548 .I57 2022
616.849 8--dc23

Table of Contents

Preface.. IX

Chapter 1   Orexin, orexin receptor antagonists and central cardiovascular control 1
             Pascal Carrive

Chapter 2   Distinct effects of IPSU and suvorexant on mouse sleep architecture........................... 8
             Daniel Hoyer, Thomas Dürst, Markus Fendt, Laura H. Jacobson, Claudia Betschart,
             Samuel Hintermann, Dirk Behnke, Simona Cotesta, Grit Laue, Silvio Ofner,
             Eric Legangneux and Christine E. Gee

Chapter 3   Dual orexin receptor antagonists show distinct effects on locomotor performance,
             ethanol interaction and sleep architecture relative to gamma-aminobutyric
             acid-A receptor modulators.. 14
             Andres D. Ramirez, Anthony L. Gotter, Steven V. Fox, Pamela L. Tannenbaum,
             Lih angYao, Spencer J. Tye, Terrence McDonald, Joseph Brunner, Susan L. Garson,
             Duane R. Reiss, Scott D. Kuduk, Paul J. Coleman, Jason M. Uslaner, Robert Hodgson,
             Susan E. Browne, John J. Renger and Christopher J. Winrow

Chapter 4   Orexin receptor antagonists as therapeutic agents for insomnia 25
             Ana C. Equihua, Alberto K. De La Herrán-Arita and Rene Drucker-Colin

Chapter 5   Orexin 1 receptor antagonists in compulsive behavior and anxiety: possible
             therapeutic use 35
             Emilio Merlo Pich and Sergio Melotto

Chapter 6   Hypocretin (orexin) regulation of sleep-to-wake transitions...................................... 41
             Luis de Lecea and Ramón Huerta

Chapter 7   Synaptic interactions between perifornical lateral hypothalamic area, locus
             coeruleus nucleus and the oral pontine reticular nucleus are implicated in the
             stage succession during sleep-wakefulness cycle... 48
             Silvia Tortorella, Margarita L. Rodrigo-Angulo, Angel Núñez and Miguel Garzón

Chapter 8   Orexin-1 and orexin-2 receptor antagonists reduce ethanol self-administration in
             high-drinking rodent models.. 57
             Rachel I. Anderson, Howard C. Becker, Benjamin L. Adams,
             Cynthia D. Jesudason and Linda M. Rorick-Kehn

Chapter 9   Orexin antagonists for neuropsychiatric disease: progress and potential pitfalls 66
             Jiann Wei Yeoh, Erin J. Campbell, Morgan H. James,
             Brett A. Graham and Christopher V. Dayas

Chapter 10   Orexin-1 receptor blockade dysregulates REM sleep in the presence
of orexin-2 receptor antagonism 78
Christine Dugovic, Jonathan E. Shelton, Sujin Yun, Pascal Bonaventure,
Brock T. Shireman and Timothy W. Lovenberg

Chapter 11   The hypocretin/orexin antagonist almorexant promotes sleep without impairment
of performance in rats 86
Stephen R. Morairty, Alan J. Wilk, Webster U. Lincoln, Thomas C. Neylan and
Thomas S. Kilduff

Chapter 12   The selective orexin receptor 1 antagonist ACT-335827 in a rat model of
diet-induced obesity associated with metabolic syndrome 94
Michel A. Steiner, Carla Sciarretta, Anne Pasquali and Francois Jenck

Chapter 13   Kinetic properties of "dual" orexin receptor antagonists at OX_1R and OX_2R
orexin receptors 106
Gabrielle E. Callander, Morenike Olorunda, Dominique Monna, Edi Schuepbach,
Daniel Langenegger, Claudia Betschart, Samuel Hintermann, Dirk Behnke,
Simona Cotest, Markus Fendt, Grit Laue, Silvio Ofner, Emmanuelle Briard,
Christine E. Gee, Laura H. Jacobson and Daniel Hoyer

Chapter 14   Cannabinoid-hypocretin cross-talk in the central nervous system: what we
know so far 116
África Flores, Rafael Maldonado and Fernando Berrendero

Chapter 15   LSN2424100: a novel, potent orexin-2 receptor antagonist with selectivity over
orexin-1 receptors and activity in an animal model predictive of
antidepressant-like efficacy 133
Thomas E. Fitch, Mark J. Benvenga, Cynthia D. Jesudason, Charity Zink,
Amy B. Vandergriff, Michelle M. Menezes, Douglas A. Schober and
Linda M. Rorick-Kehn

Chapter 16 OX_1 and OX_2 orexin/hypocretin receptor pharmacogenetics 144
Miles D. Thompson, Henri Xhaard, Takeshi Sakurai, Innocenzo Rainero and
Jyrki P. Kukkonen

Chapter 17   Orexin A and orexin receptor 1 axonal traffic in dorsal roots at the
CNS/PNS interface 156
Damien Colas, Annalisa Manca, Jean-Dominique Delcroix and Philippe Mourrain

Chapter 18   Effects of a newly developed potent orexin-2 receptor-selective
antagonist, compound 1 m, on sleep/wakefulness states in mice 163
Keishi Etori, Yuki C. Saito, Natsuko Tsujino and Takeshi Sakurai

Chapter 19   Orexin, cardio-respiratory function, and hypertension 176
Aihua Li and Eugene Nattie

Chapter 20   **Differential actions of orexin receptors in brainstem cholinergic and monoaminergic neurons revealed by receptor knockouts: implications for orexinergic signalling in arousal and narcolepsy**... 194
Kristi A. Kohlmeier, Christopher J. Tyler, Mike Kalogiannis, Masaru Ishibashi, Morten P. Kristensen, Iryna Gumenchuk, Richard M. Chemelli, Yaz Y. Kisanuki, Masashi Yanagisawa and Christopher S. Leonard

Permissions

List of Contributors

Index

Preface

This book was inspired by the evolution of our times; to answer the curiosity of inquisitive minds. Many developments have occurred across the globe in the recent past which has transformed the progress in the field.

Insomnia or sleeplessness is a sleep disorder which causes difficulty in falling asleep, or staying asleep as long as desired. It also leads to excessive daytime sleepiness, low energy and a depressed mood. Treatment for insomnia usually involves sleep-inducing medication, cognitive behavioral therapy for insomnia (CBT-i), or a combination of both. Orexins are neurotransmitters in the body that regulate feelings of sleepiness and wakefulness. An orexin antagonist inhibits the effects of orexin, and can be used to treat insomnia. This book provides comprehensive insights into the field of insomnia treatments. It is compiled in such a manner, that it will provide in-depth knowledge about the therapeutic potential of orexin antagonist. This book will serve as a reference to a broad spectrum of readers.

This book was developed from a mere concept to drafts to chapters and finally compiled together as a complete text to benefit the readers across all nations. To ensure the quality of the content we instilled two significant steps in our procedure. The first was to appoint an editorial team that would verify the data and statistics provided in the book and also select the most appropriate and valuable contributions from the plentiful contributions we received from authors worldwide. The next step was to appoint an expert of the topic as the Editor-in-Chief, who would head the project and finally make the necessary amendments and modifications to make the text reader-friendly. I was then commissioned to examine all the material to present the topics in the most comprehensible and productive format.

I would like to take this opportunity to thank all the contributing authors who were supportive enough to contribute their time and knowledge to this project. I also wish to convey my regards to my family who have been extremely supportive during the entire project.

Editor

Orexin, orexin receptor antagonists and central cardiovascular control

Pascal Carrive *

Blood Pressure, Brain and Behavior Laboratory, School of Medical Sciences, University of New South Wales, Sydney, NSW, Australia

Edited by:
Michel A. Steiner, Actelion
Pharmaceuticals Ltd., Switzerland

Reviewed by:
Giovanna Zoccoli, University of
Bologna, Italy
Tomoyuki Kuwaki, Kagoshima
University Graduate School of
Medical and Dental Sciences, Japan

*Correspondence:
Pascal Carrive, School of Medical
Sciences, University of New South
Wales, Sydney, NSW 2052, Australia
e-mail: p.carrive@unsw.du.au

Orexin makes an important contribution to the regulation of cardiovascular function. When injected centrally under anesthesia, orexin increases blood pressure, heart rate and sympathetic nerve activity. This is consistent with the location of orexin neurons in the hypothalamus and the distribution of orexin terminals in the central autonomic network. Thus, the two orexin receptors, Ox1R and Ox2R, which have partly overlapping distributions in the brain, are expressed in the sympathetic preganglionic neurons (SPN) of the thoracic cord as well as in regions such as the pressor area of the rostral ventrolateral medulla (RVLM). Both Ox1R and Ox2R appear to contribute to the cardiovascular effects of orexin, although Ox1R is probably more important. Blockade of orexin receptors reduces the cardiovascular response to certain stressors, especially psychogenic stressors such as novelty, aggressive conspecifics and induced panic. Blockade of orexin receptors also reduces basal blood pressure and heart rate in spontaneous hypertensive rats, a model of essential hypertension. Thus, there is a link between psychogenic stress, orexin and elevated blood pressure. The use of dual orexin receptor antagonists (DORAs) and selective orexin receptor antagonists (SORAs) may be beneficial in the treatment of certain forms of hypertension.

Keywords: Ox1R, Ox2R, blood pressure, heart rate, sympathetic, rostral ventrolateral medulla, psychological stress, SHR

INTRODUCTION

Orexin contributes to the central regulation of cardiovascular function because it is a key player in the control of wakefulness and arousal. Indeed, to stay awake and interacting with the environment requires autonomic and cardiovascular adjustments not only to support muscle activity but also to prepare for muscle activity, as is the case for motivated behaviors and emotions. This link with arousal and motivated behavior makes orexin a significant new player in the field of central cardiovascular control. Most of our knowledge of central cardiovascular control is based on brainstem-mediated short-term homeostatic regulation that has been studied in the anesthetized preparation, while comparatively little is known about suprabulbar regulation in relation to behavior and emotions. In other words, orexin reveals another dimension of central cardiovascular control, one that could lead to new therapeutic interventions in some forms of cardiovascular diseases, such as for example, stress related hypertension or essential hypertension.

EARLY STUDIES

The cardiovascular effects of orexin were first demonstrated in 1999 by Samson et al. (1999) and Shirasaka et al. (1999). Both studies showed that orexin A and orexin B (OxA, OxB, 1–5 nmol) could evoke marked and sustained increases in blood pressure when injected in the lateral ventricle of freely moving rats. Both reported a stronger effect with OxA than OxB. Most importantly, Shirasaka et al. showed (i) that this pressor effect was associated with an increase in heart rate and renal sympathetic nerve activity and (ii) that the same effects could still be evoked under

anesthesia. The later two findings established without doubt that the cardiovascular effect of orexin was due to a direct central sympathoexcitatory action. This was confirmed shortly after in a series of three papers by Dun and collaborators (Chen et al., 2000; Dun et al., 2000; Antunes et al., 2001). They showed that the same cardiovascular effects were still evoked (i) by intracisternal and intrathecal (T2–T3) injections of OxA and OxB and (ii) by microinjections of OxA in the vasopressor area of the rostral ventrolateral medulla [RVLM, (Chen et al., 2000; Dun et al., 2000)]. They also demonstrated that OxA and OxB directly depolarize vasopressor neurons of the RVLM and sympathetic preganglionic neurons (SPN) in the thoracic cord (Dun et al., 2000; Antunes et al., 2001).

Pharmacological blockade studies were not possible at the time due to lack of receptor antagonists. However, a seminal study by Kayaba et al. (2003) showed that orexin knock out mice had (i) a reduced basal blood pressure and (ii) a reduced cardiovascular response to a psychosocial stressor (resident-intruder test), but not to a noxious stimulus (tail pinch). This study suggested an important role of orexin in the cardiovascular response to motivated behavior.

ANATOMY OF THE OREXIN SYSTEM IN RELATION TO THE CENTRAL AUTONOMIC NETWORK
OREXIN NEURONS AND THEIR CONNECTIONS

The neurons that make orexin are found in the dorsal part of the tuberal hypothalamus, nowhere else in the brain. The group is centered on the perifornical area (PeF) and extends medially into the dorsomedial hypothalamic nucleus and laterally into the lateral hypothalamic area (Peyron et al., 1998; Nambu et al., 1999). Interestingly, this region corresponds relatively well to the classic hypothalamic defense area, a region identified more than 50 years ago and from which powerful behavioral and cardiovascular responses can be evoked (Hilton, 1982; Carrive, 2011).

Specific inputs to orexin neurons, identified with a genetically encoded retrograde tracer (Sakurai et al., 2005) or from appositions of anterogradely labeled terminals (Yoshida et al., 2006), originate mostly from forebrain areas, either limbic [lateral septum, bed nucleus of the stria terminalis (BNST), amygdala, infralimbic cortex] or hypothalamic (preoptic area, posterior hypothalamus). These regions are also well known for their role in emotions and autonomic control (Saper, 2004).

On the output side, orexin terminals can be seen not only in the limbic structures described above where they make reciprocal connections, but also in all the autonomic centers of the hypothalamus and brainstem, including the periaqueductal gray (PAG), parabrachial nucleus, nucleus of the solitary tract (Sol), the premotor sympathetic centers of the paraventricular nucleus of the hypothalamus (Pa), rostral ventrolateral and ventromedial medulla (RVLM, RVMM) and medullary raphe (**Figure 1**) (Peyron et al., 1998; Nambu et al., 1999; Baldo et al., 2003; Ciriello

and De Oliveira, 2003; Ciriello et al., 2003; Zheng et al., 2005; Shahid et al., 2012). Orexin neurons are also themselves premotor sympathetic neurons since they directly innervate SPN (Van Den Pol, 1999; Date et al., 2000; Llewellyn-Smith et al., 2003). Projections are also found in the dorsal motor nucleus of the vagus although the projection may be weak (Peyron et al., 1998; De Oliveira et al., 2003). Thus, orexin neurons can act at all levels of the central autonomic network, from limbic structures to premotor autonomic centers to the SPNs themselves.

OREXIN RECEPTORS AND THEIR DISTRIBUTION

There are two orexin receptors, Ox1R and Ox2R (Gotter et al., 2012). OxA can act on both Ox1R and Ox2R while OxB acts primarily on Ox2R. The two receptors have a differential, partly overlapping distribution in the brain, including within the central autonomic network (**Figure 1**). However, it is not clear how the two receptors relate to the cardiovascular functions of orexin.

Three main *in situ* hybridization studies have compared the distribution of the two receptors in the brain and hypothalamus (Trivedi et al., 1998; Lu et al., 2000; Marcus et al., 2001). They show that the BNST expresses both receptors while the amygdala primarily expresses Ox1R and the septum primarily Ox2R. In the hypothalamus, most areas express both receptors,

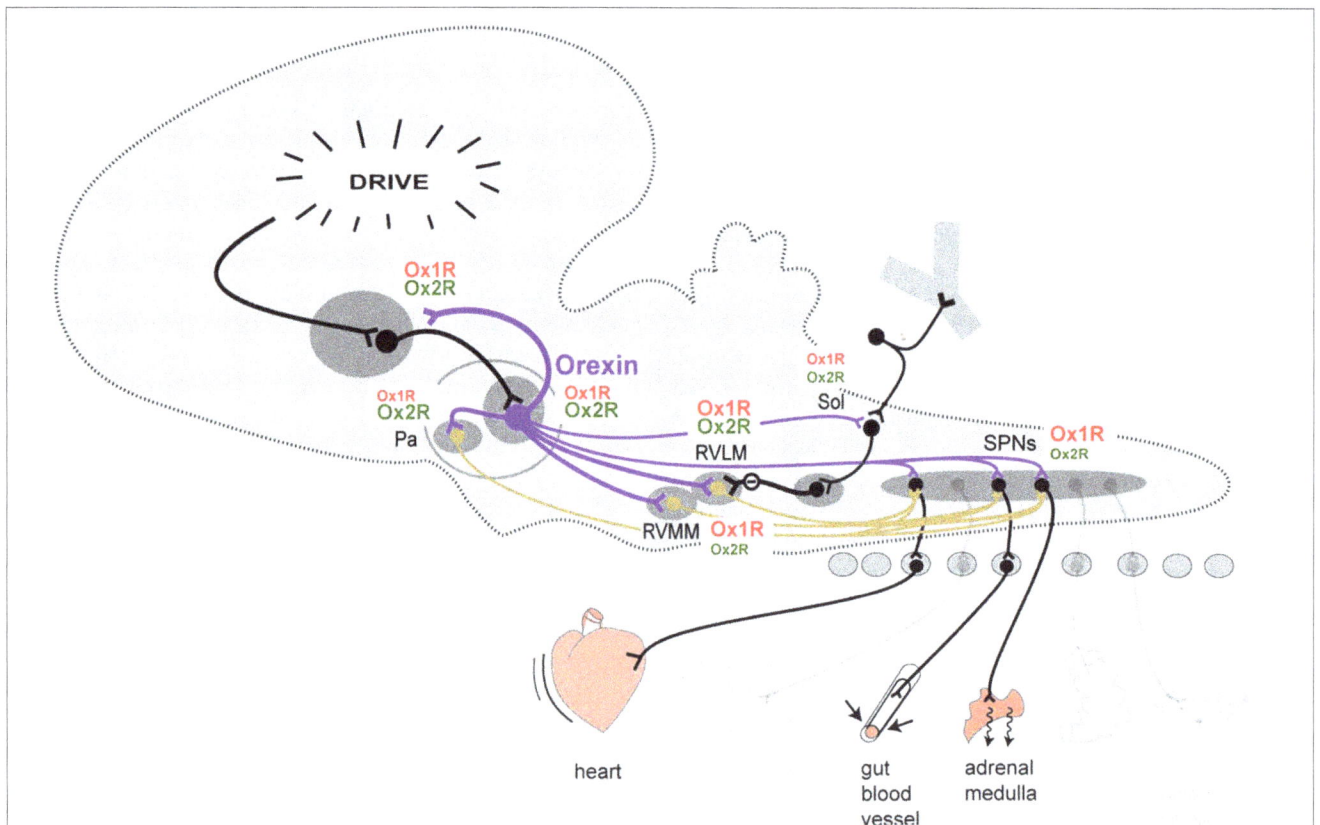

FIGURE 1 | Schematic overview of the orexinergic pathways involved in the descending control of sympathetic output to cardiovascular effectors. The contribution of Ox1R and Ox2R at each level is represented by the relative size of the Ox1R and Ox2R labels. This is a tentative representation only, reflecting the current stage of our knowledge. Abbreviations: Pa, paraventricular nucleus of the hypothalamus; RVLM, rostral ventrolateral medulla; RVMM, rostral ventromedial medulla (plus medullary raphe); Sol, solitary nucleus; SPN, sympathetic preganglionic neurons.

except Pa, which appears to exclusively express Ox2R. In the brainstem, most of the autonomic areas described above also express both receptors, except for the A5 catecholaminergic cell group, which like the A6 group of the locus coeruleus exclusively expresses Ox1R. Single cell RT-PCR in SPNs show that Ox1R is easier to detect than Ox2R (Van Den Top et al., 2003).

Immunohistochemical studies of Ox1R and Ox2R distribution (Hervieu et al., 2001; Cluderay et al., 2002) have confirmed the overall distribution of the two receptors, but they also show more overlap than suggested by the *in situ* hybridization studies. For instance, the amygdala also contains Ox2R and the septum Ox1R. More importantly, Pa also contains a significant amount of Ox1R in both its magno- and parvocellular areas, which colocalizes with vasopressin/oxytocin and CRF, respectively (Hervieu et al., 2001; Bäckberg et al., 2002). Interestingly, orexin neurons themselves have both receptors as autoreceptors (Bäckberg et al., 2002; Yamanaka et al., 2010). Other reports confirm dense Ox1R labeling in the RVMM area (Ciriello and De Oliveira, 2003; Ciriello et al., 2003) and both Ox1R and Ox2R in C1 neurons of the RVLM (Shahid et al., 2012). The presence of Ox1R and Ox2R in SPNs remains to be verified by immunohistochemistry.

OREXIN RECEPTORS MEDIATING THE CARDIOVASCULAR EFFECTS OF CENTRALLY INJECTED EXOGENOUS OREXIN

Given the partly overlapping distribution of Ox1R and Ox2R in central autonomic structures, it is not clear if one receptor or the other or both mediate(s) the cardiovascular effect of orexin. This question can be answered by challenging the effect of exogenous OxA (which acts on both receptors) with selective orexin receptor antagonists (SORA) or by using selective agonists. The two Ox1R SORA are SB334867, the most popular, and SB408124 (Scammell and Winrow, 2011; Gotter et al., 2012; Morairty et al., 2012). So far the only Ox2R SORA to have been used in this field of research is TCS-OX229 (Hirose et al., 2003), although a number of studies have also used the selective Ox2R agonist, [Ala11,D-Leu15]-OxB (Asahi et al., 2003).

OREXIN MICROINJECTED IN THE VENTRICLES OR SUBARACHNOID SPACE

Hirota et al. (2003) were the first to demonstrate that prior blockade of Ox1R with intracerebroventricular (icv) injections of the Ox1R antagonist SB334867 (50 nmol) could almost completely block the cardiovascular response of icv OxA (50 nmol). This was confirmed in the awake rat using smaller doses of icv OxA (3 nmol) and another Ox1R antagonist, SB408124 (3 nmol) (Samson et al., 2007). Similarly, spinal intrathecal injections of SB334867 (200 nmol) almost completely blocked the pressor, tachycardic, and sympathetic nerve response to intrathecal OxA (50 nmol) (Shahid et al., 2011). However, Huang et al. (2010) showed that the Ox2R antagonist TCS-OX229 (3 and 10 nmol) was more potent than SB334867 (3 and 10 nmol) in reducing the pressor and tachycardic effect of OxA (3 nmol) when injected in the cisterna magna. These studies suggest that Ox1R is important, but Ox2R, which has not been challenged as much as Ox1R, might be equally as important.

OREXIN MICROINJECTED WITHIN REGIONS OF THE CENTRAL AUTONOMIC NETWORK
SPN

Injection of OxA and OxB on identified SPN evokes strong depolarization due to a direct postsynaptic action (Antunes et al., 2001; Van Den Top et al., 2003). The response was as strong with OxA as with OxB, and OxA's effect was only reduced by 60% after blockade with SB334867 (Van Den Top et al., 2003). It led these authors to suggest that both receptors might be involved.

RVLM

A similar study on neonate RVLM pressor neurons by Huang et al. (2010) revealed equipotent depolarizing effect of OxA, OxB and the specific OxB agonist [Ala11,D-Leu15]-OxB. These authors further showed that TCS-OX229 was more potent than SB334867 in reducing the effect of OxA (Huang et al., 2010). Similar observations were reported by Shahid et al. (2012) who showed that OxA and [Ala11,D-Leu15]-OxB had equipotent cardiovascular effects when injected in the RVLM and that SB334867 reduced OxA's effect by half.

Sol

Injections of low doses (2.5–5 pmol) of OxA and OxB in the nucleus of the solitary nucleus evokes equipotent bradycradic and depressor responses (De Oliveira et al., 2003; Shih and Chuang, 2007; Ciriello et al., 2013), however at higher dose (>40 pmol) both evoke tachycardic and pressor responses, with OxA more potent than OxB. The effects appear to be mediated by both Ox1R and Ox2R (Shih and Chuang, 2007).

Others

When injected in the medullary raphe area, OxA produces tachycardic effects at low dose (2.5 pmol) and pressor and tachycardic effects at high dose (30 pmol) (Luong and Carrive, 2012). In contrast, OxA evokes bradycardic effects when injected in the external part of the Ambiguus nucleus, presumably by activating vagal preganglionic neurons (Ciriello and De Oliveira, 2003). However, it is not known what receptor mediates these effects, although these two areas have been shown to contain Ox1R.

To summarize, the cardiovascular effect of exogenous orexin can in large part be explained by an action through Ox1R at almost all levels (**Figure 1**). However, in the RVLM, one of the most important vasopressor center in the brain, an action through Ox2R appears as important, ifnot more. Ox2R may also contribute at the level of SPNs themselves.

OREXIN RECEPTORS MEDIATING THE CARDIOVASCULAR RESPONSES OF CENTRALLY RELEASED, ENDOGENOUS OREXIN

Orexin microinjections may reveal important properties of orexin's loci and mode of action, but the main question is how endogenous orexin acts in the behaving animal, where and through which receptors. Coordinated release of orexin at multiple levels of the neuraxis in synchrony with activation of other non-orexinergic system would have far more subtle effects than those of a ventricular or intracerebral injection. The approach therefore consists in first identifying behavioral conditions or pathological states associated with orexin release and then challenging these responses or states with systemic injections of dual and selective orexin receptor antagonists (DORA and SORA). Almorexant (Brisbare-Roch et al., 2007; Morairty et al., 2012) is the main DORA that has been used so far in relation to central autonomic control. The SORAs are the same as those described above.

CENTRALLY EVOKED RESPONSES

Disinhibition of the PeF is one way of inducing an orexin-mediated response. Remarkably, although orexin neurons (i) contain other peptides and use glutamate as their main neurotransmitter and (ii) only represent a fraction of the output neurons of the perifornical area, still, 50% of the tachycardic and pressor response obtained by bicuculline injection in the perifornical hypothalamus is blocked by systemic administration of Almorexant (15 mg/kg, iv) (Iigaya et al., 2012). This indicates that the peptide plays an important role in the output of this area. As suggested by the cardiovascular effects of OxA in the medulla and spinal cord described above, it is likely that Almorexant will exert its effect via an action on the targets of orexin neurons, however, part of its action maybe in the perifornical area itself since Almorexant microinjections in the PeF can reduce the tachycardic and pressor responses to perifornical disinhibition (Stettner and Kubin, 2013).

Similar results have been reported with Ox1R SORAs. In the rabbit, SB334867 and SB408124 (7 mg/kg, iv) markedly reduced the pressor response evoked by electrical stimulation of the dorsal hypothalamus and PAG (Nisimaru et al., 2013). In conscious rat SB334867 (10 mg/kg, iv) also reduced by about 40–50% the tachycardic, pressor and hyperthermic response to muscimol injection in the medial preoptic area, an area that exerts a tonic inhibition of the dorsal hypothalamic area (Rusyniak et al., 2011).

PSYCHOLOGICAL STRESSORS AND INDUCED PANIC

A number of psychological stressors have been challenged with Almorexant or Ox1R SORAs. Novelty, conditioned fear to context, restraint and cold exposure, all evoke tachycardic and pressor responses, however, Almorexant (300 mg/kg, io) affected only novelty and contextual fear (Furlong et al., 2009). The pressor responses to novelty and conditioned fear, the tachycardic response to novelty and the cardiac sympathetic response to conditioned fear were reduced by 45% or more, but restraint and cold exposure were not significantly affected by Almorexant (Furlong et al., 2009). This led the authors to suggest that the stress responses to which orexin contribute might be more psychological than physical, reminiscent of the observation by Kayaba et al. (2003), that the cardiovascular response to pinch was not affected in knock out orexin mice, whereas that to social stress was.

The other studies have used Ox1R SORAs, mainly SB334867. A major study by Johnson et al. (2009) showed that both the pressor and tachycardic responses evoked by sodium lactate in panic prone rats were markedly reduced by systemic SB334867 (30 mg/kg, ip). A similar effect was observed with SB408124 (30 mg/kg, ip also). The same high dose of SB334867 also reduced the pressor (but not bradycardic) response to hypercapnia (20% CO2, a suffocation signal) as well as the tachycardic (but not

pressor) response to the anxiogenic partial inverse benzodiazepine agonist FG7142 (Johnson et al., 2012a,b). SB334867 (10 mg/kg, iv) also reduces the pressor but not tachycardic response to a moderate dose of metamphetamine (Rusyniak et al., 2012). Finally, a recent study with a new selective Ox1R antagonist (ACT335827, 100–300 mg/kg, io) reported a significant reduction of the tachycardic (but not pressor) response to social stress (Steiner et al., 2013).

This indicates that orexin contributes to the cardiovascular components of some forms of stress as initially shown in orexin knock-out mice by Kayaba et al. (2003). The Ox1R appears to play an important part in this, however the dose of Ox1R antagonists used in these studies is very high. They could be acting on Ox2R as well. Unfortunately, the contribution of Ox2R is not yet known as no study has tried to challenge these responses with Ox2R antagonists.

CHRONIC STRESS-INDUCED AND SPONTANEOUS HYPERTENSION

Recent work has revealed a potentially important role of orexin in stress-induced or spontaneous forms of hypertension.

Xiao et al. (2012) used electric shocks over a period of 14 days to produce a stress-induced hypertensive state (+30 mmHg). Remarkably, this treatment doubled the number of orexin neurons and almost doubled the amount of Ox1R in the RVLM (Ox2R was not investigated). Consistent with this effect, unilateral microinjections of OxA in RVLM produced greater pressor and tachycardic responses in these animals. Conversely, RVLM injections of the Ox1R SORA SB408124 reduced systolic pressure and heart rate in those hypertensive animals but not in the normotensive non-stressed controls. Interestingly, Ox2R was also involved since the Ox2R SORA TCS-OX229 reduced systolic pressure in these hypertensive animals. This study shows that chronic stress can upregulate the orexin system and that both receptors, with possibly a dominance of the Ox1R, mediate the resulting hypertension. Most remarkable is the increase in orexin neurons as a result of chronic stress.

Finally, two recent studies suggest that essential hypertension in the Spontaneously hypertensive rat (SHR) may in part be due to an overactive orexin system. Thus, Li et al. (2013) have shown that oral administration of Almorexant in the conscious SHR reduces mean arterial blood pressure (~30 mmHg), heart rate and plasma noradrenaline during both wakefulness and NREM sleep, but has no significant effect in normotensive WKY rats. Lee et al. (2013) further showed in the anaesthetized SHR that icv TCS-OX229 (10 and 30 nmol) but not SB334867 (100 nmol) reduced MAP and HR. Surprisingly, there was a reduction of Ox2R density in the RVLM, but no change in PVN, DMH/PeF, and caudal NTS. Ox1R was also the same as in WKY in all four regions. Finally, bilateral injections of TCS-OX229 in the RVLM markedly lowered MAP (~30 mmHg), suggesting that the cause of the hypertensive phenotype in these animals could be an over-activation of Ox2R.

BASAL BLOOD PRESSURE AND HEART RATE IN OREXIN DEFICIENT HUMANS AND MICE

If orexin upregulation leads to hypertension, then one would expect orexin downregulation or deficiency to lead to hypotension. Indeed, a reduced baseline blood pressure during wakefulness has been reported in orexin knock-out and orexin neuron-ablated mice (orexin-ataxin3 transgene) (Kayaba et al., 2003; Lo Martire et al., 2012). However, other studies have found no difference between these mice and wild type controls (Bastianini et al., 2011; Silvani et al., 2013). Interestingly, in human, patients with narcolepsy with cataplexy, which have reduced levels of orexin and orexin neurons, also have normal basal blood pressure when awake (Grimaldi et al., 2010, 2012; Dauvilliers et al., 2012). In contrast, and somewhat unexpectedly, baseline blood pressure during sleep tends to be higher than in controls. Thus, in both patients and transgenic mice, the circadian variation in blood pressure is consistently reduced. The dip in blood pressure that is normally seen between wakefulness and sleep is reduced, as is the rise in blood pressure when waking up from sleep (Bastianini et al., 2011; Dauvilliers et al., 2012; Grimaldi et al., 2012; Lo Martire et al., 2012; Silvani et al., 2013).

In terms of heart rate, the same studies in mice report either no change (Kayaba et al., 2003; Lo Martire et al., 2012) or an increase (Bastianini et al., 2011; Silvani et al., 2013) during wakefulness, whereas in patients both increases (Grimaldi et al., 2010, 2012; Sorensen et al., 2013) and decreases have been reported (Dauvilliers et al., 2012). During sleep, heart rate may be higher (Bastianini et al., 2011) or the same (Bastianini et al., 2011; Lo Martire et al., 2012; Silvani et al., 2013) in transgenic mice, and higher (Grimaldi et al., 2012) or the same (Dauvilliers et al., 2012) in patients. Nevertheless, as observed with blood pressure, the rise in heart rate at the transition between sleep and arousal is reduced in both transgenic mice and narcoleptic patients (Silvani et al., 2013; Sorensen et al., 2013).

To summarize, a chronic lack of orexin does not necessarily lead to a lower blood pressure and heart rate, but it will result in a blunted circadian variation of these parameters. There may be a simple explanation to this. As suggested by Grimaldi et al. (2012), the altered sleep/wake regulation could have a confounding effect opposing the direct sympatholytic effect of orexin deficiency. Simply put, trying not to fall asleep during the active period or conversely, being regularly awaken during the inactive period, will both increase sympathetic activity. Nevertheless, a more relevant observation with respect to narcoleptic patients is their reduced autonomic response to emotional stimuli, especially aversive ones (Tucci et al., 2003). In contrast, their cardiovascular response to basic homeostatic challenges such as head-up tilt, Valsalva maneuver and cold pressor test are unaffected (Grimaldi et al., 2010), which is consistent with orexin's primary role in motivated behavior.

CONCLUSION

The orexinergic system plays an important role in central cardiovascular control. It is excitatory and contributes to the sympathetic response associated with motivated behavior, including some forms of stress. However, the mode of action of orexin is far from clear. Orexin terminals and orexin receptors are found in all the regions known to regulate cardiovascular function from sympathetic motor to premotor autonomic to limbic levels. So far anatomical and pharmacological evidences point toward a primary role for Ox1R, however this view is biased by the fact that most studies have used Ox1R SORAs (i.e., SB334867). Ox2R is also found in most central cardiovascular centers and when challenged is often found to be as important as Ox1R. Thus, it is not clear how the two receptors interact and if their effects are additive or synergistic. Nevertheless, blockade of orexin receptors can reduce the hypertension that is evoked by some acute psychological stressors, induced by chronic stress or simply spontaneous as in the case of adult SHR, a model of essential hypertension. Clearly there is an interesting link between psychogenic stress, orexin, and elevated blood pressure. Further research in SORAs and DORAs may well lead to the development of new anti-hypertensive drugs.

ACKNOWLEDGMENTS

Supported by grants from the National Health of Medical Research Council of Australia.

REFERENCES

Antunes, V. R., Brailoiu, G. C., Kwok, E. H., Scruggs, P., and Dun, N. J. (2001). Orexins/hypocretins excite rat sympathetic preganglionic neurons *in vivo* and *in vitro. Am. J. Physiol.* 281, R1801–R1807.

Asahi, S., Egashira, S.-I., Matsuda, M., Iwaasa, H., Kanatani, A., Ohkubo, M., et al. (2003). Development of an orexin-2 receptor selective agonist, [Ala(11), D-Leu(15)]orexin-B. *Bioorg. Med. Chem. Lett.* 13, 111–113.

Bäckberg, M., Hervieu, G., Wilson, S., and Meister, B. (2002). Orexin receptor-1 (OX-R1) immunoreactivity in chemically identified neurons of the hypothalamus: focus on orexin targets involved in control of food and water intake. *Eur. J. Neurosci.* 15, 315–328. doi: 10.1046/j.0953-816x.2001.01859.x

Baldo, B. A., Daniel, R. A., Berridge, C. W., and Kelley, A. E. (2003). Overlapping distributions of orexin/hypocretin- and dopamine-beta-hydroxylase immunoreactive fibers in rat brain regions mediating arousal, motivation, and stress. *J. Comp. Neurol.* 464, 220–237. doi: 10.1002/cne.10783

Bastianini, S., Silvani, A., Berteotti, C., Elghozi, J.-L., Franzini, C., Lenzi, P., et al. (2011). Sleep related changes in blood pressure in hypocretin-deficient narcoleptic mice. *Sleep* 34, 213–218.

Brisbare-Roch, C., Dingemanse, J., Koberstein, R., Hoever, P., Aissaoui, H., Flores, S., et al. (2007). Promotion of sleep by targeting the orexin system in rats, dogs and humans. *Nat. Med.* 13, 150–155. doi: 10.1038/nm1544

Carrive, P. (2011). "Central circulatory control. Psychological stress and the defense reaction," in *Central Regulation of Autonomic Function, 2nd Edn.,* eds I. J. Llewellyn-Smith and A. Verberne (New York, NY: Oxford University Press), 220–237. doi: 10.1093/acprof:oso/9780195306637.003.0012

Chen, C. T., Hwang, L. L., Chang, J. K., and Dun, N. J. (2000). Pressor effects of orexins injected intracisternally and to rostral ventrolateral medulla of anesthetized rats. *Am. J. Physiol.* 278, R692–R697.

Ciriello, J., Caverson, M. M., McMurray, J. C., and Bruckschwaiger, E. B. (2013). Co-localization of hypocretin-1 and leucine-enkephalin in hypothalamic neurons projecting to the nucleus of the solitary tract and their effect on arterial pressure. *Neuroscience* 250, 599–613. doi: 10.1016/j.neuroscience.2013.07.054

Ciriello, J., and De Oliveira, C. V. R. (2003). Cardiac effects of hypocretin-1 in nucleus ambiguus. *Am. J. Physiol.* 284, R1611–R1620. doi: 10.1152/ajpregu.00719.2002

Ciriello, J., Li, Z., and De Oliveira, C. V. R. (2003). Cardioacceleratory responses to hypocretin-1 injections into rostral ventromedial medulla. *Brain Res.* 991, 84–95. doi: 10.1016/j.brainres.2003.08.009

Cluderay, J. E., Harrison, D. C., and Hervieu, G. J. (2002). Protein distribution of the orexin-2 receptor in the rat central nervous system. *Regul. Peptides* 104, 131–144. doi: 10.1016/S0167-0115(01)00357-3

Date, Y., Mondal, M. S., Matsukura, S., and Nakazato, M. (2000). Distribution of orexin-A and orexin-B (hypocretins) in the rat spinal cord. *Neurosci. Lett.* 288, 87–90. doi: 10.1016/S0304-3940(00)01195-2

Dauvilliers, Y., Jaussent, I., Krams, B., Scholz, S., Lado, S., Levy, P., et al. (2012). Non-dipping blood pressure profile in narcolepsy with cataplexy. *PLoS ONE* 7:e38977. doi: 10.1371/journal.pone.0038977

De Oliveira, C. V. R., Rosas-Arellano, M. P., Solano-Flores, L. P., and Ciriello, J. (2003). Cardiovascular effects of hypocretin-1 in nucleus of the solitary tract. *Am. J. Physiol.* 284, H1369–H1377. doi: 10.1152/ajpheart.00877.2002

Dun, N. J., Le Dun, S., Chen, C. T., Hwang, L. L., Kwok, E. H., and Chang, J. K. (2000). Orexins: a role in medullary sympathetic outflow. *Regul. Peptides* 96, 65–70. doi: 10.1016/S0167-0115(00)00202-0

Furlong, T. M., Vianna, D. M. L., Liu, L., and Carrive, P. (2009). Hypocretin/orexin contributes to the expression of some but not all forms of stress and arousal. *Eur. J. Neurosci.* 30, 1603–1614. doi: 10.1111/j.1460-9568.2009.06952.x

Gotter, A. L., Webber, A. L., Coleman, P. J., Renger, J. J., and Winrow, C. J. (2012). International union of basic and clinical pharmacology. LXXXVI. orexin receptor function, nomenclature and pharmacology. *Pharmacol. Rev.* 64, 389–420. doi: 10.1124/pr.111.005546

Grimaldi, D., Calandra-Buonaura, G., Provini, F., Agati, P., Pierangeli, G., Franceschini, C., et al. (2012). Abnormal sleep-cardiovascular system interaction in narcolepsy with cataplexy: effects of hypocretin deficiency in humans. *Sleep* 35, 519–528. doi: 10.5665/sleep.1738

Grimaldi, D., Pierangeli, G., Barletta, G., Terlizzi, R., Plazzi, G., Cevoli, S., et al. (2010). Spectral analysis of heart rate variability reveals an enhanced sympathetic activity in narcolepsy with cataplexy. *Clin. Neurophysiol.* 121, 1142–1147. doi: 10.1016/j.clinph.2010.01.028

Hervieu, G. J., Cluderay, J. E., Harrison, D. C., Roberts, J. C., and Leslie, R. A. (2001). Gene expression and protein distribution of the orexin-1 receptor in the rat brain and spinal cord. *Neuroscience* 103, 777–797. doi: 10.1016/S0306-4522(01)00033-1

Hilton, S. M. (1982). The defence-arousal system and its relevance for circulatory and respiratory control. *J. Exp. Biol.* 100, 159–174.

Hirose, M., Egashira, S.-I., Goto, Y., Hashihayata, T., Ohtake, N., Iwaasa, H., et al. (2003). N-acyl 6,7-dimethoxy-1,2,3,4-tetrahydroisoquinoline: the first orexin-2 receptor selective non-peptidic antagonist. *Bioorg. Med. Chem. Lett.* 13, 4497–4499. doi: 10.1016/j.bmcl.2003.08.038

Hirota, K., Kushikata, T., Kudo, M., Kudo, T., Smart, D., and Matsuki, A. (2003). Effects of central hypocretin-1 administration on hemodynamic responses in young-adult and middle-aged rats. *Brain Res.* 981, 143–150. doi: 10.1016/S0006-8993(03)03002-6

Huang, S.-C., Dai, Y.-W. E., Lee, Y.-H., Chiou, L.-C., and Hwang, L.-L. (2010). Orexins depolarize rostral ventrolateral medulla neurons and increase arterial pressure and heart rate in rats mainly via orexin 2 receptors. *J. Pharmacol. Exp. Ther.* 334, 522–529. doi: 10.1124/jpet.110.167791

Iigaya, K., Horiuchi, J., McDowall, L. M., Lam, A. C. B., Sediqi, Y., Polson, J. W., et al. (2012). Blockade of orexin receptors with Almorexant reduces cardiorespiratory responses evoked from the hypothalamus but not baro- or chemoreceptor reflex responses. *Am. J. Physiol.* 303, R1011–R1022. doi: 10.1152/ajpregu.00263.2012

Johnson, P. L., Samuels, B. C., Fitz, S. D., Federici, L. M., Hammes, N., Early, M. C., et al. (2012a). Orexin 1 receptors are a novel target to modulate panic responses and the panic brain network. *Physiol. Behav.* 107, 733–742. doi: 10.1016/j.physbeh.2012.04.016

Johnson, P. L., Samuels, B. C., Fitz, S. D., Lightman, S. L., Lowry, C. A., and Shekhar, A. (2012b). Activation of the orexin 1 receptor is a critical component of CO(2)-mediated anxiety and hypertension but not bradycardia. *Neuropsychopharmacology* 37, 1911–1922. doi: 10.1038/npp.2012.38.

Johnson, P. L., Truitt, W., Fitz, S. D., Minick, P. E., Dietrich, A., Sanghani, S., et al. (2009). A key role for orexin in panic anxiety. *Nat. Med.* 16, 111–115. doi: 10.1038/nm.2075

Kayaba, Y., Nakamura, A., Kasuya, Y., Ohuchi, T., Yanagisawa, M., Komuro, I., et al. (2003). Attenuated defense response and low basal blood pressure in orexin knockout mice. *Am. J. Physiol.* 285, R581–R593. doi: 10.1152/ajpregu.00671.2002

Lee, Y.-H., Dai, Y.-W. E., Huang, S.-C., Li, T. L., and Hwang, L.-L. (2013). Blockade of central orexin 2 receptors reduces arterial pressure in spontaneously hypertensive rats. *Exp. Physiol.* 98, 1145–1155. doi: 10.1113/expphysiol.2013.072298

Li, A., Hindmarch, C. C. T., Nattie, E. E., and Paton, J. F. R. (2013). Antagonism of orexin receptors significantly lowers blood pressure in spontaneously hypertensive rats. *J. Physiol.* doi: 10.1113/jphysiol.2013.256271. [Epub ahead of print].

Llewellyn-Smith, I. J., Martin, C. L., Marcus, J. N., Yanagisawa, M., Minson, J. B., and Scammell, T. E. (2003). Orexin-immunoreactive inputs to rat sympathetic

preganglionic neurons. *Neurosci. Lett.* 351, 115–119. doi: 10.1016/S0304-3940(03)00770-5

Lo Martire, V., Silvani, A., Bastianini, S., Berteotti, C., and Zoccoli, G. (2012). Effects of ambient temperature on sleep and cardiovascular regulation in mice: the role of hypocretin/orexin neurons. *PLoS ONE* 7:e47032. doi: 10.1371/journal.pone.0047032

Lu, X. Y., Bagnol, D., Burke, S., Akil, H., and Watson, S. J. (2000). Differential distribution and regulation of OX1 and OX2 orexin/hypocretin receptor messenger RNA in the brain upon fasting. *Horm. Behav.* 37, 335–344. doi: 10.1006/hbeh.2000.1584

Luong, L. N. L., and Carrive, P. (2012). Orexin microinjection in the medullary raphe increases heart rate and arterial pressure but does not reduce tail skin blood flow in the awake rat. *Neuroscience* 202, 209–217. doi: 10.1016/j.neuroscience.2011.11.073

Marcus, J. N., Aschkenasi, C. J., Lee, C. E., Chemelli, R. M., Saper, C. B., Yanagisawa, M., et al. (2001). Differential expression of orexin receptors 1 and 2 in the rat brain. *J. Comp. Neurol.* 435, 6–25. doi: 10.1002/cne.1190

Morairty, S. R., Revel, F. G., Malherbe, P., Moreau, J.-L., Valladao, D., Wettstein, J. G., et al. (2012). Dual hypocretin receptor antagonism is more effective for sleep promotion than antagonism of either receptor alone. *PLoS ONE* 7:e39131. doi: 10.1371/journal.pone.0039131

Nambu, T., Sakurai, T., Mizukami, K., Hosoya, Y., Yanagisawa, M., and Goto, K. (1999). Distribution of orexin neurons in the adult rat brain. *Brain Res.* 827, 243–260. doi: 10.1016/S0006-8993(99)01336-0

Nisimaru, N., Mittal, C., Shirai, Y., Sooksawate, T., Anandaraj, P., Hashikawa, T., et al. (2013). Orexin-neuromodulated cerebellar circuit controls redistribution of arterial blood flows for defense behavior in rabbits. *Proc. Natl. Acad. Sci. U.S.A.* 110, 14124–14131. doi: 10.1073/pnas.1312804110

Peyron, C., Tighe, D. K., Van Den Pol, A. N., De Lecea, L., Heller, H. C., Sutcliffe, J. G., et al. (1998). Neurons containing hypocretin (orexin) project to multiple neuronal systems. *J. Neurosci.* 18, 9996–10015.

Rusyniak, D. E., Zaretsky, D. V., Zaretskaia, M. V., and Dimicco, J. A. (2011). The role of orexin-1 receptors in physiologic responses evoked by microinjection of PgE2 or muscimol into the medial preoptic area. *Neurosci. Lett.* 498, 162–166. doi: 10.1016/j.neulet.2011.05.006

Rusyniak, D. E., Zaretsky, D. V., Zaretskaia, M. V., Durant, P. J., and Dimicco, J. A. (2012). The orexin-1 receptor antagonist SB-334867 decreases sympathetic responses to a moderate dose of methamphetamine and stress. *Physiol. Behav.* 107, 743–750. doi: 10.1016/j.physbeh.2012.02.010

Sakurai, T., Nagata, R., Yamanaka, A., Kawamura, H., Tsujino, N., Muraki, Y., et al. (2005). Input of orexin/hypocretin neurons revealed by a genetically encoded tracer in mice. *Neuron* 46, 297–308. doi: 10.1016/j.neuron.2005.03.010

Samson, W. K., Bagley, S. L., Ferguson, A. V., and White, M. M. (2007). Hypocretin/orexin type 1 receptor in brain: role in cardiovascular control and the neuroendocrine response to immobilization stress. *Am. J. Physiol.* 292, R382–R387. doi: 10.1152/ajpregu.00496.2006

Samson, W. K., Gosnell, B., Chang, J. K., Resch, Z. T., and Murphy, T. C. (1999). Cardiovascular regulatory actions of the hypocretins in brain. *Brain Res.* 831, 248–253.

Saper, C. B. (2004). "Central autonomic nervous system," in *The Rat Nervous System, 3rd Edn.*, ed G. Paxinos (San Diego, CA: Elsevier), 761–794.

Scammell, T. E., and Winrow, C. J. (2011). Orexin receptors: pharmacology and therapeutic opportunities. *Annu. Rev. Pharmacol. Toxicol.* 51, 243–266. doi: 10.1146/annurev-pharmtox-010510-100528

Shahid, I. Z., Rahman, A. A., and Pilowsky, P. M. (2011). Intrathecal orexin A increases sympathetic outflow and respiratory drive, enhances baroreflex sensitivity and blocks the somato-sympathetic reflex. *Br. J. Pharmacol.* 162, 961–973. doi: 10.1111/j.1476-5381.2010.01102.x

Shahid, I. Z., Rahman, A. A., and Pilowsky, P. M. (2012). Orexin A in rat rostral ventrolateral medulla is pressor, sympatho-excitatory, increases barosensitivity and attenuates the somato-sympathetic reflex. *Br. J. Pharmacol.* 165, 2292–2303. doi: 10.1111/j.1476-5381.2011.01694.x

Shih, C.-D., and Chuang, Y.-C. (2007). Nitric oxide and GABA mediate bi-directional cardiovascular effects of orexin in the nucleus tractus solitarii of rats. *Neuroscience* 149, 625–635. doi: 10.1016/j.neuroscience.2007.07.016

Shirasaka, T., Nakazato, M., Matsukura, S., Takasaki, M., and Kannan, H. (1999). Sympathetic and cardiovascular actions of orexins in conscious rats. *Am. J. Physiol.* 277, R1780–R1785.

Silvani, A., Bastianini, S., Berteotti, C., Cenacchi, G., Leone, O., Lo Martire, V., et al. (2013). Sleep and cardiovascular phenotype in middle-aged hypocretin-deficient narcoleptic mice. *J. Sleep Res.* doi: 10.1111/jsr.12081. [Epub ahead of print].

Sorensen, G. L., Knudsen, S., Petersen, E. R., Kempfner, J., Gammeltoft, S., Sorensen, H. B. D., et al. (2013). Attenuated heart rate response is associated with hypocretin deficiency in patients with narcolepsy. *Sleep* 36, 91–98. doi: 10.5665/sleep.2308

Steiner, M. A., Gatfield, J., Brisbare-Roch, C., Dietrich, H., Treiber, A., Jenck, F., et al. (2013). Discovery and characterization of ACT-335827, an orally available, brain penetrant orexin receptor type 1 selective antagonist. *ChemMedChem* 8, 898–903. doi: 10.1002/cmdc.201300003

Stettner, G. M., and Kubin, L. (2013). Antagonism of orexin receptors in the posterior hypothalamus reduces hypoglossal and cardiorespiratory excitation from the perifornical hypothalamus. *J. Appl. Physiol.* 114, 119–130. doi: 10.1152/japplphysiol.00965.2012

Trivedi, P., Yu, H., Macneil, D. J., Van Der Ploeg, L. H., and Guan, X. M. (1998). Distribution of orexin receptor mRNA in the rat brain. *FEBS Lett.* 438, 71–75. doi: 10.1016/S0014-5793(98)01266-6

Tucci, V., Stegagno, L., Vandi, S., Ferrillo, F., Palomba, D., Vignatelli, L., et al. (2003). Emotional information processing in patients with narcolepsy: a psychophysiologic investigation. *Sleep* 26, 558–564.

Van Den Pol, A. N. (1999). Hypothalamic hypocretin (orexin): robust innervation of the spinal cord. *J. Neurosci.* 19, 3171–3182.

Van Den Top, M., Nolan, M. F., Lee, K., Richardson, P. J., Buijs, R. M., Davies, C. H., et al. (2003). Orexins induce increased excitability and synchronisation of rat sympathetic preganglionic neurones. *J. Physiol.* 549, 809–821. doi: 10.1113/jphysiol.2002.033290

Xiao, F., Jiang, M., Du, D., Xia, C., Wang, J., Cao, Y., et al. (2012). Orexin A regulates cardiovascular responses in stress-induced hypertensive rats. *Neuropharmacology* 67C, 16–24. doi: 10.1016/j.neuropharm.2012.10.021

Yamanaka, A., Tabuchi, S., Tsunematsu, T., Fukazawa, Y., and Tominaga, M. (2010). Orexin directly excites orexin neurons through orexin 2 receptor. *J. Neurosci.* 30, 12642–12652. doi: 10.1523/JNEUROSCI.2120-10.2010

Yoshida, K., McCormack, S., España, R. A., Crocker, A., and Scammell, T. E. (2006). Afferents to the orexin neurons of the rat brain. *J. Comp. Neurol.* 494, 845–861. doi: 10.1002/cne.20859

Zheng, H., Patterson, L. M., and Berthoud, H.-R. (2005). Orexin-A projections to the caudal medulla and orexin-induced c-Fos expression, food intake, and autonomic function. *J. Comp. Neurol.* 485, 127–142. doi: 10.1002/cne.20515

Conflict of Interest Statement: The author declares that the research was conducted in the absence of any commercial or financial relationships that could be construed as a potential conflict of interest.

Distinct effects of IPSU and suvorexant on mouse sleep architecture

Daniel Hoyer[1,2], Thomas Dürst[1], Markus Fendt[1,3], Laura H. Jacobson[1,4], Claudia Betschart[5], Samuel Hintermann[5], Dirk Behnke[5], Simona Cotesta[5], Grit Laue[6], Silvio Ofner[5], Eric Legangneux[7] and Christine E. Gee[1,8]*

[1] Neuroscience, Novartis Institutes for BioMedical Research, Basel, Switzerland
[2] Department of Pharmacology and Therapeutics, Faculty of Medicine, Dentistry and Health Sciences, The University of Melbourne, Parkville, VIC, Australia
[3] Center of Behavioral Brain Sciences, Institute for Pharmacology and Toxicology, Otto-von-Guericke University Magdeburg, Magdeburg, Germany
[4] The Florey Institute of Neuroscience and Mental Health, The University of Melbourne, Parkville, VIC, Australia
[5] Global Discovery Chemistry, Novartis Institutes for BioMedical Research, Basel, Switzerland
[6] Metabolism and Pharmacokinetics, Novartis Institutes for BioMedical Research, Basel, Switzerland
[7] Translational Medicine, Novartis Institutes for BioMedical Research, Basel, Switzerland
[8] Center for Molecular Neuroscience Hamburg, Institute for Synaptic Physiology, Hamburg, Germany

Edited by:
Michel A. Steiner, Actelion
Pharmaceuticals Ltd., Switzerland

Reviewed by:
Michihiro Mieda, Kanazawa
University, Japan
Brock T. Shireman, Janssen, USA

*Correspondence:
Christine E. Gee, Center for
Molecular Neurobiology Hamburg,
Institute for Synaptic Physiology,
Falkenried 94, 20251 Hamburg,
Germany
e-mail: christine.gee@
zmnh.uni-hamburg.de

Dual orexin receptor (OXR) antagonists (DORAs) such as almorexant, SB-649868, suvorexant (MK-4305), and filorexant (MK-6096), have shown promise for the treatment of insomnias and sleep disorders. Whether antagonism of both OX_1R and OX_2R is necessary for sleep induction has been a matter of some debate. Experiments using knockout mice suggest that it may be sufficient to antagonize only OX_2R. The recent identification of an orally bioavailable, brain penetrant OX_2R preferring antagonist 2-((1H-Indol-3-yl)methyl)-9-(4-methoxypyrimidin-2-yl)-2,9-diazaspiro[5.5]undecan-1-one (IPSU) has allowed us to test whether selective antagonism of OX_2R may also be a viable strategy for induction of sleep. We previously demonstrated that IPSU and suvorexant increase sleep when dosed during the mouse active phase (lights off); IPSU inducing sleep primarily by increasing NREM sleep, suvorexant primarily by increasing REM sleep. Here, our goal was to determine whether suvorexant and IPSU affect sleep architecture independently of overall sleep induction. We therefore tested suvorexant (25 mg/kg) and IPSU (50 mg/kg) in mice during the inactive phase (lights on) when sleep is naturally more prevalent and when orexin levels are normally low. Whereas IPSU was devoid of effects on the time spent in NREM or REM, suvorexant substantially disturbed the sleep architecture by selectively increasing REM during the first 4 h after dosing. At the doses tested, suvorexant significantly decreased wake only during the first hour and IPSU did not affect wake time. These data suggest that OX_2R preferring antagonists may have a reduced tendency for perturbing NREM/REM architecture in comparison with DORAs. Whether this effect will prove to be a general feature of OX_2R antagonists vs. DORAs remains to be seen.

Keywords: orexin receptor antagonist, insomnia, pharmacology, REM and NREM sleep

INTRODUCTION

Since the link between the hypocretin/orexin system and sleep disorders was discovered (Chemelli et al., 1999; Lin et al., 1999; Nishino et al., 2000), there has been much interest in developing orexin receptor antagonists (ORAs) for the treatment of insomnia. Several dual orexin receptor antagonists (DORAs) have now been tested in the clinic and have demonstrated sleep inducing properties in healthy volunteers and/or in patients suffering from insomnia (Brisbare-Roch et al., 2007; Winrow et al., 2011; Bettica et al., 2012a). Whereas ORAs are expected to be without the side effects characteristic of currently available treatments, questions about mechanism related safety have accompanied their development. As the lack of orexin signaling causes narcolepsy with cataplexy, there is concern that DORAs may induce sudden loss of motor control or sleep attacks. Whereas the therapeutic potential

for treating insomnia with ORAs is undisputedly high, there is less consensus regarding the necessity of targeting both receptors and whether selective antagonists might reduce potential safety concerns without loss of efficacy (Mieda et al., 2013).

Several lines of evidence suggest that selective OX_2R antagonists may be sufficient for sleep induction and may have a reduced tendency for induction of cataplexy and/or narcolepsy in comparison with DORAs. In knockout mice, the sleep inducing properties of the DORA almorexant require intact OX_2Rs but not OX_1Rs (Mang et al., 2012). Also, selective OX_2R antagonists induce sleep in rats and mice, whereas OX_1R selective antagonists do not [(Dugovic et al., 2009; Steiner et al., 2013); but see Morairty et al. (2012)]. Together these findings strongly suggest that antagonizing OX_2R may be sufficient for sleep induction.

In humans, orexin deficiency leads to narcolepsy with cataplexy (Nishino et al., 2000). The narcolepsy/cataplexy phenotype is mimicked in mice lacking orexin peptides, lacking orexinergic neurons or mice lacking both orexin receptors (OXR) (Chemelli et al., 1999; Hara et al., 2001; Kalogiannis et al., 2011). Although mice lacking OX$_2$R also have sleep attacks, the incidence of cataplexy in these mice is close to null (Willie et al., 2003). Thus, there may be a reduced risk of inducing cataplectic events when only OX$_2$R are antagonized. In dogs, mutations in OX$_2$R alone are sufficient to cause narcolepsy with cataplexy. Interestingly, sporadic narcolepsy with cataplexy in dogs is associated with orexin deficiency resulting in more severe symptoms than the OX$_2$R mutations (Baker et al., 1982; Ripley et al., 2001). It is tempting to speculate that OX$_2$R antagonists might be less prone to induce symptoms similar to either narcolepsy or cataplexy than DORAs even in this very sensitive species. To date, although functionally relevant polymorphisms of the OXRs have been described in humans (Thompson et al., 2004; Rainero et al., 2008; Annerbrink et al., 2011), mutations of the receptors have not been linked to narcolepsy/cataplexy. Rather loss of the orexinergic neurons or, extremely rarely, mutations resulting in loss of the peptides have been reported to be the underlying cause (Peyron et al., 2000; Thannickal et al., 2000). Together, such findings suggest it may be a general rule that loss of OX$_2$R signaling has a reduced propensity for inducing narcolepsy and/or cataplexy as compared to loss of the entire orexin signaling pathway.

We have therefore been interested in determining whether antagonists of OX$_2$R are comparable to DORAs in their ability to induce sleep. Recently, we identified the orally bioavailable, brain penetrating OX$_2$R preferring antagonist IPSU that induces sleep when administered at the start of the active (dark) phase in mice (Betschart et al., 2013). The aim of the present study was to investigate whether IPSU and the DORA suvorexant affect the natural sleep architecture, by testing low doses of the two compounds during the light phase when mice are primarily inactive and spend a high proportion of the time sleeping.

METHODS

All experiments were performed according to Swiss guidelines and law and were approved by the Veterinary Authority of Basel-Stadt, Switzerland. Every effort was made to minimize the number of animals used and to minimize any pain or discomfort. Male C57Bl/6 mice weighing 25–35 g were single or group-housed on wood shavings in type II ($14 \times 16 \times 22$ cm) and type III ($15 \times 22 \times 37$ cm) cages, respectively. Each cage contained a nest box, a piece of wood and tissue paper nesting materials, and animals had access to food and water *ad libitum*. The housing cages were placed in a temperature and humidity controlled room (20–24°C, 45% humidity) with a light/dark cycle of 12:12 (lights on at 03:00, max 80 Lux).

Suvorexant and IPSU were both synthesized and purified *in house* according to published procedures (Cox et al., 2008; Betschart et al., 2013). We selected doses that were effective at promoting sleep in mice for the first 4 h when administered at the start of the dark phase [Betschart et al. (2013) and unpublished observations]. At the mouse OXRs, IPSU has about 6.2×

higher affinity at OX$_2$R than OX$_1$R (pKd OX$_1$R 6.34, OX$_2$R 7.23) whereas suvorexant is about 6.5× more potent at OX$_1$R than OX$_2$R [pKd OX$_1$R 8.77, OX$_2$R 8.06; FLIPR assay Callander et al. (2013)]. Both compounds are highly brain penetrant. One hour after oral dosing of 50 mg/kg, brain levels reached 8778 pmol/g for IPSU and 10329 pmol/g for suvorexant giving free levels of 53.6 and 67.0 pmol/g, respectively (Betschart et al., 2013). In the present study we decided to dose IPSU at the previously effective dose of 50 mg/kg and to reduce suvorexant to 25 mg/kg to better match the estimated OX$_2$R occupancy. At 1 h following 25 mg/kg suvorexant brain levels reached 3605 pmol/g and free levels were therefore 23.4 pmol/g. Estimating the available antagonist concentrations to be 53.6 and 23.4 nM for IPSU and suvorexant, we estimated receptor occupancies according to:

$$\text{Bound} = \text{Bmax}/(1 + \text{Kd}/\text{L})$$

where Bmax is 100%, Kd the affinity from the FLIPR assay, and L the free brain concentrations at the doses tested.

The expected occupancies of suvorexant are therefore 93% at OX$_1$R, 73% at OX$_2$R and for IPSU 11% at OX$_1$R and 48% at OX$_2$R. These values are similar to the effective values for sleep induction at OX$_2$R reported by Gotter et al. (2013).

IMPLANTATION OF ELECTROCORTICOGRAM/ ELECTROENCEPHALOGRAM (EEG) AND ELECTROMYOGRAM (EMG) ELECTRODES

Mice were administered buprenorphine (0.05 mg/kg s.c.) 1 h before surgery, anesthetized with ketamine/xylazine (110 mg/kg, 10:1, i.p.) and placed in a stereotaxic frame. The skull was exposed and four miniature stainless steel screws (SS-5/TA Science Products GmbH, Hofheim, Germany) attached to 36-gauge, Teflon-coated solid silver wires were placed in contact with the frontal and parietal cortex (3 mm posterior to bregma, ±2 mm from the sagittal suture) through bore holes. The frontal electrodes served as reference. The wires were crimped to a small 6-channel connector (CRISTEK Micro Strip Connector) that was affixed to the skull with dental acrylic. Electromyograph (EMG) signals were acquired by a pair of multistranded stainless steel wires (7SS-1T, Science Products GmbH, Hofheim, Germany) inserted into the neck muscles and also crimped to the headmount. After surgery, mice were kept singly in cages and allowed to recover on a heating pad. Buprenorphine, 0.05 mg/kg, s.c. was given 8 and 16 h after surgery to control pain. After 24 h, the mice were housed with their former cage mates and allowed to recover for 2 weeks.

SLEEP STUDIES

Mice were habituated to individual cages in a sound-attenuated recording chamber for 6–10 days (lights on 03:00, lights off 15:00, max 80 lux) at a temperature of about 23°C. During the studies, mice had access to food and water *ad libitum*, to one sheet of nesting paper and a piece of wood but no nesting box. Mice were weighed and attached to recording cables that connected their headmounts to a commutator (G-4-E, Gaueschi) allowing free movement in the experiment boxes, 1 day before beginning the experiment. The recording chamber was opened each day during the light period between 08:00 and 09:00 to care for the mice and all experimental manipulations and oral applications were performed in a time window of 5–15 min before the start of the recordings at 09:00, exactly 6 h after lights on. Day 1, the mice were manipulated and habituated to the oral application syringe. Day 2, they received vehicle (methylcellulose 0.5%, 10 mL/kg, per os). Day 3, 50 mg/kg IPSU or 25 mg/kg suvorexant was administered per os. Recordings began at 09:00 (hour 0) and continued for 23 h. The experimental chamber was secured about 5 min prior to start of the recordings and the mice remained undisturbed for the next 23 h. On Day 4, the mice were returned to their normal housing cages for at least 2 weeks before returning to the experiment.

EEG/EMG signals were amplified using a Grass Model 78D amplifier (Grass Instrument CO., Quincy, MA, USA), analog filtered (EEG: 0.3–30 Hz, EMG: 5–30 Hz) and acquired using Harmonie V5.2 (acquisition frequency: 200 Hz with calibration the first day, record duration: 23h). Animals were video recorded during data collection, using an infrared video camera and locomotor activity was detected using infrared sensors (InfraMot Infrared Activity Sensor 30-2015 SENS, TSE Systems) placed in the roof of the boxes. Activity signals were acquired in 10 s intervals by the software Labmaster V2.4.4. EEG/EMG and activity recordings were imported into and scored in 10 s epochs using the rodent scoring module of Somnologica into wake, NREM

sleep and REM sleep. Epochs during which there were state transitions were scored as the state present for at least 50% of the epoch. The time in each state per hour was calculated and mean ± s.e.m. is shown. Restricted maximum likelihood analysis (REML) was applied to the data from the first 6 h to determine if there was a statistically significant effect of treatment or a significant interaction between treatment and hour. When either treatment or the interaction was significant ($p < 0.05$), post-hoc Fisher's Least Significant Difference (LSD) tests were applied to determine hour by hour where there were significant differences between the vehicle and compound days.

The first 2 h following drug treatment were, in addition, manually scored to assess sleep-wake transitions including very short awakenings i.e., those with durations of 1–5 s that are often seen in mice and which would not be detected using 10 s epochs.

RESULTS

The ORA IPSU (50 mg/kg) had no effect on the sleep architecture of mice when administered during the middle of the light phase (**Figures 1A,C**). The amount of time spent in wake, NREM and REM were unchanged following administration of IPSU relative to the previous day when vehicle was administered [treatment: wake $F_{(1, 120)} = 0.002$, $p = 0.96$, NREM $F_{(1, 120)} = 0.002$, $p = 0.97$, REM $F_{(1, 120)} = 0.001$, $p = 0.97$, treatment × hour: wake $F_{(5, 120)} = 0.59$, $p = 0.71$, NREM $F_{(5, 120)} = 0.56$, $p = 0.73$, REM $F_{(5, 120)} = 0.44$, $p = 0.82$, REML].

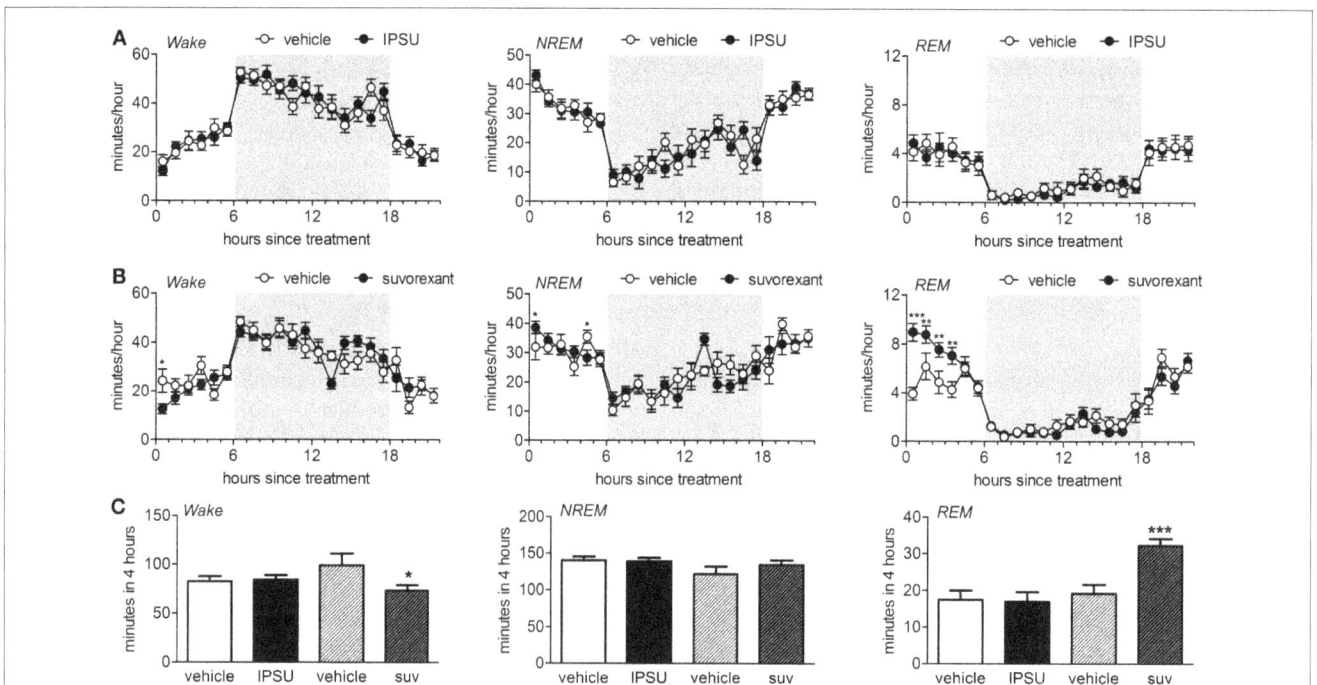

FIGURE 1 | **Sleep architecture during the inactive period is perturbed by a DORA but not by an OX$_2$R antagonist in C57Bl/6 mice. (A)** EEG/EMG/motility signals were used to score vigilance states into wake, NREM and REM beginning from time 0, 6 h into the light period. Vehicle (0.5% methylcellulose in water) or 50 mg/kg IPSU were applied per os 5–15 min prior to start of the recordings on successive days ($n = 11$). The mean ± s.e.m. minutes per hour spent in each stage are shown. Shading indicates the dark period. **(B)** Vehicle (0.5% methylcellulose in water) or 25 mg/kg suvorexant were applied per os 5–15 min prior to start of the recordings on successive days ($n = 11$). *$p < 0.05$, **$p < 0.01$, ***$p < 0.001$ Fisher's LSD. **(C)** Quantification of the effect of IPSU and suvorexant on wake, NREM and REM during the first 4 h post-treatment. *$p < 0.05$, ***$p < 0.001$ paired t-test drug vs. vehicle.

In contrast, the DORA suvorexant (25 mg/kg) slightly decreased time spent in wake, had weak effects on time in NREM but strongly increased the amount of time spent in REM sleep during the first 4 h immediately following application [**Figures 1B,C**, treatment: wake $F_{(1, 120)} = 3.4, p = 0.066$, NREM $F_{(1, 120)} = 0.44, p = 0.51$, REM $F_{(1, 120)} = 28.9, p < 0.001$, treatment × hour: wake $F_{(5, 120)} = 2.31, p = 0.048$, NREM $F_{(5, 120)} = 1.76, p = 0.13$, REM $F_{(5, 120)} = 3.37, p = 0.007$, REML].

Manual rescoring of the first 2 h after vehicle or drug application confirmed that the automatic scoring was in excellent agreement when amount of time in each stage was compared, better than 90% as previously reported by us and others (Pick et al., 2011; Mang et al., 2012). The number of awakenings was, however, different. Very short awakenings were found within epochs scored as NREM (Léna et al., 2004). We therefore used the results from the manual scoring to quantify the latency to NREM or REM and the sleep-wake transitions (**Table 1**).

Both IPSU and suvorexant showed a tendency to shorten the latency to NREM and REM sleep but only the shortening of latency to REM by suvorexant was significantly different from the vehicle. Awakenings from NREM were unaffected by either compound. Whereas awakenings from REM were significantly increased by suvorexant, the OX_2R antagonist IPSU had no effect.

DISCUSSION

Whereas IPSU did not perturb the normal sleep pattern of mice during the inactive period, suvorexant profoundly altered the sleep pattern, doubling the time spent in REM. The latency to REM and number of awakenings from REM was also selectively increased by suvorexant but not by IPSU. This pattern is similar to that found when these compounds were dosed at the start of the dark (active) period in mice (Betschart et al., 2013). Suvorexant promoted sleep primarily by increasing REM with small effects on NREM and IPSU promoted sleep primarily by promoting NREM and to a lesser degree REM (Betschart et al., 2013). The stronger enhancement of REM vs. NREM by suvorexant has also been seen in rats and in both healthy humans and humans suffering from insomnia (Winrow et al., 2011; Herring et al., 2012; Sun et al., 2013). Interestingly, our findings indicate that this DORA influences REM independently of the circadian dosing time, increasing the time in REM during both the light (active) phase and dark (active) phase whereas, at the dose tested, the OX_2R preferring

antagonist IPSU influences sleep only during the active phase in mice.

Influencing the balance between REM and NREM is an area of potential differentiation between OX_2R preferring antagonists and DORAs. Classic benzodiazepines, "Z drugs" such as zolpidem, and antidepressants are well known for suppressing REM sleep whereas ORAs certainly lack this property. Although IPSU is not highly selective for OX_2R vs. OX_1R at mouse receptors ($\sim6.2\times$), the opposite is true for suvorexant, which prefers mouse OX_1R vs. OX_2R ($\sim6.5\times$, Betschart et al., 2013; Callander et al., 2013). Thus, the balance between antagonism of OX_1R and OX_2R may contribute to the differential effects of ORAs on sleep architecture. Our findings suggest that reducing the level of OX_1R antagonism shifts the sleep balance toward NREM. Supporting this hypothesis, almorexant induces a greater REM increase in $OX_1R^{-/-}$ than in wildtype mice (Mang et al., 2012). Likewise, whereas both almorexant and the OX_2R antagonist JNJ-10397049 increased NREM during the light phase in rats, only almorexant also increased REM, and co-application of an OX_1R antagonist significantly reduced the NREM induced by the OX_2R antagonist (Dugovic et al., 2009). For the most part, DORAs increase REM more than NREM in rodent studies when % increase is considered (Brisbare-Roch et al., 2007; Winrow et al., 2011; Betschart et al., 2013; Black et al., 2013). However, the contribution of REM as a proportion of total sleep time varies for different compounds. For example, in mice almorexant-induced increases in REM remain within the proportion seen during normal sleep, even at high doses (Mang et al., 2012), whereas suvorexant increases REM proportion much above that seen during normal sleep (Betschart et al., 2013). Almorexant is unusual among the DORAs in that it appears to become a somewhat OX_2R preferring antagonist *in vivo*. The *ex vivo* occupancy of almorexant was found to be about 2x higher and much longer lasting at OX_2Rs (>12 h) vs. OX_1Rs (Morairty et al., 2012). This preference is most likely driven by the unusual kinetics (Malherbe et al., 2009; Mang et al., 2012; Callander et al., 2013) so that with short exposures the compound may act as a DORA, and when equilibrium is allowed to be reached almorexant has functional selectivity for OX_2Rs. Evidence against our hypothesis includes the description of a newer DORA that increases NREM preferentially in rats (Sifferlen et al., 2013). The structure of this compound is quite similar to that of almorexant but whether the kinetics also bias it toward OX_2R selectivity when equilibrated

---

Table 1 | Effect of the OX_2R preferring antagonist IPSU and the DORA, suvorexant on latency to sleep and sleep to wake transitions during the first 2 h after administration during the inactive period.

	Vehicle	IPSU	Diff	Vehicle	Suvorexant	Diff
Latency to NREM (minutes)	9.5 ± 3.0	2.6 ± 1.0	-7.0 ± 3.3	13.1 ± 5.9	4.8 ± 1.9	-8.3 ± 6.3
Latency to REM (minutes)	22.1 ± 3.4	14.5 ± 2.3	-7.6 ± 4.5	37.0 ± 10.1	$8.4 \pm 2.3^*$	-28.6 ± 8.8
Awakenings from NREM	25.1 ± 2.6	25.3 ± 2.0	0.2 ± 2.4	19.4 ± 1.6	18.6 ± 1.9	-0.8 ± 2.4
Awakenings from REM	10.2 ± 0.9	10.8 ± 1.1	0.6 ± 1.1	8.2 ± 1.4	$15.6 \pm 1.2^{**}$	7.4 ± 1.6
Short awakenings from NREM (<5 s)	23.55 ± 2.8	26.5 ± 4.3	2.9 ± 1.9	25.7 ± 4.0	26.6 ± 3.1	0.9 ± 2.1
Total awakenings	58.8 ± 4.7	62.6 ± 5.1	3.7 ± 2.7	53.3 ± 4.9	$60.8 \pm 3.8^{***}$	7.5 ± 1.9

*$p < 0.05$, **$p < 0.01$, ***$p < 0.001$, paired t-test.

is unknown. Interestingly, species differences also exist in the effects of DORAs on sleep architecture. In dogs, suvorexant predominately increased NREM (Winrow et al., 2011). The effects of DORAs on REM in humans appear to more closely mimic the effects in rodents rather than dogs as in the clinical settings, REM was preferentially enhanced with SB-649868 (Bettica et al., 2012a,b,c) and suvorexant (Herring et al., 2012; Sun et al., 2013). With the limited data available, whether the differential effects of the DORAs and OX2R antagonists on sleep architecture are in fact due to differences in receptor affinity/occupancy or are due to other factors such as compound class and species, remains to be seen as more compounds from different chemical classes are developed.

Why might a DORA be expected to influence REM more strongly than an OX_2R preferring antagonist? Intracerebroventicular or local application of orexin-A in the highly OX_1R expressing locus coeruleus reduces REM sleep, an effect that is blocked by the OX_1R antagonist SB-334867 (Smith et al., 2003; Mieda et al., 2011). Additionally, knock-down of OX_1R receptors in the locus coeruleus selectively increases REM, without affecting NREM during the active phase (Chen et al., 2010). Interestingly, we did not see a similar dependence of circadian time on the REM enhancement by suvorexant. REM sleep is not however, exclusively modulated by OX_1Rs. OX_2R knockdown in the lateral pontomesencephalic tegmentum increased REM both during the active and inactive phases (Chen et al., 2013) and while OX_1R antagonists alone generally do not induce REM (Steiner et al., 2013), they may increase REM on top of the effects of OX_2R antagonists (Dugovic et al., 2009). Overall, both OX_1R and OX_2R when activated or down regulated in the appropriate regions appear to be able to modulate REM sleep. However, the modulatory role of OX_1R on REM may be greater than that of OX_2R.

In conclusion, we hypothesize that selective OX_2R antagonists have potential for the treatment of insomnia and may prove to perturb sleep architecture to a lesser degree than some of the DORAs. More highly selective antagonists from different chemical classes will be required to test this hypothesis further.

AUTHOR CONTRIBUTIONS

All authors read and commented on the manuscript. Daniel Hoyer and Claudia Betschart led the team and participated in writing the manuscript. Thomas Dürst planned and performed experiments and analyzed data. Claudia Betschart, Samuel Hintermann, Dirk Behnke, Silvio Ofner, and Simona Cotesta synthesized and/or designed compounds. Grit Laue performed in vivo analyses related to pharmacokinetics. Markus Fendt, Laura H. Jacobson, and Eric Legangneux contributed to experimental design and writing the manuscript. Christine E. Gee designed the study, performed analysis, and wrote the manuscript.

ACKNOWLEDGMENTS

This study was entirely funded by the Novartis Institutes for BioMedical Research, Novartis AG.

REFERENCES

Annerbrink, K., Westberg, L., Olsson, M., Andersch, S., Sjödin, I., Holm, G., et al. (2011). Panic disorder is associated with the Val308Iso polymorphism in the hypocretin receptor gene. Psychiatr. Genet. 21, 85–89. doi: 10.1097/YPG.0b013e328341a3db

Baker, T. L., Foutz, A. S., McNerney, V., Mitler, M. M., and Dement, W. C. (1982). Canine model of narcolepsy: genetic and developmental determinants. Exp. Neurol. 75, 729–742. doi: 10.1016/0014-4886(82)90038-3

Betschart, C., Hintermann, S., Behnke, D., Cotesta, S., Fendt, M., Gee, C. E., et al. (2013). Identification of a novel series of orexin receptor antagonists with a distinct effect on sleep architecture for the treatment of insomnia. J. Med. Chem. 56, 7590–7607. doi: 10.1021/jm4007627

Bettica, P., Nucci, G., Pyke, C., Squassante, L., Zamuner, S., Ratti, E., et al. (2012a). Phase I studies on the safety, tolerability, pharmacokinetics and pharmacodynamics of SB-649868, a novel dual orexin receptor antagonist. J. Psychopharmacol. 26, 1058–1070. doi: 10.1177/0269881111408954

Bettica, P., Squassante, L., Groeger, J. A., Gennery, B., Winsky-Sommerer, R., and Dijk, D.-J. (2012b). Differential effects of a dual orexin receptor antagonist (SB-649868) and zolpidem on sleep initiation and consolidation, SWS, REM sleep, and EEG power spectra in a model of situational insomnia. Neuropsychopharmacology 37, 1224–1233. doi: 10.1038/npp.2011.310

Bettica, P., Squassante, L., Zamuner, S., Nucci, G., Danker-Hopfe, H., and Ratti, E. (2012c). The orexin antagonist SB-649868 promotes and maintains sleep in men with primary insomnia. Sleep 35, 1097–1104. doi: 10.5665/sleep.1996

Black, S. W., Morairty, S. R., Fisher, S. P., Chen, T.-M., Warrier, D. R., and Kilduff, T. S. (2013). Almorexant promotes sleep and exacerbates cataplexy in a murine model of narcolepsy. Sleep 36, 325–336. doi: 10.5665/sleep.2442

Brisbare-Roch, C., Dingemanse, J., Koberstein, R., Hoever, P., Aissaoui, H., Flores, S., et al. (2007). Promotion of sleep by targeting the orexin system in rats, dogs and humans. Nat. Med. 13, 150–155. doi: 10.1038/nm1544

Callander, G. E., Olorunda, M., Monna, D., Schuepbach, E., Langenegger, D., Betschart, C., et al. (2013). Kinetic properties of "dual" orexin receptor antagonists at OX1R and OX2R orexin receptors. Front. Neuropharmacol. Rev. 7:230. doi: 10.3389/fnins.2013.00230

Chemelli, R. M., Willie, J. T., Sinton, C. M., Elmquist, J. K., Scammell, T., Lee, C., et al. (1999). Narcolepsy in orexin knockout mice: molecular genetics of sleep regulation. Cell 98, 437–451. doi: 10.1016/S0092-8674(00)81973-X

Chen, L., McKenna, J. T., Bolortuya, Y., Brown, R. E., and McCarley, R. W. (2013). Knockdown of orexin type 2 receptor in the lateral pontomesencephalic tegmentum of rats increases REM sleep. Eur. J. Neurosci. 37, 957–963. doi: 10.1111/ejn.12101

Chen, L., McKenna, J. T., Bolortuya, Y., Winston, S., Thakkar, M. M., Basheer, R., et al. (2010). Knockdown of orexin type 1 receptor in rat locus coeruleus increases REM sleep during the dark period. Eur. J. Neurosci. 32, 1528–1536. doi: 10.1111/j.1460-9568.2010.07401.x

Cox, C. D., Breslin, M. J., and Coleman, P. J. (2008). Substituted diazepan orexin receptor antagonists. Patent No. WO2008/008158.

Dugovic, C., Shelton, J. E., Aluisio, L. E., Fraser, I. C., Jiang, X., Sutton, S. W., et al. (2009). Blockade of orexin-1 receptors attenuates orexin-2 receptor antagonism-induced sleep promotion in the rat. J. Pharmacol. Exp. Ther. 330, 142–151. doi: 10.1124/jpet.109.152009

Gotter, A. L., Winrow, C. J., Brunner, J., Garson, S. L., Fox, S. V., Binns, J., et al. (2013). The duration of sleep promoting efficacy by dual orexin receptor antagonists is dependent upon receptor occupancy threshold. BMC Neurosci. 14:90. doi: 10.1186/1471-2202-14-90

Hara, J., Beuckmann, C. T., Nambu, T., Willie, J. T., Chemelli, R. M., Sinton, C. M., et al. (2001). Genetic ablation of orexin neurons in mice results in narcolepsy, hypophagia, and obesity. Neuron 30, 345–354. doi: 10.1016/S0896-6273(01)00293-8

Herring, W. J., Snyder, E., Budd, K., Hutzelmann, J., Snavely, D., Liu, K., et al. (2012). Orexin receptor antagonism for treatment of insomnia: a randomized clinical trial of suvorexant. Neurology 79, 2265–2274. doi: 10.1212/WNL.0b013e31827688ee

Kalogiannis, M., Hsu, E., Willie, J. T., Chemelli, R. M., Kisanuki, Y. Y., Yanagisawa, M., et al. (2011). Cholinergic modulation of narcoleptic attacks in double orexin receptor knockout mice. PLoS ONE 6:e18697. doi: 10.1371/journal.pone.0018697

Léna, C., Popa, D., Grailhe, R., Escourrou, P., Changeux, J.-P., and Adrien, J. (2004). Beta2-containing nicotinic receptors contribute to the organization of sleep and regulate putative micro-arousals in mice. *J. Neurosci.* 24, 5711–5718. doi: 10.1523/JNEUROSCI.3882-03.2004

Lin, L., Faraco, J., Li, R., Kadotani, H., Rogers, W., Lin, X., et al. (1999). The sleep disorder canine narcolepsy is caused by a mutation in the hypocretin (orexin) receptor 2 gene. *Cell* 98, 365–376. doi: 10.1016/S0092-8674(00)81965-0

Malherbe, P., Borroni, E., Pinard, E., Wettstein, J. G., and Knoflach, F. (2009). Biochemical and electrophysiological characterization of almorexant, a dual orexin 1 receptor (OX1)/orexin 2 receptor (OX2) antagonist: comparison with selective OX1 and OX2 antagonists. *Mol. Pharmacol.* 76, 618–631. doi: 10.1124/mol.109.055152

Mang, G. M., Dürst, T., Bürki, H., Imobersteg, S., Abramowski, D., Schuepbach, E., et al. (2012). The dual orexin receptor antagonist almorexant induces sleep and decreases orexin-induced locomotion by blocking orexin 2 receptors. *Sleep* 35, 1625–1635. doi: 10.5665/sleep.2232

Mieda, M., Hasegawa, E., Kisanuki, Y. Y., Sinton, C. M., Yanagisawa, M., and Sakurai, T. (2011). Differential roles of orexin receptor-1 and -2 in the regulation of non-REM and REM sleep. *J. Neurosci.* 31, 6518–6526. doi: 10.1523/JNEUROSCI.6506-10.2011

Mieda, M., Tsujino, N., and Sakurai, T. (2013). Differential roles of orexin receptors in the regulation of sleep/wakefulness. *Front. Endocrinol. (Lausanne).* 4:57. doi: 10.3389/fendo.2013.00057

Morairty, S. R., Revel, F. G., Malherbe, P., Moreau, J.-L., Valladao, D., Wettstein, J. G., et al. (2012). Dual hypocretin receptor antagonism is more effective for sleep promotion than antagonism of either receptor alone. *PLoS ONE* 7:e39131. doi: 10.1371/journal.pone.0039131

Nishino, S., Ripley, B., Overeem, S., Lammers, G. J., and Mignot, E. (2000). Hypocretin (orexin) deficiency in human narcolepsy. *Lancet* 355, 39–40. doi: 10.1016/S0140-6736(99)05582-8

Peyron, C., Faraco, J., Rogers, W., Ripley, B., Overeem, S., Charnay, Y., et al. (2000). A mutation in a case of early onset narcolepsy and a generalized absence of hypocretin peptides in human narcoleptic brains. *Nat. Med.* 6, 991–997. doi: 10.1038/79690

Pick, J., Chen, Y., Moore, J. T., Sun, Y., Wyner, A. J., Friedman, E. B., et al. (2011). Rapid eye movement sleep debt accrues in mice exposed to volatile anesthetics. *Anesthesiology* 115, 702–712. doi: 10.1097/ALN.0b013e31822ddd72

Rainero, I., Gallone, S., Rubino, E., Ponzo, P., Valfre, W., Binello, E., et al. (2008). Haplotype analysis confirms the association between the HCRTR2 gene and cluster headache. *Headache* 48, 1108–1114. doi: 10.1111/j.1526-4610.2008.01080.x

Ripley, B., Fujiki, N., Okura, M., Mignot, E., and Nishino, S. (2001). Hypocretin levels in sporadic and familial cases of canine narcolepsy. *Neurobiol. Dis.* 8, 525–534. doi: 10.1006/nbdi.2001.0389

Sifferlen, T., Koberstein, R., Cottreel, E., Boller, A., Weller, T., Gatfield, J., et al. (2013). Structure-activity relationship studies and sleep-promoting activity of novel 1-chloro-5,6,7,8-tetrahydroimidazo[1,5-a]pyrazine derivatives as dual orexin receptor antagonists. Part 2. *Bioorg. Med. Chem. Lett.* 23, 3857–3863. doi: 10.1016/j.bmcl.2013.04.071

Smith, M. I., Piper, D. C., Duxon, M. S., and Upton, N. (2003). Evidence implicating a role for orexin-1 receptor modulation of paradoxical sleep in the rat. *Neurosci. Lett.* 341, 256–258. doi: 10.1016/S0304-3940(03)00066-1

Steiner, M. A., Gatfield, J., Brisbare-Roch, C., Dietrich, H., Treiber, A., Jenck, F., et al. (2013). Discovery and characterization of ACT-335827, an orally available, brain penetrant orexin receptor type 1 selective antagonist. *ChemMedChem* 8, 898–903. doi: 10.1002/cmdc.201300003

Sun, H., Kennedy, W. P., Wilbraham, D., Lewis, N., Calder, N., Li, X., et al. (2013). Effects of suvorexant, an orexin receptor antagonist, on sleep parameters as measured by polysomnography in healthy men. *Sleep* 36, 259–267. doi: 10.5665/sleep.2386

Thannickal, T. C., Moore, R. Y., Nienhuis, R., Ramanathan, L., Gulyani, S., Aldrich, M., et al. (2000). Reduced number of hypocretin neurons in human narcolepsy. *Neuron* 27, 469–474. doi: 10.1016/S0896-6273(00)00058-1

Thompson, M. D., Comings, D. E., Abu-Ghazalah, R., Jereseh, Y., Lin, L., Wade, J., et al. (2004). Variants of the orexin2/hcrt2 receptor gene identified in patients with excessive daytime sleepiness and patients with Tourette's syndrome comorbidity. *Am. J. Med. Genet. B Neuropsychiatr. Genet.* 129B, 69–75. doi: 10.1002/ajmg.b.30047

Willie, J. T., Chemelli, R. M., Sinton, C. M., Tokita, S., Williams, S. C., Kisanuki, Y. Y., et al. (2003). Distinct narcolepsy syndromes in Orexin receptor-2 and Orexin null mice: molecular genetic dissection of Non-REM and REM sleep regulatory processes. *Neuron* 38, 715–730. doi: 10.1016/S0896-6273(03)00330-1

Winrow, C. J., Gotter, A. L., Cox, C. D., Doran, S. M., Tannenbaum, P. L., Breslin, M. J., et al. (2011). Promotion of sleep by suvorexant-a novel dual orexin receptor antagonist. *J. Neurogenet.* 25, 52–61. doi: 10.3109/01677063.2011.566953

Conflict of Interest Statement: All authors were or are employees of Novartis AG and may own stock in the company.

Dual orexin receptor antagonists show distinct effects on locomotor performance, ethanol interaction and sleep architecture relative to gamma-aminobutyric acid-A receptor modulators

Andres D. Ramirez[1], Anthony L. Gotter[1], Steven V. Fox[2], Pamela L. Tannenbaum[2], Lihang Yao[2], Spencer J. Tye[2], Terrence McDonald[1], Joseph Brunner[1], Susan L. Garson[1], Duane R. Reiss[1], Scott D. Kuduk[3], Paul J. Coleman[3], Jason M. Uslaner[2], Robert Hodgson[2], Susan E. Browne[2], John J. Renger[1] and Christopher J. Winrow[1]*

[1] Merck Research Laboratories, Department of Neuroscience, Merck & Co., Inc., West Point, PA, USA
[2] Merck Research Laboratories, Department of In Vivo Pharmacology, Merck & Co., Inc., West Point, PA, USA
[3] Merck Research Laboratories, Department of Medicinal Chemistry, Merck & Co., Inc., West Point, PA, USA

Edited by:
Michel A. Steiner, Actelion
Pharmaceuticals Ltd., Switzerland

Reviewed by:
Enrico Sanna, University of Cagliari,
Italy
Robyn M. Brown, Florey
Neuroscience Institutes, Australia
Yong Lu, Northeast Ohio Medical
University, USA

*Correspondence:
Christopher J. Winrow, Merck &
Co., Inc. 770 Sumneytown Pike,
WP26-265 West Point, PA
19486-0004, USA
e-mail: christopher_winrow@
merck.com

Dual orexin receptor antagonists (DORAs) are a potential treatment for insomnia that function by blocking both the orexin 1 and orexin 2 receptors. The objective of the current study was to further confirm the impact of therapeutic mechanisms targeting insomnia on locomotor coordination and ethanol interaction using DORAs and gamma-aminobutyric acid (GABA)-A receptor modulators of distinct chemical structure and pharmacological properties in the context of sleep-promoting potential. The current study compared rat motor co-ordination after administration of DORAs, DORA-12 and almorexant, and GABA-A receptor modulators, zolpidem, eszopiclone, and diazepam, alone or each in combination with ethanol. Motor performance was assessed by measuring time spent walking on a rotarod apparatus. Zolpidem, eszopiclone and diazepam [0.3–30 mg/kg administered orally (PO)] impaired rotarod performance in a dose-dependent manner. Furthermore, all three GABA-A receptor modulators potentiated ethanol- (0.25–1.5 g/kg) induced impairment on the rotarod. By contrast, neither DORA-12 (10–100 mg/kg, PO) nor almorexant (30–300 mg/kg, PO) impaired motor performance alone or in combination with ethanol. In addition, distinct differences in sleep architecture were observed between ethanol, GABA-A receptor modulators (zolpidem, eszopiclone, and diazepam) and DORA-12 in electroencephalogram studies in rats. These findings provide further evidence that orexin receptor antagonists have an improved motor side-effect profile compared with currently available sleep-promoting agents based on preclinical data and strengthen the rationale for further evaluation of these agents in clinical development.

Keywords: orexin, dual orexin receptor antagonist, locomotor performance, sleep, insomnia, GABA, ethanol, rats

INTRODUCTION

Orexin neurons are a cluster of cells located in the perifornical lateral hypothalamic area. The neuropeptides orexin A and B bind to and activate the orexin 1 and 2 receptors (OX_1R and OX_2R, respectively) with differential selectivity; orexin A binds both receptors with similar affinity while orexin B exhibits approximately 10-fold selectivity for OX_2R (Sakurai et al., 1998). Recent advances have been made in the development of pharmacological agents that antagonize orexin receptors and interest in their potential clinical application has increased (Scammell and Winrow, 2011). The most salient role for orexin signaling is its regulation of arousal and vigilance stage control, but it has also been implicated in several other processes including feeding, reward, stress, and mood (Gotter et al., 2012). The neuronal networks underlying these processes are becoming better understood as orexin receptor antagonists with greater selectivity have been developed (Ohno and Sakurai, 2008).

Orexin neurons are active during the waking phase in animals, but are largely quiescent during the sleep phase (Yoshida et al., 2001; Kiyashchenko et al., 2002). Genetic loss of orexin signaling in canines and rodents and orexin deficiency in humans causes symptoms of narcolepsy (Chemelli et al., 1999; Lin et al., 1999; Nishino et al., 2000), indicating the importance of orexin neurons in regulating sleep-arousal mechanisms. For example, damaging orexin neurons using the neurotoxin hypocretin-2-saporin alters sleep behavior in rats (Gerashchenko et al., 2003) and acute optogenetic silencing of these cells *in vivo* induces slow-wave sleep in mice (Tsunematsu et al., 2011). Orexin neurons of the lateral hypothalamus project to nuclei involved in regulating arousal and vigilance state. OX_1R and OX_2R have overlapping expression in these regions, with OX_2R having selective expression in tuberomammillary nuclei of the hypothalamus, primarily responsible for driving histamine-mediated arousal (Lin et al., 1988; Trivedi et al., 1998; Marcus et al., 2001). Both receptors are expressed in brainstem nuclei involved in sleep regulation, the exception being the selective expression of OX_1R in the locus coeruleus, most notably involved in the regulation of REM sleep (Trivedi et al., 1998; Marcus et al., 2001). Regulation of orexin neuron activity is provided both by excitatory projections from the dorsomedial nucleus of the hypothalamus and by inhibitory gamma-aminobutyric acid (GABA) inputs arising from the ventrolateral preoptic area (Thompson et al., 1996; Yoshida et al., 2006). Increased inhibitory GABA activity on orexin neurons and other sleep-related nuclei suppresses arousal and promotes sleep (Saper et al., 2005).

Currently available sleep agents (including benzodiazepines and related compounds) are typically GABA-A receptor modulators, which are believed to mediate sedative effects through their high affinity for the GABA-A α1 receptor subunit (Graham et al., 1996; Rudolph et al., 1999; McKernan et al., 2000). Hypnotics do not bind to the GABA-A receptor active site but instead potentiate the affinity of GABA for the receptor via allosteric modulation and result in increased inhibitor activity of the receptor (Bianchi, 2010). GABA-A receptors are located throughout the central nervous system (CNS), and have a role not only in sleep induction, but in numerous other brain functions as well (Sieghart and Sperk, 2002). This broad functionality can lead to a variety of undesirable side effects such as unsteady gait, next-day sedation, cognition deficits, lost balance and confusion (Barker et al., 2004; Hindmarch et al., 2006; Otmani et al., 2008; Vermeeren and Coenen, 2011). In an attempt to boost their sleep-promoting effects, some chronic users of GABA-A receptor modulators combine these agents with alcohol (Johnson et al., 1998).

Ethanol acts, at least partially, by enhancing GABA transmission at GABA-A receptors (Hanchar et al., 2005; Lovinger and Roberto, 2013) and chronic consumption of alcohol can result in cross-tolerance to benzodiazepines (Devaud et al., 1996; Cagetti et al., 2003). The actions of alcohol and benzodiazepines therefore converge mechanistically at GABA-A receptors, synergistically increasing their activity and potentially amplifying next-day hangover effects. It is well-documented that co-administration of alcohol and benzodiazepines/benzodiazepine receptor modulators can precipitate toxicities and accidents (Tanaka, 2002; Kurzthaler et al., 2005), emphasizing the unmet need for novel sleep-promoting agents with improved adverse-event profiles.

Recently, a number of orexin receptor antagonists including SB-649868 (Bettica et al., 2012a), almorexant (Brisbare-Roch et al., 2007), suvorexant (Winrow et al., 2011) and MK-6096 (Winrow et al., 2012) have demonstrated sleep-promoting properties in both animal and in clinical studies (Herring et al., 2012a; Hoever et al., 2012; Bettica et al., 2012b). As these antagonists target orexin receptors directly, we were interested in comparing structurally distinct orexin receptor antagonists with a variety of GABA-A receptor modulators, to evaluate their effects on sleep architecture and potential for ethanol interactions. In foundational studies, Steiner et al. (Steiner et al., 2011) compared the effects of almorexant and zolpidem both alone and when co-administered with ethanol in the context of rat locomotor performance and myorelaxation in rotarod and grip strength assays. Zolpidem affected both locomotor performance and grip strength

in a dose-dependent manner and was exacerbated by ethanol, whereas neither of these changes were observed with almorexant at dosages up to 300 mg/kg (PO). The earlier study examined one representative compound from each class, specifically in rotarod and grip assays. In order to make a thorough assessment of the mechanistic differences between the two drug classes, the current study evaluated the locomotor performance and ethanol interaction not only of almorexant, but also a chemically distinct dual orexin receptor antagonists (DORA) of diverse structure, DORA-12, as well as benzodiazepine and non-benzodiazepine GABA-A modulators diazepam, eszopiclone and zolpidem. Further, locomotor performance was evaluated directly in the context of sleep-promoting efficacy. These results demonstrate a distinct difference between these sleep-promoting mechanisms, orexin antagonism and GABA-A receptor activation, in terms of locomotor performance in the presence or absence of ethanol and in the context of effects on sleep architecture.

MATERIALS AND METHODS
ANIMALS
All animal studies were performed in accordance with the National Research Council Institute of Laboratory Animal Resources Guide for the Care and Use of Laboratory Animals and were approved by the Merck Institutional Animal Care and Use Committee. Male Sprague-Dawley rats (180–225 g) were maintained under normal laboratory conditions (controlled temperature and food plus water *ad libitum*) under a regular 12-h light/dark cycle (18:00 lights off and 06:00 lights on). Male animals were used to avoid variability due to time-dependent changes in estrus and rat sex-dependent differences in metabolic enzyme activity. All behavioral tests were performed during the light phase of the cycle, which in nocturnal rats is the normal resting phase. Animals were fasted overnight, housed two per cage prior to testing and acclimated to the testing room for 30 min before testing. All studies used a between-subjects design.

COMPOUNDS AND FORMULATIONS
All pharmacological agents were synthesized by Merck chemists or purchased from Sigma Company (Cream Ridge, NJ, USA) and diluted in 20% Vitamin E-TPGS (d-alpha-tocopheryl polyethylene glycol 1000 succinate) vehicle to a dose volume of 2 mL/kg, to be administered orally using standard stainless steel gavage needles affixed to a 5 cc syringe (PO). Ethanol was diluted in distilled water to a dose volume of 2 mL/kg to be administered intra-peritoneally (IP). After the acclimation period, rats were administered compound or vehicle PO and tested after 30 min or were administered compound PO followed immediately by ethanol IP and tested after 30 min.

ROTAROD TEST
The rotarod apparatus (IITC Life Sciences, Woodland Hills, CA, USA) consisted of a rod 60 mm in diameter suspended 25.4 cm from the floor of the apparatus. The speed of the rod could be varied as desired. Rats were first trained over 2 days (2–3 trials) to walk on the rod rotating at a constant speed (12 rpm). Rats were then selected for inclusion in assays if they were able to remain on the rod for 120 s as it was accelerated from 4 to 20 rpm (over

150 s). Animals unable to perform the training task were excluded from further testing. Roughly 10% of the animals failed to meet this criterion.

During compound testing, rats were administered the test compound and then returned to their home cage for the duration of the pretreatment period. The rats were then placed on the rotarod at a speed that accelerated from 4 to 40 rpm over 300 s. Latency to fall (time to the rat falling from the apparatus, up to 300 s) for each animal was digitally recorded by trip plates in the platform which were triggered as soon as the rat fell from the rod. One testing trial was performed for each animal.

PLASMA CONCENTRATIONS AND ETHANOL BLOOD LEVELS
At the end of the rotarod testing, which lasted approximately 35–40 min, rats were immediately euthanized by carbon dioxide overdose and blood samples were drawn via cardiac puncture for compound level and/or blood alcohol content (BAC) testing. Blood was centrifuged at 1300 RCF for 10 min at 4°C to obtain serum for determination of compound plasma concentration and BAC. Ethanol analysis was performed using the Siemens Ethanol_2 method on the Siemens Advia 1800 clinical chemistry analyzer. The method utilizes alcohol dehydrogenase to catalyze the oxidation of ethanol to acetaldehyde as well as reducing nicotinamide adenine dinucleotide (NAD) to NADH. This causes an increase in absorbance at 340 nm which is proportional to the BAC (Clinical Pathology Diagnostic Group at Merck West Point).

Data were analyzed using a one-way analysis of variance followed by a *post-hoc* Newmans-Keuls multiple comparison test; $p < 0.05$ was considered significant. Data in the results tables were normalized to controls.

RAT AMBULATORY POLYSOMNOGRAPHY
Male Sprague-Dawley rats (Charles Rivers Laboratory, Raleigh, NC; $n = 8$–16/study, weight: 450–600 g) were singly housed in polycarbonate cages (48.3 × 25.4 × 20.3 cm; LabProducts, Seaford, DE) with free access to food and water in a 12:12 light:dark cycle. Prior to testing, adult rats of sufficient weight were implanted with radio telemetric devices (TL10M3-F50-EEE, Data Sciences International, Arden Hills, MN) and mean time in vigilance states [active wake, light sleep, delta sleep, rapid eye movement (REM) sleep] was determined as detailed previously (Renger et al., 2004; Winrow et al., 2011, 2012). For these experiments, vehicle and drug treatments were administered on three consecutive days during the middle of the active or dark phase (Zeitgeber Time 18:00–18:30) in a balanced cross-over design such that each animal received both vehicle and drug in alternate arms of the experiment. Mean within-subject change from vehicle was determined for time spent in each vigilance state for the 2 h following treatment. Population t-tests were used to determine significance from vehicle under each condition.

RESULTS
INDIVIDUAL ACUTE EFFECTS ON MOTOR PERFORMANCE OF GABA-A RECEPTOR MODULATORS, ETHANOL AND OREXIN RECEPTOR ANTAGONISTS
The chemical structures of the orexin receptor antagonists included in this study are shown in **Figure 1**.

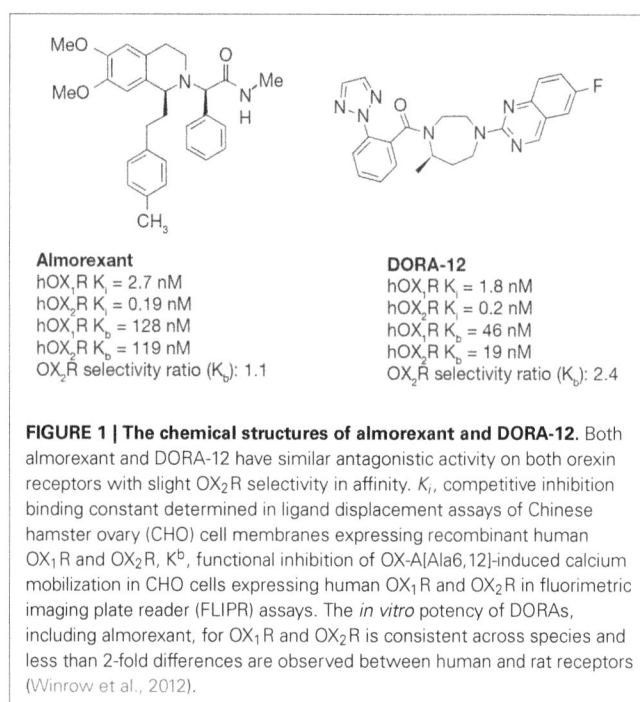

Almorexant
$hOX_1R K_i = 2.7$ nM
$hOX_2R K_i = 0.19$ nM
$hOX_1R K_b = 128$ nM
$hOX_2R K_b = 119$ nM
OX_2R selectivity ratio (K_b): 1.1

DORA-12
$hOX_1R K_i = 1.8$ nM
$hOX_2R K_i = 0.2$ nM
$hOX_1R K_b = 46$ nM
$hOX_2R K_b = 19$ nM
OX_2R selectivity ratio (K_b): 2.4

FIGURE 1 | **The chemical structures of almorexant and DORA-12.** Both almorexant and DORA-12 have similar antagonistic activity on both orexin receptors with slight OX_2R selectivity in affinity. K_i, competitive inhibition binding constant determined in ligand displacement assays of Chinese hamster ovary (CHO) cell membranes expressing recombinant human OX_1R and OX_2R, K^b, functional inhibition of OX-A[Ala6,12]-induced calcium mobilization in CHO cells expressing human OX_1R and OX_2R in fluorimetric imaging plate reader (FLIPR) assays. The *in vitro* potency of DORAs, including almorexant, for OX_1R and OX_2R is consistent across species and less than 2-fold differences are observed between human and rat receptors (Winrow et al., 2012).

Time spent walking on the rotarod by rats treated with either GABA-A receptor modulators, orexin receptor antagonists, ethanol or vehicles was measured to assess the compounds' individual effects on motor performance. Rotarod performance 30 min after drug administration was impaired in a dose-dependent manner by all the GABA-A receptor modulators tested (**Figure 2A**). Zolpidem [$F_{(4, 38)} = 14.26, p < 0.01$], eszopiclone [$F_{(4, 45)} = 38.19, p < 0.01$] and diazepam [$F_{(4, 44)} = 18.1, p < 0.01$] all had a significant effect on rotarod performance. The highest doses of zolpidem, eszopiclone and diazepam (10, 30, and 10 mg/kg, respectively) reduced motor ability by 48.2, 56.1, and 57.8%, respectively, compared with vehicle treatment ($p < 0.001$; **Table 1**). The lowest dose to result in significant impairment compared with vehicle-treated animals was 3.0 mg/kg for all of the GABA-A receptor modulators [19.7, 15.1, and 30.2% impairment for zolpidem, eszopiclone, and diazepam, respectively; $p < 0.01$ for all (**Table 1**)].

Ethanol administration dose-dependently impaired motor performance in the rats [$F_{(4, 30)} = 11.83, p < 0.01$] with doses of 0.5, 1.0 and 1.5 g/kg significantly decreasing latency to fall relative to vehicle (**Figure 2B**). The highest ethanol dose (1.5 g/kg) produced a 64.6% decrease in motor ability in the rotarod compared with vehicle-treated animals ($p < 0.001$, **Table 1**).

Almorexant doses ranging from 30 to 300 mg/kg PO did not affect the rats' ability to walk on the rotarod [$F_{(3, 36)} = 0.23, p > 0.05$] (**Figure 2C** and **Table 1**). Similarly, DORA-12 did not affect rotarod performance over doses ranging from 10 to 100 mg/kg, PO [$F_{(3, 38)} = 0.54, p > 0.05$] (**Figure 2C** and **Table 1**).

BAC and compound plasma concentrations were monitored to ensure that levels increased concomitantly with increasing doses of ethanol or sleep-promoting compounds, respectively. Plasma levels of the GABA-A receptor modulators increased with higher

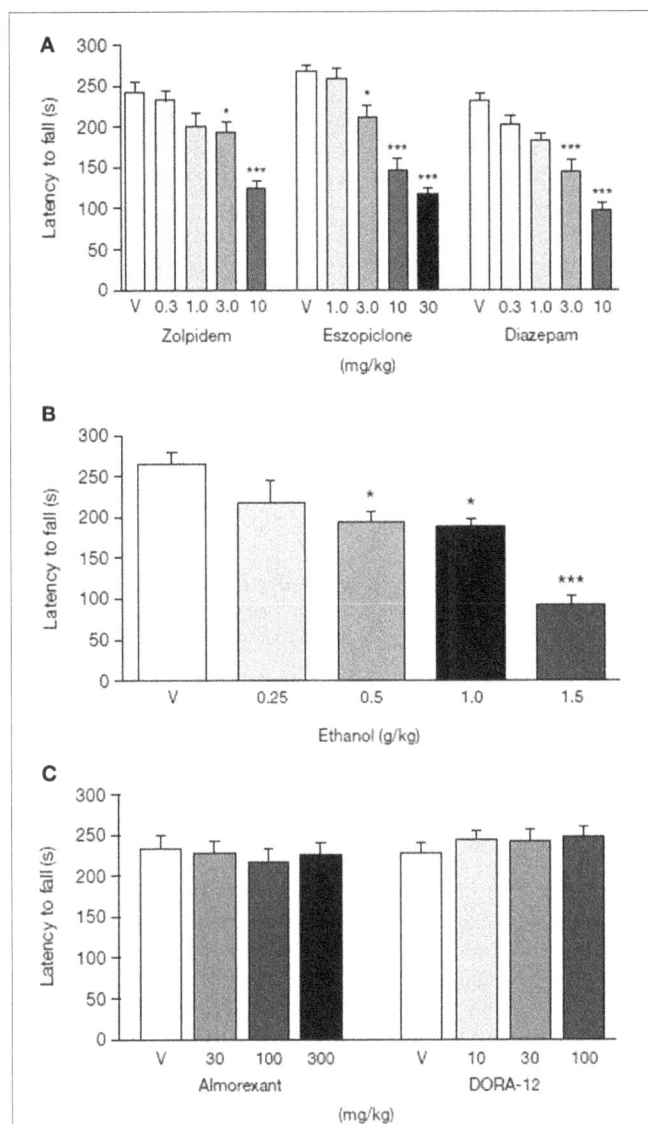

FIGURE 2 | Dose-response curve for latency to fall from rotarod for rats administered (A) GABA-A receptor modulators, (B) ethanol, and (C) orexin receptor antagonists. Comparison of GABA-A receptor modulators, ethanol and orexin receptor antagonists in terms of latency to fall using rotarod as a measure of motor performance. Paraoral acute administration of zolpidem, eszopiclone, diazepam, and IP administration of ethanol dose-dependently impairs rotarod performance. Paraoral doses of orexin receptor antagonists, almorexant and DORA-12, do not impair locomotor performance after acute administration. Data are shown as mean ± standard error of the mean. *p < 0.05, ***p < 0.001 for the level of significance vs. the vehicle-treated group. ANOVA post-hoc Newman-Keuls multiple comparison tests (n = 7–12). ANOVA, analysis of variance; PO, per oral; V, vehicle.

Table 1 | Dose-response effects of ethanol, GABA-A receptor modulators and orexin receptor antagonists on compound plasma or blood alcohol concentrations and latency to fall from the rotarod.

Treatment	Dose[a]	[Compound]$_{plasma}$/ BAC(μM) / (mg/dL)[b]	Rotarod performance (% change)	Latency to fall (s)[b]
ETHANOL TESTS				
Vehicle	V	–	0	264.8 ± 15.5
Ethanol	0.25	<10	−17.2	219.1 ± 27.6
	0.50	35.4 ± 4.8	−26.2*	195.4 ± 12.9*
	1.0	107.0 ± 8.8	−28.2*	189.7 ± 9.9*
	1.5	204.1 ± 11.3	−64.6***	93.7 ± 10.6***
ZOLPIDEM TESTS				
Vehicle	V	–	0	242.5 ± 12.3
Zolpidem	0.3	0.036 ± 0.004	−3.7	233.6 ± 10.4
	1.0	0.115 ± 0.020	−16.9	201.4 ± 15.9
	3.0	0.333 ± 0.040	−19.7*	194.6 ± 11.0*
	10	0.878 ± 0.121	−48.2***	125.6 ± 8.4***
ESZOPICLONE TESTS				
Vehicle	V	–	0	267.9 ± 6.9
Eszopiclone	1.0	0.090 ± 0.01	−3.4	258.9 ± 12.1
	3.0	0.400 ± 0.03	−15.1*	212.6 ± 8.2*
	10	1.100 ± 0.12	−45.1***	147.1 ± 13.0***
	30	3.15 ± 0.53	−56.1***	117.5 ± 7.0***
DIAZEPAM TESTS				
Vehicle	V	–	0	231.8 ± 26.5
Diazepam	0.3	0.04 ± 0.01	−8.4	203.6 ± 10.4
	1.0	0.05 ± 0.02	−15.7	182.3 ± 9.6
	3.0	0.13 ± 0.08	−30.2***	145.1 ± 13.9***
	10	0.31 ± 0.15	−57.8***	97.8 ± 7.9***
ALMOREXANT TESTS				
Vehicle	V	–	0	235.4 ± 16.3
almorexant	30	0.62 ± 0.12	−2.6	229.3 ± 14.0
	100	4.81 ± 0.37	−7.1	218.7 ± 14.0
	300	11.81 ± 1.38	−3.2	227.9 ± 13.0
DORA-12 TESTS				
Vehicle	V	–	0	229.0 ± 13.3
DORA-12	10	0.43 ± 0.04	+7.4	246.0 ± 9.8
	30	0.97 ± 0.09	+6.4	243.6 ± 10.2
	100	4.06 ± 0.40	+8.3	247.9 ± 13.8

ANOVA, analysis of variance; SEM, standard error of the mean; V, vehicle
Plasma/alcohol levels refer to time points between 35 and 40 min after dosing of compounds.
[a] Doses of zolpidem, eszopiclone and diazepam are given in mg/kg; doses of ethanol are given as g/kg.
[b] Mean ± SEM shown for compound concentrations in plasma, blood alcohol concentrations (BAC) and Latency to fall.
*p < 0.05, ***p < 0.001 significance versus vehicle treatment group. ANOVA post-hoc Newman-Keuls multiple comparison test.

doses (**Table 1**) and were accompanied by a greater reduction in latency to fall. Similarly, BAC increased with increased doses of ethanol (**Table 1**). In contrast, latency to fall was not reduced by increasing doses of almorexant and DORA-12, despite concomitant increases in the plasma concentrations of these orexin receptor antagonists (**Table 1** and **Figure 2**).

DIFFERENTIAL SLEEP-PROMOTING EFFECTS OF ETHANOL, GABA-A RECEPTOR MODULATORS AND DORA-12

To evaluate the effects of these compounds on locomotor activity in the context of sleep promotion, the benzodiazepine (diazepam) and non-benzodiazepine (eszopiclone and zolpidem) GABA-A receptor modulators, the orexin receptor antagonist DORA-12 and ethanol, were assessed for their ability to promote sleep in rats at the highest doses tested in rotarod experiments. Almorexant has been well-documented to promote sleep at dosages ranging from 30 to 300 mg/kg, the approximate maximum effect level (Brisbare-Roch et al., 2007), and has been previously shown in our lab to attenuate active wake at 100 mg/kg for as long as 7 h (Gotter et al., 2013). As seen in **Figure 3**, all treatments with the exception of zolpidem 30 mg/kg significantly attenuated active wake during the 2 h following treatment (-6.0 min $\pm$ 3.6 min, $p = 0.118$, paired t-test for individual animals relative to vehicle). DORA-12 reduced the time spent in active wake to a similar extent as eszopiclone (30 mg/kg) and ethanol (1.5 g/kg) (reductions of 13.5 ± 2.3, 14.0 ± 2.7, 12.7 ± 4.4 min, respectively), while diazepam 10 mg/kg had the greatest effect (20.4 ± 5.0 min). Relative to vehicle, all treatments significantly increased delta sleep time during the 2-h analysis period to similar magnitudes, with increases ranging from 9.6 ± 4.6 min in the

case of diazepam to 12.8 ± 2.9 min for eszopiclone. DORA-12 increased delta sleep by 10.9 ± 1.4 min. Light sleep, which is a minor component of rat sleep, was only significantly affected by diazepam in these studies. The most striking differences were on REM sleep changes. Ethanol and diazepam had no effect on REM, but eszopiclone and zolpidem both attenuated REM sleep relative to vehicle (-4.2 ± 0.8 and -5.1 ± 0.9 min, respectively), despite the fact that zolpidem was not effective in significantly reducing active wake in this experiment. DORA-12, on the other hand, significantly increased REM sleep time relative to vehicle (by 6.6 ± 1.1 min). We have recently shown that almorexant, dosed at 100 mg/kg during the active phase, has similar effects in terms of the magnitude of active wake reduction as a 30 mg/kg dose of DORA-12 (Gotter et al., 2013), consistent with previous observations (Brisbare-Roch et al., 2007). These results demonstrate a clear difference between the sleep promoted by the standard of care for insomnia and the effects of DORA-12.

ACUTE EFFECT ON MOTOR PERFORMANCE OF GABA-A RECEPTOR MODULATORS IN COMBINATION WITH ETHANOL

Sub-threshold doses (below the doses observed to impair motor performance) of the GABA-A receptor modulators zolpidem, eszopiclone, and diazepam were identified from their respective dose–response curves (**Figure 2A**). A minimum effective dose of ethanol (1 g/kg) was identified that produced BAC ranging from 106.9 ± 7.7 mg/dL-139.1 ± 2.42 mg/dL (**Figure 2B**). Sub-threshold doses of the GABA-A receptor modulators were then co-administered with the minimum effective dose of ethanol to assess whether ethanol may have additive motor impairments associated with GABA-A receptor modulators.

Diazepam 3.0 mg/kg co-administered with ethanol reduced rats' latencies to fall from the rotarod by 63.4% compared with vehicle (**Figure 4A** and **Table 2**). By way of comparison, rats administered ethanol or diazepam alone demonstrated 30.8 and 15.5% decreases, respectively, in latency to fall (**Table 2**). In these animals, there was a significant main effect of diazepam and ethanol [$F_{(1, 32)} = 10.8$ and 49.7, respectively, $p < 0.001$] as well as a significant diazepam by ethanol interaction [$F_{(1, 32)} = 4.8$, $p = 0.036$]. *Post-hoc* analysis showed that animals administered ethanol alone differed significantly from animals given only vehicle ($p < 0.05$). *Post-hoc* tests also revealed that animals given diazepam with ethanol differed from animals given diazepam or ethanol alone ($p < 0.05$).

A similar pattern of effect was observed with eszopiclone. Both eszopiclone and ethanol produced a main effect of treatment [$F_{(1, 34)} = 7.78$ and 12.58, $p = 0.001$ and 0.009, respectively]; however, there was no interaction when the two compounds were given together, suggesting an additive effect. The percent decrease in rotarod latency when eszopiclone was given without and with alcohol was 12.1% and 34.5%, respectively. *Post-hoc* analysis showed that animals administered ethanol ($p > 0.05$) did not differ significantly from vehicle-vehicle group (**Figure 4A** and **Table 2**).

Zolpidem also negatively impacted rotarod performance, as indicated by a main effect of zolpidem treatment [$F_{(1, 29)} = 14.53$, $p < 0.001$]. Ethanol likewise produced an effect in this experiment, as indicated by a main effect [$F_{(1, 29)} = 25.49$, $p <$

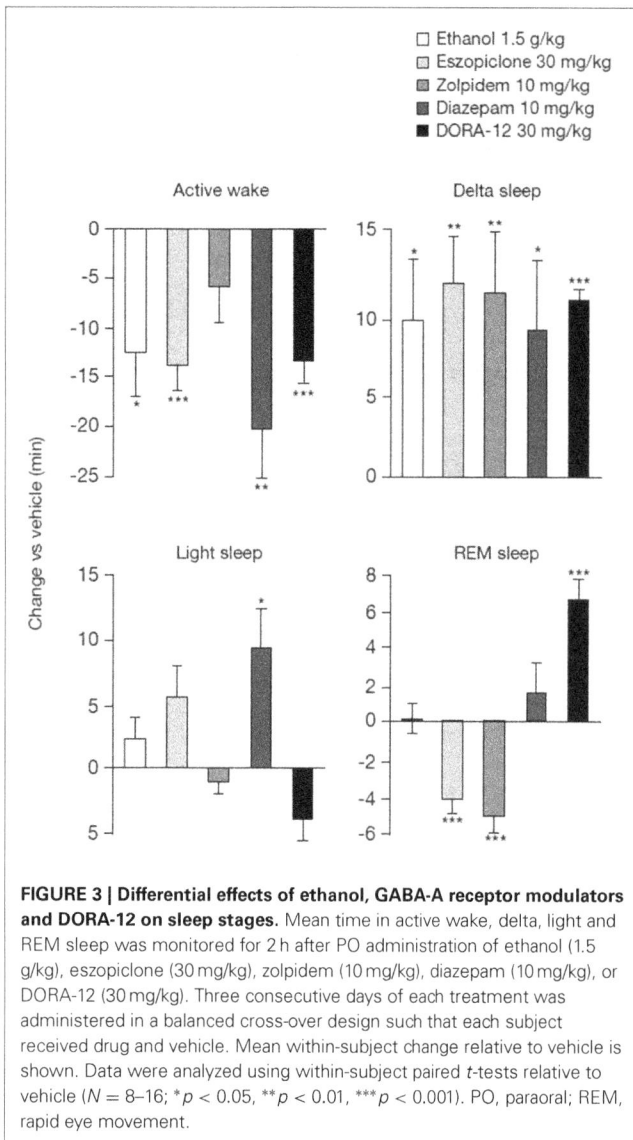

FIGURE 3 | Differential effects of ethanol, GABA-A receptor modulators and DORA-12 on sleep stages. Mean time in active wake, delta, light and REM sleep was monitored for 2 h after PO administration of ethanol (1.5 g/kg), eszopiclone (30 mg/kg), zolpidem (10 mg/kg), diazepam (10 mg/kg), or DORA-12 (30 mg/kg). Three consecutive days of each treatment was administered in a balanced cross-over design such that each subject received drug and vehicle. Mean within-subject change relative to vehicle is shown. Data were analyzed using within-subject paired t-tests relative to vehicle ($N = 8$–16; $*p < 0.05$, $**p < 0.01$, $***p < 0.001$). PO, paraoral; REM, rapid eye movement.

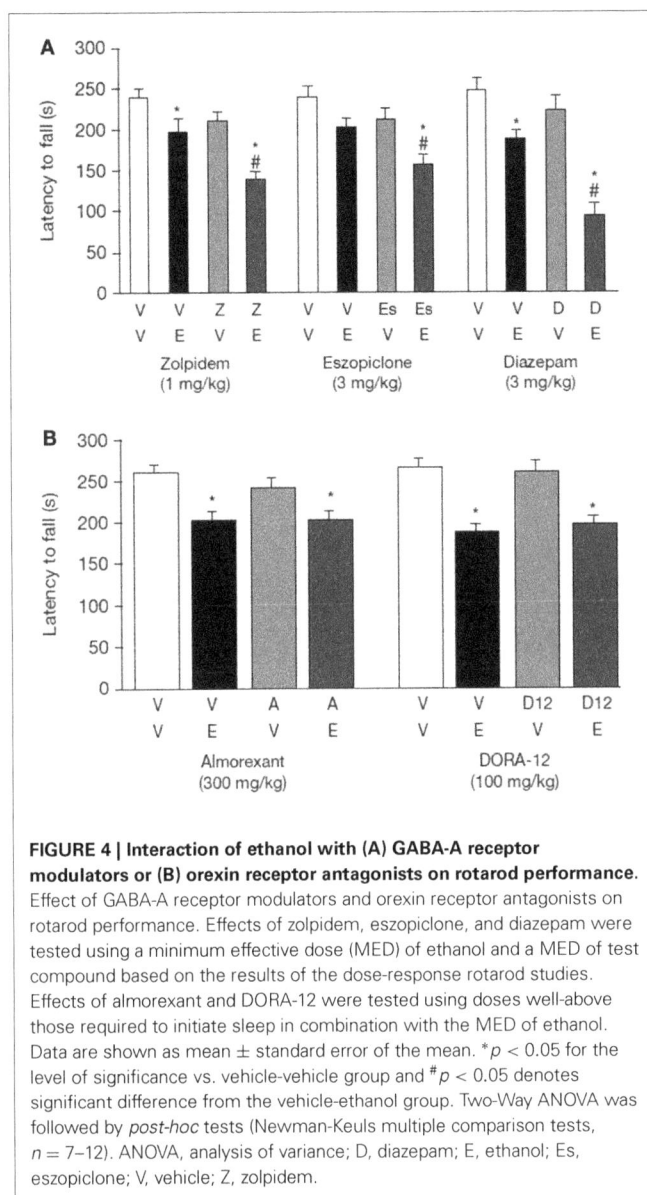

FIGURE 4 | Interaction of ethanol with (A) GABA-A receptor modulators or (B) orexin receptor antagonists on rotarod performance. Effect of GABA-A receptor modulators and orexin receptor antagonists on rotarod performance. Effects of zolpidem, eszopiclone, and diazepam were tested using a minimum effective dose (MED) of ethanol and a MED of test compound based on the results of the dose-response rotarod studies. Effects of almorexant and DORA-12 were tested using doses well-above those required to initiate sleep in combination with the MED of ethanol. Data are shown as mean ± standard error of the mean. *$p < 0.05$ for the level of significance vs. vehicle-vehicle group and #$p < 0.05$ denotes significant difference from the vehicle-ethanol group. Two-Way ANOVA was followed by *post-hoc* tests (Newman-Keuls multiple comparison tests, $n = 7–12$). ANOVA, analysis of variance; D, diazepam; E, ethanol; Es, eszopiclone; V, vehicle; Z, zolpidem.

0.001]. The interaction between ethanol and zolpidem was not significant, indicating that the effects of these two compounds on rotarod performance was additive [$F_{(1, 29)} = 1.53, p = 0.23$]. The percent decrease in rotarod latency when zolpidem was given without and with ethanol was 12.3 and 42.3%, respectively (**Figure 4A** and **Table 2**).

ACUTE EFFECT ON MOTOR PERFORMANCE OF OREXIN RECEPTOR ANTAGONISTS ADMINISTERED IN COMBINATION WITH ETHANOL

By contrast with the GABA-A receptor modulators, neither almorexant nor DORA-12 potentiated motor performance impairment when co-administered with ethanol (**Figure 4B** and **Table 2**). In both the almorexant and DORA-12 experiments, ethanol produced a main effect of treatment [$F_{(1, 35 \text{ and } 36)} = 7.84$ and 36.5, $p = 0.008$ and <0.001, respectively]. However, neither almorexant nor DORA-12 produced a main effect of treatment, and there was no interaction between either of the

two DORAs and ethanol. Rotarod performance was impaired to a similar extent when given with and without almorexant (22.5 and 22.3%, respectively). Likewise, rotarod performance was impaired to a similar extent when ethanol was given with and without DORA-12 (25.1 and 29.1%, respectively). BACs were similar when ethanol was administered alone or in combination with either one of the orexin receptor antagonists (**Table 2**), demonstrating that neither DORA-12 nor almorexant had a measureable impact on ethanol metabolism.

DORA-12 and almorexant plasma concentrations were stable when administered alone but fluctuated when co-administered with ethanol. Co-administration of ethanol also resulted in fluctuations in the drug–plasma concentrations of the GABA-A receptor modulators (**Table 2**).

DISCUSSION

The aim of the current study was to evaluate the potential impact of different insomnia therapeutic mechanisms on locomotor coordination in the presence or absence of ethanol relative to doses effective in promoting sleep. The current work goes beyond that of others (Steiner et al., 2011), by evaluating locomotor performance following treatment with multiple, distinct compounds within each class—two orexin receptor antagonists, a benzodiazepine and two non-benzodiazepine GABA-A receptor modulators—in order to determine if these results were due to pathway-dependent effects and not due to individual compound idiosyncrasies. In addition, locomotor impairment was evaluated in the context of sleep-promoting effects and sleep architecture. These results demonstrate that, at equally effective sleep-promoting doses, GABA-A receptor modulators induce substantial locomotor impairment and ethanol interaction relative to that observed in response to DORAs. This analysis also illustrates fundamental differences in sleep architecture induced by orexin receptor antagonists compared with GABA-A receptor modulators.

The use of multiple, pharmacologically distinct compounds from the orexin receptor antagonist and GABA-A receptor modulator classes indicates that the observed differences in locomotor impairment are due to the different sleep-promoting mechanisms. Studies in animals and humans have demonstrated consistent sleep-promoting effects of orexin receptor antagonists with distinct structural and pharmacological properties (Brisbare-Roch et al., 2007; Winrow et al., 2011, 2012; Bettica et al., 2012c; Herring et al., 2012b). Almorexant has been shown previously not to impair locomotor performance or to interact with ethanol (Steiner et al., 2011). We have further demonstrated that DORA-12 did not disrupt locomotor activity in the presence or absence of ethanol. DORA-12 is chemically distinct from almorexant, has greater *in vivo* potency, a distinct pharmacokinetic profile and faster binding kinetics despite similar *in vitro* activity at the receptor (Brisbare-Roch et al., 2007; Gotter et al., 2013). These results indicate that antagonism of orexin signaling promotes sleep, but does not significantly impair motor function. Contrary to the effects seen with orexin receptor antagonists, three different GABA-A receptor modulators of distinct chemical structure—a classic benzodiazepine, diazepam, and the

Table 2 | Interaction of GABA-A receptor modulators and orexin receptor antagonists combined with a minimum effective dose of ethanol on drug plasma concentration, blood alcohol concentrations and latency to fall from the rotarod.

Treatment	Compound dose (mg/kg)	Ethanol dose (g/kg)	[Compound]$_{plasma}$ (μM)[a]	BAC (mg/dL)[a]	% Change in rotarod performance	Latency to fall (s)[a]
ZOLPIDEM TESTS						
Vehicle	V	V	–	–	0	242.7 ± 10.0
Zolpidem	1.0	V	0.102 ± 0.02	–	−12.3	212.9 ± 10.9
	V	1.0	–	121.5 ± 14.2	−18.2*	198.6 ± 16.2*
	1.0	1.0	0.086 ± 0.04	124.4 ± 11.7	−42.3*	140.1 ± 9.1*#
ESZOPICLONE TESTS						
Vehicle	V	V	–	–	0	242.9 ± 12.4
Eszopiclone	3.0	V	0.42 ± 0.04	–	−12.1	213.4 ± 15.6
	V	1.0	–	106.9 ± 7.7	−16.3	203.4 ± 11.4
	3.0	1.0	0.20 ± 0.07	114.8 ± 5.4	−34.5*	159.0 ± 12.1*#
DIAZEPAM TESTS						
Vehicle	V	V	–	–	0	250.4 ± 13.8
Diazepam	3.0	V	0.103 ± 0.03	–	−15.5	226.5 ± 15.8
	V	1.0	–	139.1 ± 2.42	−30.8*	188.7 ± 12.5*
	3.0	1.0	0.145 ± 0.04	119.8 ± 12.6	−63.4*#	94.6 ± 15.7*#
ALMOREXANT TESTS						
Vehicle	V	V	–	–	0	263.4 ± 9.12
Almorexant	300	V	9.67 ± 0.95	–	−7.2	244.3 ± 11.4
	V	1.0	–	109.2 ± 6.7	−22.3	204.7 ± 10.6*
	300	1.0	7.77 ± 0.75	105.6 ± 7.12	−2.5	204.2 ± 11.1*
DORA-12 TESTS						
Vehicle	V	V	–	–	0	267.2 ± 12.9
DORA-12	100	V	3.03 ± 0.37	–	−1.5	263.1 ± 13.5
	V	1.0	–	130.6 ± 2.8	−29.1	189.4 ± 10.5*
	100	1.0	1.25 ± 0.36	123.5 ± 5.0	−25.1	200.1 ± 9.1*

ANOVA, analysis of variance; SEM, standard error of the mean; V, vehicle.

[a] Mean ± SEM.

*p < 0.05, significance versus vehicle-vehicle; #p < 0.05, significance versus vehicle-ethanol. Two-Way ANOVA was followed by post-hoc tests (Newman-Keuls multiple comparison test).

non-benzodiazepines, zolpidem and eszopiclone—all impaired rotarod performance and potentiated the effects of ethanol in the current study. While all three compounds interact with the same allosteric benzodiazepine binding site on GABA-A receptors to increase their activity, the subunit specificity and pharmacokinetic properties of each differ, particularly that of diazepam which has an extended plasma half-life relative to zolpidem and eszopiclone (Graham et al., 1996; Rudolph et al., 1999; McKernan et al., 2000; Bianchi, 2010; Gotter et al., 2013). This impairment is observed across benzodiazepine and non-benzodiazepine compounds and is likely a result of the widespread expression of GABA-A receptors throughout the CNS (Sieghart and Sperk, 2002). Taken together, the results reveal that the distinct effects on locomotor performance mediated by orexin receptor antagonists vs. GABA-A receptor modulators are due to pathway-dependent effects.

The differences between orexin antagonism and GABA-receptor activation on locomotor performance were also highlighted in the context of sleep-promoting efficacy. DORA-12, which promoted sleep at 30 mg/kg to a similar or greater extent relative to high doses of eszopiclone, zolpidem and

ethanol, exhibited no locomotor impairment. Even at 100 mg/kg, DORA-12 induced no locomotor impairment or ethanol interaction. Almorexant administered at 300 mg/kg, a dose well-above that required for sleep-promoting effects (Brisbare-Roch et al., 2007; Gotter et al., 2013), also left locomotor performance unaffected. Comparative clinical studies will be needed to confirm the translatability of these differences observed in the rat rotarod assay.

In addition to comparing the magnitude of sleep promotion, as measured by active wake reduction, the current work also demonstrates clear differences in the sleep architecture induced by GABA-A receptor modulators, DORA-12 and ethanol. At the doses tested, both classes of drugs as well as ethanol significantly promoted delta sleep to similar levels in the 2 h following treatment. In the case of zolpidem, this was despite insignificant effects on active wake reduction. This difference relative to prior studies (e.g., Renger et al., 2004) was likely due to the 2-h quantification performed here. The most striking difference between these classes of compounds was their effects upon REM sleep. The highly significant increase in REM induced by DORA-12 was diametrically opposed to the REM-suppressing effects of eszopiclone and zolpidem. These effects were consistent with prior studies separately evaluating other DORAs (Brisbare-Roch et al., 2007; Bettica et al., 2012a; Winrow et al., 2012) and GABA-A modulators (Brunner et al., 1991; Renger et al., 2004). Differential effects on REM sleep were also observed in a recent study comparing several GABA-A modulators with the orexin antagonist DORA-22; the GABA-A receptor modulators eszopiclone and zolpidem were associated with dose-responsive disruptions in EEG spectral profiles during sleep, while DORA-22 produced only marginal changes in EEG measures during compound-induced sleep (Fox et al., 2013). In the present study, diazepam was highly effective in attenuating active wake; however, this GABA-A modulator did not attenuate REM. This may be due to either GABA-A receptor subtype specificity differences from other compounds in this class (Arbilla et al., 1985), or more likely the limited 2-h analysis used here relative to this longer half-life compound, since diazepam has been noted to attenuate REM in prior studies (Renger et al., 2004). Ethanol attenuated active wake and promoted delta sleep to a similar extent as eszopiclone and DORA-12, but neither increased nor decreased REM sleep.

GABA is the principal inhibitory neurotransmitter in the nervous system, and as a consequence, GABA-A receptor modulators impact neurons throughout the CNS and modulate numerous signaling events, many of which are not involved with sleep promotion. Some of these additional CNS activities may be responsible for the unwanted effects associated with GABA-A receptor agonists, including drowsiness at arousal and induction of seemingly non-restorative sleep (Mohler, 2006). Consequently, some patients use alcohol in conjunction with GABA-A receptor modulators in an attempt to assist with falling asleep. Indeed, aged Finnish males who use anxiolytics and sedatives (mainly benzodiazepines) are reportedly more likely to be binge drinkers and heavy alcohol consumers than those who do not take psychotropics (Ilomaki et al., 2008).

Orexin neurons project to many regions in the brain including discrete brain centers that are part of the sleep-arousal system (Peyron et al., 1998; Marcus et al., 2001). Orexin receptor antagonists may therefore become an important new class of therapeutics that treat insomnia using a novel mechanism (Winrow and Renger, 2013). Even though orexin receptor antagonists are effective at promoting sleep at moderate doses, the observation that they did not impair motor performance in rats (as measured on the accelerating rotarod), or exacerbate the motor impairment induced by alcohol, suggests that the potential for negative motor side effects may be lower with orexin receptor antagonists than with GABA-A receptor modulators. The lowest dose of GABA-A receptor modulators to attenuate motor activity significantly on the rotarod was 3 mg/kg for zolpidem, eszopiclone, and diazepam, corresponding with ranges reported by other studies to promote sleep 1–3 mg/kg for zolpidem, 3–10 mg/kg for eszopiclone and 1–3 mg/kg for diazepam (Renger et al., 2004; Fox et al., 2013; Gotter et al., 2013). Neither almorexant nor DORA-12 affected latency to fall from the rotarod at doses ranging from 30 to 300 mg/kg and from 10 to 100 mg/kg, respectively DORA-12.30 mg/kg induced similar or greater sleep-promoting

efficacy relative to highly impairing doses of eszopiclone and zolpidem in the current work, and the sleep-promoting effects were consistent with prior experiments (Fox et al., 2013). Given that the animals treated with DORA-12 or almorexant were able to perform without impairment, it appears that these compounds induce sleep without affecting motor co-ordination in rats.

The potential risks associated with combining GABA-A receptor modulators (including benzodiazepines and benzodiazepine receptor agonists) and alcohol are perhaps best underscored by examining the links between their consumption and impaired driving skills. It is well-established that alcohol alone disrupts sleep, and can induce grogginess and decrease alertness (Stein and Friedmann, 2005). Benzodiazepine use is associated with an increased risk of on-the-road traffic accidents (Barbone et al., 1998; Woratanarat et al., 2009; Chang et al., 2013), and individuals combining alcohol with long-acting benzodiazepines are significantly more likely to be unsafe drivers than persons driving under the influence of alcohol alone (Maxwell et al., 2010). Furthermore, studies have demonstrated that drivers involved in motor vehicle accidents often had detectable levels of benzodiazepines alone and in combination with alcohol (Christophersen and Morland, 2008; Ricci et al., 2008; Legrand et al., 2013). Benzodiazepine use also increases the risk of falls in the elderly (Leipzig et al., 1999; Ray et al., 2000; Ensrud et al., 2002; Allain et al., 2005; Titler et al., 2011). When alcohol is combined with hypnotics, the frequency of falls and hip fractures in the elderly increases further (Allain et al., 2005). Interestingly, a recent study of next-day driving performance, balance and cognitive tests in elderly (65–80 years) healthy volunteers found no impairment by the orexin receptor antagonist, suvorexant, whereas the GABA-A receptor modulator, zopiclone, impaired these parameters (Vermeeren et al., 2012).

In conclusion, these results demonstrate distinct differences between the orexin antagonist and GABA-A receptor mechanisms on sleep architecture and locomotor performance, and their interaction with ethanol. When administered at sleep-inducing doses, structurally distinct orexin receptor antagonists had no effect on rat rotarod performance and did not potentiate the effect of ethanol, whereas benzodiazepine and non-benzodiazepine GABA-A receptor modulators impaired locomotor function and exacerbated the impairing effects of ethanol on this task at doses well-below that required to induce sleep. Furthermore, REM sleep differences were observed between these classes of compounds where DORA-12 induced significant increases in REM sleep as opposed to the REM-suppressing effects of eszopiclone and zolpidem. Our results corroborate the findings of Steiner and colleagues (Steiner et al., 2011) who also reported an absence of motor disruption with the orexin receptor antagonist almorexant and a lack of additive effects when almorexant was co-administered with ethanol, and align with data in human subjects demonstrating that almorexant does not potentiate ethanol-induced motor or cognitive deficits (Hoch et al., 2013). Clinical evaluation of the effects of suvorexant and alcohol in combination in humans is currently underway.

AUTHOR CONTRIBUTIONS

Susan E. Browne, Joseph Brunner, Susan L. Garson, Andres D. Ramirez, Duane R. Reiss, John J. Renger, Jason M. Uslaner, and Christopher J. Winrow conceived, designed or planned the study. Steven V. Fox, Susan L. Garson, Anthony L. Gotter, Robert Hodgson, Terrence McDonald, Andres D. Ramirez, Duane R. Reiss, Pamela L. Tannenbaum and Jason M. Uslaner collected or assembled the data. Susan E. Browne, Steven V. Fox, Susan L. Garson, Robert Hodgson, Andres D. Ramirez, John J. Renger, Jason M. Uslaner, Christopher J. Winrow, and Lihang Yao performed or supervised analyses. Susan E. Browne, Paul J. Coleman, Steven V. Fox, Susan L. Garson, Anthony L. Gotter, Robert Hodgson, Scott D. Kuduk, Terrence McDonald, Andres D. Ramirez, John J. Renger, Pamela L. Tannenbaum, Spencer J. Tye, Jason M. Uslaner, Christopher J. Winrow, and Lihang Yao interpreted the results. Susan E. Browne, Susan L. Garson, Anthony L. Gotter, Robert Hodgson, Andres D. Ramirez, and John J. Renger wrote sections of the initial draft of the manuscript. All authors provided substantive suggestions for revision or critically reviewed iterations of the manuscript and reviewed and approved the final version of the manuscript.

ACKNOWLEDGMENTS

This study was sponsored by Merck & Co., Inc., Whitehouse Station, NJ, USA. Editorial assistance was provided by Jane Bryant, Ph.D. of Complete Medical Communications. This assistance was funded by Merck & Co., Inc., Whitehouse Station, NJ. The authors would like to thank Shannon Nguyen for technical contributions and expertise, as well as the Clinical Pathology Diagnostic Group at Merck & Co., Inc., West Point, for its analysis of compound plasma concentrations and BAC.

REFERENCES

Allain, H., Bentue-Ferrer, D., Polard, E., Akwa, Y., and Patat, A. (2005). Postural instability and consequent falls and hip fractures associated with use of hypnotics in the elderly: a comparative review. *Drugs Aging* 22, 749–765. doi: 10.2165/00002512-200522090-00004

Arbilla, S., Depoortere, H., George, P., and Langer, S. Z. (1985). Pharmacological profile of the imidazopyridine zolpidem at benzodiazepine receptors and electrocorticogram in rats. *Naunyn Schmiedebergs. Arch. Pharmacol.* 330, 248–251. doi: 10.1007/BF00572441

Barbone, F., McMahon, A. D., Davey, P. G., Morris, A. D., Reid, I. C., McDevitt, D. G., et al. (1998). Association of road-traffic accidents with benzodiazepine use. *Lancet* 352, 1331–1336. doi: 10.1016/S0140-6736(98)04087-2

Barker, M. J., Greenwood, K. M., Jackson, M., and Crowe, S. F. (2004). Cognitive effects of long-term benzodiazepine use: a meta-analysis. *CNS Drugs* 18, 37–48. doi: 10.2165/00023210-200418010-00004

Bettica, P., Nucci, G., Pyke, C., Squassante, L., Zamuner, S., Ratti, E., et al. (2012a). Phase I studies on the safety, tolerability, pharmacokinetics and pharmacodynamics of SB-649868, a novel dual orexin receptor antagonist. *J. Psychopharmacol.* 26, 1058–1070. doi: 10.1177/026988111 1408954

Bettica, P., Squassante, L., Zamuner, S., Nucci, G., Danker-Hopfe, H., and Ratti, E. (2012b). The orexin antagonist SB-649868 promotes and maintains sleep in men with primary insomnia. *Sleep* 35, 1097–1104. doi: 10.5665/sleep.1996

Bettica, P., Squassante, L., Groeger, J. A., Gennery, B., Winsky-Sommerer, R., and Dijk, D. J. (2012c). Differential effects of a dual orexin receptor antagonist (SB-649868) and zolpidem on sleep initiation and consolidation, SWS, REM sleep, and EEG power spectra in a model of situational insomnia. *Neuropsychopharmacology* 37, 1224–1233. doi: 10.1038/npp.2011.310

Bianchi, M. T. (2010). Context dependent benzodiazepine modulation of GABA(A) receptor opening frequency. *Curr. Neuropharmacol.* 8, 10–17. doi: 10.2174/157015910790909467

Brisbare-Roch, C., Dingemanse, J., Koberstein, R., Hoever, P., Aissaoui, H., Flores, S., et al. (2007). Promotion of sleep by targeting the orexin system in rats, dogs and humans. *Nat. Med.* 13, 150–155. doi: 10.1038/nm1544

Brunner, D. P., Dijk, D. J., Munch, M., and Borbely, A. A. (1991). Effect of zolpidem on sleep and sleep EEG spectra in healthy young men. *Psychopharmacology (Berl.)* 104, 1–5. doi: 10.1007/BF02244546

Cagetti, E., Liang, J., Spigelman, I., and Olsen, R. W. (2003). Withdrawal from chronic intermittent ethanol treatment changes subunit composition, reduces synaptic function, and decreases behavioral responses to positive allosteric modulators of GABAA receptors. *Mol. Pharmacol.* 63, 53–64. doi: 10.1124/mol.63.1.53

Chang, C. M., Wu, E. C., Chen, C. Y., Wu, K. Y., Liang, H. Y., Chau, Y. L., et al. (2013). Psychotropic drugs and risk of motor vehicle accidents: a population-based case-control study. *Br. J. Clin. Pharmacol.* 75, 1125–1133. doi: 10.1111/j.1365-2125.2012.04410.x

Chemelli, R. M., Willie, J. T., Sinton, C. M., Elmquist, J. K., Scammell, T., Lee, C., et al. (1999). Narcolepsy in orexin knockout mice: molecular genetics of sleep regulation. *Cell* 98, 437–451. doi: 10.1016/S0092-8674(00) 81973-X

Christophersen, A. S., and Morland, J. (2008). Frequent detection of benzodiazepines in drugged drivers in Norway. *Traffic Inj. Prev.* 9, 98–104. doi: 10.1080/15389580701869190

Devaud, L. L., Purdy, R. H., Finn, D. A., and Morrow, A. L. (1996). Sensitization of gamma-aminobutyric acidA receptors to neuroactive steroids in rats during ethanol withdrawal. *J. Pharmacol. Exp. Ther.* 278, 510–517.

Ensrud, K. E., Blackwell, T. L., Mangione, C. M., Bowman, P. J., Whooley, M. A., Bauer, D. C., et al. (2002). Central nervous system-active medications and risk for falls in older women. *J. Am. Geriatr. Soc.* 50, 1629–1637. doi: 10.1046/j.1532-5415.2002.50453.x

Fox, S. V., Gotter, A. L., Tye, S. J., Garson, S. L., Savitz, A. T., Uslaner, J. M., et al. (2013). Quantitative electroencephalography within sleep/wake states differentiates GABA-A modulators eszopiclone and zolpidem from dual orexin receptor antagonists in rats. *Neuropsychopharmacology* 38, 2401–2408. doi: 10.1038/npp. 2013.139

Gerashchenko, D., Blanco-Centurion, C., Greco, M. A., and Shiromani, P. J. (2003). Effects of lateral hypothalamic lesion with the neurotoxin hypocretin-2-saporin on sleep in Long-Evans rats. *Neuroscience* 116, 223–235. doi: 10.1016/S0306-4522(02)00575-4

Gotter, A. L., Webber, A. L., Coleman, P. J., Renger, J. J., and Winrow, C. J. (2012). International Union of Basic and Clinical Pharmacology. LXXXVI. Orexin receptor function, nomenclature and pharmacology. *Pharmacol. Rev.* 64, 389–420. doi: 10.1124/pr.111.005546

Gotter, A. L., Winrow, C. J., Brunner, J., Garson, S. L., Fox, S. V., Binns, J., et al. (2013). The duration of sleep promoting efficacy by dual orexin receptor antagonists is dependent upon receptor occupancy threshold. *BMC Neurosci.* 14:90. doi: 10.1186/1471-2202-14-90

Graham, D., Faure, C., Besnard, F., and Langer, S. Z. (1996). Pharmacological profile of benzodiazepine site ligands with recombinant GABAA receptor subtypes. *Eur. Neuropsychopharmacol.* 6, 119–125. doi: 10.1016/0924-977X(95) 00072-W

Hanchar, H. J., Dodson, P. D., Olsen, R. W., Otis, T. S., and Wallner, M. (2005). Alcohol-induced motor impairment caused by increased extrasynaptic GABA(A) receptor activity. *Nat. Neurosci.* 8, 339–345. doi: 10.1038/ nn1398

Herring, W. J., Connor, K., Ivgy-May, N., Snavely, D., Snyder, E., Liu, K., et al. (2012a). "Efficacy and safety of suvorexant, a dual orexin receptor antagonist, in patients with primary insomnia: results from two pivotal trials," in *26th Annual Meeting of the Associated Professional Sleep Societies*, (Boston, MA).

Herring, W. J., Snyder, E., Budd, K., Hutzelmann, J., Snavely, D., Liu, K., et al. (2012b). Orexin receptor antagonism for treatment of insomnia: A randomized clinical trial of suvorexant. *Neurology* 79, 2265–2274. doi: 10.1212/WNL.0b013e31827688ee

Hindmarch, I., Legangneux, E., Stanley, N., Emegbo, S., and Dawson, J. (2006). A double-blind, placebo-controlled investigation of the residual psychomotor and cognitive effects of zolpidem-MR in healthy elderly volunteers. *Br. J. Clin. Pharmacol.* 62, 538–545. doi: 10.1111/j.1365-2125.2006.02705.x

Hoch, M., Hay, J. L., Hoever, P., de Kam, M. L., Te Beek, E. T., van Gerven, J. M., et al. (2013). Dual orexin receptor antagonism by almorexant does not potentiate impairing effects of alcohol in humans. *Eur. Neuropsychopharmacol.* 23, 107–117. doi: 10.1016/j.euroneuro.2012.04.012

Hoever, P., Dorffner, G., Benes, H., Penzel, T., Danker-Hopfe, H., Barbanoj, M. J., et al. (2012). Orexin receptor antagonism, a new sleep-enabling paradigm: a proof-of-concept clinical trial. *Clin. Pharmacol. Ther.* 91, 975–985. doi: 10.1038/clpt.2011.370

Ilomaki, J., Korhonen, M. J., Enlund, H., Hartzema, A. G., and Kauhanen, J. (2008). Risk drinking behavior among psychotropic drug users in an aging Finnish population: the FinDrink study. *Alcohol* 42, 261–267. doi: 10.1016/j.alcohol.2008.02.002

Johnson, E. O., Roehrs, T., Roth, T., and Breslau, N. (1998). Epidemiology of alcohol and medication as aids to sleep in early adulthood. *Sleep* 21, 178–186.

Kiyashchenko, L. I., Mileykovskiy, B. Y., Maidment, N., Lam, H. A., Wu, M. F., John, J., et al. (2002). Release of hypocretin (orexin) during waking and sleep states. *J. Neurosci.* 22, 5282–5286. Available online at: http://www.jneurosci.org/content/22/13/5282.long

Kurzthaler, I., Wambacher, M., Golser, K., Sperner, G., Sperner-Unterweger, B., Haidekker, A., et al. (2005). Alcohol and/or benzodiazepine use: different accidents–different impacts? *Hum. Psychopharmacol.* 20, 583–589. doi: 10.1002/hup.736

Legrand, S. A., Gjerde, H., Isalberti, C., Van der Linden, T., Lillsunde, P., Dias, M. J., et al. (2013). Prevalence of alcohol, illicit drugs and psychoactive medicines in killed drivers in four European countries. *Int. J. Inj. Contr. Saf. Promot.* doi: 10.1080/17457300.2012.748809. [Epub ahead of print].

Leipzig, R. M., Cumming, R. G., and Tinetti, M. E. (1999). Drugs and falls in older people: a systematic review and meta-analysis: I. Psychotropic drugs. *J. Am. Geriatr. Soc.* 47, 30–39.

Lin, J. S., Sakai, K., and Jouvet, M. (1988). Evidence for histaminergic arousal mechanisms in the hypothalamus of cat. *Neuropharmacology* 27, 111–122. doi: 10.1016/0028-3908(88)90159-1

Lin, L., Faraco, J., Li, R., Kadotani, H., Rogers, W., Lin, X. Y., et al. (1999). The sleep disorder canine narcolepsy is caused by a mutation in the hypocretin (orexin) receptor 2 gene. *Cell* 98, 365–376. doi: 10.1016/S0092-8674(00)81965-0

Lovinger, D. M., and Roberto, M. (2013). Synaptic effects induced by alcohol. *Curr. Top. Behav. Neurosci.* 13, 31–86. doi: 10.1007/7854_2011_143

Marcus, J. N., Aschkenasi, C. J., Lee, C. E., Chemelli, R. M., Saper, C. B., Yanagisawa, M., et al. (2001). Differential expression of orexin receptors 1 and 2 in the rat brain. *J. Comp. Neurol.* 435, 6–25. doi: 10.1002/cne.1190

Maxwell, H. G., Dubois, S., Weaver, B., and Bedard, M. (2010). The additive effects of alcohol and benzodiazepines on driving. *Can. J. Public Health* 101, 353–357. Available online at: http://journal.cpha.ca/index.php/cjph/article/view/1975

McKernan, R. M., Rosahl, T. W., Reynolds, D. S., Sur, C., Wafford, K. A., Atack, J. R., et al. (2000). Sedative but not anxiolytic properties of benzodiazepines are mediated by the GABA(A) receptor alpha1 subtype. *Nat. Neurosci.* 3, 587–592. doi: 10.1038/75761

Mohler, H. (2006). GABA(A) receptor diversity and pharmacology. *Cell Tissue Res.* 326, 505–516. doi: 10.1007/s00441-006-0284-3

Nishino, S., Ripley, B., Overeem, S., Lammers, G. J., and Mignot, E. (2000). Hypocretin (orexin) deficiency in human narcolepsy. *Lancet* 355, 39–40. doi: 10.1016/S0140-6736(99)05582-8

Ohno, K., and Sakurai, T. (2008). Orexin neuronal circuitry: role in the regulation of sleep and wakefulness. *Front. Neuroendocrinol.* 29, 70–87. doi: 10.1016/j.yfrne.2007.08.001

Otmani, S., Demazieres, A., Staner, C., Jacob, N., Nir, T., Zisapel, N., et al. (2008). Effects of prolonged-release melatonin, zolpidem, and their combination on psychomotor functions, memory recall, and driving skills in healthy middle aged and elderly volunteers. *Hum. Psychopharmacol.* 23, 693–705. doi: 10.1002/hup.980

Peyron, C., Tighe, D. K., van den Pol, A. N., de Lecea, L., Heller, H. C., Sutcliffe, J. G., et al. (1998). Neurons containing hypocretin (orexin) project to multiple neuronal systems. *J. Neurosci.* 18, 9996–10015.

Ray, W. A., Thapa, P. B., and Gideon, P. (2000). Benzodiazepines and the risk of falls in nursing home residents. *J. Am. Geriatr. Soc.* 48, 682–685. Available onine at: http://onlinelibrary.wiley.com/journal/10.1111/%28ISSN%291532-5415/issues

Renger, J. J., Dunn, S. L., Motzel, S. L., Johnson, C., and Koblan, K. S. (2004). Sub-chronic administration of zolpidem affects modifications to

rat sleep architecture. *Brain Res.* 1010, 45–54. doi: 10.1016/j.brainres.2004.02.067

Ricci, G., Majori, S., Mantovani, W., Zappaterra, A., Rocca, G., and Buonocore, F. (2008). Prevalence of alcohol and drugs in urine of patients involved in road accidents. *J. Prev. Med. Hyg.* 49, 89–95. Available online at: http://www.jpmh.org/issues.htm

Rudolph, U., Crestani, F., Benke, D., Brunig, I., Benson, J. A., Fritschy, J. M., et al. (1999). Benzodiazepine actions mediated by specific gamma-aminobutyric acid(A) receptor subtypes. *Nature* 401, 796–800. doi: 10.1038/44579

Sakurai, T., Amemiya, A., Ishii, M., Matsuzaki, I., Chemelli, R. M., Tanaka, H., et al. (1998). Orexins and orexin receptors: A family of hypothalamic neuropeptides and G protein-coupled receptors that regulate feeding behavior. *Cell* 92, 573–585. doi: 10.1016/S0092-8674(00)80949-6

Saper, C. B., Scammell, T. E., and Lu, J. (2005). Hypothalamic regulation of sleep and circadian rhythms. *Nature* 437, 1257–1263. doi: 10.1038/nature04284

Scammell, T. E., and Winrow, C. J. (2011). Orexin receptors: pharmacology and therapeutic opportunities. *Annu. Rev. Pharmacol. Toxicol.* 51, 243–266. doi: 10.1146/annurev-pharmtox-010510-100528

Sieghart, W., and Sperk, G. (2002). Subunit composition, distribution and function of GABA(A) receptor subtypes. *Curr. Top. Med. Chem.* 2, 795–816. doi: 10.2174/1568026023393507

Stein, M. D., and Friedmann, P. D. (2005). Disturbed sleep and its relationship to alcohol use. *Subst. Abus.* 26, 1–13. doi: 10.1300/J465v26n01_01

Steiner, M. A., Lecourt, H., Strasser, D. S., Brisbare-Roch, C., and Jenck, F. (2011). Differential effects of the dual orexin receptor antagonist almorexant and the GABA(A)-alpha1 receptor modulator zolpidem, alone or combined with ethanol, on motor performance in the rat. *Neuropsychopharmacology* 36, 848–856. doi: 10.1038/npp.2010.224

Tanaka, E. (2002). Toxicological interactions between alcohol and benzodiazepines. *J. Toxicol. Clin. Toxicol.* 40, 69–75. doi: 10.1081/CLT-120002887

Thompson, R. H., Canteras, N. S., and Swanson, L. W. (1996). Organization of projections from the dorsomedial nucleus of the hypothalamus: a PHA-L study in the rat. *J. Comp. Neurol.* 376, 143–173. doi: 10.1002/(SICI)1096-9861(19961202)376:1<143::AID-CNE9>3.0.CO;2-3

Titler, M. G., Shever, L. L., Kanak, M. F., Picone, D. M., and Qin, R. (2011). Factors associated with falls during hospitalization in an older adult population. *Res. Theory Nurs. Pract.* 25, 127–148. doi: 10.1891/1541-6577.25.2.127

Trivedi, P., Yu, H., MacNeil, D. J., Van der Ploeg, L. H. T., and Guan, X. M. (1998). Distribution of orexin receptor mRNA in the rat brain. *FEBS Lett.* 438, 71–75. doi: 10.1016/S0014-5793(98)01266-6

Tsunematsu, T., Kilduff, T. S., Boyden, E. S., Takahashi, S., Tominaga, M., and Yamanaka, A. (2011). Acute optogenetic silencing of orexin/hypocretin neurons induces slow-wave sleep in mice. *J. Neurosci.* 31, 10529–10539. doi: 10.1523/JNEUROSCI.0784-11.2011

Vermeeren, A., and Coenen, A. M. (2011). Effects of the use of hypnotics on cognition. *Prog. Brain Res.* 190, 89–103. doi: 10.1016/B978-0-444-53817-8.00005-0

Vermeeren, A., Vuurman, E., Bautmans, A., Li, X., Vets, E., Lewis, N., et al. (2012). Suvorexant, a dual orexin receptor antagonist, does not impair next day driving performance in healthy elderly subjects. *J. Sleep Sleep Disord. Res.* 35, A226, 0670 (Abstract).

Winrow, C. J., Gotter, A. L., Cox, C. D., Doran, S. M., Tannenbaum, P. L., Breslin, M. J., et al. (2011). Promotion of sleep by suvorexant - a novel dual orexin receptor antagonist. *J. Neurogenet.* 25, 52–61. doi: 10.3109/01677063.2011.566953

Winrow, C. J., Gotter, A. L., Cox, C. D., Tannenbaum, P. L., Garson, S. L., Doran, S. M., et al. (2012). Pharmacological characterization of MK-6096 - a dual orexin receptor antagonist for insomnia. *Neuropharmacology* 62, 978–987. doi: 10.1016/j.neuropharm.2011.10.003

Winrow, C. J., and Renger, J. J. (2013). Discovery and development of orexin receptor antagonists as therapeutics for insomnia. *Br. J. Pharmacol.* doi: 10.1111/bph.12261. [Epub ahead of print].

Woratanarat, P., Ingsathit, A., Suriyawongpaisal, P., Rattanasiri, S., Chatchaipun, P., Wattayakorn, K., et al. (2009). Alcohol, illicit and non-illicit psychoactive drug use and road traffic injury in Thailand: a case-control study. *Accid. Anal. Prev.* 41, 651–657. doi: 10.1016/j.aap.2009.03.002

Yoshida, K., McCormack, S., Espana, R. A., Crocker, A., and Scammell, T. E. (2006). Afferents to the orexin neurons of the rat brain. *J. Compar. Neurol.* 494, 845–861. doi: 10.1002/cne.20859

Yoshida, Y., Fujiki, N., Nakajima, T., Ripley, B., Matsumura, H., Yoneda, H., et al. (2001). Fluctuation of extracellular hypocretin-1 (orexin A) levels in the rat in relation to the light-dark cycle and sleep-wake activities. *Eur. J. Neurosci.* 14, 1075–1081. doi: 10.1046/j.0953-816x.2001.01725.x

Conflict of Interest Statement: All authors are employed by Merck Sharp & Dohme Corp., a subsidiary of Merck & Co., Inc., Whitehouse Station, NJ, USA, and receive salary from, research support from and potentially own stock in Merck & Co., Inc.

4

Orexin receptor antagonists as therapeutic agents for insomnia

Ana C. Equihua[1], Alberto K. De La Herrán-Arita[2] and Rene Drucker-Colin[1]*

[1] Neuropatología Molecular, Instituto de Fisiología Celular, Universidad Nacional Autónoma de México, Mexico City, México
[2] Center for Sleep Sciences and Medicine, Stanford University, Palo Alto, CA, USA

Edited by:
Christopher J. Winrow, Merck, USA

Reviewed by:
Matthew R. Ebben, Weill Medical College of Cornell University, USA
Gabriella Gobbi, McGill University, Canada
Matt Carter, University of Washington, USA
Michihiro Mieda, Kanazawa University, Japan

*Correspondence:
Rene Drucker-Colin, Departamento de Neurociencias, Instituto de Fisiología Celular, Universidad Nacional Autónoma de México, Circuito exterior S/N, Apdo. Postal 70-600, 04510 Mexico City, D.F, México
e-mail: drucker@unam.mx

Insomnia is a common clinical condition characterized by difficulty initiating or maintaining sleep, or non-restorative sleep with impairment of daytime functioning. Currently, treatment for insomnia involves a combination of cognitive behavioral therapy (CBTi) and pharmacological therapy. Among pharmacological interventions, the most evidence exists for benzodiazepine (BZD) receptor agonist drugs (GABA$_A$ receptor), although concerns persist regarding their safety and their limited efficacy. The use of these hypnotic medications must be carefully monitored for adverse effects. Orexin (hypocretin) neuropeptides have been shown to regulate transitions between wakefulness and sleep by promoting cholinergic/monoaminergic neural pathways. This has led to the development of a new class of pharmacological agents that antagonize the physiological effects of orexin. The development of these agents may lead to novel therapies for insomnia without the side effect profile of hypnotics (e.g., impaired cognition, disturbed arousal, and motor balance difficulties). However, antagonizing a system that regulates the sleep-wake cycle may create an entirely different side effect profile. In this review, we discuss the role of orexin and its receptors on the sleep-wake cycle and that of orexin antagonists in the treatment of insomnia.

Keywords: orexin receptor antagonist, insomnia, hypocretins/orexins, therapy-related, sleep disorders

INTRODUCTION

Insomnia is the most common sleep disorder in the world. In the US alone, as much as 48% of the population reports experiencing transitory insomnia, while 22% suffers from insomnia almost every night as mentioned on the National Sleep Foundation website.

According to the second International Classification of Sleep Disorders (ICSD-2), insomnia is characterized by disturbed sleep that leads to impaired daytime functioning (e.g., fatigue, memory impairment, poor school performance, irritability, daytime sleepiness and proneness to errors, among other symptoms). Disturbed sleep can manifest as a difficulty in initiating/maintaining sleep, early morning awakening, or sleep that is chronically non-restorative or poor in quality, despite adequate opportunity for sleep to occur. Insomnia becomes a chronic problem when symptoms have been present for at least a month (NIH State-of-the-Science Conference Statement on Manifestations and Management of Chronic Insomnia in Adults, 2005).

The definition for insomnia disorder in the Diagnostic and Statistical Manual of Mental Disorders, 5th Edition, does not differ much from that of the ICSD-2 as it also includes complaints of dissatisfaction with sleep quantity or quality despite adequate opportunity to sleep and low performance in daytime functioning. In addition, the manual also includes a more specific timeframe where complaints occur at least three nights per week for at least 3 months.

The National Institutes of Health classifies insomnia as either primary (PI) or comorbid (previously referred to as secondary insomnia). PI refers to insomnia without comorbid conditions, whereas comorbid insomnia is employed when complaints arise in the context of another condition, such as depression, Parkinson's disease, rheumatoid arthritis, or restless leg syndrome; or as the side effect of a drug, such as caffeine, nicotine, alcohol or beta-blockers.

The etiology of PI is thought to be related to sustained physiological hyperarousal throughout the day. Management of insomnia can be achieved using cognitive behavioral therapy (CBTi) and/or pharmacological therapy. Common prescription medications for insomnia are benzodiazepine (BZD) receptor agonists (both BZDs and nonBZDs), sedating antidepressants and melatonin receptor agonists. Pharmaceutical intervention is often the first-line approach for the treatment of insomnia but still has many pitfalls, such as the development of tolerance, addiction and undesired side effects (including complex sleep related behaviors and abnormal thoughts).

Orexin (hypocretin) receptor antagonists are a new, promising pharmacological treatment for PI. The orexinergic system (otherwise known as the hypocretinergic system) has been strongly linked to the sleep/wake cycle (SWC) for its role in promoting and sustaining arousal (Piper et al., 2000; Xi et al., 2001). In addition, the antagonism of orexinergic receptors has been shown to induce somnolence in different species (Brisbare-Roch et al., 2007). In clinical trials orexin receptor antagonists have performed well, and subjects have reported improved quality of sleep with few side effects, the most common being complaints of mild headaches and dizziness.

In the first part of this review we discuss the current state of PI and the research that has led to the use of orexin receptor antagonists as therapy for PI. In the second part we focus on existing orexin receptor antagonists and their effectiveness in promoting sleep in animal models and managing insomnia in humans.

OVERVIEW OF THE CURRENT TREATMENT OF INSOMNIA
CBTi

The main objective of CBTi is to tackle the cognitive and behavioral factors that could be perpetuating insomnia. The most frequent factors are excessive worrying about not sleeping enough and maladaptive behaviors such as spending excessive time in bed awake, excessive use of caffeine, and napping. Common techniques applied in CBTi include sleep hygiene education, cognitive restructuring, stimulus control, sleep restriction therapy and relaxation training (Morin et al., 1994; NIH State-of-the-Science Conference Statement on Manifestations and Management of Chronic Insomnia in Adults, 2005). Several studies have found that CBTi is an effective approach with long-term results for the treatment of insomnia (Morin, 1999; Jacobs et al., 2004).

The shortcomings of CBTi are related to access and adherence to treatment. Patients need to be trained by specialized medical practitioners, who are not readily available, and to stay highly motivated, as the therapy requires them to devote time to practicing and carrying out the techniques.

PHARMACOLOGICAL TREATMENTS FOR INSOMNIA

Pharmacological treatments for insomnia can broadly be classified as prescription FDA approved and non-prescription, over-the-counter (OTC), treatments.

Prescription FDA approved

Contemporary FDA approved pharmacological treatment includes $GABA_A$ receptor agonists (BZDs and nonBZDs), sedating antidepressants and melatonin agonists. The use of a pharmacological therapy for the treatment of insomnia is somewhat easier than CBTi, but presupposes other difficulties, such as unresponsiveness to treatment, limited therapeutic potential, a poor side effect profile, tolerance and addiction. FDA medicines approved for the treatment of insomnia are listed in **Table 1**.

BZDs and nonBZDs. The first FDA approved drugs for insomnia were BZDs (estazolam, quazepam, triazolam, flurazepam and temazepam) and nonBZDs, also known as z-drugs (zaleplon, zolpidem, and eszopiclone). These drugs, with the exception of eszopiclone, are effective for the short-term management of insomnia. Eszopiclone on the other hand, has been found to have sustained efficacy for up to 6 months (**Table 1**).

BZD and nonBZD compounds are $GABA_A$ agonists. $GABA_A$ receptors are pentameric receptors conformed of combinations of α (1–6), β (1–3), γ (1–3), δ (1), ϵ (1), π (1), and θ (1) subunits. The endogenous ligand GABA binds at the active site located at the interface of α- and β-subunits, instead, the binding site for BZDs and nonBZDs is located between α- and γ-subunits of α- and γ-subunit containing $GABA_A$ receptors. Differences among BZDs and nonBZDs relate to their selectivity for different types of $GABA_A$ receptors, while BZDs can bind to subunits of the α1, α2,

α3, and α5 classes, nonBZDs preferentially bind to the α1 subclass (Rudolph and Knoflach, 2011).

Activation of $GABA_A$ receptors tends to stabilize or hyperpolarize the resting potential, and can make it more difficult for excitatory neurotransmitters to depolarize the neuron and generate an action potential. The net effect is typically inhibitory, reducing the activity of the neuron. The $GABA_A$ channel opens quickly and thus contributes to the early part of the inhibitory post-synaptic potential. This can lead to several undesired side effects that range from cognitive and psychomotor impairment, rebound insomnia, and anterograde amnesia, to increased risk of motor collisions and falls (Lader, 2012; Gunja, 2013).

Sedating antidepressants. For a long time, antidepressants were used to treat insomnia in an off-label manner. Among these, the serotonin antagonist and reuptake inhibitor trazodone was the most popular. Then, in 2010, the FDA approved the tricyclic antidepressant (TCA) doxepin for the treatment of sleep maintenance insomnia (frequent nighttime or early morning awakenings).

There are different classes of antidepressants with sedating properties; in particular doxepin is classified as a serotonin and norepinephrine reuptake inhibitor TCA. Despite this, the sleep-promoting effects of doxepin are thought to relate mainly to its antihistaminergic properties (Risberg et al., 1975). In this regard, doxepin is a potent histamine H_1 receptor antagonist (Richelson, 1979).

Therapeutic effects of doxepin are observed at very low dosages (3–6 mg/day), improving sleep maintenance without rebound insomnia or physical dependence. Common side effects include sedation, nasopharyngitis, gastrointestinal effects, and hypertension (Weber et al., 2010).

Melatonin agonists. Melatonin is a natural hormone produced by the pineal gland following a circadian rhythm. The production of melatonin peaks when the lights go out, which signals the organism that it is nighttime (Reiter, 1986). In humans, melatonin has sleep-promoting effects as it has been found to induce sedation, lower core body temperature, reduce sleep latencies and increase total sleep time (Dollins et al., 1994; Zhdanova et al., 1996; Erman et al., 2006).

Ramelteon is an FDA approved melatonin agonist that acts upon MT_1 and MT_2 receptors improving sleep-onset latency at a recommended dose of 8 mg/day. The most common complaints users have described are headache, somnolence, dizziness and sore throat (Pandi-Perumal et al., 2011). Overall, ramelteon is very well tolerated, and unlike BZDs, residual effects such as cognitive and psychomotor impairments are absent (Johnson et al., 2006) (**Table 1**).

Non-prescription (OTC)

The most commonly used OTC sleep aids are antihistamines; other OTC include alcohol, valerian and l-tryptophan. Histaminergic neurons are mainly localized in the tuberomammillary nucleus (TMN) from where they project to many regions of the (CNS) system including the wake-promoting basal forebrain (BF) and orexinergic neurons in the lateral hypothalamus

Table 1 | FDA approved medications for the treatment of insomnia.

Generic name		Therapeutic indication	Dosage (mg)	Known side effects	Mechanism of action
BENZODIAZEPINE RECEPTOR AGONISTS					
BDZs	Estazolam	Insomnia	0.5–2	Dizziness, drowsiness, next day sedation, memory loss, anxiety, loss of coordination.	Positive allosteric modulator of $GABA_A$ receptors
	Quazepam		7.5–15	Rebound insomnia. Allergic reactions.	
	Triazolam		0.125–0.50	Complex sleep related behaviors: sleep-driving, making phone calls, eating.	
	Flurazepam		15–30	Abnormal thoughts and behavior: worsening of depression, suicidal thoughts or actions, increased aggressiveness.	
	Temazepam		7.5–30		
NonBDZs	Zaleplon	Sleep-onset insomnia	2.5–10	Dizziness, headache, drowsiness, nausea, vomiting.	
	Zolpidem	Sleep-onset and sleep maintenance insomnia	5–20	Complex sleep related behaviors. Abnormal thoughts and behavior.	
	Eszopiclone		1–3	Physical dependence.	
SEDATING ANTIDEPRESSANTS					
Doxepin		Sleep-maintenance insomnia	3–6	Sedation, nasopharyngitis, gastrointestinal effects, hypertension. Complex sleep related behaviors. Abnormal thoughts and behavior.	5-HT & NE reuptake inhibitor H_1 receptor antagonist
MELATONIN RECEPTOR AGONISTS					
Ramelteon		Sleep-onset insomnia	8	Drowsiness, tiredness, dizziness. Allergic reactions. Complex sleep related behaviors Abnormal thoughts and behavior. Hormone effects: decreased interest in sex, problems getting pregnant.	MT_1 & MT_2 receptor agonist

All information was obtained from the FDA website (www.fda.gov). Abbreviations: BDZs, benzodiazepines; 5-HT, serotonin; NE, norepinephrine; H, histamine; MT, melatonin.

(LH) (Köhler et al., 1985; Panula et al., 1989). The sedating effects of antihistamines have been known for a long time (Risberg et al., 1975) and are thought to be related to inhibition of H_1 receptor activity (Saitou et al., 1999).

Despite the popularity of OCT sedating antihistamines, these agents have several undesirable side effects that limit their usefulness as sleep aids (NIH State-of-the-Science Conference Statement on Manifestations and Management of Chronic Insomnia in Adults, 2005). In addition to antagonizing histamine receptors, these compounds often display anticholinergic effects (dry mouth, blurred vision, constipation, tachycardia, urinary retention, and memory deficits) and next-day impairment (Kay, 2000; Meoli et al., 2005).

NEUROBIOLOGICAL MODEL OF INSOMNIA

PI, though classified as a sleep disorder, is thought to be a consequence of physiological hyperarousal during sleep and wakefulness. For example, objective sleepiness measures such as the Multiple Sleep Latency Test (MSLT), have failed to show increased sleepiness in insomniacs when compared to healthy controls (Edinger et al., 2003). Furthermore, insomniacs appear to be more alert following a night of poor sleep when compared to control subjects (Stepanski et al., 1988) and during sleep exhibit a surge of beta and gamma activity (Perlis et al., 2001), suggesting a generalized disorder that persists throughout the SWC. This model has been supported by studies that have detected physiological differences between insomniacs and controls. Monroe was the first to document that poor sleepers have increased physiological activity, which includes augmented heart rate, body temperature, oxygen consumption, secretion of cortisol, adrenocorticotropic hormone (ACTH) and adrenaline (Monroe, 1967; Adam et al., 1986; Vgontzas et al., 2001; Bonnet and Arand, 2010).

Elevated levels of free cortisol and ACTH in the urine are indicators of the overactivation of the hypothalamic-pituitary-adrenal axis (HPA) that could account for some of the symptoms of PI, including arousal, fragmented sleep and increased sleep latency (Steiger et al., 1991; Richardson and Roth, 2001).

The HPA plays a fundamental role in the stress response; increased levels of cortisol after a night of sleep loss have been interpreted as reflecting the stress of maintaining a state of vigilance (Chapotot et al., 2001). In normal conditions, cortisol levels somewhat parallel arousal throughout the day, reaching peak levels after waking and decreasing around midnight (Pruessner et al., 1997; Bartter et al., 2006). In contrast, chronic insomniacs have significantly higher cortisol levels during the evening (Spath-Schwalbe, 1992).

The hypothalamic nucleus that comprises the HPA is the paraventricular nucleus (PVN) where corticotropin-releasing hormone (CRH) release is key to inducing stress responses and augmenting the levels of ACTH and cortisol. A reciprocal excitatory interaction between the HPA and the orexinergic system has recently been revealed to occur. First, an anatomical interface between these two nuclei has been observed: orexin neurons extensively innervate the PVN, whereas CRH neurons innervate the LH (Winsky-Sommerer et al., 2004). Second, a physiological association has also been reported: there is an enhanced release of CRH that follows the intracerebroventricular (ICV) infusion of orexins (Al-Barazanji et al., 2001; Sakamoto et al., 2004), as well as an activation of orexinergic neurons after CRH administration (Winsky-Sommerer et al., 2004). This anatomical and functional overlap has raised the question of whether or not the orexinergic system is involved in the modulation of stress.

To study the response of orexinergic neurons in stressful situations, experiments have been carried out. In one trial, the activity of orexin-producing neurons in rats was evaluated after they were subjected to a swimming stress test known to increase the amount of ACTH in plasma. During this test the activation of orexinergic cells, measured by c-Fos immunoreactivity, significantly increased, suggesting orexinergic activation associated with stress. Furthermore, the study also showed that pretreatment with an orexin antagonist significantly reduced the amount of ACTH released to plasma (Chang et al., 2007), revealing a role for orexins in this particular stress response. However, it seems that orexin-producing neurons are not activated by all kinds of stress; instead they appear to be specifically recruited by stressful scenarios that require increased attention to environmental cues (Furlong et al., 2009).

The HPA also directly influences the activity of the locus coeruleus (LC), a major source of norepinephrine in the CNS and a very important wake-promoting nucleus (Buckley and Schatzberg, 2005). Orexinergic neurons also have an excitatory influence on the LC, as they activate it during the waking hours of the SWC (Hagan et al., 1999; Bourgin et al., 2000; Del Cid-Pellitero and Garzón, 2011). Although it has not yet been tested, it is possible that repetitive stressful events, requiring attention to environmental cues, activate the HPA and induce the release of CRH, subsequently activating the LC and orexinergic neurons. This would promote attention and inhibit sleep, setting in motion a vicious cycle that could develop into chronic insomnia.

RATIONALE FOR OREXIN ANTAGONISM AIMED AT THE TREATMENT OF INSOMNIA

The orexinergic system was first described in the 1990s (de Lecea et al., 1998; Peyron et al., 1998; Sakurai et al., 1998). Shortly thereafter it was linked to the development of the sleep disorder narcolepsy (Chemelli et al., 1999; Lin et al., 1999; Thannickal et al., 2000). Since then, orexins have been intensely studied for their role in the SWC primarily as wake-promoting neurotransmitters (Alexandre et al., 2013).

Orexin producing neurons are found in the LH. These neurons synthesize two excitatory neuropeptides called orexin A and B (OX_A and OX_B, alternatively known as hypocretin 1 and 2) cleaved from a common protein precursor called prepro-orexin (prepro-hypocretin). Orexinergic neurons extensively innervate the CNS (Peyron et al., 1998), specifically areas known for their role in promoting arousal like the LC, TMN, BF, cerebral cortex and dorsal raphe (DR).

Several studies have corroborated the role of the orexinergic system in sustaining wakefulness. For instance, it has been shown that orexinergic neuronal activity is a function of the degree of wakefulness, and is highest during active waking, and decreases during quiet waking and sleep (Kiyashchenko et al., 2002; Lee et al., 2005; Mileykovskiy et al., 2005). In addition, both ICV infusions (Piper et al., 2000; De la Herrán-Arita et al., 2011) and microinjections in sleep control related nuclei (Bourgin et al., 2000; España et al., 2001; Xi et al., 2001) of OX_A lengthen the amount of time spent awake in a dose dependent manner. Moreover, the use of optogenetics to activate orexinergic neurons in the LH has been shown to increase the probability of a transition from nREM or REM sleep to waking (Adamantidis et al., 2007).

Orexins exert their actions through their interaction with two G protein-coupled receptors called OX_1R and OX_2R (hcrt1R and hcrt2R, respectively). These receptors have different affinities for the orexin peptides, while OX_A binds to both receptors, OX_B selectively binds to OX_2R (Sakurai et al., 1998) (**Figure 1**). In addition, orexin receptors are differentially located throughout the CNS; the LC mainly expresses OX_1R, the TMN and the PVN exclusively express OX_2R, while the DR, BF and cortex express both receptors (Marcus et al., 2001) (**Figure 1**).

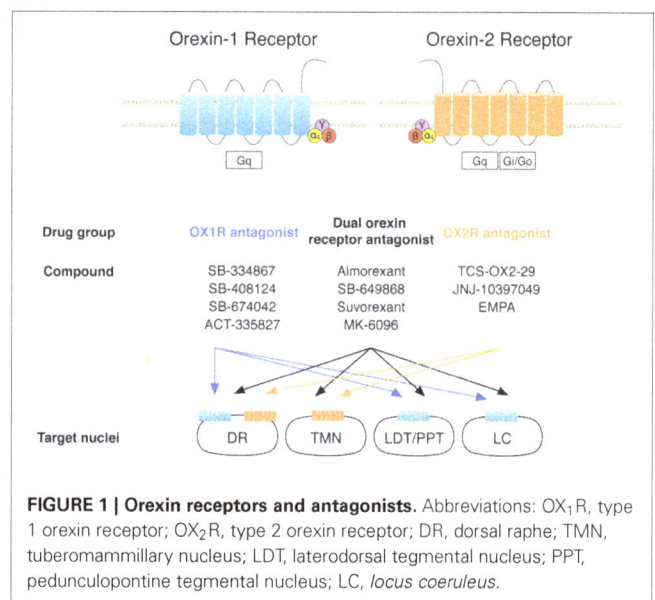

FIGURE 1 | Orexin receptors and antagonists. Abbreviations: OX_1R, type 1 orexin receptor; OX_2R, type 2 orexin receptor; DR, dorsal raphe; TMN, tuberomammillary nucleus; LDT, laterodorsal tegmental nucleus; PPT, pedunculopontine tegmental nucleus; LC, *locus coeruleus*.

The distinct distribution and affinities of orexin receptors suggest they play different roles in the maintenance of wakefulness (**Table 2**). This has been studied using different strains of transgenic mice, such as Knockouts (KO) for either one of the orexin receptors, or both (DKO). These mice show varying degrees of sleep disturbance. While OX_1R KO mice do not exhibit any obvious behavioral alterations (Sakurai, 2007), OX_2R KO mice manifest some features of narcolepsy, including an inability to sustain wakefulness (Willie et al., 2003). DKO mice display the most profoundly disturbed sleep phenotype of all three models: narcolepsy with cataplexy (transient episodes of behavioral arrest) (Kalogiannis et al., 2011). The robust narcoleptic phenotype in DKO mice indicates a synergistic role between OX_1R and OX_2R in the maintenance of wakefulness.

To further characterize the role of orexin receptors, selective orexin receptor KO mice were stimulated with ICV infusions of OX_A. Specific stimulation of OX_1R in OX_2R KO mice produced a moderate improvement in wakefulness and suppression of nREM, whereas the stimulation of OX_2R in OX_1R KO mice resulted in a greatly enhanced wakefulness (Mieda et al., 2011). This suggests that OX_1R plays an important role in suppressing the instigation of nREM sleep, while OX_2R has a major role in promoting wakefulness.

In another direction, overexpression of components of the orexinergic system also disrupts the SWC. For example in the zebrafish, overexpression of orexinergic neurons has been shown to induce an insomnia-like phenotype (Prober et al., 2006). Mice that overexpress prepro-orexin display sleep abnormalities which include fragmentation of nREM sleep, reduced REM sleep, and increased motor activity during REM sleep, suggesting an inability to maintain sleep states (Willie et al., 2011).

If we take into consideration that the activation of the orexinergic system promotes wakefulness and that its disruption brings about sleep disturbances, orexin antagonists could offer a very effective therapeutic alternative for insomnia.

OREXIN ANTAGONISTS FOR TREATING INSOMNIA

The newest molecules in the pipeline for the treatment of insomnia are orexin antagonists. There are many orexin antagonists currently being studied for the treatment of insomnia and they fall into one of two categories: single orexin receptor antagonists (SORAs) and dual orexin receptor antagonists (DORAs).

In the following part of this review, we evaluate the effectiveness of these drugs for the treatment of insomnia. A summary of orexin antagonists is provided in **Table 2**.

SORAs

Evidence from experiments conducted in transgenic models of orexin receptor KO mice suggests that SORAs targeting OX_1R will not promote sleep as effectively as those aimed at OX_2R.

OX_1R

Of the available SORAs, SB-334867 was the first drug designed to selectively antagonize OX_1R (Smart et al., 2001). This SORA is able to counteract the suppression of REM sleep after ICV infusion of OX_A in rats. However, it does not decrease wakefulness, or increase the amount of time spent in sleep, nor does it reduce sleep latency by itself at any given dose (Smith et al., 2003). Morairty and colleagues, later noted that SB-334867 at 3 and 30 mg/kg increased cumulative nREM during the first 4 and 6 h following administration (Morairty et al., 2012). SB-334867 is classified as a selective OX_1R antagonist, but unspecific binding to adenosine and serotonin receptors has been reported; it also affects monoamine and norepinephrine transporters at high concentrations (Lebold et al., 2013).

Although the effect of SB-334867 on sleep induction was poor, this molecule has proven to be useful for the treatment of other conditions, such as substance abuse, withdrawal, obesity and panic disorder (White et al., 2005; Johnson et al., 2010; Jupp et al., 2011; Smith and Aston-Jones, 2012).

Other selective OX_1R antagonists include SB-408124, SB-674042 and the newest AK-335827. So far, neither SB-408124 nor AK-335827 have been found to promote sleep (Dugovic et al., 2009; Steiner et al., 2013). In the case of SB-408124 however, insufficient brain penetration was found and this could account in part for the absence of observable effects (Morairty et al., 2012).

There are few studies characterizing the effect of these antagonists; nonetheless, there is some evidence that they can be useful in the treatment of substance abuse and withdrawal, and have potential for treating obesity and panic disorder. For example, it has been shown that subcutaneous administration of SB-408124 lowers the release of dopamine in the *nucleus accumbens* (Dugovic et al., 2009), and orally administered AK-335827 has anxiolytic effects (Steiner et al., 2013).

It is interesting that despite the lack of sleep-promoting effects of OX_1R SORAs on their own, these compounds have the capacity to thwart the sleep inhibiting effects of ICV orexin infusion

Table 2 | Summary of orexin receptor antagonists.

Name	Affinity (K_i, nM)		Possible applications
	OX_1R	OX_2R	
SINGLE OREXIN RECEPTOR ANTAGONIST		**SELECTIVITY**	
SB-334867	28	1704	OX_1R	Withdrawal, substance abuse, obesity, panic disorder
SB-408124	22	1405		
SB-674042	1.1	129		
ACT-335827	6	417 (IC_{50})		
TCS-OX2-29	–	7.4 (pKi)	OX_2R	Sleep promotion
JNJ-10397049	1644	6		
EMPA	900	1.1		
Antagonist 26	6.34	7.23 (pKi)		
DUAL OREXIN RECEPTOR ANTAGONIST		**FDA PHASE**	
Almorexant	13	8	III (discontinued)	Treatment of insomnia
SB-649868	0.3	0.4	II (completed)	
Suvorexant	0.6	0.4	III (pending approval)	
MK-6096	2.5	0.3	–	–
DORA 30	18	7 (IC_{50})	–	Sleep promotion

(Smith et al., 2003). Strikingly, they can also reduce the sleep-promoting effects of other antagonists; as observed under the coadministration of OX_1R and OX_2R antagonists which has a milder sleep-promoting effect than when the OX_2R antagonist is administered by itself (Dugovic et al., 2009). This could be due to the high concentrations used in these experiments (30 mg/kg) and the unspecific binding that follows.

OX_2R

Type 2 orexin receptors are selectively expressed both in the PVN and the TMN. As mentioned above, the PVN is part of the HPA, and the overactivation of the HPA has been proposed to be involved in the etiology of PI. Withholding the orexinergic stimuli to the HPA could help prevent the development of the vicious cycle proposed earlier. Additionally, the TMN, a histaminergic nucleus, has a major role in the arousal effect observed after orexinergic stimulation (Huang et al., 2001). Inhibition of the TMN with orexinergic antagonists could, facilitate the induction of sleep by allowing the sleep promoting nuclei to prevail.

OX_2R antagonists are less common than the other classes. Among the few available molecules that have been studied in the context of sleep promotion are EMPA, TCS-OX2-29 and JNJ-10397049. These antagonists have been more successful at diminishing wakefulness than OX_1R antagonists.

EMPA is the least effective sleep-promoting OX_2R SORA studied. While intraperitoneal administration of EMPA (100 mg/kg) has been shown to selectively increase cumulative nREM sleep during the first 4 and 6 h after administration, these increases are not accompanied by any significant increase in REM sleep or reduction in latencies for either sleep stage (Morairty et al., 2012). On the other hand, rats that received an ICV infusion of TCS-OX2-29 (40 nmol) increased their total sleep time by 7% in comparison to controls that received saline infusions. Interestingly, this effect was secondary to a selective increase in REM sleep (Kummangal et al., 2013).

Intraperitoneal administration (5, 25 or 50 mg/kg) of JNJ-10397049 6 h into the dark phase, produced a robust increase in total sleep time, traced to increases in both REM and nREM sleep (Gozzi et al., 2011). Similar results have been observed with subcutaneous injections (Dugovic et al., 2009). Starting at doses of 3 mg/kg, administration of JNJ-10397049 2 h into the light phase significantly decreased the latency to nREM sleep while increasing the length of each bout. At higher concentrations (30 mg/kg), this drug also induced a decrease in REM sleep latency without noticeable changes in its duration. Overall, 3 mg/kg of JNJ-10397049 increased total sleep time by 42% while keeping the proportion of nREM/REM sleep observed in vehicle treated animals.

Furthermore, microdialysis assays showed that this compound reduces histamine release in the LH (Dugovic et al., 2009). As mentioned earlier, release of histamine in the TMN is fundamental for the wake-promoting effects of OX_A ICV infusions (Huang et al., 2001).

Animal studies support the notion that OX_2R antagonists are helpful as sleep inducing agents. Further research is needed to determine the degree of sleep generation achieved by these compounds in different species, including humans. It is possible that the sleep-promoting effect of selectively antagonizing OX_2R is less

pronounced than the one observed with DORAs, but it may also be more specific, which would be worth investigating.

DORAs

It had been long suspected that antagonizing both orexin receptors would elicit the most powerful sleep-promoting effects; therefore, many of the studies around orexin antagonists have focused on DORAs. So far, evidence has proven this to be the case (Morairty et al., 2012), to the point that DORAs are the only orexin antagonists currently undergoing clinical trials in the hope that they will be approved by the FDA for the treatment of insomnia.

Almorexant

ACT-078573 (almorexant) is the most widely studied DORA and one of the first to enter phase III clinical trials (NCT00608985).

In wild type mice, the administration of almorexant 15 min before lights-out reduced the amount of time spent awake, while increasing the length of nREM and REM sleep bouts in a dose dependent manner (Mang et al., 2012). Notably, the proportion of REM sleep observed after almorexant administration during the dark phase was in the range of that observed during the light phase with vehicle treatment.

Further studies in KO mice determined that the sleep-inducing effect of almorexant was related to the stimulation of OX_2R and not OX_1R. This conclusion was reached after the authors did not observe any changes in the amount of sleep in OX_2R KO, but did for OX_1R KO mice. Interaction with sites other than orexin receptors that could account for the changes in sleep times was discarded when no changes were observed in the SWC of DKO mice.

When administered in healthy humans, almorexant was well tolerated. Doses of and above 200 mg elicited decreased alertness, with increased reports of fatigue, drowsiness, sleepiness, and sleep efficiency, measured as an increase in SWS and REM sleep (Brisbare-Roch et al., 2007). In PI patients, it proved to be effective for boosting sleep, increasing total sleep time, and reducing both REM sleep latency and the frequency of awakening (Hoever et al., 2012). This effect was dose dependent, with the most notorious effect on sleep architecture achieved at doses of 400 mg; doses of 100 and 200 mg had modest effects on sleep, with fewer adverse effects (e.g., headache, dizziness, blurred vision).

Although almorexant appeared to be well tolerated, the pharmaceutical companies sponsoring this drug discontinued the clinical trials in 2011 citing "safety observations" that required further evaluation. Currently, almorexant is in a new phase of clinical trials in order to evaluate its effect on cognitive performance (NCT01243060).

SB-649868

SB-649868 is a potent orally active DORA manufactured by the same pharmaceutical company as almorexant. There is also evidence for the effectiveness of SB-649868 in promoting sleep, both in animal studies and human trials.

When dispensed to rats, it elicited an increase in total sleep time (related to increases of both nREM and REM sleep) and reduced sleep latencies at doses of 10 and 30 mg. Moreover, the effect of SB-649868 on motor coordination was null, given that the rotarod model of coordination failed to reveal any motor impairment in rats treated with this compound, even when the orexin antagonist was administered concurrently with ethanol (Di Fabio et al., 2011). Compared to almorexant, the *in vivo* efficacy of this compound is excellent, thus it has been moved on to clinical trials.

The administration of SB-649868 to healthy volunteers who participated in a noise-disturbed sleep study showed that this compound is effective at inducing somnolence and fatigue at 10 and 30 mg doses (Bettica et al., 2012). Furthermore, patients diagnosed with PI reported that SB-649868 significantly improved the quality of sleep (10, 30, and 60 mg) while objectively increasing total sleep time, reducing sleep latency and suppressing nighttime awakenings (Bettica et al., 2012). During this study, the most common complaints were headaches, dry mouth and nasopharyngitis; the number of complaints increased in a dose dependent manner. Phase II clinical trials of SB-649868 have been completed (NCT00426816).

Suvorexant

Another promising DORA is the potent MK-4305 (suvorexant), a compound variation from the diazepane series. Animal studies have shown that suvorexant reduces active wake time by increasing nREM and REM sleep in rats, dogs, and monkeys (Winrow et al., 2011). In all cases, these effects were achieved at much lower doses (10 mg) than with almorexant.

This molecule is also in phase III clinical trials (NCT01097616) and is currently under evaluation for approval by the FDA. In healthy humans, the lowest dose (10 mg) reduced the number of awakenings after sleep onset; and at higher doses (50 mg) it reduced sleep latency, while increasing sleep efficiency and total sleep time (Sun et al., 2013). High doses (50 and 100 mg) elicit undesirable side effects such as an increase in reaction time, difficulty waking up and reduced alertness following awakening; in addition it leads to mild complaints of headaches and somnolence.

When administered to PI patients, suvorexant reduced sleep latency and increased the time patients spent asleep after a single administration without reducing the number of awakenings after sleep onset. The increase in total sleep time was mostly attributable to an increase in REM sleep. The most frequent adverse effects were somnolence, headaches, dizziness and abnormal dreams, all of which occurred in a dose dependent manner. In addition, there were no next-day residual effects, no rebound insomnia, complex sleep-related behaviors or withdrawal effects after 4 weeks. Instead, during this study there were a few reports of sleep paralysis (1, $n = 59$, at 40 mg), and at high doses (80 mg), excessive daytime sleepiness (1, $n = 61$), and hypnagogic hallucinations (1, $n = 61$) (Herring et al., 2012). These are symptoms of narcolepsy, and should be carefully monitored due to the close association between narcolepsy and the orexinergic system.

In general, suvorexant was well tolerated and, because the most consistently effective dosages were 30 and 40 mg, the pharmaceutical company manufacturing suvorexant submitted a dose range of 15–40 mg for FDA approval. To date, suvorexant has not been approved and the FDA has requested a lower starting dose of 10 mg for the general population and a 5 mg dose for those taking concomitant CYP3A4 inhibitors.

One potential advantage of DORAs over classic insomnia treatments, such as BZDs, is the possibility of inducing a more physiological sleep. For instance, while DORAs enhance REM sleep, BZDs have proven to suppress this sleep stage (Lanoir and Killam, 1968; Borbély et al., 1985; Gaillard et al., 2009). In addition, orexin antagonists appear to have a better side effect profile, with mild complaints of headaches and dizziness being the most common. The only exception appears to be almorexant, given the surprising suspension of clinical trials. Although the reasons for halting clinical trials have not been disclosed to the public, it is conceivable that the high doses required to achieve therapeutic effects could also cause more severe adverse effects, not observed in other drugs that require doses 10 times smaller.

One of the most important questions when characterizing an orexin antagonist is whether or not it elicits narcoleptic symptoms. Thus far, orexin antagonists have not been observed to cause cataplexy in animal models or in human patients. Up until now, reports of human patients complaining of sleep paralysis or hypnagogic hallucinations have been scarce, only occurring with high doses of suvorexant. As clinical trials progress, medical practitioners should still be on the alert for symptoms of narcolepsy.

DISCUSSION

The research and evaluation of new insomnia treatments is often complex, given that insomnia is usually of multifactorial etiology. Understanding the molecular and receptor mechanisms involved in promoting sleep in a variety of disorders could provide future approaches to new drug development.

An abundance of current research data has demonstrated the importance of the orexin system in the regulation of the SWC. Excitement over the potential of orexin receptor antagonists for treating insomnia peaked in 2007 when Actelion Pharmaceuticals Ltd. revealed that almorexant significantly decreased wakefulness in rats, dogs and humans, without evidence of cataplexy; unfortunately, clinical trials were discontinued in 2011 due to safety concerns that required further evaluation. Second generation inhibitors with improved pharmaceutical properties are currently being developed and tested for the potential treatment of insomnia and other disorders linked to dysfunction in the orexin system.

Orexin antagonism may offer improved avenues for combining medications with non-drug treatments such as CBTi for insomnia. However, more randomized controlled trials are needed to assess both the short- and long-term effects of these medications, as well as their efficacy in comorbid diseases that affect the quality and quantity of sleep.

ACKNOWLEDGMENTS

We would like to express our appreciation to Diana Millán Aldaco, Francisco Perez Eugenio and Marcela Palomero Rivero for their technical assistance and to Bianca Delfosse for her help in revising this manuscript. This work was supported by the following grants: CONACyT-179927 and DGAPA-PAPIIT-IN204612 to

Dr. Drucker-Colín, and DGAPA-PAPIIT-IB202112 and SECITI-PINV11-30 to Dr. Guerra-Crespo. Alberto K De La Herrán-Arita is a recipient of the Stanford School of Medicine Dean's Postdoctoral Fellowship Award and Ana C. Equihua receives a grant from CONACyT.

REFERENCES

Adam, K., Tomeny, M., and Oswald, I. (1986). Physiological and psychological differences between good and poor sleepers. *J. Psychiatr. Res.* 20, 301–316. doi: 10.1016/0022-3956(86)90033-6

Adamantidis, A. R., Zhang, F., Aravanis, A. M., Deisseroth, K., and de Lecea, L. (2007). Neural substrates of awakening probed with optogenetic control of hypocretin neurons. *Nature* 450, 420–424. doi: 10.1038/nature06310

Al-Barazanji, K. A., Wilson, S., Baker, J., Jessop, D. S., and Harbuz, M. S. (2001). Central orexin-A activates hypothalamic-pituitary-adrenal axis and stimulates hypothalamic corticotropin releasing factor and arginine vasopressin neurones in conscious rats. *J. Neuroendocrinol.* 13, 421–424. doi: 10.1046/j.1365-2826.2001.00655.x

Alexandre, C., Andermann, M. L., and Scammell, T. E. (2013). Control of arousal by the orexin neurons. *Curr. Opin. Neurobiol.* 23, 1–8. doi: 10.1016/j.conb.2013.04.008

Bartter, F. C., Delea, C. S., and Halberg, F. (2006). A map of blood and urinary changes related to circadian variations in adrenal cortical function in normal subjects. *Ann. N.Y. Acad. Sci.* 98, 969–983. doi: 10.1111/j.1749-6632.1962.tb30612.x

Bettica, P., Squassante, L., Zamuner, S., Nucci, G., Danker-Hopfe, H., and Ratti, E. (2012). The orexin antagonist SB-649868 promotes and maintains sleep in men with primary insomnia. *Sleep* 35, 1097–1104. doi: 10.5665/sleep.1996

Bonnet, M. H., and Arand, D. L. (2010). Hyperarousal and insomnia: state of the science. *Sleep Med. Rev.* 14, 9–15. doi: 10.1016/j.smrv.2009.05.002

Borbély, A. A., Mattmann, P., Loepfe, M., Strauch, I., and Lehmann, D. (1985). Effect of benzodiazepine hypnotics on all-night sleep EEG spectra. *Hum Neurobiol.* 4, 189–194.

Bourgin, P., Huitrón-Résendiz, S., Spier, A. D., Fabre, V., Morte, B., Criado, J. R., et al. (2000). Hypocretin-1 modulates rapid eye movement sleep through activation of locus coeruleus neurons. *J. Neurosci.* 20, 7760–7765.

Brisbare-Roch, C., Dingemanse, J., Koberstein, R., Hoever, P., Aissaoui, H., Flores, S., et al. (2007). Promotion of sleep by targeting the orexin system in rats, dogs and humans. *Nat. Med.* 13, 150–155. doi: 10.1038/nm1544

Buckley, T. M., and Schatzberg, A. F. (2005). On the interactions of the hypothalamic-pituitary-adrenal (HPA) axis and sleep: normal HPA axis activity and circadian rhythm, exemplary sleep disorders. *J. Clin. Endocrinol. Metab.* 90, 3106–3114. doi: 10.1210/jc.2004-1056

Chang, H., Saito, T., Ohiwa, N., Tateoka, M., Deocaris, C. C., Fujikawa, T., et al. (2007). Inhibitory effects of an orexin-2 receptor antagonist on orexin A- and stress-induced ACTH responses in conscious rats. *Neurosci. Res.* 57, 462–466. doi: 10.1016/j.neures.2006.11.009

Chapotot, F., Buguet, A., Gronfier, C., and Brandenberger, G. (2001). Hypothalamo-pituitary-adrenal axis activity is related to the level of central arousal: effect of sleep deprivation on the association of high-frequency waking electroencephalogram with cortisol release. *Neuroendocrinology* 73, 312–321. doi: 10.1159/000054648

Chemelli, R., Willie, J., and Sinton, C. M. (1999). Narcolepsy in orexin knockout mice: molecular genetics of sleep regulation. *Cell* 98, 437–451. doi: 10.1016/S0092-8674(00)81973-X

De la Herrán-Arita, A. K., Zomosa-Signoret, V. C., Millán-Aldaco, D. A., Palomero-Rivero, M., Guerra-Crespo, M., et al. (2011). Aspects of the narcolepsy-cataplexy syndrome in O/E3-null mutant mice. *Neuroscience* 183, 134–143. doi: 10.1016/j.neuroscience.2011.03.029

Del Cid-Pellitero, E., and Garzón, M. (2011). Hypocretin1/OrexinA-containing axons innervate locus coeruleus neurons that project to the Rat medial prefrontal cortex. Implication in the sleep-wakefulness cycle and cortical activation. *Synapse* 65, 843–857. doi: 10.1002/syn.20912

de Lecea, L., Kilduff, T., Peyron, C., Gao, X., Foye, P., Danielson, P., et al. (1998). The hypocretins: hypothalamus-specific peptides with neuroexcitatory activity. *Proc. Natl. Acad. Sci. U.S.A.* 95, 322–327. doi: 10.1073/pnas.95.1.322

Di Fabio, R., Pellacani, A., Faedo, S., Roth, A., Piccoli, L., Gerrard, P., et al. (2011). Discovery process and pharmacological characterization of a novel dual orexin 1 and orexin 2 receptor antagonist useful for treatment of sleep disorders. *Bioorg. Med. Chem. Lett.* 21, 5562–5567. doi: 10.1016/j.bmcl.2011.06.086

Dollins, A. B., Zhdanova, I. V., Wurtman, R. J., Lynch, H. J., and Deng, M. H. (1994). Effect of inducing nocturnal serum melatonin concentrations in daytime on sleep, mood, body temperature, and performance. *Proc. Natl. Acad. Sci. U.S.A.* 91, 1824–1828. doi: 10.1073/pnas.91.5.1824

Dugovic, C., Shelton, J. E., Aluisio, L. E., Fraser, I. C., Jiang, X., Sutton, S. W., et al. (2009). Blockade of orexin-1 receptors attenuates orexin-2 receptor antagonism-induced sleep promotion in the rat. *J. Pharmacol. Exp. Ther.* 330, 142–151. doi: 10.1124/jpet.109.152009

Edinger, J. D., Glenn, D. M., Bastian, L. A., Marsh, G. R., Dailey, D., Hope, T. V., et al. (2003). Daytime testing after laboratory or home-based polysomnography: comparisons of middle-aged insomnia sufferers and normal sleepers. *J. Sleep Res.* 12, 43–52. doi: 10.1046/j.1365-2869.2003.00335.x

Erman, M., Seiden, D., Zammit, G., Sainati, S., and Zhang, J. (2006). An efficacy, safety, and dose-response study of Ramelteon in patients with chronic primary insomnia. *Sleep Med.* 7, 17–24. doi: 10.1016/j.sleep.2005.09.004

España, R. A., Baldo, B. A., Kelley, A. E., and Berridge, C. W. (2001). Wake-promoting and sleep-suppressing actions of hypocretin (orexin): basal forebrain sites of action. *Neuroscience* 106, 699–715. doi: 10.1016/S0306-4522(01)00319-0

Furlong, T. M., Vianna, D. M. L., Liu, L., and Carrive, P. (2009). Hypocretin/orexin contributes to the expression of some but not all forms of stress and arousal. *Eur. J. Neurosci.* 30, 1603–1614. doi: 10.1111/j.1460-9568.2009.06952.x

Gaillard, J.-M., Schulz, P., and Tissot, R. (2009). Effects of three Benzodiazepines (Nitrazepam, Flunitrazepam and Bromazepam) on sleep of normal subjects, studied with an automatic sleep scoring system. *Pharmacopsychiatry* 6, 207–217. doi:10.1055/s-0028-1094383

Gozzi, A., Turrini, G., Piccoli, L., Massagrande, M., Amantini, D., Antolini, M., et al. (2011). Functional magnetic resonance imaging reveals different neural substrates for the effects of orexin-1 and orexin-2 receptor antagonists. *PLoS ONE* 6:e16406. doi: 10.1371/journal.pone.0016406

Gunja, N. (2013). In the Zzz zone: the effects of z-drugs on human performance and driving. *J. Med. Toxicol.* 9, 163–171. doi: 10.1007/s13181-013-0294-y

Hagan, J. J., Leslie, R. A., Patel, S., Evans, M. L., Wattam, T. A., Holmes, S., et al. (1999). Orexin A activates locus coeruleus cell firing and increases arousal in the rat. *Proc. Natl. Acad. Sci. U.S.A.* 96, 10911–10916. doi: 10.1073/pnas.96.19.10911

Herring, W. J., Snyder, E., Budd, K., Hutzelmann, J., Snavely, D., Liu, K., et al. (2012). Orexin receptor antagonism for treatment of insomnia: a randomized clinical trial of suvorexant. *Neurology* 79, 2265–2274. doi: 10.1212/WNL.0b013e31827688ee

Hoever, P., Dorffner, G., Beneš, H., Penzel, T., Danker-Hopfe, H., Barbanoj, M. J., et al. (2012). Orexin receptor antagonism, a new sleep-enabling paradigm: a proof-of-concept clinical trial. *Clin. Pharmacol. Ther.* 91, 975–985. doi: 10.1038/clpt.2011.370

Huang, Z. L., Qu, W. M., Li, W. D., Mochizuki, T., Eguchi, N., Watanabe, T., et al. (2001). Arousal effect of orexin A depends on activation of the histaminergic system. *Proc. Natl. Acad. Sci. U.S.A.* 98, 9965–9970. doi: 10.1073/pnas.181330998

Jacobs, G. D., Pace-Schott, E. F., Stickgold, R., and Otto, M. W. (2004). Cognitive behavior therapy and pharmacotherapy for insomnia: a randomized controlled trial and direct comparison. *Arch. Intern. Med.* 164, 1888–1896. doi: 10.1001/archinte.164.17.1888

Johnson, M. W., Suess, P. E., and Griffiths, R. R. (2006). Ramelteon: a novel hypnotic lacking abuse liability and sedative adverse effects. *Arch. Gen. Psychiatry* 63, 1149–1157. doi: 10.1001/archpsyc.63.10.1149

Johnson, P. L., Truitt, W., Fitz, S. D., Minick, P. E., Dietrich, A., Sanghani, S., et al. (2010). A key role for orexin in panic anxiety. *Nat. Med.* 16, 111–115. doi: 10.1038/nm.2075

Jupp, B., Krivdic, B., Krstew, E., and Lawrence, A. J. (2011). The orexin receptor antagonist SB-334867 dissociates the motivational properties of alcohol and sucrose in rats. *Brain Res.* 1391, 54–59. doi: 10.1016/j.brainres.2011.03.045

Kalogiannis, M., Hsu, E., Willie, J. T., Chemelli, R. M., Kisanuki, Y. Y., Yanagisawa, M., et al. (2011). Cholinergic modulation of narcoleptic attacks in double orexin receptor knockout mice. *PLoS ONE* 6:e18697. doi: 10.1371/journal.pone.0018697

Kay, G. G. (2000). The effects of antihistamines on cognition and performance. *J. Allergy Clin. Immunol.* 105, S622–S627. doi: 10.1067/mai.2000.106153

Kiyashchenko, L., Mileykovskiy, B., Maidment, N., Lam, H. A., Wu, M.-F., John, J., et al. (2002). Release of Hypocretin (Orexin) during waking and sleep states. *J. Neurosci.* 22, 5282–5286.

Köhler, C., Swanson, L. W., Haglund, L., and Wu, J. Y. (1985). The cytoarchitecture, histochemistry and projections of the tuberomammillary nucleus in the rat. *Neuroscience* 16, 85–110. doi: 10.1016/0306-4522(85)90049-1

Kummangal, B. A., Kumar, D., and Mallick, H. N. (2013). Intracerebroventricular injection of orexin-2 receptor antagonist promotes REM sleep. *Behav. Brain Res.* 237, 59–62. doi: 10.1016/j.bbr.2012.09.015

Lader, M. (2012). Benzodiazepine harm: how can it be reduced? *Br. J. Clin. Pharmacol.* 1–19. doi: 10.1111/j.1365-2125.2012.04418.x

Lanoir, J., and Killam, E. K. (1968). Alteration in the sleep-wakefulness patterns by benzodiazepines in the cat. *Electroencephalogr. Clin. Neurophysiol.* 25, 530–542. doi: 10.1016/0013-4694(68)90232-0

Lebold, T. P., Bonaventure, P., and Shireman, B. T. (2013). Selective orexin receptor antagonists. *Bioorg. Med. Chem. Lett.* 23, 4761–4769. doi: 10.1016/j.bmcl.2013.06.057

Lee, M. G., Hassani, O. K., and Jones, B. E. (2005). Discharge of identified orexin/hypocretin neurons across the sleep-waking cycle. *J. Neurosci.* 25, 6716–6720. doi: 10.1523/JNEUROSCI.1887-05.2005

Lin, L., Faraco, J., Li, R., Kadotani, H., Rogers, W., Lin, X., et al. (1999). The sleep disorder canine narcolepsy is caused by a mutation in the hypocretin (orexin) receptor 2 gene. *Cell* 98, 365–376. doi: 10.1016/S0092-8674(00)81965-0

Mang, G. M., Dürst, T., Bürki, H., Imobersteg, S., Abramowski, D., Schuepbach, E., et al. (2012). The dual orexin receptor antagonist almorexant induces sleep and decreases orexin-induced locomotion by blocking orexin 2 receptors. *Sleep* 35, 1625–1635. doi: 10.5665/sleep.2232

Marcus, J. N., Aschkenasi, C. J., Lee, C. E., Chemelli, R. M., Saper, C. B., Yanagisawa, M., et al. (2001). Differential expression of orexin receptors 1 and 2 in the rat brain. *J. Comp. Neurol.* 435, 6–25. doi: 10.1002/cne.1190

Meoli, A., Rosen, C., Kristo, D., Kohrman, M., Gooneratne, N., Aguillard, R., et al. (2005). Oral nonprescription treatment for insomnia: an evaluation of products with limited evidence. *J. Clin. Sleep Med.* 1, 173–187.

Mieda, M., Hasegawa, E., Kisanuki, Y. Y., Sinton, C. M., Yanagisawa, M., and Sakurai, T. (2011). Differential roles of orexin receptor-1 and -2 in the regulation of non-REM and REM sleep. *J. Neurosci.* 31, 6518–6526. doi: 10.1523/JNEUROSCI.6506-10.2011

Mileykovskiy, B. Y., Kiyashchenko, L. I., and Siegel, J. M. (2005). Behavioral correlates of activity in identified hypocretin/orexin neurons. *Neuron* 46, 787–798. doi: 10.1016/j.neuron.2005.04.035

Monroe, L. (1967). Psychological and physiological differences between good and poor sleepers. *J. Abnorm. Psychol.* 72, 255–264. doi: 10.1037/h0024563

Morairty, S. R., Revel, F. G., Malherbe, P., Moreau, J.-L., Valladao, D., Wettstein, J. G., et al. (2012). Dual hypocretin receptor antagonism is more effective for sleep promotion than antagonism of either receptor alone. *PLoS ONE* 7:e39131. doi: 10.1371/journal.pone.0039131

Morin, C. M. (1999). Behavioral and pharmacological therapies for late-life insomnia: a randomized controlled trial. *JAMA* 281, 991. doi: 10.1001/jama.281.11.991

Morin, C. M., Culbert, J., and Schwartz, S. (1994). Nonpharmacological interventions for insomnia: a meta-analysis of treatment efficacy. *Am. J. Psichiatr.* 151, 1172–1180.

NIH State-of-the-Science Conference Statement on Manifestations and Management of Chronic Insomnia in Adults. (2005). *NIH Consens Sci Statements*, Vol. 22.

Pandi-Perumal, S. R., Spence, D. W., Verster, J. C., Srinivasan, V., Brown, G. M., Cardinali, D. P., et al. (2011). Pharmacotherapy of insomnia with ramelteon: safety, efficacy and clinical applications. *J. Cent. Nerv. Syst. Dis.* 3, 51–65. doi: 10.4137/JCNSD.S1611

Panula, P., Pirvola, U., Auvinen, S., and Airaksinen, M. (1989). Histamine-immunoreactive nerve fibers in the rat brain. *Neuroscience* 28, 585–610. doi: 10.1016/0306-4522(89)90007-9

Perlis, M. L., Smith, M. T., Andrews, P. J., Orff, H., and Giles, D. E. (2001). Beta/Gamma EEG activity in patients with primary and secondary insomnia and good sleeper controls. *Sleep* 24, 110–117.

Peyron, C., Tighe, D. K., van den Pol, A., de Lecea, L., Heller, H. C., Sutcliffe, J. G., et al. (1998). Neurons containing hypocretin (orexin) project to multiple neuronal systems. *J. Neurosci.* 18, 9996–10015.

Piper, D. C., Upton, N., Smith, M. I., and Hunter, A. J. (2000). The novel brain neuropeptide, orexin-A, modulates the sleep-wake cycle of rats. *Eur. J. Neurosci.* 12, 726–730. doi: 10.1046/j.1460-9568.2000.00919.x

Prober, D. A., Rihel, J., Onah, A. A., Sung, R.-J., and Schier, A. F. (2006). Hypocretin/orexin overexpression induces an insomnia-like phenotype in zebrafish. *J. Neurosci.* 26, 13400–13410. doi: 10.1523/JNEUROSCI.4332-06.2006

Pruessner, J., Wolf, O., Hellhammer, D., Buske-Kirschbaum, A., von Auer, K., Jobst, S., et al. (1997). Free cortisol levels after awakening: a reliable biological marker for the assessment of adrenocortical activity. *Life Sci.* 61, 2539–2549. doi: 10.1016/S0024-3205(97)01008-4

Reiter, R. J. (1986). Normal patterns of melatonin levels in the pineal gland and body fluids of humans and experimental animals. *J. Neural Transm. Suppl.* 21, 35–54.

Richardson, G. S., and Roth, T. (2001). Future directions in the management of insomnia. *J. Clin. Psychiatry* 62, 39–45.

Richelson, E. (1979). Tricyclic antidepressants and histamine H1 receptors. *Mayo Clin. Proc.* 54, 669–674.

Risberg, A., Risberg, J., and Ingvar, D. (1975). Effects of promethazine on nocturnal sleep in normal man. *Psychopharmacologia* 43, 279–284. doi: 10.1007/BF00429264

Rudolph, U., and Knoflach, F. (2011). Beyond classical benzodiazepines: novel therapeutic potential of GABAA receptor subtypes. *Nat. Rev. Drug Discov.* 10, 685–697. doi: 10.1038/nrd3502

Saitou, K., Kaneko, Y., Sugimoto, Y., Chen, Z., and Kamei, C. (1999). Slow wave sleep-inducing effects of first generation H1-antagonists. *Biol. Pharm. Bull.* 22, 1079–1082. doi: 10.1248/bpb.22.1079

Sakamoto, F., Yamada, S., and Ueta, Y. (2004). Centrally administered orexin-A activates corticotropin-releasing factor-containing neurons in the hypothalamic paraventricular nucleus and central amygdaloid nucleus of rats: possible involvement of central orexins on stress-activated central CRF neurons. *Regul. Pept.* 118, 183–191. doi: 10.1016/j.regpep.2003.12.014

Sakurai, T. (2007). The neural circuit of orexin (hypocretin): maintaining sleep and wakefulness. *Nat. Rev. Neurosci.* 8, 171–181. doi: 10.1038/nrn2092

Sakurai, T., Amemiya, A., Ishii, M., Matsuzaki, I., Chemelli, R. M., Tanaka, H., et al. (1998). Orexins and orexin receptors: a family of hypothalamic neuropeptides and G protein-coupled receptors that regulate feeding behavior. *Cell* 92, 573–585. doi: 10.1016/S0092-8674(00)80949-6

Smart, D., Sabido-David, C., Brough, S. J., Jewitt, F., Johns, A., Porter, R. A., et al. (2001). SB-334867-A: the first selective orexin-1 receptor antagonist. *Br. J. Pharmacol.* 132, 1179–1182. doi: 10.1038/sj.bjp.0703953

Smith, M. I., Piper, D. C., Duxon, M. S., and Upton, N. (2003). Evidence implicating a role for orexin-1 receptor modulation of paradoxical sleep in the rat. *Neurosci. Lett.* 341, 256–258. doi: 10.1016/S0304-3940(03)00066-1

Smith, R. J., and Aston-Jones, G. (2012). Orexin / hypocretin 1 receptor antagonist reduces heroin self-administration and cue-induced heroin seeking. *Eur. J. Neurosci.* 35, 798–804. doi: 10.1111/j.1460-9568.2012.08013.x

Spath-Schwalbe, E. (1992). Nocturnal adrenocorticotropin and cortisol secretion depends on sleep duration and decreases in association with spontaneous awakening in the morning. *J. Clin. Endocrinol. Metab.* 75, 1431–1435. doi: 10.1210/jc.75.6.1431

Steiger, A., Guldner, J., Knisatschek, H., Rothe, B., Lauer, C., and Holsboer, F. (1991). Effects of an ACTH/MSH(4-9) analog (HOE 427) on the sleep EEG and nocturnal hormonal secretion in humans. *Peptides* 12, 1007–1010. doi: 10.1016/0196-9781(91)90051-P

Steiner, M. A., Gatfield, J., Brisbare-Roch, C., Dietrich, H., Treiber, A., Jenck, F., et al. (2013). Discovery and characterization of ACT-335827, an orally available, brain penetrant orexin receptor type 1 selective antagonist. *ChemMedChem* 8, 898–903. doi: 10.1002/cmdc.201300003

Stepanski, E., Zorick, F., Roehrs, T., Young, D., and Roth, T. (1988). Daytime alertness in patients with chronic insomnia compared with asymptomatic control subjects. *Sleep* 11, 54–60.

Sun, H., Kennedy, W. P., Wilbraham, D., Lewis, N., Calder, N., Li, X., et al. (2013). Effects of suvorexant, an orexin receptor antagonist, on sleep parameters as measured by polysomnography in healthy men. *Sleep* 36, 259–267. doi: 10.5665/sleep.2386

Thannickal, T. C., Moore, R. Y., Nienhuis, R., Ramanathan, L., Gulyani, S., Aldrich, M. S., et al. (2000). Reduced number of hypocretin neurons in human narcolepsy. *Neuron* 27, 469–474. doi: 10.1016/S0896-6273(00)00058-1

Vgontzas, A. N., Bixler, E. O., Lin, H. M., Prolo, P., Mastorakos, G., Vela-Bueno, A., et al. (2001). Chronic insomnia is associated with nyctohemeral activation of the hypothalamic-pituitary-adrenal axis: clinical implications. *J. Clin. Endocrinol. Metab.* 86, 3787–3794. doi: 10.1210/jc.86.8.3787

Weber, J., Siddiqui, M. A., Wagstaff, A. J., and McCormack, P. L. (2010). Low-dose doxepin: in the treatment of insomnia. *CNS Drugs* 24, 713–720. doi: 10.2165/11200810-000000000-00000

White, C. L., Ishii, Y., Mendoza, T., Upton, N., Stasi, L. P., Bray, G. A., et al. (2005). Effect of a selective OX1R antagonist on food intake and body weight in two strains of rats that differ in susceptibility to dietary-induced obesity. *Peptides* 26, 2331–2338. doi: 10.1016/j.peptides.2005.03.042

Willie, J. T., Chemelli, R. M., Sinton, C. M., Tokita, S., Williams, S. C., Kisanuki, Y. Y., et al. (2003). Distinct narcolepsy syndromes in orexin receptor-2 and orexin null mice. *Neuron* 38, 715–730. doi: 10.1016/S0896-6273(03)00330-1

Willie, J. T., Takahira, H., Shibahara, M., Hara, J., Nomiyama, M., Yanagisawa, M., et al. (2011). Ectopic overexpression of orexin alters sleep/wakefulness states and muscle tone regulation during REM sleep in mice. *J. Mol. Neurosci.* 43, 155–161. doi: 10.1007/s12031-010-9437-7

Winrow, C. J., Gotter, A. L., Cox, C. D., Doran, S. M., Tannenbaum, P. L., Breslin, M. J., et al. (2011). Promotion of sleep by suvorexant-a novel dual orexin receptor antagonist. *J. Neurogenet.* 25, 52–61. doi: 10.3109/01677063.2011.566953

Winsky-Sommerer, R., Yamanaka, A., Diano, S., Borok, E., Roberts, A. J., Sakurai, T., et al. (2004). Interaction between the corticotropin-releasing factor system and hypocretins (orexins): a novel circuit mediating stress response. *J. Neurosci.* 24, 11439–11448. doi: 10.1523/JNEUROSCI.3459-04.2004

Xi, M., Morales, F. R., and Chase, M. H. (2001). Effects on sleep and wakefulness of the injection of hypocretin-1 (orexin-A) into the laterodorsal tegmental nucleus of the cat. *Brain Res.* 901, 259–264. doi: 10.1016/S0006-8993(01)02317-4

Zhdanova, I., Wurtman, R., Morabito, C., Piotrovska, V., and Lynch, H. (1996). Effects of low oral doses of melatonin, given 2–4 h before habitual bedtime, on sleep in normal young humans. *Sleep* 19, 423–431.

Conflict of Interest Statement: The authors declare that the research was conducted in the absence of any commercial or financial relationships that could be construed as a potential conflict of interest.

5

Orexin 1 receptor antagonists in compulsive behavior and anxiety: possible therapeutic use

Emilio Merlo Pich[1]* and Sergio Melotto[2]

[1] Neuroscience DTA, F. Hoffman – La Roche, Basel, Switzerland
[2] Legnago, Italy

Edited by:
Michel A. Steiner, Actelion Pharmaceuticals Ltd., Switzerland

Reviewed by:
G. Koob, The Scripps Research Institute, USA
Jonathan Hollander, The Scripps Research Institute, USA
William A. Truitt, Indiana University School of Medicine, USA

*Correspondence:
Emilio Merlo Pich, Neuroscience DTA, F. Hoffman – La Roche, Granzacherstrasse 126, Basel 4070 Switzerland
e-mail: emilio.merlo_pich@ roche.com;
emilio.merlopich@gmail.com

Fifteen years after the discovery of hypocretin/orexin a large body of evidence has been collected supporting its critical role in the modulation of several regulatory physiological functions. While reduced levels of hypocretin/orexin were initially associated with narcolepsy, increased levels have been linked in recent years to pathological states of hypervigilance and, in particular, to insomnia. The filing to FDA of the dual-activity orexin receptor antagonist (DORA) suvorexant for the indication of insomnia further corroborates the robustness of such evidences. However, as excessive vigilance is also typical of anxiety and panic episodes, as well as of abstinence and craving in substance misuse disorders. In this review we briefly discuss the evidence supporting the development of hypocretin/orexin receptor 1 (OX1) antagonists for these indications. Experiments using the OX1 antagonist SB-334867 and mutant mice have involved the OX1 receptor in mediating the compulsive reinstatement of drug seeking for ethanol, nicotine, cocaine, cannabinoids and morphine. More recently, data have been generated with the novel selective OX1 antagonists GSK1059865 and ACT-335827 on behavioral and cardiovascular response to stressors and panic-inducing agents in animals. Concluding, while waiting for pharmacologic data to become available in humans, risks and benefits for the development of an OX1 receptor antagonist for Binge Eating and Anxiety Disorders are discussed.

Keywords: drug addiction, relapse, binge eating, repetitive behavior, emotion, OX1 receptor antagonist, GSK1059865

INTRODUCTION

Hypocretin/orexin is an hypothalamic neuropeptide consisting of two forms, A and B, containing 33 and 28 amino acids respectively, and binding to two G-protein coupled receptors, OX1 (or hcrt-1) and OX2 (or hcrt-2) (de Lecea et al., 1998; Sakurai et al., 1998).

The hypocretin/orexin peptide is produced in a small population of neurons located in the dorsomedial—perifornical hypothalamic area (DMH/PeF) and in the lateral hypothalamic nucleus (LH). Positive nerve fibers and terminals can be found in several areas of the central and peripheral nervous system, including vagus nerve, spinal cord, brainstem, hypothalamus, thalamus, limbic system, and some cortical regions (Peyron et al., 1998; Heinonen et al., 2008). OX/hcrt receptors show a similarly extended distribution (Marcus et al., 2001), suggesting a potential relevant role of hypocretins/orexins as regulatory peptides for several adaptive and limbic system-controlled functions (Johnson et al., 2012a,b; Mahler et al., 2012; Boutrel et al., 2013; Tsujino and Sakurai, 2013).

The OX1 receptor contains 425 amino acids while the OX2 receptor contains 444 amino acids with a sequence similarity between the two receptors of 68% (Sakurai et al., 1998). While both receptors are coupled with Gq-protein, only the OX1 receptor is additionally coupled with Gs-protein.

Receptor activation increases intracellular calcium levels via a Gq–dependent phospholipase C (PLC)-mediated increase of inositol-1,4,5-triphosphate (Lund et al., 2000) and diacylglycerol, resulting in the activation of the δ form of the protein kinase C, eventually engaging the ERK phosphorylation pathway (Ekholm et al., 2007).

OX1 and OX2 receptors are differentially distributed throughout the mammalian brain (Marcus et al., 2001), matching the distribution of hypocretin/orexin terminals. Evidence for a functional segregation of the two receptors was recently obtained using pharmacological magnetic resonance imaging (phMRI) in rats. The activating effects of amphetamine were differentially attenuated by pre-treatment with the selective OX2 receptor antagonist JNJ-1037049 or with the novel OX1 receptor antagonist GSK1059865: JNJ-1037049 attenuated the amphetamine effects in frontal cortex and thalamus, areas involved in arousal, while GSK1059865 reduced the activation in the extended amygdala, BNST and ventral striatum; all brain areas involved in stress and motivation (Gozzi et al., 2011). These differences in functional maps, together with differences in behavioral profiles support a rationale for exploring different indications for novel therapeutics that selectively target either OX1 or OX2 receptors. However, while the role of the OX2 receptor in sleep and arousal is strongly supported by the available experimental evidence

(Gatfield et al., 2010), the therapeutic potential of selective antagonism of the OX1 receptor is still under evaluation (Gotter et al., 2012).

The better understanding of the biology of the hypocretin/orexin system has promoted drug discovery programs in several pharmaceutical companies, resulting in a series of patents and compounds with different selectivity and in vitro characteristics (Faedo et al., 2012; Lebold et al., 2013). As shown above, some compounds were used as pharmacologic tools to explore OX1- and OX2-dependent neurotransmission in vivo. Few compounds were successfully progressed in humans, in particular the dual OX1-OX2 receptor antagonist (DORA) almorexant (Hoever et al., 2012), SB-649868 (Bettica et al., 2012), and suvorexant (Herring et al., 2012). Only suvorexant went successfully through Phase 3 development and it was filed in USA as new treatment for insomnia in 2013.

The first pharmacological tool used as OX1 receptor antagonist was SB-334867 (Jones et al., 2001; Smart et al., 2001). Recently, other compounds have been proposed: GSK1059865 (Alvaro et al., 2009; Gozzi et al., 2011), 2,5 di-substituted piperidines (Jiang et al., 2012) and ACT-335827 (Steiner et al., 2013).

In this review we address the evidence, mostly collected with pharmacologic tools, for a preferential role of the OX1-mediated neurotransmission in compulsive behavior, particularly in relation to addiction and binge eating, and in anxiety.

HYPOCRETIN/OREXIN AND THE OX1 RECEPTOR IN DRUG ADDICTION-LIKE AND COMPULSIVE EATING BEHAVIORS

Several preclinical findings indicated the involvement of the hypocretin/orexin system in compulsive and repetitive behavior as well as in the control of goal-oriented behavior. Recent excellent reviews summaries the evidence collected in more than hundred articles indicting that the hypocretin/orexin system in the lateral hypothalamus (Harris et al., 2005) is involved in the behavioral addiction-like dysregulations associated with exposure to cocaine, amphetamine, morphine, heroin, nicotine, ethanol and cannabinoids in rodents (Espana et al., 2011; Mahler et al., 2012; Boutrel et al., 2013; Flores et al., 2013), as well as in the excessive intake of palatable food associated with binge eating (Tsujino and Sakurai, 2013).

Data supporting the hypocretin/orexin involvement in the effects of addictive drugs was initially obtained in mice carrying a null mutation (KO) of the hypocretin/orexin peptide, showing reduced signs of withdrawal from morphine (Georgescu et al., 2003). Subsequently, impaired conditioned place preference for morphine (Narita et al., 2006) and for nicotine (Plaza-Zabala et al., 2012) was demonstrated in rodents. More recently, studies in KO mice with deletion of the OX1 receptor showed reduced cocaine and cannabinoid self-administration and the blockade of reinstatement of drug taking after abstinence (Hollander et al., 2012; Flores et al., 2013), indicating a critical role for OX1 receptors in mediating reinstatement of drug seeking.

In rodents SB-334867, a preferential OX1 receptor antagonist, reduced sensitization, drug seeking behavior and withdrawal syndrome in rodents exposed to ethanol, nicotine, morphine, and cocaine. These and other findings were extensively described in recent reviews (Mahler et al., 2012; Boutrel et al., 2013). Of particular interest is the fact that SB-334867 consistently attenuated the compulsive behavior associated with the reinstatement of drug seeking, induced by either acute stress or cues associated previously with drug taking, a phenomenon observed for ethanol, nicotine, cocaine, cannabinoids and morphine.

Recently, the highly selective OX1 receptor antagonist GSK 1059865 (5-bromo-N-[(2S,5S)-1-(3-fluoro-2-methoxybenzoyl)-5-methylpiperidin-2-yl]methyl-pyridin-2-amine) was characterized within the GSK collection (Alvaro et al., 2009). GSK1059865 at the dose of 25 mg/kg i.p. (estimated to fully occupy the OX1 receptors in the brain of the rat) only marginally modified the physiological sleep of rats, indicating a weak hypnotic effect (Gozzi et al., 2011; Piccoli et al., 2012) and confirming difference vs. OX2 receptor blockade (Mieda et al., 2011). Conversely, at 10 and 30 mg/kg i.p. doses, GSK1059865 significantly antagonized the cocaine effect in a conditioned place-preference paradigm (Gozzi et al., 2011). These results are in line with the proposed role of selective OX1 receptor antagonism in preventing relapse to drug seeking but not inducing sleep.

OX1 receptors were also recently involved in mediating the binge episodes of compulsive eating (Avena and Bocarsly, 2012), also defined as "food addiction," another compulsive behavior increasingly common among obese individuals (Volkow and Wise, 2005; Pedram et al., 2013). Although it was initially shown that the acute central administration of orexin-A stimulates feeding behavior by acting on specific hypothalamic circuits (Friederich et al., 2013), hypocretin/orexin-induced food intake appears to be influenced by several other factors, including the palatability of the food, the energy balance, the level of arousal and the emotional status (Yamanaka et al., 2003; Zheng et al., 2007; Choi et al., 2010; Tsujino and Sakurai, 2013). This suggests that the hypocretin/orexin system can activate more complex behavioral patterns than the sole increase of food intake (Mahler et al., 2012). Indeed, recent studies indicate a possible involvement of hypocretin/orexin dysregulation in compulsive intake of palatable food (Smith and Robbins, 2013).

Compulsive eating can be elicited in rodents by alternating periods of regular access to food with periods of food restriction over a few weeks, a specific chronic stressful condition that can produce binge episodes when a large amount of palatable food becomes suddenly available. The model was pharmacologically validated in rats, showing an inhibitory effect of topiramate on the compulsive food intake (Cifani et al., 2009) similar to that observed in human binge eaters (McElroy et al., 2003). Although data regarding the involvement of the hypocretin/orexin pathway in this experimental procedure of binge eating were not available, we studied the effect of GSK1059865 as a tool to assess the relevance of the OX1 receptors (Piccoli et al., 2012). Interestingly, GSK1059865, at the doses of 10 and 30 mg/kg, was not able to inhibit highly palatable food intake in control animals (not exposed to cyclic food restriction), confirming the minor effect of OX1 receptor blockade on natural reward when it occurs under physiological conditions. On the contrary, GSK1059865 potently inhibited the compulsive eating behavior in rats exposed to chronic stress/food restriction (Piccoli et al., 2012). Interestingly, regular food intake was also inhibited by the OX1 antagonist

SB-334867 in rats genetically prone to obesity but not in control rats (White et al., 2005). These findings confirmed the role of the OX1 receptor-mediated transmission in attenuating the excessive drive produced by craving associated to distress that was also observed with addictive drugs.

Interestingly binge eating was also inhibited by the DORA SB-649868, but not by the selective OX2 receptor antagonist JNJ-10397049, suggesting that the effects of SB-649868 are probably due to the OX1 component of its mechanism of action (Piccoli et al., 2012). Intriguingly, the lack of effect of almorexant in animals exposed only to acute stress suggested that the procedure of alternating periods of food restriction is critical for the engagement of the hypocretin/orexin system in promoting compulsive eating of highly palatable food (Funabashi et al., 2009; Pankevich et al., 2010). This observation suggests that in this paradigm DORA and OX1 antagonists do not work primarily via an anti-stress effect. This is not surprising, given the complex role of hypocretin/orexin in the maintenance of energy balance and the sensitivity of hypocretin/orexin neurons to directly respond to the changes of circulating glucose levels and to endocrine signals (Tsujino and Sakurai, 2013).

Overall, the results obtained with GSK1059865 confirm that selective OX1 receptor antagonism is not directly affecting the reward pathways involved in hedonic eating, but rather support a role in the compulsive aspect of food intake, those that probably account for the development and persistence of abnormal eating behaviors in binge eaters and, possibly, in bulimic patients. In addition, these data highlight the need to re-evaluate the putative OX1 receptor antagonism profile, so far based mostly on SB-334867 (Haynes et al., 2000), a compound whose selectivity at high dose and stability have been under discussion (Hollander et al., 2012; McElhinny et al., 2012).

To date a limited number of human biomarker studies support a role for the hypocretin/orexin system in the behavioral dysregulation that characterizes addiction, and none of them used pharmacologic agents. Changes of hypocretin/orexin levels in blood were observed in alcoholics during alcohol withdrawal, showing positive association with distress scores (von der Goltz et al., 2011), while negative association was observed with craving scores in abstinent smokers (von der Goltze et al., 2010). Increased expression of hypocretin/orexin levels was also found in the in peripheral blood of cigarette smokers and cannabis abusers (Rotter et al., 2012). While the interpretation of these finding is still unclear, subjects affected by narcolepsy were studied for their liability to addiction with the hope to get more informative results. Accordingly, narcolepsy is commonly associated with mutations in the hypocretin/orexin gene (Peyron et al., 1998), resulting in a constitutive deficiency of the peptide, similar to that obtained in hypocretin/orexin KO mice. Subtle differences in reward processing and risk-taking behavior were reported in narcoleptic subjects, but the prevalence of tobacco smoking in these patients was not different from that of the normal population (Bayard and Dauvilliers, 2013). There results can be seen at variance with evidence of reduced effects of addictive drugs in hypocretin/orexin KO mice (for review see Mahler et al., 2012; Boutrel et al., 2013). Interestingly, narcoleptic subjects declared using cigarette smoking and nicotine patches as self-medication to reduce sleepiness and increase arousal (Ebben and Krieger,

2012). Altogether, the findings indicate complexity in the relationship between addictive behaviors and dysfunctional hypocretin/orexin system in humans, supporting the need of additional, more focused translational studies.

HYPOCRETIN/OREXIN AND THE OX1 RECEPTOR IN ANXIETY

Textbooks of physiology describe the posterior and perifornical regions of the hypothalamus as the part of the limbic circuit that controls "fight-or-flight" reactions in response to an imminent threat (Hess and Akert, 1955). As mentioned above, neurons that produce hypocretin/oirexin are located in the perifornical region (Peyron et al., 1998) and project to the majority of the limbic brain structures involved in the fear, stress and anxiety circuit (Shin and Liberzon, 2009), suggesting a possible role of hypocretin/orexin in controlling not only wakefulness and arousal, but also fear, anxiety, and stress responses (Johnson et al., 2012a; Sears et al., 2013).

This hypothesis was explored over the years and summarized in recent articles and reviews (Bisetti et al., 2006; Mathew et al., 2008; Johnson et al., 2010, 2012a). In these contributions interested readers can find the evidence supporting the role of hypocretin/orexin neurons in orchestrating the autonomic, respiratory, cardiovascular and behavioral responses to stressful and panic-inducing stimuli.

The working hypothesis implies that stressful stimuli (or high endogenous levels of anxiogenic mediators) would increase the activity on hypocretin/orexin neurons, which in turn will release more hypocretin/orexin in their terminal fields located in brain limbic regions that regulate emotion and stress response. Then hypocretin/orexin will be shifting the level of activation of the fear, stress and anxiety circuit toward a higher level of arousal, which includes vegetative, endocrine and behavioral phenomena typical of anxiety and panic states. An abnormal persistence of excessive release of hypocretin/orexin could be seen as a critical factor in the maintenance of high arousal and anxiety, as well as a liability to relapse into panic episodes in predisposed individuals, suggesting a potential critical pathophysiological role for anxiety.

Data in humans showed an increased release of extracellular hypocretin/orexin driven by emotional stimuli in the amygdala of subjects suffering from treatment-resistant temporal lobe epilepsy that were implanted with microdialysis probes (Blouin et al., 2013). In this study the levels of hypocretin/orexin increased during wake and decreased during sleep, but the highest peaks were observed during acute emotional activations of both positive and negative valence. The amygdala is considered a key structure for processing salience and negative emotion, which is associated with pathologic anxiety. In rodents microinjection of hypocretin/orexin into the amygdala increases anxiety-like behavior (Avolio et al., 2011). Interestingly, abnormal high levels of hypocretin/orexin were found in the cerebro-spinal fluid (CSF) of patients with Panic Anxiety Disorders, suggesting a possible hyperactivity state (Johnson et al., 2010). In another study increased levels of hypocretin/orexin were measured in the peripheral blood of subjects with chronic obstructive pulmonary disorder (COPD), a condition associated with hypercapnia, acidosis and a 10-fold increased risk of panic attacks (Zhu et al., 2011).

Converging findings suggest that the anxiogenic properties of hypocretin/orexin are primarily mediated by the engagement of OX1 receptors. In rodents the autonomic and behavioral responses to stress were attenuated by pre-treatments with OX1 receptor antagonists, such as SB-334867 (Johnson et al., 2010, 2012b), GSK 1034865 (Gozzi et al., 2011) and ACT-335827 (Steiner et al., 2013), or with a DORA, such as almorexant (Steiner et al., 2012). Significant attenuation of anxiety-like responses was observed in paradigms including fear conditioning (Sears et al., 2013; Steiner et al., 2013), panicogenic lactate infusion (Johnson et al., 2010), hypercapnia (Li et al., 2010; Johnson et al., 2012b), administration of FG-7142 (Johnson et al., 2012a), high dose nicotine (Plaza-Zabala et al., 2010), and yohimbine (Richards et al., 2008). Recent evidence using OX1 and OX2 KO mice showed a critical role of OX1 receptors located in the locus coeruleus in mediating cued fear-conditioning learning and threat memory formation (Sears et al., 2013; Soya et al., 2013).

Evidence that hypocretin/orexin-containing neurons receive inputs from other neurons producing the anxiogenic peptide corticotropin releasing factor (CRF) and that hypocretin/orexin neurons projects to CRF-rich brain regions suggested the possibility that these two peptidergic systems are functionally entangled in the control of the stress response (Ida et al., 2000; Pañeda et al., 2005). However, if this hypothesis is correct, the anxiolytic properties of CRF-1 antagonists (Zorrilla and Koob, 2004) and those of OX1 antagonists would overlap, showing similar profiles. Interestingly, a recent study using phMRI in rats suggests that the involvement of CRF-1 and OX1 in stress responses can be functionally segregated. In this experiment a phMRI activation brain map was elicited in rats with yohimbine at doses known to produce anxiogenic effects. Pre-treatments with either CP-154,526, a selective CRF-1 antagonist (Seymour et al., 2003), or the selective OX1 receptor antagonist GSK1059865 (Gozzi et al., 2011) were performed. The yohimbine activation brain map was attenuated by CP-154,526 in the motor, cingulate, retrosplenial, dorsal prefrontal cortex, dorsal portions of the caudate-putamen, and in the amygdala. Differently, GSK1059865 attenuated the yohimbine activation map in the nucleus accumbens, septum, dorsal thalamus, amygdala, ventral hippocampus, orbitofrontal, prefrontal, insular, cingulate retrosplenial, and piriform cortex (Gozzi et al., 2013). Overall, the OX1 receptor antagonist exerted a more extensive effect on the fear, stress and anxiety circuit than the CRF1 antagonist, attenuating the activations of regions of the dopaminergic mesolimbic system. In line with the latter observation, a dissociation was found between the effects of OX1 and CRF-1 antagonists on the rat mesolimbic dopamine system in stress-induced cocaine (Wang et al., 2009) and nicotine seeking (Plaza-Zabala et al., 2012).

Interestingly, in some studies both OX1 antagonists and DORAs did not show anxiolytic effects in specific behavioral tests (e.g., the elevated plus maze) (Steiner et al., 2012; Rodgers et al., 2013). These data are in line with the hypothesis that hypocretin/orexin receptor antagonists do not alter basal anxiety levels in rodents, but exert anxiolytic-like properties when anxiety levels are transiently exacerbated by potent stimuli such as acidosis/hypercapnia.

LIMITATIONS AND CONCLUSION

The rationale for considering OX1 receptors as a possible target in conditions such as Anxiety Disorders, Drug Addiction, and Binge Eating was reviewed. Based on the current knowledge on mechanism of action, OX1 receptor antagonists should have fewer development risks than DORAs. As highlighted by Scammell and Winrow (2011) and Boutrel et al. (2013) for DORAs, the chronic simultaneous blockade of both hypocretin/orexin receptors can potentially: (1) induce narcoleptic-like symptoms, including catalepsy; (2) impair goal oriented decision-making; (3) reduce pleasure associated with rewarding activities; (4) induce sedation, sleepiness and impaired coping responses under acute emergency or stress; (5) impact on basal metabolism with increased body weight. However, so far the human experience with the DORAs suvorexant, SB-649868 and almorexant is very encouraging, showing minimal occurrence of the above mentioned adverse events and, in particular, no induction of narcoleptic eoisodes or impairment of decision making performance when tested within the dose range currently proposed. However, more data on larger populations and higher doses are required to reach a final conclusion.

Interestingly, treatments with selective OX1 antagonists are not expected to share the same risks of DORAs since only the OX2 receptor is primarily associated with narcolepsy which was demonstrated for dogs carrying a disruptive genetic mutation of this receptor (Wu et al., 2011). The additional potential benefits of an OX1 antagonist include: (1) A preclinical anxiolytic profile that differentiates it from benzodiazepines, serotonin-uptake inhibitors, and CRF-1 antagonists; (2) The capacity of reducing hyper-arousal states associated to acute and severe anxiety episodes with relevant physical symptoms, such as panic attacks or withdrawal from addictive drugs; (3) The attenuation of compulsive and repetitive behaviors associated with sensitization, stress-relieve, or drug seeking; (4) The lack of effects on desire of natural rewards, and (5) the lack of sleep-inducing effects.

These considerations are based on a limited dataset of preclinical studies, only recently conducted with the new generation of selective compounds. Chronic dosing studies are missing and therefore information of long term risks and benefits are not available yet. In addition, no selective OX1 receptor antagonists have been tested in humans so far and the translational barrier is still unclear. However, the promising therapeutic potential in the modulation of anxiety and compulsive behaviors is stimulating further basic research and is encouraging active investments of pharmaceutical companies.

REFERENCES

Alvaro, G., Amantini, D., and Stasi, L. (2009). *Pyridine Derivatives Used to Treat Orexin Related Disorders*. WO 2009124956. PCT Int. Appl.

Avena, N. M., and Bocarsly, M. E. (2012). Dysregulation of brain reward systems in eating disorders: neurochemical information from animal models of binge eating, bulimia nervosa, and anorexia nervosa. *Neuropharmacology* 63, 87–96. doi: 10.1016/j.neuropharm.2011.11.010

Avolio, E., Alò, R., Carelli, A., and Canonaco, M. (2011). Amygdalar orexinergic-GABAergic interactions regulate anxiety behaviors of the Syrian golden hamster. *Behav. Brain Res.* 218, 288–295. doi: 10.1016/j.bbr.2010.11.014

Bayard, S., and Dauvilliers, Y. A. (2013). Reward-based behaviors and emotional processing in human with narcolepsy-cataplexy. *Front. Behav. Neurosci.* 7:50. doi: 10.3389/fnbeh.2013.00050

Bettica, P., Squassante, L., Zamuner, S., Nucci, G., Danker-Hopfe, D., and Ratti, E. (2012). The orexin antagonist SB-649868 promotes and maintain sleep in men with primary insomnia. *Sleep* 35, 1097–1104. doi: 10.5665/sleep.1996

Bisetti, A., Cvetkovic, V., Serafin, M., Bayer, L., Machard, D., Jones, B. E., et al. (2006). Excitatory action of hypocretin/orexin on neurons of the central medial amygdala. *Neuroscience* 142, 999–1004. doi: 10.1016/j.neuroscience.2006.07.018

Blouin, A. M., Fried, I., Wilson, C. L., Staba, R. J., Behnke, E. J., Lam, H. A., et al. (2013). Human hypocretin and melanin-concentrating hormone levels are linked to emotion and social interaction. *Nat. Commun.* 4, 1547–1553. doi: 10.1038/ncomms2461

Boutrel, B., Steiner, N., and Halfon, O. (2013). The hypocretins and the reward function: what have we learned so far? *Front. Behav. Neurosci.* 7:59. doi: 10.3389/fnbeh.2013.00059

Choi, D. L., Davis, J. F., Fitzgerald, M. E., and Benoit, S. C. (2010). The role of orexin-A in food motivation, reward-based feeding behavior and food-induced neuronal activation in rats. *Neuroscience* 167, 11–20. doi: 10.1016/j.neuroscience.2010.02.002

Cifani, C., Polidori, C., Melotto, S., Ciccocioppo, R., and Massi, M. (2009). A preclinical model of binge eating elicited by yo-yo dieting and stressful exposure to food: effect of sibutramine, fluoxetine, topiramate, and midazolam. *Psychopharmacology (Berl.)* 204, 113–125. doi: 10.1007/s00213-008-1442-y

de Lecea, L., Kilduff, T. S., Peyron, C., Gao, X. B., Foye, P. E., Danielson, P. E., et al. (1998). The hypocretins: hypothalamus-specific peptides with neuroexcitatory activity. *Proc. Natl. Acad. Sci. U.S.A.* 95, 322–327. doi: 10.1073/pnas.95.1.322

Ebben, M. R., and Krieger, A. C. (2012). Narcolepsy with cataplexy masked by the use of nicotine. *J. Clin. Sleep Med.* 8, 195–196. doi: 10.5664/jcsm.1780

Ekholm, M. E., Johansson, L., and Kukkonen, J. P. (2007). IP3 independent signalling of OX1 orexin/hypocretin receptor to Ca2+ influx and ERK. *Biochem. Biophys. Res. Commun.* 353, 475–480. doi: 10.1016/j.bbrc.2006.12.045

Espana, R. A., Melchior, J. R., Roberts, D. C., and Jones, S. R. (2011). Hypocretin 1/orexin A in the ventral tegmental area enhances dopamine responses to cocaine and promotes cocaine self-administration. *Psychopharmacology (Berl.)* 214, 415–426. doi: 10.1007/s00213-010-2048-8

Faedo, S., Perdonà, E., Antolini, M., di Fabio, R., Merlo Pich, E., and Corsi, M. (2012). Functional and binding kinetic studies make a distinction between OX 1 and OX2 orexin receptor antagonists. *Eur. J. Pharmacol.* 692, 1–9. doi: 10.1016/j.ejphar.2012.07.007

Flores, A., Maldonado, R., and Berrendero, F. (2013). The hypocretin/orexin receptor-1 as a novel target to modulate cannabinoid reward. *Biol. Psychiatry* 3223, 590–598. doi: 10.1016/j.biopsych.2013.06.012

Friederich, H. C., Wu, M., Simon, J. J., and Herzog, W. (2013). Neurocircuit function in eating disorders. *Int. J. Eat. Disord.* 46, 425–432. doi: 10.1002/eat.22099

Funabashi, T., Hagiwara, H., Mogi, K., Mitsushima, D., Shinohara, K., and Kimura, F. (2009). Sex differences in the responses of orexin neurons in the lateral hypothalamic area and feeding behavior to fasting. *Neurosci. Lett.* 463, 31–34. doi: 10.1016/j.neulet.2009.07.035

Gatfield, J., Brisbare-Roch, C., Jenck, F., and Boss, C. (2010). Orexin receptor antagonists: a new concept in CNS disorders? *ChemMedChem* 5, 1197–1214. doi: 10.1002/cmdc.201000132

Georgescu, D., Zachariou, V., Barrot, M., Mieda, M., Willie, J. T., and Eisch, A. J. (2003). Involvement of the lateral hypothalamic peptide orexin in morphine dependence and with- drawal. *J. Neurosci.* 23, 3106–3111. doi: 10.1002/micr.10128

Gotter, A. L., Roecker, A. J., Hargreaves, R., Coleman, P. J., Winrow, C. J., and Renger, J. J. (2012). Orexin receptors as therapeutic drug targets. *Prog. Brain Res.* 198, 163–188. doi: 10.1016/B978-0-444-59489-1.00010-0

Gozzi, A., Lepore, S., Vicentini, E., Merlo-Pich, E., and Bifone, A. (2013). Differential effect of orexin-1 and CRF-1 antagonism on stress circuits: a fMRI study in the rat with the pharmacological stressor yohimbine. *Neuropsychopharmacology* 38, 2120–2130. doi: 10.1038/npp.2013.109

Gozzi, A., Turrini, G., Piccoli, L., Massagrande, M., Amantini, D., Antolini, M., et al. (2011). Functional magnetic resonance imaging reveals different neural substrates for the effects of orexin-1 and orexin-2 receptor antagonists. *PLoS ONE* 6:e16406. doi: 10.1371/journal.pone.0016406

Harris, G. C., Wimmer, M., and Aston-Jones, G. (2005). A role for lateral hypothalamic orexin neurons in reward seeking. *Nature* 437, 556–559. doi: 10.1038/nature04071

Haynes, A. C., Jackson, B., Chapman, H., Tadayyon, M., Johns, A., Porter, R. A., et al. (2000). A selective orexin-1 receptor antagonist reduces food consumption

in male and female rats. *Regul. Pept.* 96, 45–51. doi: 10.1016/S0167-0115(00)00199-3

Heinonen, M. V., Purhonen, A. K., Makela, K. A., and Herzig, K. H. (2008). Functions of orexin in peripheral tissue. *Acta Physiol. (Oxf.)* 192, 471–485. doi: 10.1111/j.1748-1716.2008.01836.x

Herring, W. J., Snyder, E., Budd, K., Hutzelmann, J., Snavely, D., Liu, K., et al. (2012). Orexin receptor antagonism for treatment of insomnia: a randomized clinical trial of suvorexant. *Neurology* 79, 2265–2274. doi: 10.1212/WNL.0b013e31827688ee

Hess, W. R., and Akert, K. (1955). Experimental data on role of hypothalamus in mechanism of emotional behavior. *AMA Arch. Neurol. Psychiatry* 73, 127–129. doi: 10.1001/archneurpsyc.1955.02330080005003

Hoever, P., Dorffner, G., Bene, H., Penzel, T., Danker-Hopfe, H., Barbanoj, M. J., et al. (2012). Orexin receptor antagonism, a new sleep-enabling paradigm: a proof-of-concept clinical trial. *Clin. Pharmacol. Ther.* 91, 975–985. doi: 10.1038/clpt.2011.370

Hollander, J. A., Pham, D., Fowler, C. D., and Kenny, P. J. (2012). Hypocretin-1 receptors regulate the reinforcing and reward-enhancing effects of cocaine: pharmacological and behavioral genetics evidence. *Front. Behav. Neurosci.* 6:47. doi: 10.3389/fnbeh.2012.00047

Ida, T., Nakahara, K., Murakami, T., Hanada, R., Nakazato, M., and Murakami, N. (2000). Possible involvement of orexin in the stress reaction in rats. *Biochem. Biophys. Res. Commun.* 270, 318–323. doi: 10.1006/bbrc.2000.2412

Jiang, R., Song, X., Bali, P., Smith, A., Bayona, C. R., Lin, L., et al. (2012). Disubstituted piperidines as potent orexin (hypocretin) receptor antagonists. *Bioorg. Med. Chem. Lett.* 12, 3890–3894. doi: 10.1016/j.bmcl.2012.04.122

Johnson, P. L., Molosh, A., Fitz, S. D., Truitt, W. A., and Shekhar, A. (2012a). Orexin, stress, and anxiety/panic states. *Prog. Brain Res.* 198, 133–161. doi: 10.1016/B978-0-444-59489-1.00009-4

Johnson, P. L., Samuels, B. C., Fitz, S. D., Federici, L. M., Hammes, N., Early, M. C., et al. (2012b). Orexin 1 receptors are a novel target to modulate panic responses and the panic brain network. *Physiol. Behav.* 107, 733–742. doi: 10.1016/j.physbeh.2012.04.016

Johnson, P. L., Truitt, W., Fitz, S. D., Minick, P. E., Dietrich, A., Sanghani, S., et al. (2010). A key role for orexin in panic anxiety. *Nat. Med.* 16, 111–115. doi: 10.1038/nm.2075

Jones, D. N. C., Gartlon, J., Parker, F., Taylor, S. G., Routledge, C., Hemmati, P., et al. (2001). Effects of centrally administered orexin-B and orexin-A: a role for orexin-1 receptors in orexin-B-induced hyperactivity. *Psychopharmacology* 153, 210–218. doi: 10.1007/s002130000551

Lebold, T. P., Bonaventure, P., and Shireman, B. T. (2013). Selective orexin receptor antagonists. *Bioorg. Med. Chem. Lett.* 223, 4761–4769. doi: 10.1016/j.bmcl.2013.06.057

Li, Y., Li, S., Wei, C., Wang, H., Sui, N., and Kirouac, G. J. (2010). Orexins in the paraventricular nucleus of the thalamus mediate anxiety-like responses in rats. *Psychopharmacology* 212, 251–265. doi: 10.1007/s00213-010-1948-y

Lund, P. E., Sariatmadari, R., Uustare, A., Detheux, M., Parmentier, M., and Kukkonen, J. P. (2000). The orexin OX1 receptor activates a novel CA2+ influx pathway necessary for coupling to phospholipase C. *J. Biol. Chem.* 275, 30806–30812. doi: 10.1074/jbc.M002603200

Mahler, S. V., Smith, R. J., Moorman, D. E., Sartor, G. C., and Aston-Jones, G. (2012). Multiple roles for orexin/hypocretin in addiction. *Prog. Brain Res.* 198, 79–121. doi: 10.1016/B978-0-444-59489-1.00007-0

Marcus, J. N., Aschkenasi, C. J., Lee, C. E., Chemelli, R. M., Saper, C. B., Yanagisawa, M., et al. (2001). Differential expression of orexin receptors 1 and 2 in the rat brain. *J. Comp. Neurol.* 435, 6–25. doi: 10.1002/cne.1190

Mathew, S. J., Price, R. B., and Charney, D. S. (2008). Recent advances in the neurobiology of anxiety disorders: implications for novel therapeutics. *Am. J. Med. Genet. C Semin. Med. Genet.* 148C, 89–98. doi: 10.1002/ajmg.c.30172

McElhinny, C. J. Jr., Lewin, A. H., Mascarella, S. W., Runyon, S., Brieaddy, L., and Carroll, F. I. (2012). Hydrolytic instability of the important orexin 1 receptor antagonist SB-334867: possible confounding effects on *in vivo* and *in vitro* studies. *Bioorg. Med. Chem. Lett.* 22, 6661–6664. doi: 10.1016/j.bmcl.2012.08.109

McElroy, S. L., Arnold, L. M., Shapira, N. A., Keck, P. E. Jr., Rosenthal, N. R., Karim, M. R., et al. (2003). Topiramate in the treatment of binge eating disorder associated with obesity: a randomized, placebo-controlled trial. *Am. J. Psychiatry* 160, 255–261. doi: 10.1176/appi.ajp.160.2.255

Mieda, M., Hasegawa, E., Kisanuki, Y. Y., Sinton, C. M., Yanagisawa, M., and Sakurai, T. (2011). Differential roles of orexin receptor-1 and -2 in the regulation of non-REM and REM sleep. *J. Neurosci.* 31, 6518–6526. doi: 10.1523/JNEUROSCI.6506-10.2011

Narita, M., Nagumo, Y., Hashimoto, S., Khotib, J., Miyatake, M., and Sakurai, T. (2006). Direct involvement of orexinergic systems in the activation of the mesolimbic dopamine pathway and related behaviours induced by morphine. *J. Neurosci.* 26, 398–405. doi: 10.1523/JNEUROSCI.2761-05.2006

Pañeda, C., Winsky-Sommerer, R., Boutrel, B., and de Lecea, L. (2005). The corticotropin-releasing factor-hypocretin connection: implications in stress response and addiction. *Drug News Perspect.* 18, 250–255. doi: 10.1358/dnp.2005.18.4.908659

Pankevich, D. E., Teegarden, S. L., Hedin, A. D., Jensen, C. L., and Bale, T. L. (2010). Caloric restriction experience reprograms stress and orexigenic pathways and promotes binge eating. *J. Neurosci.* 30, 16399–16407. doi: 10.1523/JNEUROSCI.1955-10.2010

Pedram, P., Wadden, D., Amini, P., Gulliver, W., Randell, E., Cahill, F., et al. (2013). Food addiction: its prevalence and significant association with obesity in the general population. *PLoS ONE* 8:e74832. doi: 10.1371/journal.pone.0074832

Peyron, C., Tighe, D. K., van den Pol, A. N., de Lecea, L., Heller, H. C., Sutcliffe, J. G., et al. (1998). Neurons containing hypocretin (orexin) project to multiple neuronal systems. *J. Neurosci.* 18, 9996–10015.

Piccoli, L., Micioni Di Bonaventura, M. V., Cifani, C., Costantini, V. J., Massagrande, M., Montanari, D., et al. (2012). Role of orexin-1 receptor mechanisms on compulsive food consumption in a model of binge eating in female rats. *Neuropsychopharmacology* 37, 1999–2011. doi: 10.1038/npp.2012.48

Plaza-Zabala, A., Flores, A., Maldonado, R., and Berrendero, F. (2012). Hypocretin/Orexin signaling in the hypothalamic paraventricular nucleus is essential for the expression of nicotine withdrawal. *Biol. Psychiatry* 71, 214–223. doi: 10.1016/j.biopsych.2011.06.025

Plaza-Zabala, A., Martín-García, E., de Lecea, L., Maldonado, R., and Berrendero, F. (2010). Hypocretins regulate the anxiogenic-like effects of nicotine and induce reinstatement of nicotine-seeking behavior. *J. Neurosci.* 30, 2300–2310. doi: 10.1523/JNEUROSCI.5724-09.2010

Richards, J. K., Simms, J. A., Steensland, P., Taha, S. A., Borgland, S. L., Bonci, A., et al. (2008). Inhibition of orexin-1/hypocretin-1 receptors inhibits yohimbine-induced reinstatement of ethanol and sucrose seeking in long-evans rats. *Psychopharmacology (Berl.)* 199, 109–117. doi: 10.1007/s00213-008-1136-5

Rodgers, R. J., Wright, F. L., Snow, N. F., and Taylor, L. J. (2013). Orexin-1 receptor antagonism fails to reduce anxiety-like behaviour in either plus-maze-naïve or plus-maze-experienced mice. *Behav. Brain Res.* 243, 213–219. doi: 10.1016/j.bbr.2012.12.064

Rotter, A., Bayerlein, K., Hansbauer, M., Weiland, J., Sperling, W., Kornhuber, J., et al. (2012). Orexin A expression and promoter methylation in patients with cannabis dependence in comparison to nicotine-dependent cigarette smokers and nonsmokers. *Neuropsychobiology* 66, 126–133. doi: 10.1159/000339457

Sakurai, T., Amemiya, A., Ishii, M., Matsuzaki, I., Chemelli, R. M., Tanaka, H., et al. (1998). Orexins and orexin receptors: a family of hypothalamic neuropeptides and G protein-coupled receptors that regulate feeding behavior. *Cell* 92, 573–585. doi: 10.1016/S0092-8674(00)80949-6

Scammell, T. E., and Winrow, C. J. (2011). Orexin receptors: pharmacology and therapeutic opportunities. *Annu. Rev. Pharmacol. Toxicol.* 51, 243–266. doi: 10.1146/annurev-pharmtox-010510-100528

Sears, R. M., Fink, A. E., Wigestrand, M. B., Farb, C. R., de Lecea, L., and Ledoux, J. E. (2013). Orexin/hypocretin system modulates amygdala-dependent threat learning through the locus coeruleus. *Proc. Natl. Acad. Sci. U.S.A.* 110, 20260–20265. doi: 10.1073/pnas.1320325110

Seymour, P. A., Schmidt, A. W., and Schulz, D. W. (2003). The pharmacology of CP-154,526, a non-peptide antagonist of the CRH1 receptor: a review. *CNS Drug Rev.* 9, 57–96. doi: 10.1111/j.1527-3458.2003.tb00244.x

Shin, L. M., and Liberzon, I. (2009). The neurocircuitry of fear, stress, and anxiety disorders. *Neuropsychopharmacology* 35, 169–191. doi: 10.1038/npp.2009.83

Smart, D., Sabido-David, C., Brough, S. J., Jewitt, F., Johns, A., Porter, R. A., et al. (2001). SB-334867-A: the first selective orexin-1 receptor antagonist. *Br. J. Pharmacol.* 132, 1179–1182. doi: 10.1038/sj.bjp.0703953

Smith, D. G., and Robbins, T. W. (2013). The neurobiological underpinnings of obesity and binge eating: a rationale for adopting the food addiction model. *Biol. Psychiatry* 73, 804–810. doi: 10.1016/j.biopsych.2012.08.026

Soya, S., Shoji, H., Hasegawa, E., Hondo, M., Miyakawa, T., Yanagisawa, M., et al. (2013). Orexin receptor-1 in the locus coeruleus plays an important role in cue-dependent fear memory consolidation. *J. Neurosci.* 33, 14549–14557. doi: 10.1523/JNEUROSCI.1130-13.2013

Steiner, M. A., Gatfield, J., Brisbare-Roch, C., Dietrich, H., Treiber, A., Jenck, F., et al. (2013). Discovery and characterization of ACT-335827, an orally available, brain penetrant orexin receptor type1 selective antagonist. *ChemMedChem* 8, 898–903. doi: 10.1002/cmdc.201300003

Steiner, M. A., Lecourt, H., and Jenck, F. (2012). The brain orexin system and almorexant in fear-conditioned startle reactions in the rat. *Psychopharmacology (Berl.)* 223, 465–475. doi: 10.1007/s00213-012-2736-7

Tsujino, N., and Sakurai, T. (2013). Role of orexin in modulating arousal, feeding, and motivation. *Front. Behav. Neurosci.* 7:28. doi: 10.3389/fnbeh.2013.00028

Volkow, N. D., and Wise, R. A. (2005). How can drug addiction help us understand obesity? *Nat. Neurosci.* 8, 555–560. doi: 10.1038/nn1452

von der Goltz, C., Koopmann, A., Dinter, C., Richter, A., Grosshans, M., Fink, T., et al. (2011). Involvement of orexin in the regulation of stress, depression and reward in alcohol dependence. *Horm. Behav.* 60, 644–650. doi: 10.1016/j.yhbeh.2011.08.017

von der Goltz, C., Koopmann, A., Dinter, C., Richter, A., Rockenbach, C., Grosshans, M., et al. (2010). Orexin and leptin are associated with nicotine craving: a link between smoking, appetite and reward. *Psychoneuroendocrinology* 35, 570–577. doi: 10.1016/j.psyneuen.2009.09.005

Wang, B., You, Z. B., and Wise, R. A. (2009). Reinstatement of cocaine seeking by hypocretin/orexin in the ventral tegmental area: independence from the local corticotropin-releasing factor network. *Biol. Psychiatry* 65, 857–862. doi: 10.1016/j.biopsych.2009.01.018

White, C. L., Ishii, Y., Mendoza, T., Upton, N., Stasi, L. P., Bray, G. A., et al. (2005). Effect of a selective OX1R antagonist on food intake and body weight in two strains of rats that differ in susceptibility to dietary-induced obesity. *Peptides* 26, 2331–2338. doi: 10.1016/j.peptides.2005.03.042

Wu, M. F., Nienhuis, R., Maidment, N., Lam, H. A., and Siegel, J. M. (2011). Role of the hypocretin (orexin) receptor 2 (Hcrt-r2) in the regulation of hypocretin level and cataplexy. *J. Neurosci.* 31, 6305–6310. doi: 10.1523/JNEUROSCI.0365-11.2011

Yamanaka, A., Beuckmann, C. T., Willie, J. T., Hara, J., Tsujino, N., Mieda, M., et al. (2003). Hypothalamic orexin neurons regulate arousal according to energy balance in mice. *Neuron* 38, 701–713. doi: 10.1016/S0896-6273(03)00331-3

Zheng, H., Patterson, L. M., and Berthoud, H. R. (2007). Orexin signaling in the ventral tegmental area is required for high-fat appetite induced by opioid stimulation of the nucleus accumbens. *J. Neurosci.* 27, 11075–11082. doi: 10.1523/JNEUROSCI.3542-07.2007

Zhu, L. Y., Summah, H., Jiang, H. N., and Qu, J. M. (2011). Plasma orexin-a levels in COPD patients with hypercapnic respiratory failure. *Mediators Inflamm.* 2011, 754847. doi: 10.1155/2011/754847

Zorrilla, E. P., and Koob, G. F. (2004). The therapeutic potential of CRF1 antagonists for anxiety. *Expert Opin. Investig. Drugs* 13, 799–828. doi: 10.1517/13543784.13.7.799

Conflict of Interest Statement: Emilio Merlo Pich is full time employee of F. Hoffman-La Roche. The other author declares that the research was conducted in the absence of any commercial or financial relationships that could be construed as a potential conflict of interest.

6

Hypocretin (orexin) regulation of sleep-to-wake transitions

Luis de Lecea[1] * and Ramón Huerta[2]

[1] *Department of Psychiatry and Behavioral Sciences, Stanford University School of Medicine, Stanford, CA, USA*
[2] *BioCircuits Institute, University of California, San Diego, La Jolla, CA, USA*

Edited by:
Christopher J. Winrow, Merck, USA

Reviewed by:
Juan Mena-Segovia, University of Oxford, UK
Michael M. Halassa, Massachusetts Institute of Technology, USA
Dipesh Chaudhury, Mount Sinai School of Medicine, USA

*Correspondence:
Luis de Lecea, Department of Psychiatry and Behavioral Sciences, Stanford University School of Medicine, 1201 Welch Road, Stanford, CA 94305, USA
e-mail: llecea@stanford.edu

The hypocretin (Hcrt), also known as orexin, peptides are essential for arousal stability. Here we discuss background information about the interaction of Hcrt with other neuromodulators, including norepinephrine and acetylcholine probed with optogenetics. We conclude that Hcrt neurons integrate metabolic, circadian and limbic inputs and convey this information to a network of neuromodulators, each of which has a different role on the dynamic of sleep-to-wake transitions. This model may prove useful to predict the effects of orexin receptor antagonists in sleep disorders and other conditions.

Keywords: hypothalamus, orexin, sleep, optogenetics, hypervigilance/avoidance

INTRODUCTION

Transitions between states of vigilance have long been associated with changes in cortical excitability associated with changes in the activity of monoamines and neuromodulators (Steriade, 2003). Steriade and McCarley (1990), Steriade et al. (1993), Steriade (2003) performed intracellular recordings of cortical neurons in different brain states and proposed that the concerted activity of norepinephrine, histamine, acetylcholine, and glutamate was sufficient to induce a sleep-to-wake transition. However, the mechanisms underlying the precise coordination of sleep states have remained poorly understood. The discovery of the hypocretins (Hcrts), also known as orexins, has provided a missing link in the regulation of states of vigilance.

THE HYPOCRETINS/OREXINS: CRITICAL REGULATORS OF AROUSAL STABILITY

Soon after their discovery in 1998 (de Lecea et al., 1998; Sakurai et al., 1998), two groups described the association between Hcrt deficiency and the sleep disorder narcolepsy (Chemelli et al., 1999; Lin et al., 1999; Nishino et al., 2000, 2001; Peyron et al., 2000; Thannickal et al., 2000). Several studies have shown that the Hcrt knockout (KO) or Hcrt-R2 deficient (Mochizuki et al., 2011) mice have normal amounts of sleep and wakefulness across the light/dark cycle (Mochizuki et al., 2004) but exhibit an increased instability of behavior states. Dogs with mutations in Hcrt R2 exhibit narcolepsy with cataplexy (Lin et al., 1999). Patients that suffer from narcolepsy with cataplexy have very low levels of Hcrt-1 in their CSF (Nishino et al., 2000; Peyron et al., 2000; Thannickal et al., 2000). These deficits are likely caused by selective degeneration of Hcrt cells (rather than down regulation of the Hcrt gene) because other markers that colocalize with Hcrt are also reduced in narcoleptic patients (Crocker et al., 2005). Indeed, a recent study has revealed epitopes in the Hcrt precursor sequence that trigger activation of

CD4 T-cells (De la Herran-Arita et al., 2013). All of these data clearly demonstrate that Hcrt signaling is necessary for arousal stability.

The first recordings of Hcrt neurons *in vitro* indicated that these cells are spontaneously active and responsive to multiple stimuli. Studies by Fujiki et al. (2001) using microdialysis and Estabrooke et al. (2001) using c-fos mapping revealed a circadian modulation of Hcrt peptide concentration in brain tissue. Parallel studies using juxtacellular recordings in head-fixed or freely moving animals showed that, surprisingly, Hcrt activity is mostly phasic, and precedes sleep-to-wake transitions by 10–20 s (Lee et al., 2005; Mileykovskiy et al., 2005). The question remained as to whether this phasic activity of Hcrt neurons was permissive or instructive for awakenings. In the first *in vivo* application of optogenetics in behaving animals, Adamantidis et al. (2007) found the photostimulation-induced activation of Hcrt neurons specifically increases the probability of transitions from sleep to wake (Adamantidis et al., 2007). This induction was frequency-dependent as only frequencies > 5Hz increased awakening probability. Semi-chronic stimulation of Hcrt neurons did not result in significant increases in the amount of non-rapid eye movement (NREM) sleep suggesting that phasic activation of Hcrt cells is involved in the transition to wake, but not in wake maintenance. Optogenetic silencing of Hcrt neurons induces sleep during the light phase, but not during the dark phase (Tsunematsu et al., 2011). These findings were further validated using a newly developed pharmacogenetic technology designer receptors exclusively activated by designer drugs (DREADDs; Sasaki et al., 2011) that allows the modulation of neural activity with temporal resolution of several hours. Therefore, the Hcrt system acts as a regulator of behavior states by modulating the arousal threshold (Sutcliffe and de Lecea, 2002), so that the organism can keep appropriate and adequate wakefulness to cope with fluctuations of the external and internal environments.

Then, does the existence of two subtypes of receptors account for these two aspects of functions of Hcrt? Hcrt-R2 deficient mice display fragmented wakefulness similar to the narcoleptic phenotype whereas Hcrt-R1-knockout mice only show a mild sleep disorder (Willie et al., 2001; Mieda et al., 2011). However, the double Hcrt-R1 and Hcrt-R2 receptor knockout mice suffer a more severe deficit in sleep–wake cycle than Hcrt-R2-knockouts, which exhibit a low degree of cataplexy and rapid eye movement sleep (REM) sleep intrusion (Chemelli et al., 1999; Willie et al., 2003; Mieda et al., 2011). Therefore, both the Hcrt-R1 and Hcrt-R2 are essential in the process of keeping a stable sleep/wakefulness cycle, with a larger contribution of Hcrt-R2. On the other hand, a recent study revealed that the Hcrt-1-mediated promotion of wakefulness was attenuated in both Hcrt-R1 and Hcrt-R2-knockout mice, and both receptors seem to be associated with the suppression of REM sleep (Mieda et al., 2011). However, a recently functional magnetic resonance imaging (fMRI) study revealed that the antagonist of Hcrt-R2 but not Hcrt-R1 increased REM, non-REM and total sleep-time, suggesting the distinct roles of the two receptors (Gozzi et al., 2011). Also, the recent development of Hcrt receptor selective antagonists showed that Hcrtr-1 blockade attenuates Hcrt-R2 antagonism and revealed complex interactions between Hcrt-R1 and Hcrt-R2 (Dugovic et al., 2009). Selective and non-selective Hcrt receptor antagonists have recently completed Phase III clinical trials for the treatment of insomnia (Herring et al., 2012), a remarkable development from a gene product discovered only 15 years ago.

AFFERENTS TO HCRT NEURONS
Anatomical and electrophysiological evidence accumulated over the last decade has shown that at least 10 other transmitters and hormone are sensed by Hcrt cells (Inutsuka and Yamanaka, 2013). *Most notably, NE, 5HT, NPY, CCK, ghrelin, nicotinic, and muscarinic acetylcholine, AMPA, NMDA Glutamate, GABAa, and GABAb receptors are expressed by Hcrt cells* (Sakurai, 2007). In the absence of co-localization studies, it is assumed that most of these receptors are randomly distributed within the Hcrt population. *Thus, as a network, Hcrt neurons receive information about the general excitability and arousal (Glu, GABA, ACh, NE, 5HT), feeding and metabolic state (NPY, Ghrelin, Leptin, and CCK).* Interestingly, Hcrt neurons may change their sensitivity to NE after sleep deprivation (Grivel et al., 2005), thus providing a mechanism through which Hcrt cells sense previous sleep history and homeostatic balance. Anatomical afferents have revealed several key areas that send axons to Hcrt cells (Sakurai et al., 2005; Yoshida et al., 2006) including the bed nucleus of the stria terminalis, the amygdala, and the medial septum, supporting a role of the limbic system in regulating Hcrt responses.

EFFECTORS OF HCRT NEURONS: THE MONOAMINES
The flip/flop model of sleep–wake cycle (Saper et al., 2010) posits that monoamines stimulate neocortical neurons and inhibit sleep centers to promote wakefulness. Importantly, these monoaminergic neurons in tuberomammillary nucleus (TMN, Histaminergic), locus coeruleus (LC, noradrenergic), dorsal raphe nuclei (DRN, serotoninergic), ventral periaqueductal gray matter (vPAG, dopaminergic) receive dense projections of Hcrt neurons (Peyron

et al., 1998; Saper et al., 2005), consist with the distribution of HcrtRs (Marcus et al., 2001). LC neurons mainly express Hcrt-R1, TMN neurons mostly Hcrt-R2 whereas DRN express both Hcrt-R1 and Hcrt-R2. Moreover, Hcrt neurons exhibit parallel firing patterns with monoaminergic neurons that represent tonic firing during wakefulness especially during active wakefulness, mild firing during slow wave sleep, and then silent during REM sleep (Estabrooke et al., 2001; Lee et al., 2005; Mileykovskiy et al., 2005), except its intensive firing at the transition to wakefulness. These data are also consistent with the oscillation of extracellular Hcrt-1 concentration that peak during the waking state and fall down to about half their max levels during sleep (Yoshida et al., 2001; Zeitzer et al., 2003). These observations suggest that Hcrt system stabilizes wakefulness through driving the arousal system during the arousal state (Saper et al., 2010).

Indeed, *in vitro* electrophysiological studies showed that Hcrt activates the TMN histaminergic (Bayer et al., 2001; Eriksson et al., 2001; Huang et al., 2001; Schone et al., 2012), LC noradrenergic (Hagan et al., 1999) and DRN serotoninergic (Liu et al., 2002) neurons, and *in vivo* experiments revealed the involvement of LC and the Hcrt-R1 in LC (Bourgin et al., 2000), as well as the histamine 1R (H1R; Huang et al., 2001) and the Hcrt-R2 signaling in TMN (Mochizuki et al., 2011) in Hcrt-induced arousal (Schone et al., 2012). However, recent reports found that Hcrt-mediated sleep-to-wake transition in mice did not depend on the histaminergic system (Carter et al., 2009a) and the mice could display a normal sleep/wake pattern in the condition that both H1R and Hcrt-R1 are deficient (Hondo et al., 2010). The role of Histaminergic cells may be more related to maintenance of the awake state, as histamine-deficient HDC knockout mice only show decreased arousal in new environments

Moreover, Lu and Greco (2006) demonstrated that loss of dopaminergic neurons in vPAG, a rostral extension of the ventral tegmental area (VTA), results in a reduction of wakefulness by 20% accompanied by increase of NREM, REM sleep. This finding is supported by a recent report (Kaur et al., 2009) that identified the Hcrt -vPAG circuit, whose activity suppresses REM sleep but not non- REM sleep. On the other hand, Hcrt neurons receive inhibition innervation from noradrenergic (Li et al., 2002), serotoninergic (Yamanaka et al., 2003; Kumar et al., 2007) and dopaminergic (Yamanaka et al., 2006) inputs whereas the histamine has little, if any, effect (Yamanaka et al., 2003). The role of noradrenergic innervation to Hcrt cells remains controversial, as some reports show excitatory effects in rats and others demonstrate inhibitory action (Grivel et al., 2005).

Cholinergic neurons in pedunculopontine tegmental nucleus/laterodorsal tegmental nucleus (PPT/LDT) fire most rapidly during wakefulness and REM sleep but slowly during NREM sleep (Saper et al., 2005), suggesting that they help to maintain the cortical activation in the states of wakefulness and REM sleep. Application of Hcrt-1 into LDT results in a significant increase of wakefulness but a decrease of amount rather than the duration of REM sleep (Xi et al., 2001). *In vitro* studies have shown that carbachol, a cholinergic agonist, excites Hcrt neurons (Bayer et al., 2005). In addition, intracerebroventricular (ICV) administration of Hcrt -1 (Piper et al., 2000) or local application into the LC (Bourgin et al., 2000) basal forebrain (Espana et al., 2001;

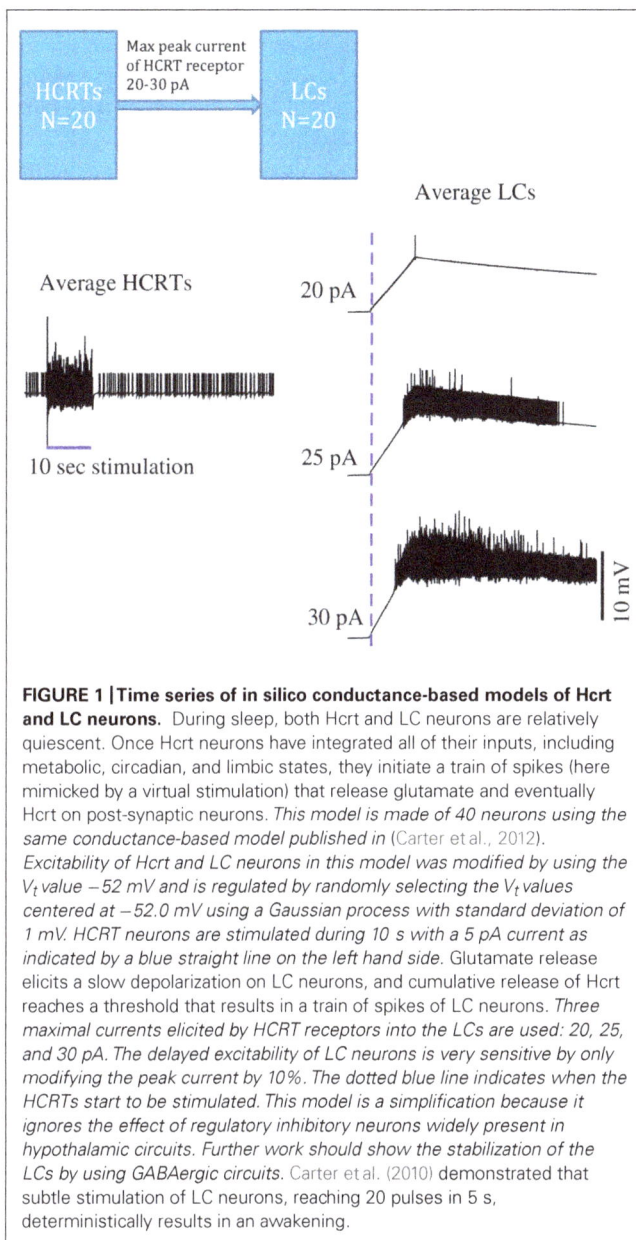

FIGURE 1 | Time series of in silico conductance-based models of Hcrt and LC neurons. During sleep, both Hcrt and LC neurons are relatively quiescent. Once Hcrt neurons have integrated all of their inputs, including metabolic, circadian, and limbic states, they initiate a train of spikes (here mimicked by a virtual stimulation) that release glutamate and eventually Hcrt on post-synaptic neurons. *This model is made of 40 neurons using the same conductance-based model published in* (Carter et al., 2012). *Excitability of Hcrt and LC neurons in this model was modified by using the V_t value −52 mV and is regulated by randomly selecting the V_t values centered at −52.0 mV using a Gaussian process with standard deviation of 1 mV. HCRT neurons are stimulated during 10 s with a 5 pA current as indicated by a blue straight line on the left hand side.* Glutamate release elicits a slow depolarization on LC neurons, and cumulative release of Hcrt reaches a threshold that results in a train of spikes of LC neurons. *Three maximal currents elicited by HCRT receptors into the LCs are used: 20, 25, and 30 pA. The delayed excitability of LC neurons is very sensitive by only modifying the peak current by 10%. The dotted blue line indicates when the HCRTs start to be stimulated. This model is a simplification because it ignores the effect of regulatory inhibitory neurons widely present in hypothalamic circuits. Further work should show the stabilization of the LCs by using GABAergic circuits.* Carter et al. (2010) demonstrated that subtle stimulation of LC neurons, reaching 20 pulses in 5 s, deterministically results in an awakening.

Thakkar et al., 2001), lateral preoptic area (Methippara et al., 2000) increases the waking time at the expense of sleep. In summary, Hcrt-induced arousal is modulated not only by monoaminergic neurons, but also needs the participation of cholinergic neurons in the PPT/LDT and basal forebrain.

Importantly, the Hcrt system may be modulated by the circadian clock and homeostatic states (Deboer et al., 2004; Carter et al., 2009b; Appelbaum et al., 2010). Even though there is no evidence of a direct synaptic connection between the Suprachiasmatic nucleus (SCN) and Hcrt cells, the circadian clock drives Hcrt system through the output circuits of the Suprachiasmatic nucleus (SCN) (Deurveilher and Semba, 2005). *The internal clock molecular machinery in Hcrt neurons (i.e., per, CLOCK, BMAL1, etc.) may also influence neuronal excitability during the light/dark*

cycle, effectively integrating circadian cues without direct Suprachiasmatic nucleus (SCN) connectivity. Additionally, local modulation of Hcrt neurons by Hcrt release (Li et al., 2002; Yamanaka et al., 2010), melanin-concentrating hormone (MCH; Rao et al., 2008; Hassani et al., 2009) or LepRB neurons (Leinninger et al., 2011) may also be important in the circadian stabilization of proper sleep–wake cycle. Intrinsic plasticity mechanisms may regulate the firing probability of Hcrt cells during day and night (Appelbaum et al., 2010). During the wakefulness period, tonic excitation of Hcrt neurons may be enhanced when the organism faces certain stressors like emotional stimulation, which involves the limbic input (Tsujino and Sakurai, 2009). Horvath and Gao (2005) *proposed that plasticity mechanisms in Hcrt cells are critical players in the connection between arousal, metabolism, and brain reward function.* Adamantidis and de Lecea (2008a,b) have suggested that Hcrt exerts different functions on different timescales: phasic activity lasting 1–10 s that would be mostly responsible for the state transitions, and a clock-regulated oscillation that would encode superimposed information about metabolic and circadian state.

TRANSLATIONAL CONSIDERATIONS
The Hcrt system has been involved in a myriad of pathological processes, including Parkinson's (PD; Drouot et al., 2003; Asai et al., 2008; Baumann et al., 2008; Fronczek et al., 2008), Alzheimer's (AD; Kang et al., 2009; Scammell et al., 2012), anxiety and panic disorders (Johnson et al., 2010) and depression (Salomon et al., 2003; Borgland and Labouebe, 2010). The mechanisms of these associations vary broadly, particularly in the neurodegenerative diseases. For instance, some studies have shown that a Hcrt receptor antagonist can reduce plaque formation in animal models of AD. However, other reports have shown the same prevalence of AD in narcoleptics and control patients. The role of Hcrt in panic and anxiety may be mediated through several of its connections to the paraventricular hypothalamus and brainstem nuclei. Similarly, the projections of Hcrt cells to serotonergic dorsal raphe neurons and periaqueductal gray suggest a possible mechanism of modulation of 5HT release and mood. Hcrt R1 knockout animals and pharmacological inhibition reduces time of immobility in the tail suspension test (Scott et al., 2011). In contrast, Hcrt r2 knockout animals showed increased despair. Future development of Hcrtr1 selective antagonists may thus proof useful in the treatment of depression.

OUTPUT OF HCRT NEURONS
Peyron et al. (1998) described a broad distribution of Hcrt fibers throughout the brain. Very few Hcrt projections have been studied in detail. The LC receives a very dense network of Hcrt-immunopositive axon terminals, and the connectivity between Hcrt and LC neurons has been shown to be monosynaptic. *Recently,* Carter et al. (2012) *have suggested a conductance-based computational model by which a short (> 10 s) period of phasic Hcrt activity enhances the excitability of post-synaptic LC neurons through conductances that elevate the concentration of intracellular calcium (***Figure 1***). Hcrt action on post-synaptic targets is remarkably slow* (Burlet et al., 2002; Kohlmeier et al., 2008), *lasting several seconds, a dynamic that is consistent with the wake latencies observed after optogenetic stimulation of Hcrt cells in vivo* (Mileykovskiy et al.,

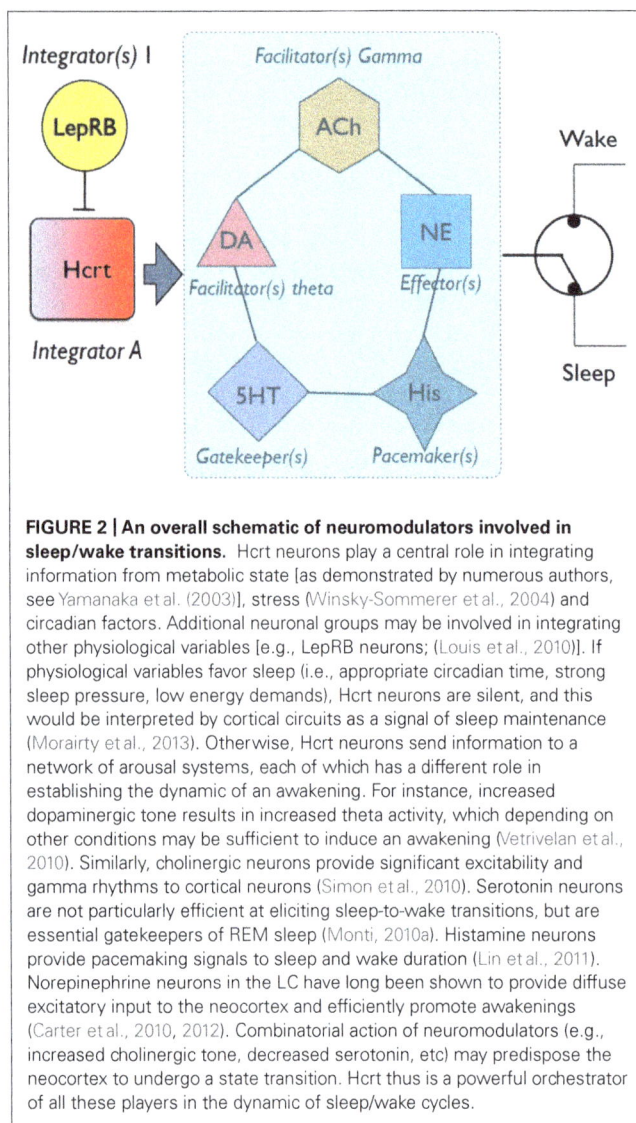

FIGURE 2 | An overall schematic of neuromodulators involved in sleep/wake transitions. Hcrt neurons play a central role in integrating information from metabolic state [as demonstrated by numerous authors, see Yamanaka et al. (2003)], stress (Winsky-Sommerer et al., 2004) and circadian factors. Additional neuronal groups may be involved in integrating other physiological variables [e.g., LepRB neurons; (Louis et al., 2010)]. If physiological variables favor sleep (i.e., appropriate circadian time, strong sleep pressure, low energy demands), Hcrt neurons are silent, and this would be interpreted by cortical circuits as a signal of sleep maintenance (Morairty et al., 2013). Otherwise, Hcrt neurons send information to a network of arousal systems, each of which has a different role in establishing the dynamic of an awakening. For instance, increased dopaminergic tone results in increased theta activity, which depending on other conditions may be sufficient to induce an awakening (Vetrivelan et al., 2010). Similarly, cholinergic neurons provide significant excitability and gamma rhythms to cortical neurons (Simon et al., 2010). Serotonin neurons are not particularly efficient at eliciting sleep-to-wake transitions, but are essential gatekeepers of REM sleep (Monti, 2010a). Histamine neurons provide pacemaking signals to sleep and wake duration (Lin et al., 2011). Norepinephrine neurons in the LC have long been shown to provide diffuse excitatory input to the neocortex and efficiently promote awakenings (Carter et al., 2010, 2012). Combinatorial action of neuromodulators (e.g., increased cholinergic tone, decreased serotonin, etc) may predispose the neocortex to undergo a state transition. Hcrt thus is a powerful orchestrator of all these players in the dynamic of sleep/wake cycles.

2005). *Release of Hcrt, either synaptic or extrasynaptic, increases the excitability of LC neurons.* Since optogenetic studies have showed that only a few light pulses (~20) to LC neurons are sufficient to induce behavioral sleep-to-wake transitions, mild excitation of LC neurons by other afferents within ~10 s of Hcrt-enhanced excitability would reach the threshold of an awakening with high probability (**Figure 1**).

In addition to the LC, alternative pathways such as dopaminergic, serotonergic or cholinergic systems also result in enhanced probability of arousal (**Figure 2**). Slow dynamics of neuromodulators (between 1 and 30 s) are consistent with a behavioral state transition that needs time to integrate and decide the most physiologically sensible solution. Hcrt neurons integrate multiple variables from circadian, metabolic and limbic structures. This integration is non-redundant, as Hcrt dysfunction results in uncoordinated intrusions of sleep into wakefulness associated with narcolepsy. However, other redundant integrators may exist (e.g., GABAergic systems in the lateral hypothalamus including Leptin-sensitive neurons). Information from the integrating systems is

conveyed into an array of systems that have different roles in the dynamics of sleep to wake transitions. For instance, high serotonergic tone inhibits REM sleep (Monti, 2010b). Histamine neurons in the TMN fire during waking and set the length of wake bouts. Cholinergic neurons in the basal forebrain (Arrigoni et al., 2010) and dopaminergic cells provide direct innervation to the neocortex, whereas norepinephrine is a powerful arousal-promoting factor as described above. It is noteworthy that Hcrt neurons are silent during REM sleep, as it suggests that activation of Hcrt neurons is dispensable for cortical desynchronization and cholinergic excitation. Also, the fact that Hcrt stimulation suppresses REM sleep suggests several possible mechanisms: (i) direct excitation of serotoninergic neurons in the raphe; (ii) a state-dependent modulation of cholinergic activity; (iii) reciprocal excitation/inhibition of MCH neurons recently shown to be involved in REM sleep maintenance. Thus, we underscore the relevance of Hcrt neurons in coordinating arousal centers as key elements of a switchboard, not master switches as has been proposed elsewhere in the literature. Future use of optogenetic and other state-of-the art methods to interrogate combinations of neuromodulators will provide a much more detailed mechanistic description of the role of Hcrt and effectors in the modulation of sleep/wake cycles.

REFERENCES

Adamantidis, A., and de Lecea, L. (2008a). Physiological arousal: a role for hypothalamic systems. *Cell. Mol. Life. Sci.* 65, 1475–1488. doi: 10.1007/s00018-008-7521-8

Adamantidis, A., and de Lecea, L. (2008b). Sleep and metabolism: shared circuits, new connections. *Trends Endocrinol. Metab.* 19, 362–370. doi: 10.1016/j.tem.2008.08.007

Adamantidis, A. R., Zhang, F., Aravanis, A. M., Deisseroth, K., and De Lecea, L. (2007). Neural substrates of awakening probed with optogenetic control of hypocretin neurons. *Nature* 450, 420–424. doi: 10.1038/nature06310

Appelbaum, L., Wang, G., Yokogawa, T., Skariah, G. M., Smith, S. J., Mourrain, P., et al. (2010). Circadian and homeostatic regulation of structural synaptic plasticity in hypocretin neurons. *Neuron* 68, 87–98. doi: 10.1016/j.neuron.2010.09.006

Arrigoni, E., Mochizuki, T., and Scammell, T. E. (2010). Activation of the basal forebrain by the orexin/hypocretin neurones. *Acta physiol.* 198, 223–235. doi: 10.1111/j.1748-1716.2009.02036.x

Asai, H., Hirano, M., Furiya, Y., Kanbayashi, T., Ikeda, M., Kiriyama, T., et al. (2008). Cerebrospinal fluid orexin and sleep attacks in Parkinson disease. *Ann. Neurol.* 64, S50–S51.

Baumann, C. R., Scammell, T. E., and Bassetti, C. L. (2008). Parkinson's disease, sleepiness and hypocretin/orexin. *Brain* 131, e91. doi: 10.1093/brain/awm220

Bayer, L., Eggermann, E., Serafin, M., Grivel, J., Machard, D., Muhlethaler, M., et al. (2005). Opposite effects of noradrenaline and acetylcholine upon hypocretin/orexin versus melanin concentrating hormone neurons in rat hypothalamic slices. *Neuroscience* 130, 807–811. doi: 10.1016/j.neuroscience.2004.10.032

Bayer, L., Eggermann, E., Serafin, M., Saint-Mleux, B., Machard, D., Jones, B., et al. (2001). Orexins (hypocretins) directly excite tuberomammillary neurons. *Eur. J. Neurosci.* 14, 1571–1575. doi: 10.1046/j.0953-816x.2001.01777.x

Borgland, S. L., and Labouebe, G. (2010). Orexin/hypocretin in psychiatric disorders: present state of knowledge and future potential. *Neuropsychopharmacology* 35, 353–354. doi: 10.1038/npp.2009.119

Bourgin, P., Huitron-Resendiz, S., Spier, A. D., Fabre, V., Morte, B., Criado, J. R., et al. (2000). Hypocretin-1 modulates rapid eye movement sleep through activation of locus coeruleus neurons. *J. Neurosci.* 20, 7760–7765.

Burlet, S., Tyler, C. J., and Leonard, C. S. (2002). Direct and indirect excitation of laterodorsal tegmental neurons by Hypocretin/Orexin peptides: implications for wakefulness and narcolepsy. *J. Neurosci.* 22, 2862–2872.

Carter, M. E., Adamantidis, A., Ohtsu, H., Deisseroth, K., and De Lecea, L. (2009a). Sleep homeostasis modulates hypocretin-mediated sleep-to-wake transitions. *J. Neurosci.* 29, 10939–10949. doi: 10.1523/JNEUROSCI.12 05-09.2009

Carter, M. E., Adamantidis, A., Ohtsu, H., Deisseroth, K., and De Lecea, L. (2009b). Sleep homeostasis modulates hypocretin-mediated sleep-to-wake transitions. *J. Neurosci.* 29, 10939–10949. doi: 10.1523/JNEUROSCI.1205-09.2009

Carter, M. E., Brill, J., Bonnavion, P., Huguenard, J. R., Huerta, R., and De Lecea, L. (2012). Mechanism for Hypocretin-mediated sleep-to-wake transitions. *Proc. Natl. Acad. Sci. U.S.A.* 109, E2635–E2644. doi: 10.1073/pnas.120 2526109

Carter, M. E., Yizhar, O., Chikahisa, S., Nguyen, H., Adamantidis, A., Nishino, S., et al. (2010). Tuning arousal with optogenetic modulation of locus coeruleus neurons. *Nat. Neurosci.* 13, 1526–1533. doi: 10.1038/nn.2682

Chemelli, R. M., Willie, J. T., Sinton, C. M., Elmquist, J. K., Scammell, T., Lee, C., et al. (1999). Narcolepsy in orexin knockout mice: molecular genetics of sleep regulation. *Cell* 98, 437–451. doi: 10.1016/S0092-8674(00) 81973-X

Crocker, A., Espana, R. A., Papadopoulou, M., Saper, C. B., Faraco, J., Sakurai, T., et al. (2005). Concomitant loss of dynorphin, NARP, and orexin in narcolepsy. *Neurology* 65, 1184–1188. doi: 10.1212/01.wnl.0000168173. 71940.ab

De la Herran-Arita, A. K., Kornum, B. R., Mahlios, J., Jiang, W., Lin, L., Hou, T., et al. (2013). CD4+ T cell autoimmunity to hypocretin/orexin and cross-reactivity to a 2009 H1N1 influenza a epitope in narcolepsy. *Sci. Transl. Med.* 5, 216ra176. doi: 10.1126/scitranslmed.3007762

de Lecea, L., Kilduff, T. S., Peyron, C., Gao, X., Foye, P. E., Danielson, P. E., et al. (1998). The hypocretins: hypothalamus-specific peptides with neuroexcitatory activity. *Proc. Natl. Acad. Sci. U.S.A.* 95, 322–327. doi: 10.1073/pnas. 95.1.322

Deboer, T., Overeem, S., Visser, N. A., Duindam, H., Frolich, M., Lammers, G. J., et al. (2004). Convergence of circadian and sleep regulatory mechanisms on hypocretin-1. *Neuroscience* 129, 727–732. doi: 10.1016/j.neuroscience.2004.07.049

Deurveilher, S., and Semba, K. (2005). Indirect projections from the suprachiasmatic nucleus to major arousal-promoting cell groups in rat: Implications for the circadian control of behavioural state. *Neuroscience* 130, 165–183. doi: 10.1016/j.neuroscience.2004.08.030

Drouot, X., Moutereau, S., Nguyen, J. P., Lefaucheur, J. P., Creange, A., Remy, P., et al. (2003). Low levels of ventricular CSF orexin/hypocretin in advanced PD. *Neurology* 61, 540–543. doi: 10.1212/01.WNL.0000078194.53210.48

Dugovic, C., Shelton, J. E., Aluisio, L. E., Fraser, I. C., Jiang, X., Sutton, S. W., et al. (2009). Blockade of orexin-1 receptors attenuates orexin-2 receptor antagonism-induced sleep promotion in the rat. *J. Pharmacol. Exp. Ther.* 330, 142–151. doi: 10.1124/jpet.109.152009

Eriksson, K. S., Sergeeva, O., Brown, R. E., and Haas, H. L. (2001). Orexin/hypocretin excites the histaminergic neurons of the tuberomammillary nucleus. *J. Neurosci.* 21, 9273–9279.

Espana, R. A., Baldo, B. A., Kelley, A. E., and Berridge, C. W. (2001). Wake-promoting and sleep-suppressing actions of hypocretin (orexin): basal forebrain sites of action. *Neuroscience* 106, 699–715. doi: 10.1016/S0306-4522(01) 00319-0

Estabrooke, I. V., Mccarthy, M. T., Ko, E., Chou, T. C., Chemelli, R. M., Yanagisawa, M., et al. (2001). Fos expression in orexin neurons varies with behavioral state. *J. Neurosci.* 21, 1656–1662.

Fronczek, R., Overeem, S., Lee, S. Y., Hegeman, I. M., Van Pelt, J., Van Duinen, S. G., et al. (2008). Hypocretin (orexin) loss and sleep disturbances in Parkinson's Disease. *Brain* 131, e88. doi: 10.1093/brain/awm222

Fujiki, N., Yoshida, Y., Ripley, B., Honda, K., Mignot, E., and Nishino, S. (2001). Changes in CSF hypocretin-1 (orexin A) levels in rats across 24 hours and in response to food deprivation. *Neuroreport* 12, 993–997. doi: 10.1097/00001756-200104170-00026

Gozzi, A., Turrini, G., Piccoli, L., Massagrande, M., Amantini, D., Antolini, M., et al. (2011). Functional magnetic resonance imaging reveals different neural substrates for the effects of orexin-1 and orexin-2 receptor antagonists. *PLoS ONE* 6:e16406. doi: 10.1371/journal.pone.0016406

Grivel, J., Cvetkovic, V., Bayer, L., Machard, D., Tobler, I., Muhlethaler, M., et al. (2005). The wake-promoting hypocretin/orexin neurons change their response to noradrenaline after sleep deprivation. *J. Neurosci.* 25, 4127–4130. doi: 10.1523/JNEUROSCI.0666-05.2005

Hagan, J. J., Leslie, R. A., Patel, S., Evans, M. L., Wattam, T. A., Holmes, S., et al. (1999). Orexin A activates locus coeruleus cell firing and increases arousal in the rat. *Proc. Natl. Acad. Sci. U.S.A.* 96, 10911–10916. doi: 10.1073/pnas.96.19. 10911

Hassani, O. K., Lee, M. G., and Jones, B. E. (2009). Melanin-concentrating hormone neurons discharge in a reciprocal manner to orexin neurons across the sleep-wake cycle. *Proc. Natl. Acad. Sci. U.S.A.* 106, 2418–2422. doi: 10.1073/pnas.0811 400106

Herring, W. J., Snyder, E., Budd, K., Hutzelmann, J., Snavely, D., Liu, K., et al. (2012). Orexin receptor antagonism for treatment of insomnia: a randomized clinical trial of suvorexant. *Neurology* 79, 2265–2274. doi: 10.1212/WNL.0b013e318 27688ee

Hondo, M., Nagai, K., Ohno, K., Kisanuki, Y., Willie, J. T., Watanabe, T., et al. (2010). Histamine-1 receptor is not required as a downstream effector of orexin-2 receptor in maintenance of basal sleep/wake states. *Acta physiol.* 198, 287–294. doi: 10.1111/j.1748-1716.2009.02032.x

Horvath, T. L., and Gao, X. B. (2005). Input organization and plasticity of hypocretin neurons: possible clues to obesity's association with insomnia. *Cell Metab.* 1, 279–286. doi: 10.1016/j.cmet.2005.03.003

Huang, Z. L., Qu, W. M., Li, W. D., Mochizuki, T., Eguchi, N., Watanabe, T., et al. (2001). Arousal effect of orexin A depends on activation of the histaminergic system. *Proc. Natl. Acad. Sci. U.S.A.* 98, 9965–9970. doi: 10.1073/pnas. 181330998

Inutsuka, A., and Yamanaka, A. (2013). The physiological role of orexin/hypocretin neurons in the regulation of sleep/wakefulness and neuroendocrine functions. *Front. Endocrinol.* 4:18. doi: 10.3389/fendo.2013.00018

Johnson, P. L., Truitt, W., Fitz, S. D., Minick, P. E., Dietrich, A., Sanghani, S., et al. (2010). A key role for orexin in panic anxiety. *Nat. Med.* 16, 111–115. doi: 10.1038/nm.2075

Kang, J. E., Lim, M. M., Bateman, R. J., Lee, J. J., Smyth, L. P., Cirrito, J. R., et al. (2009). Amyloid-beta dynamics are regulated by orexin and the sleep-wake cycle. *Science* 326, 1005–1007. doi: 10.1126/science.1180962

Kaur, S., Thankachan, S., Begum, S., Liu, M., Blanco-Centurion, C., and Shiromani, P. J. (2009). Hypocretin-2 saporin lesions of the ventrolateral periaquaductal gray (vlPAG) increase REM sleep in hypocretin knockout mice. *PLoS ONE* 4:e6346. doi: 10.1371/journal.pone.0006346

Kohlmeier, K. A., Watanabe, S., Tyler, C. J., Burlet, S., and Leonard, C. S. (2008). Dual orexin actions on dorsal raphe and laterodorsal tegmentum neurons: noisy cation current activation and selective enhancement of Ca2+ transients mediated by L-type calcium channels. *J. Neurophysiol.* 100, 2265–2281. doi: 10.1152/jn.01388.2007

Kumar, S., Szymusiak, R., Bashir, T., Rai, S., Mcginty, D., and Alam, M. N. (2007). Effects of serotonin on perifornical-lateral hypothalamic area neurons in rat. *Eur. J. Neurosci.* 25, 201–212. doi: 10.1111/j.1460-9568.2006.05268.x

Lee, M. G., Hassani, O. K., and Jones, B. E. (2005). Discharge of identified orexin/hypocretin neurons across the sleep-waking cycle. *J. Neurosci.* 25, 6716–6720. doi: 10.1523/JNEUROSCI.1887-05.2005

Leinninger, G. M., Opland, D. M., Jo, Y. H., Faouzi, M., Christensen, L., Cappellucci, L. A., et al. (2011). Leptin action via neurotensin neurons controls orexin, the mesolimbic dopamine system and energy balance. *Cell Metab.* 14, 313–323. doi: 10.1016/j.cmet.2011.06.016

Li, Y., Gao, X. B., Sakurai, T., and Van Den Pol, A. N. (2002). Hypocretin/Orexin excites hypocretin neurons via a local glutamate neuron-A potential mechanism for orchestrating the hypothalamic arousal system. *Neuron* 36, 1169–1181. doi: 10.1016/S0896-6273(02)01132-7

Lin, J. S., Sergeeva, O. A., and Haas, H. L. (2011). Histamine H3 receptors and sleep-wake regulation. *J. Pharmacol. Exp. Ther.* 336, 17–23. doi: 10.1124/jpet.110.170134

Lin, L., Faraco, J., Li, R., Kadotani, H., Rogers, W., Lin, X., et al. (1999). The sleep disorder canine narcolepsy is caused by a mutation in the hypocretin (orexin) receptor 2 gene. *Cell* 98, 365–376. doi: 10.1016/S0092-8674(00) 81965-0

Liu, R. J., Van Den Pol, A. N., and Aghajanian, G. K. (2002). Hypocretins (orexins) regulate serotonin neurons in the dorsal raphe nucleus by excitatory direct and inhibitory indirect actions. *J. Neurosci.* 22, 9453–9464.

Louis, G. W., Leinninger, G. M., Rhodes, C. J., and Myers, M. G. Jr. (2010). Direct innervation and modulation of orexin neurons by lateral hypothalamic LepRb neurons. *J. Neurosci.* 30, 11278–11287. doi: 10.1523/JNEUROSCI.1340-10.2010

Lu, J., and Greco, M. A. (2006). Sleep circuitry and the hypnotic mechanism of GABAA drugs. *J. Clin. Sleep Med.* 2, S19–S26.

Marcus, J. N., Aschkenasi, C. J., Lee, C. E., Chemelli, R. M., Saper, C. B., Yanagisawa, M., et al. (2001). Differential expression of orexin receptors 1 and 2 in the rat brain. *J. Comp. Neurol.* 435, 6–25. doi: 10.1002/cne.1190

Methippara, M. M., Alam, M. N., Szymusiak, R., and Mcginty, D. (2000). Effects of lateral preoptic area application of orexin-A on sleep- wakefulness. *Neuroreport* 11, 3423–3426. doi: 10.1097/00001756-200011090-00004

Mieda, M., Hasegawa, E., Kisanuki, Y. Y., Sinton, C. M., Yanagisawa, M., and Sakurai, T. (2011). Differential roles of orexin receptor-1 and -2 in the regulation of non-REM and REM sleep. *J. Neurosci.* 31, 6518–6526. doi: 10.1523/JNEUROSCI.6506-10.2011

Mileykovskiy, B. Y., Kiyashchenko, L. I., and Siegel, J. M. (2005). Behavioral correlates of activity in identified hypocretin/orexin neurons. *Neuron* 46, 787–798. doi: 10.1016/j.neuron.2005.04.035

Mochizuki, T., Arrigoni, E., Marcus, J. N., Clark, E. L., Yamamoto, M., Honer, M., et al. (2011). Orexin receptor 2 expression in the posterior hypothalamus rescues sleepiness in narcoleptic mice. *Proc. Natl. Acad. Sci. U.S.A.* 108, 4471–4476. doi: 10.1073/pnas.1012456108

Mochizuki, T., Crocker, A., Mccormack, S., Yanagisawa, M., Sakurai, T., and Scammell, T. E. (2004). Behavioral state instability in orexin knock-out mice. *J. Neurosci.* 24, 6291–6300. doi: 10.1523/JNEUROSCI.0586-04.2004

Monti, J. M. (2010a). The role of dorsal raphe nucleus serotonergic and non-serotonergic neurons, and of their receptors, in regulating waking and rapid eye movement (REM) sleep. *Sleep Med. Rev.* 14, 319–327. doi: 10.1016/j.smrv.2009.10.003

Monti, J. M. (2010b). The structure of the dorsal raphe nucleus and its relevance to the regulation of sleep and wakefulness. *Sleep Med. Rev.* 14, 307–317. doi: 10.1016/j.smrv.2009.11.004

Morairty, S. R., Dittrich, L., Pasumarthi, R. K., Valladao, D., Heiss, J. E., Gerashchenko, D., et al. (2013). A role for cortical nNOS/NK1 neurons in coupling homeostatic sleep drive to EEG slow wave activity. *Proc. Natl. Acad. Sci. U.S.A.* 110, 20272–20277. doi: 10.1073/pnas.1314762110

Nishino, S., Fujiki, N., Ripley, B., Sakurai, E., Kato, M., Watanabe, T., et al. (2001). Decreased brain histamine content in hypocretin/orexin receptor-2 mutated narcoleptic dogs. *Neurosci. Lett.* 313, 125–128. doi: 10.1016/S0304-3940(01)02270-4

Nishino, S., Ripley, B., Overeem, S., Lammers, G. J., and Mignot, E. (2000). Hypocretin (orexin) deficiency in human narcolepsy. *Lancet* 355, 39–40. doi: 10.1016/S0140-6736(99)05582-8.

Peyron, C., Faraco, J., Rogers, W., Ripley, B., Overeem, S., Charnay, Y., et al. (2000). A mutation in a case of early onset narcolepsy and a generalized absence of hypocretin peptides in human narcoleptic brains. *Nat. Med.* 6, 991–997. doi: 10.1038/79690

Peyron, C., Tighe, D. K., Van Den Pol, A. N., De Lecea, L., Heller, H. C., Sutcliffe, J. G., et al. (1998). Neurons containing hypocretin (orexin) project to multiple neuronal systems. *J. Neurosci.* 18, 9996–10015.

Piper, D. C., Upton, N., Smith, M. I., and Hunter, A. J. (2000). The novel brain neuropeptide, orexin-A, modulates the sleep-wake cycle of rats. *Eur. J. Neurosci.* 12, 726–730. doi: 10.1046/j.1460-9568.2000.00919.x

Rao, Y., Lu, M., Ge, F., Marsh, D. J., Qian, S., Wang, A. H., et al. (2008). Regulation of synaptic efficacy in hypocretin/orexin-containing neurons by melanin concentrating hormone in the lateral hypothalamus. *J. Neurosci.* 28, 9101–9110. doi: 10.1523/JNEUROSCI.1766-08.2008

Sakurai, T. (2007). The neural circuit of orexin (hypocretin): maintaining sleep and wakefulness. *Nat. Rev. Neurosci.* 8, 171–181. doi: 10.1038/nrn2092

Sakurai, T., Amemiya, A., Ishii, M., Matsuzaki, I., Chemelli, R. M., Tanaka, H., et al. (1998). Orexins and orexin receptors: a family of hypothalamic neuropeptides and G protein-coupled receptors that regulate feeding behavior. *Cell* 92, 573–585. doi: 10.1016/S0092-8674(00)80949-6

Sakurai, T., Nagata, R., Yamanaka, A., Kawamura, H., Tsujino, N., Muraki, Y., et al. (2005). Input of orexin/hypocretin neurons revealed by a genetically encoded tracer in mice. *Neuron* 46, 297–308. doi: 10.1016/j.neuron.2005.03.010

Salomon, R. M., Ripley, B., Kennedy, J. S., Johnson, B., Schmidt, D., Zeitzer, J. M., et al. (2003). Diurnal variation of cerebrospinal fluid hypocretin-1 (Orexin-A) levels in control and depressed subjects. *Biol. Psychiatry* 54, 96–104. doi: 10.1016/S0006-3223(02)01740-7

Saper, C. B., Fuller, P. M., Pedersen, N. P., Lu, J., and Scammell, T. E. (2010). Sleep state switching. *Neuron* 68, 1023–1042. doi: 10.1016/j.neuron.2010.11.032

Saper, C. B., Scammell, T. E., and Lu, J. (2005). Hypothalamic regulation of sleep and circadian rhythms. *Nature* 437, 1257–1263. doi: 10.1038/nature04284

Sasaki, K., Suzuki, M., Mieda, M., Tsujino, N., Roth, B., and Sakurai, T. (2011). Pharmacogenetic modulation of orexin neurons alters sleep/wakefulness states in mice. *PLoS ONE* 6:e20360. doi: 10.1371/journal.pone.0020360

Scammell, T. E., Matheson, J. K., Honda, M., Thannickal, T. C., and Siegel, J. M. (2012). Coexistence of narcolepsy and Alzheimer's disease. *Neurobiol. Aging* 33, 1318–1319. doi: 10.1016/j.neurobiolaging.2010.12.008

Schone, C., Cao, Z. F., Apergis-Schoute, J., Adamantidis, A., Sakurai, T., and Burdakov, D. (2012). Optogenetic probing of fast glutamatergic transmission from hypocretin/orexin to histamine neurons in situ. *J. Neurosci.* 32, 12437–12443. doi: 10.1523/JNEUROSCI.0706-12.2012

Scott, M. M., Marcus, J. N., Pettersen, A., Birnbaum, S. G., Mochizuki, T., Scammell, T. E., et al. (2011). Hcrtr1 and 2 signaling differentially regulates depression-like behaviors. *Behav. Brain Res.* 222, 289–294. doi: 10.1016/j.bbr.2011.02.044

Simon, C., Kezunovic, N., Ye, M., Hyde, J., Hayar, A., Williams, D. K., et al. (2010). Gamma band unit activity and population responses in the pedunculopontine nucleus. *J. Neurophysiol.* 104, 463–474. doi: 10.1152/jn.00242.2010

Steriade, M. (2003). The corticothalamic system in sleep. *Front. Biosci.* 8:d878–d899. doi: 10.2741/1043

Steriade, M., and McCarley, R. (1990). *Brainstem Control of Wakefulness and Sleep.* New York: Plenum. doi: 10.1007/978-1-4757-4669-3

Steriade, M., Mccormick, D. A., and Sejnowski, T. J. (1993). Thalamocortical oscillations in the sleeping and aroused brain. *Science* 262, 679–685. doi: 10.1126/science.8235588

Sutcliffe, J. G., and de Lecea, L. (2002). The hypocretins: setting the arousal threshold. *Nat. Rev. Neurosci.* 3, 339–349. doi: 10.1038/nrn808

Thakkar, M. M., Ramesh, V., Strecker, R. E., and Mccarley, R. W. (2001). Microdialysis perfusion of orexin-A in the basal forebrain increases wakefulness in freely behaving rats. *Arch. Ital. Biol.* 139, 313–328.

Thannickal, T. C., Moore, R. Y., Nienhuis, R., Ramanathan, L., Gulyani, S., Aldrich, M., et al. (2000). Reduced number of hypocretin neurons in human narcolepsy. *Neuron* 27, 469–474. doi: 10.1016/S0896-6273(00)00058-1

Tsujino, N., and Sakurai, T. (2009). Orexin/hypocretin: a neuropeptide at the interface of sleep, energy homeostasis, and reward system. *Pharmacol. Rev.* 61, 162–176. doi: 10.1124/pr.109.001321

Tsunematsu, T., Kilduff, T. S., Boyden, E. S., Takahashi, S., Tominaga, M., and Yamanaka, A. (2011). Acute optogenetic silencing of orexin/hypocretin neurons induces slow-wave sleep in mice. *J. Neurosci.* 31, 10529–10539. doi: 10.1523/JNEUROSCI.0784-11.2011

Vetrivelan, R., Qiu, M. H., Chang, C., and Lu, J. (2010). Role of Basal Ganglia in sleep-wake regulation: neural circuitry and clinical significance. *Front. Neuroanat.* 4:145. doi: 10.3389/fnana.2010.00145

Willie, J. T., Chemelli, R. M., Sinton, C. M., Tokita, S., Williams, S. C., Kisanuki, Y. Y., et al. (2003). Distinct narcolepsy syndromes in Orexin receptor-2 and Orexin null mice: molecular genetic dissection of Non-REM and REM sleep regulatory processes. *Neuron* 38, 715–730. doi: 10.1016/S0896-6273(03)00330-1

Willie, J. T., Chemelli, R. M., Sinton, C. M., and Yanagisawa, M. (2001). To eat or to sleep? orexin in the regulation of feeding and wakefulness. *Annu. Rev. Neurosci.* 24, 429–458. doi: 10.1146/annurev.neuro.24.1.429

Winsky-Sommerer, R., Yamanaka, A., Diano, S., Borok, E., Roberts, A. J., Sakurai, T., et al. (2004). Interaction between the corticotropin-releasing factor system and hypocretins (orexins): a novel circuit mediating stress response. *J. Neurosci.* 24, 11439–11448. doi: 10.1523/JNEUROSCI.3459-04.2004

Xi, M. C., Morales, F. R., and Chase, M. H. (2001). Effects on sleep and wakefulness of the injection of hypocretin-1 (orexin-A) into the laterodorsal tegmental nucleus of the cat. *Brain Res.* 901, 259–264. doi: 10.1016/S0006-8993(01)02317-4

Yamanaka, A., Muraki, Y., Ichiki, K., Tsujino, N., Kilduff, T. S., Goto, K., et al. (2006). Orexin neurons are directly and indirectly regulated by catecholamines in a complex manner. *J. Neurophysiol.* 96, 284–298. doi: 10.1152/jn.01361.2005

Yamanaka, A., Muraki, Y., Tsujino, N., Goto, K., and Sakurai, T. (2003). Regulation of orexin neurons by the monoaminergic and cholinergic systems. *Biochem. Biophys. Res. Commun.* 303, 120–129. doi: 10.1016/S0006-291X(03)00299-7

Yamanaka, A., Tabuchi, S., Tsunematsu, T., Fukazawa, Y., and Tominaga, M. (2010). Orexin directly excites orexin neurons through orexin 2 receptor. *J. Neurosci.* 30, 12642–12652. doi: 10.1523/JNEUROSCI.2120-10.2010

Yoshida, K., Mccormack, S., Espana, R. A., Crocker, A., and Scammell, T. E. (2006). Afferents to the orexin neurons of the rat brain. *J. Comp. Neurol.* 494, 845–861. doi: 10.1002/cne.20859

Yoshida, Y., Fujiki, N., Nakajima, T., Ripley, B., Matsumura, H., Yoneda, H., et al. (2001). Fluctuation of extracellular hypocretin-1 (orexin A) levels in the rat in relation to the light-dark cycle and sleep-wake activities. *Eur. J. Neurosci.* 14, 1075–1081. doi: 10.1046/j.0953-816x.2001.01725.x

Zeitzer, J. M., Buckmaster, C. L., Parker, K. J., Hauck, C. M., Lyons, D. M., and Mignot, E. (2003). Circadian and homeostatic regulation of hypocretin in a primate model: implications for the consolidation of wakefulness. *J. Neurosci.* 23, 3555–3560.

Conflict of Interest Statement: The authors declare that the research was conducted in the absence of any commercial or financial relationships that could be construed as a potential conflict of interest.

7

Synaptic interactions between perifornical lateral hypothalamic area, locus coeruleus nucleus and the oral pontine reticular nucleus are implicated in the stage succession during sleep-wakefulness cycle

Silvia Tortorella, Margarita L. Rodrigo-Angulo, Angel Núñez* and Miguel Garzón

Departamento de Anatomía, Histología y Neurociencia, Facultad de Medicina, Research Institute, Universidad Autonoma de Madrid, La Paz University Hospital (IDIPAZ), Madrid, Spain

Edited by:
Michel A. Steiner, Actelion
Pharmaceuticals Ltd., Switzerland

Reviewed by:
Rodrigo Espana, Drexel University
College of Medicine, USA
Hiroshi Katsuki, Kumamoto
University Graduate School of
Pharmaceutical Sciences, Japan

*Correspondence:
Angel Nuñez, Departamento de
Anatomía, Histología y
Neurociencia, Facultad de Medicina,
Research Institute, Universidad
Autonoma de Madrid, La Paz
University Hospital (IDIPAZ),
c/ Arzobispo Morcillo 4, 28029
Madrid, Spain
e-mail: angel.nunez@uam.es

The perifornical area in the posterior lateral hypothalamus (PeFLH) has been implicated in several physiological functions including the sleep-wakefulness regulation. The PeFLH area contains several cell types including those expressing orexins (Orx; also known as hypocretins), mainly located in the PeF nucleus. The aim of the present study was to elucidate the synaptic interactions between Orx neurons located in the PeFLH area and different brainstem neurons involved in the generation of wakefulness and sleep stages such as the locus coeruleus (LC) nucleus (contributing to wakefulness) and the oral pontine reticular nucleus (PnO) nucleus (contributing to REM sleep). Anatomical data demonstrated the existence of a neuronal network involving the PeFLH area, LC, and the PnO nuclei that would control the sleep-wake cycle. Electrophysiological experiments indicated that PeFLH area had an excitatory effect on LC neurons. PeFLH stimulation increased the firing rate of LC neurons and induced an activation of the EEG. The excitatory effect evoked by PeFLH stimulation in LC neurons was blocked by the injection of the Orx-1 receptor antagonist SB-334867 into the LC. Similar electrical stimulation of the PeFLH area evoked an inhibition of PnO neurons by activation of GABAergic receptors because the effect was blocked by bicuculline application into the PnO. Our data also revealed that the LC and PnO nuclei exerted a feedback control on neuronal activity of PeFLH area. Electrical stimulation of LC facilitated firing activity of PeFLH neurons by activation of catecholaminergic receptors whereas PnO stimulation inhibited PeFLH neurons by activation of GABAergic receptors. In conclusion, Orx neurons of the PeFLH area seem to be an important organizer of the wakefulness and sleep stages in order to maintain a normal succession of stages during the sleep-wakefulness cycle.

Keywords: orexin, orexin-1 receptor, GABAergic receptors, catecholaminergic receptors, wakefulness, REM sleep

INTRODUCTION

Sleep and wakefulness are two mutually exclusive states that cycle with both ultradian and circadian periods. The brain mechanisms underlying the organization of the sleep-wakefulness cycle remain unclear. Many studies have identified several populations of neurons whose activity correlates with distinct behavioral states (Carter et al., 2012, 2013). The perifornical lateral hypothalamic area (PeFLH) has been implicated in several physiological functions including sleep-wakefulness regulation (McGinty and Szymusiak, 2003; Jones, 2008); this area contains a heterogeneous population of neuronal groups as reflected by both their state-dependent discharge properties and their neurotransmitter phenotypes. Among others, these cells express hypocretin/orexin (Orx), melanin-concentrating hormone, γ-aminobutyric acid (GABA) or glutamate (Vaughan et al., 1989; Bittencourt et al., 1992; de Lecea et al., 1998; Sakurai et al., 1998; Abrahamson and Moore, 2001; Rodrigo-Angulo et al., 2008). Orx neurons, mainly located in the perifornical (PeF) nucleus, have been extensively studied and implicated in the facilitation and/or maintenance of arousal (Alam et al., 2002; Koyama et al., 2003; Siegel, 2004; Sakurai, 2005; Takahashi et al., 2005; Sasaki et al., 2011); they are maximally active during active wakefulness and virtually cease firing during both slow wave sleep and rapid eye movement (REM) sleep (Lee et al., 2005a; Mileykovskiy et al., 2005).

Hypothalamic Orx projections make asymmetrical synaptic contacts with their target neurons in numerous brain areas implicated in the control of sleep-wakefulness cycle (Peyron et al., 1998; Horvath et al., 1999). Excitatory Orx effects have been demonstrated in neurons of arousal-related structures including the locus coeruleus (LC) nucleus (Horvath et al., 1999; Eggermann et al., 2001; Marcus et al., 2001; Burlet et al., 2002; Yamanaka et al., 2002; España et al., 2005; Cid-Pellitero and Garzon, 2011) where Orx promotes wakefulness (Bourgin et al., 2000; España et al., 2001; Thakkar et al., 2001; Xi et al., 2001). This effect may be due to an excitatory effect of Orx on LC neurons, as has been demonstrated *in vitro* (Hagan et al., 1999; Horvath et al., 1999; Ivanov and Aston-Jones, 2000; Soffin et al., 2002), suggesting that the effect of Orx on LC neurons may facilitate the arousal state.

Orx axon terminals and Orx receptors have also been identified in cholinoceptive areas of the pontine reticular formation involved in REM sleep generation (Greco and Shiromani, 2001; Marcus et al., 2001; Willie et al., 2003). Cholinoceptive neurons located in the ventral part of the oral pontine reticular nucleus (PnO) are involved in the generation and maintenance of REM sleep in rats (Horner and Kubin, 1999; Kohlmeier et al., 2002; Nuñez et al., 2002) and cats (Reinoso-Suárez et al., 1994, 1999, 2001; Garzón et al., 1998). Orx receptor subtypes are expressed in PnO neurons (Greco and Shiromani, 2001; Willie et al., 2003) and activation of such receptors enhances acetyl-choline release in the rat pons (Bernard et al., 2003, 2006). However, iontophoretic application of Orx in the PnO nucleus induced an inhibition of neuronal activity in anesthetized rats (Nuñez et al., 2006a); this effect was blocked by a previous iontophoretic application of bicuculline, indicating that inhibitory action of Orx involves the activation of $GABA_A$ receptors.

The above mentioned results suggest that Orx neurons may play a crucial role in the organization of the sleep-wakefulness cycle and consequently, damage to Orx neurons could disrupt the normal succession of sleep-wake stages, as occurs in human narcolepsy and in animal models of this sleep disorder (Peyron et al., 2000; Thannickal et al., 2000). Narcolepsy is a neurological disorder characterized by severe daytime somnolence with a constellation of unusual symptoms that are best understood as intrusions of REM sleep phenomena into wakefulness (Guilleminault and Fromherz, 2005). In agreement with the hypothesis that Orx neurons play a role in narcolepsy these patients also have reduced cerebrospinal fluid levels of Orx (Nishino et al., 2000). Animal models exhibiting symptoms of narcolepsy show loss of Orx neurons or a decrease in Orx levels (Chemelli et al., 1999; Gerashchenko et al., 2001; Hara et al., 2001; Beuckmann et al., 2004). Canines with narcolepsy carry a mutation in the Orx-2 receptor (Lin et al., 1999) and mice with a deletion of this receptor (Willie et al., 2003) also show symptoms of narcolepsy.

The aim of the present study was to examine the synaptic interaction between Orx neurons located in the PeFLH area and different neuronal generators in the brainstem. We hypothesized that cross-talk among LC nucleus (contributing to wakefulness), PnO nucleus (contributing to REM sleep) and PeFLH area would orchestrate the sleep-wakefulness cycle. Anatomical and electrophysiological studies were undertaken to demonstrate this coordination of the sleep-wakefulness cycle.

MATERIALS AND METHODS

Procedures were approved by the Ethics Board of the Universidad Autonoma de Madrid in accordance with the European Communities Council guidelines (2012/63/UE) on the ethical use of animals with every effort being made to minimize the suffering and number of animals employed. Fifty-five urethane-anesthetized (1.6 g/kg i.p.) Wistar rats (from Iffa-Credo, L'Arbresle, France) weighing 250–300 g were used for the physiological experiments. Animals were placed in a stereotaxic device

with controlled body temperature (37°C). EEG activity was recorded through a macroelectrode stereotaxically placed into the frontal cortex [at 2 mm rostral to the Bregma and 2 mm from the midline (Paxinos and Watson, 2007)]. The EEG was filtered between 0.3 and 30 Hz, and amplified. Supplemental doses of the anesthetic were given when a decrease in the amplitude of the EEG delta waves was observed.

UNIT RECORDING AND DRUG APPLICATION

Single-unit recordings were obtained with tungsten microelectrodes (2 MΩ) or glass micropipettes (World Precision Instruments, Sarasota, USA) filled with 2% neurobiotin in 0.5 M NaCl (Sigma) to locate the recording site. Three-barrel glass micropipettes were also used for unit recording and simultaneous application of pharmacological agents by microiontophoresis (see below).

Recording electrodes were placed at the LC nucleus (coordinates from Bregma: A, −9.3; L, 1.5 and depth, 7.0 mm), the PnO nucleus (coordinates from Bregma: A, −8.0; L, 1.0 and depth, 8.0 mm) or at the PeFLH area (coordinates from Bregma: A, −2.1; L, 1.0 and depth, 8.0 mm) by means of micromanipulators. Extracellular recordings were filtered (0.3–3 kHz), amplified (P15; GRASS Technology, Warwick, USA) and fed into a PC computer for off-line analysis by a Cambridge Electronic Design (CED; Cambridge, UK) 1401 interface at a sampling frequency of 10 kHz for the unit recordings, together with the EEG (sampling frequency of 200 Hz). Spike 2 software (CED) was used.

When barrel micropipettes were used, one of the glass capillaries was filled with a solution of NaCl (0.5 M) in order to record unit activity. A second micropipette was filled with bicuculline-methiodide (10 mM in 0.9% NaCl, pH 3.0, Sigma, St Louis, MO, USA). The remaining micropipette was filled with 0.5 M NaCl to balance the retention and ejection currents. Each barrel of the three-barreled pipette was connected via a silver wire to a channel on a microiontophoresis current generator (World Precision Instruments) that controlled retention and ejection currents for the drug-filled micropipette. Bicuculline was ejected with a positive current using a single 30-s pulse of 50 nA and negative retaining currents of 10–20 nA were used to delay drug leakage from the micropipette.

Bipolar stimulating electrodes (120 μm diameter blunt stainless steel wire) were placed at the ipsilateral PeFLH area, LC nucleus or in the PnO nucleus (same coordinates as described above). Electrical stimulation was performed using single rectangular pulses (0.1–0.3 ms, 50–100 μA) at 0.5 Hz or pulse trains of 500-ms duration at a frequency of 50 Hz, delivered through a GRASS S88 stimulator.

DRUGS

The hypocretin-1 receptor antagonist SB-334867 (100 μM; 100 nl) was applied through a 20G cannula connected to a Hamilton syringe (flow rate: 50 nl/min). The dose was similar to previous reports (Erami et al., 2012). Reserpine (methyl reserpate 3,4,5-trimethoxybenzoic acid ester, Sigma Chemical Co., St. Louis, USA) was dissolved in 50 μl of glacial acetic acid plus 0.9% NaCl (saline). The control solution consisted of saline plus 50 μl of glacial acetic acid in saline. Reserpine doses (1.0 and 5.0 mg/kg) were administered subcutaneously (s.c.) in a volume of 1.0 ml/kg of body weight. Unit recordings were performed 48 h after the reserpine injection.

ELECTROPHYSIOLOGICAL DATA ANALYSIS

Analysis of the neocortical EEGs as well as the activity of each neuron was performed off-line in a PC computer. Spike 2 software was used to perform statistical calculations including summed peristimulus time histograms (PSTH), which were calculated using 2-ms bin widths and power spectra of the EEG. Statistical analyses were calculated with Student's two-tailed t tests for unpaired or paired data as required. Differences were considered statistically significant at a level of 95% ($p < 0.05$). All data are indicated as mean $\pm$ SEM.

ANATOMICAL STUDIES

At the end of the electrophysiological experiments animals were injected i.p. with an overdose of pentobarbital and perfused transcardially with 4% paraformaldehyde in phosphate buffer pH 7.4. Brains were frozen, sectioned at 50 μm and collected in two series. In order to confirm the location of the recording electrodes, sections from the first series were processed to reveal the neurobiotin stained neurons: after rinsing in Tris saline buffer (TS) 0.1 M at pH 7.6, sections were incubated in a 1:150 Elite ABC kit (Vector) dilution in TS and 0.25% triton X-100 for 3 h to be developed with 0.05% 3-3′ DAB and 0.003% H_2O_2. Sections of the second series were processed for Nissl staining in order to corroborate the location of the stimulating electrodes.

For the anatomical connection tracing studies, retrograde Cholera Toxin-Alexia 594 (CT-A) and 1.5% Fluoro-Gold (FG) and anterograde FluoroRuby (FR) fluorescents tracers were injected in 16 adult rats of both sexes weighing 250–280 g. Under general anesthesia (a mixture of 50% ketamine, 40% atropine, and 10% valium i.p. 1 ml/250 g) animals were placed in the stereotaxic frame, and a craniotomy was made. Fluorescent injections were performed in PnO and LC nuclei, both in the same hemispheric side by means of a 1 μl Hamilton syringe (flow rate: 40 nl/min). In order to avoid contamination and tracer overlapping, injections in PnO nucleus were made from the contralateral side in an angle of 45° at coordinates from Bregma: A, −8.4; L, 1.5, and depth, 8.5, according to the (Paxinos and Watson, 2007); 300 nl of CT-A (10 animals), 40 nl of FG (3 animals), and 450 nl of FR (3 animals) were delivered in a single pulse. Injections in LC nucleus were performed with a vertical approach using a 1 μl Hamilton syringe stereotaxicaly aimed at the coordinates from Bregma: A, −9.6; L, 1.3; and depth 6.8; 50 nl of FG (12 animals), 50 nl of FR (2 animals), and 300 nl of CT-A (2 animals) were delivered. Animals were allowed to survive for 7 days before transcardial perfusion with 4% paraformaldehyde in 0.1 M phosphate buffer at pH 7.3 followed by increasing concentrations of sucrose solutions in the same buffer. Once removed, brains were stored in 30% sucrose solution during 5 days for cryopreservation and afterwards sectioned at 40 μm on a cryostat; sections were collected in three consecutive series devoted to fluorescence and Nissl staining. The third series was processed for Orx immunolabeling using the avidin-biotin-peroxidase method; sections were incubated with 1:1000 goat anti-Orx antiserum (Santa Cruz) in

a solution containing 5% bovine serum albumin and 30% normal rabbit serum in Tris buffer 0.1 M at pH 7.6 for 48 h. After this, sections were incubated in 1:400 biotinylated rabbit anti-goat antibody solution (Chemicon) for 2 h and in 1:150 avidin-biotin-peroxidase reagent Elite ABC kit (Vector) for 1.5 h. The Orx immunoperoxidase was visualized by incubation in 0.05% 3-3′ DAB and 0.003% H_2O_2. Sections were studied under fluorescent or bright field illumination using a Zeiss Axioskop microscope.

RESULTS
ANATOMICAL RESULTS

To determine the projections from the PeF area, two retrograde tracers CT-A and FG were injected into the LC and PnO nuclei, respectively (**Figures 1A,B**). Also, the anterograde FR fluorescent tracer was used. Numerous retrograde labeled neurons were observed in several hypothalamic structures after PnO tracer injections, as we have already reported (España et al., 2005; Nuñez et al., 2006a; **Figure 1C**). The injections of the anterograde tracer in PnO nucleus labeled fibers and terminals only in the lateral sector of PeFLH area (**Figure 1E**). Neurons labeled after retrograde tracer injections in LC nucleus were located in the ventral sector of PeFLH area and intermingled with the fibers and terminals that could be observed after anterograde tracer injections in LC nucleus (**Figures 1D,F**). In all cases, the presence of double-labeled neurons was very low (<0.5% of labeled neurons).

A schematic drawing of the hypothalamic area depicting differential distribution of retrograde labeled neurons and anterograde labeled fibers after PnO and LC tracer injections is shown in **Figure 2A**. As has been previously reported (Nuñez et al., 2006a) Orx immunoreactive neurons were clustered to the PeF nucleus (**Figure 2B**). In the PeF nucleus we found double-labeled neurons projecting to PnO (data not shown) or to LC nucleus (**Figure 2C**) that were also stained for Orx.

PeF ACTIVATION OF LC

The LC neurons displayed a non-rhythmic discharge pattern with a mean spontaneous frequency of 3.4 $\pm$ 1.0 spikes/s ($n = 40$). The recording site was established by iontophoretic injection of neurobiotin through the recording micropipette (**Figure 3**, inset).

Trains of electrical stimulus delivered in the PeFLH area (50 Hz; 50 μA; 500 ms of duration) increased the mean firing rate of LC neurons from 3.4 $\pm$ 1.0 to 9.8 $\pm$ 1.7 spikes/s, measured 10 s after the stimulation train ($p < 0.001$; **Figures 3A,C**). The excitatory effect was observed in 64% of LC neurons (32 out of 50 cells), and could last up to 30 s. The EEG pattern changed from continuous slow waves evoked by the anesthetic to a faster activity evoked by PeFLH stimulation (**Figure 3A**). In spontaneous conditions the percentage of delta waves (1–4 Hz) in the EEG was 98.6 $\pm$ 1.8% and the percentage of faster (>4 Hz) waves was 1.4 $\pm$ 0.9%. During the period of 10 s after the PeFLH stimulation train the proportion of delta waves decreased to 67.3 $\pm$ 3.4% and the percentage of >4 Hz waves increased to 32.7 $\pm$ 4.6% ($p < 0.001$), indicating that the PeFLH stimulation induced an activation of the EEG.

The excitatory effect evoked by PeFLH stimulation in LC neurons was blocked by the injection of the Orx-1 receptor antagonist SB-334867 into the LC nucleus. The SB-334867 was applied by

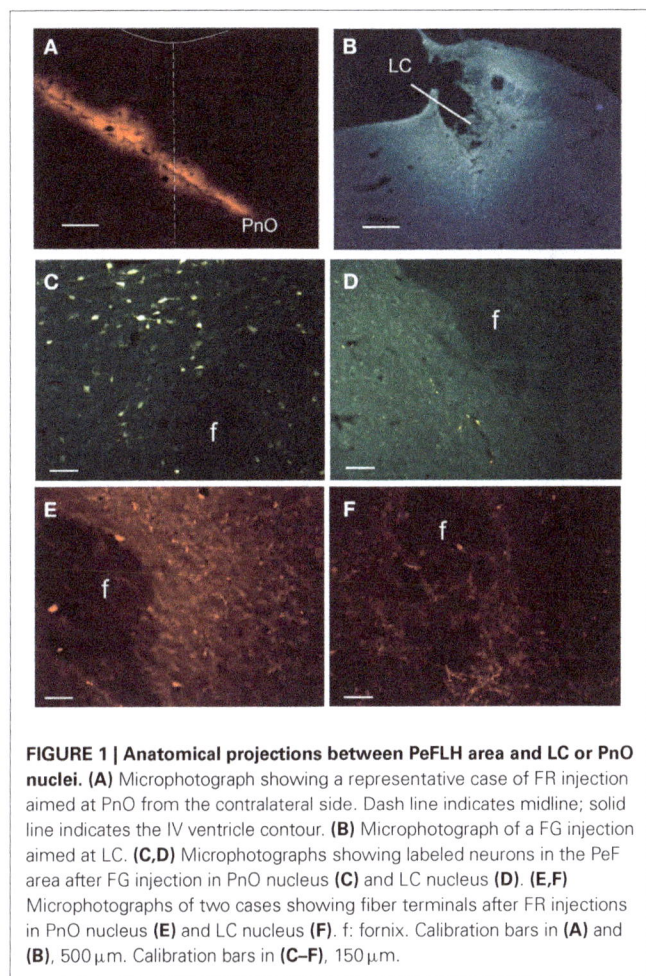

FIGURE 1 | Anatomical projections between PeFLH area and LC or PnO nuclei. (A) Microphotograph showing a representative case of FR injection aimed at PnO from the contralateral side. Dash line indicates midline; solid line indicates the IV ventricle contour. **(B)** Microphotograph of a FG injection aimed at LC. **(C,D)** Microphotographs showing labeled neurons in the PeF area after FG injection in PnO nucleus **(C)** and LC nucleus **(D)**. **(E,F)** Microphotographs of two cases showing fiber terminals after FR injections in PnO nucleus **(E)** and LC nucleus **(F)**. f: fornix. Calibration bars in **(A)** and **(B)**, 500 μm. Calibration bars in **(C–F)**, 150 μm.

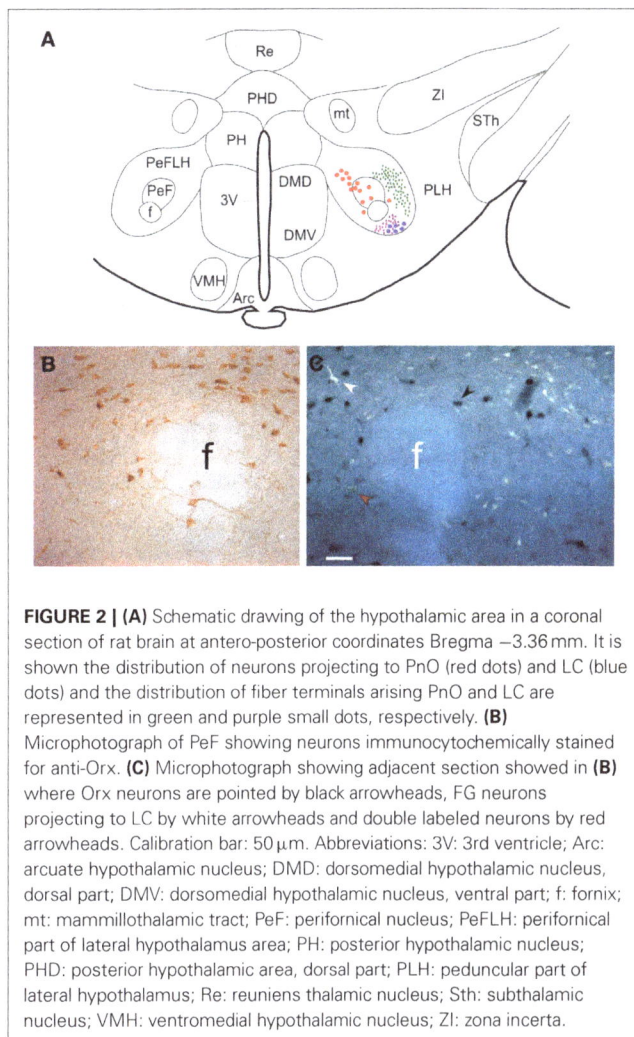

FIGURE 2 | (A) Schematic drawing of the hypothalamic area in a coronal section of rat brain at antero-posterior coordinates Bregma −3.36 mm. It is shown the distribution of neurons projecting to PnO (red dots) and LC (blue dots) and the distribution of fiber terminals arising PnO and LC are represented in green and purple small dots, respectively. **(B)** Microphotograph of PeF showing neurons immunocytochemically stained for anti-Orx. **(C)** Microphotograph showing adjacent section showed in **(B)** where Orx neurons are pointed by black arrowheads, FG neurons projecting to LC by white arrowheads and double labeled neurons by red arrowheads. Calibration bar: 50 μm. Abbreviations: 3V: 3rd ventricle; Arc: arcuate hypothalamic nucleus; DMD: dorsomedial hypothalamic nucleus, dorsal part; DMV: dorsomedial hypothalamic nucleus, ventral part; f: fornix; mt: mammillothalamic tract; PeF: perifornical nucleus; PeFLH: perifornical part of lateral hypothalamus area; PH: posterior hypothalamic nucleus; PHD: posterior hypothalamic area, dorsal part; PLH: peduncular part of lateral hypothalamus; Re: reuniens thalamic nucleus; Sth: subthalamic nucleus; VMH: ventromedial hypothalamic nucleus; ZI: zona incerta.

means of a Hamilton syringe (100 μM; 100 nl) and the effect was tested 15 min. after application when the drug concentration was stabilized. Trains of electrical stimulus delivered in the PeFLH area (50 Hz; 50 μA; 500 ms of duration) increased the mean firing rate (calculated during 10 s before and 10 s after the stimulation train) of LC neurons from 2.8 ± 0.8 to 6.3 ± 1.2 spikes/s, ($n = 12$; $p < 0.001$; **Figures 3A,C**). The excitatory responses evoked by PeFLH stimulation train in LC neurons were blocked by the SB-334867 (**Figure 3B**). Trains of electrical stimulus delivered in the PeFLH area did not increase the mean firing rate of LC neurons from 2.1 ± 0.9 to 2.8 ± 0.6 spikes/s ($n = 12$; $p = 0.12$; **Figures 3B,C**).

PeF INHIBITION OF PnO ACTIVITY

Most PnO neurons (15 out of 18 neurons; 83%) decreased their spontaneous firing rate from 1.2 ± 0.3 Hz in control conditions to 0.2 ± 0.4 Hz ($p < 0.001$) 10 s after application of a train of electrical stimuli delivered in the PeFLH area (50 Hz; 50 μA; 500 ms of duration; **Figure 4**, upper trace). To determine if the inhibitory response evoked by PeF stimulation was due to activation of GABAergic receptors, bicuculline (a GABA$_A$ receptor antagonist; 10 mM) was iontophoretically applied ($n = 8$). Bicuculline ejection increased the firing rate of PnO neurons to 4.9 ± 0.9 Hz. In

the presence of bicuculline, successive PeFLH stimulation trains did not change the firing rate of PnO neurons (**Figure 4**, lower trace), indicating that the inhibitory effect of PeF stimulation was due to activation of GABAergic receptors within the PnO nucleus, in agreement with previous reports (Nuñez et al., 2006a).

PeF NEURONAL RESPONSES TO LC OR PnO STIMULATION

Unit recordings were performed in the PeFLH area ($n = 39$). Neurons displayed a non-rhythmic discharge pattern with a mean spontaneous frequency of 1.3 ± 0.3 spikes/s. PeFLH neurons were identified by their stereotaxic coordinates after reconstruction of the electrode track.

The PeFLH area is implicated in the control of the sleep-wakefulness cycle, facilitating wakefulness (see Introduction). We study the effect on PeFLH neuronal activity of electrical stimulation of brainstem areas implicated in the generation of wakefulness (LC nucleus) or REM sleep (PnO nucleus). Trains of electrical stimuli delivered in the LC nucleus (50 Hz; 50–100 μA; 500 ms of duration) induced a 1–10 s increase in firing rate, in most PeFLH neurons (21 out of 23 cells; 91%; **Figure 5A**). The mean firing rate increased from 1.3 ± 0.3 spikes/s in spontaneous

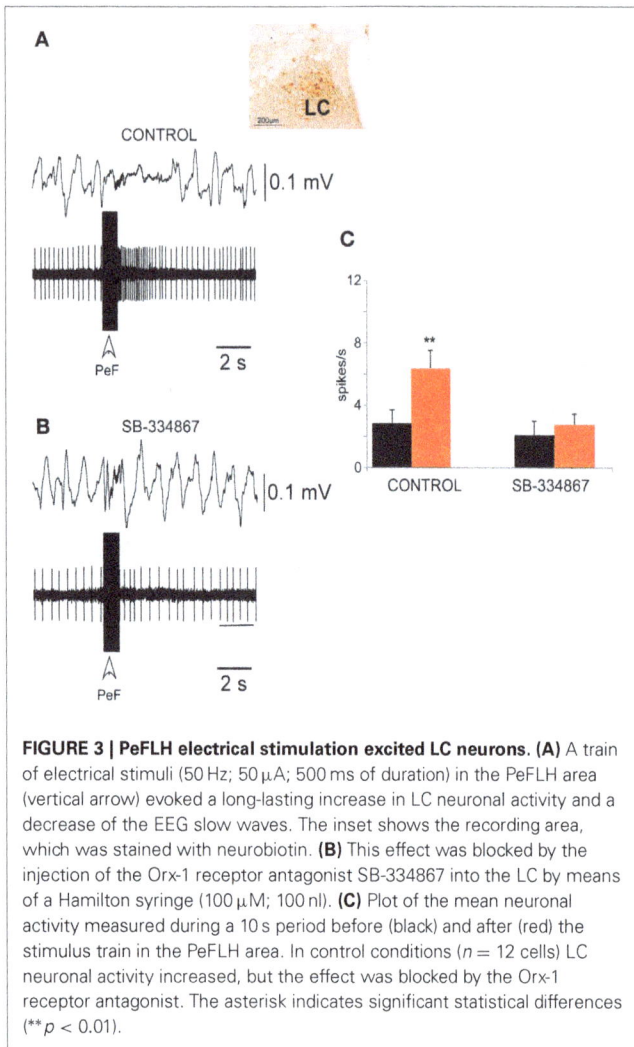

FIGURE 3 | PeFLH electrical stimulation excited LC neurons. (A) A train of electrical stimuli (50 Hz; 50 µA; 500 ms of duration) in the PeFLH area (vertical arrow) evoked a long-lasting increase in LC neuronal activity and a decrease of the EEG slow waves. The inset shows the recording area, which was stained with neurobiotin. **(B)** This effect was blocked by the injection of the Orx-1 receptor antagonist SB-334867 into the LC by means of a Hamilton syringe (100 µM; 100 nl). **(C)** Plot of the mean neuronal activity measured during a 10 s period before (black) and after (red) the stimulus train in the PeFLH area. In control conditions ($n = 12$ cells) LC neuronal activity increased, but the effect was blocked by the Orx-1 receptor antagonist. The asterisk indicates significant statistical differences (** $p < 0.01$).

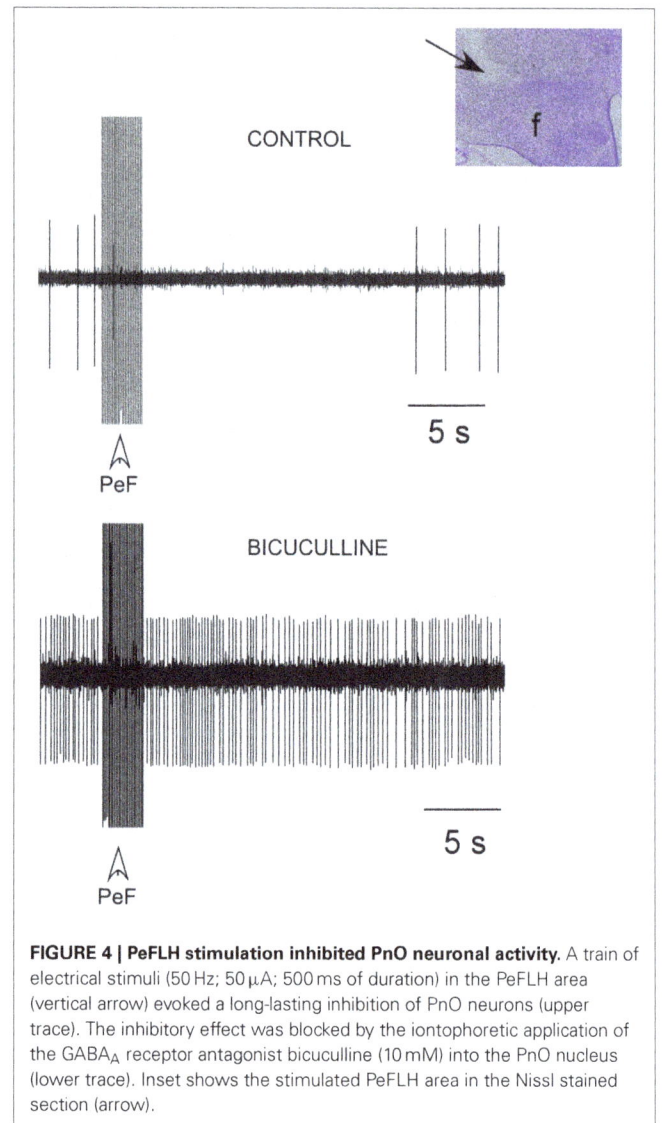

FIGURE 4 | PeFLH stimulation inhibited PnO neuronal activity. A train of electrical stimuli (50 Hz; 50 µA; 500 ms of duration) in the PeFLH area (vertical arrow) evoked a long-lasting inhibition of PnO neurons (upper trace). The inhibitory effect was blocked by the iontophoretic application of the GABA$_A$ receptor antagonist bicuculline (10 mM) into the PnO nucleus (lower trace). Inset shows the stimulated PeFLH area in the Nissl stained section (arrow).

conditions to 8.6 ± 1.4 spikes/s ($n = 21$; $p < 0.001$; **Figure 5C**). The percentage of delta waves decreased during the same time period from 96.5 ± 4.1 to $79.8 \pm 2.9\%$ ($p < 0.001$).

The alkaloid reserpine which depletes catecholamines from nerve endings have been used. Reserpine administration (1 mg/kg, once daily for three consecutive days) reduced the response of the PeFLH neurons to LC train stimulation. The LC-evoked rise in the firing rate was reduced in the presence of reserpine. Under reserpine activity rose from 1.3 ± 0.5 spikes/s before the stimulation train to 2.8 ± 1.4 spikes/s after the stimulation train; $n = 8$; $p = 0.015$; **Figures 5B,C**, indicating that the LC-evoked excitation of PeF neurons was mediated by the activation of catecholaminergic fibers.

To determine if there is a reciprocal connection between the PeFLH area and PnO nucleus, electrical stimulation of the PnO nucleus (0.5 Hz; 50–100 µA; 0.1–0.3 ms of duration) was applied during unit recordings of PeFLH neurons. Trains of electrical stimulus delivered in the PnO nucleus (50 Hz; 50–100 µA; 500 ms of duration) induced a decrease of the firing rate in 14 out of 17 PeFLH neurons during 1–8 s (82%; **Figure 6A**). The remaining neurons did not display significant changes in their firing

rate. The mean firing rate of these neurons affected by PnO train stimulation was 2.4 ± 0.5 spikes/s in spontaneous conditions and this decreased to 1.4 ± 0.6 spikes/s during 2–5 s after the stimulation train ($n = 14$; $p = 0.009$). PnO train stimulation induced a short-lasting decrease of slow waves, probably by activation of the basal forebrain through polysynaptic pathways (Camacho Evangelista and Reinoso Suarez, 1964; Nuñez et al., 2006b; Teruel-Marti et al., 2008).

The inhibition of PeFLH neuronal activity by PnO electrical stimulation was blocked by iontophoretic application of bicuculline (10 mM; $n = 8$; **Figure 6B**). **Figure 5C** shows the mean firing rate in control conditions ($n = 14$) and under bicuculline (10 mM; $n = 8$). The spontaneous firing rate of PeFLH neurons increased to 4.4 ± 1.2 spikes/s 5 min after bicuculline application and, in these conditions, PnO stimulation did not alter the firing rate of the neurons (5.0 ± 0.9 spikes/s), indicating that the PnO-evoked inhibition of PeFLH neurons was dependent on the GABA$_A$ receptor activation.

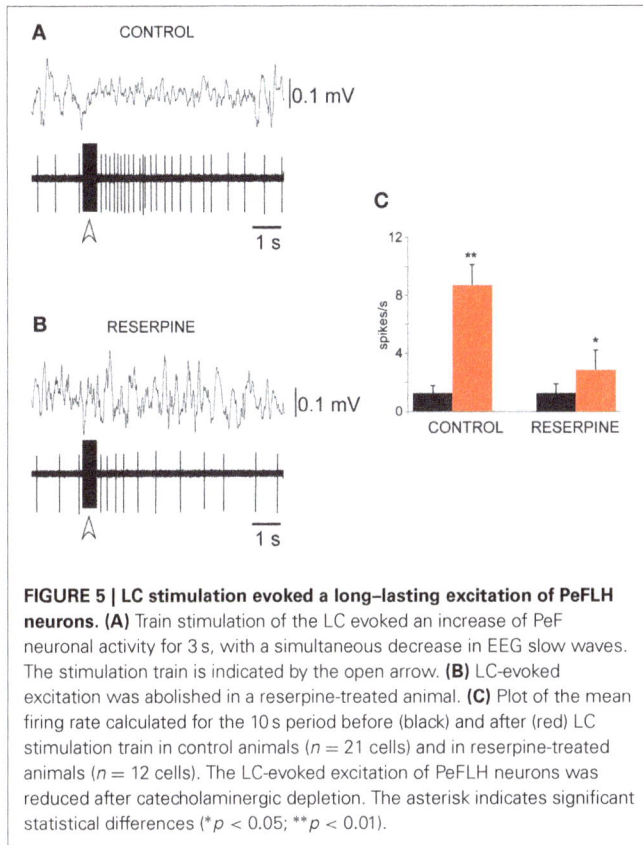

FIGURE 5 | LC stimulation evoked a long–lasting excitation of PeFLH neurons. (A) Train stimulation of the LC evoked an increase of PeF neuronal activity for 3 s, with a simultaneous decrease in EEG slow waves. The stimulation train is indicated by the open arrow. **(B)** LC-evoked excitation was abolished in a reserpine-treated animal. **(C)** Plot of the mean firing rate calculated for the 10 s period before (black) and after (red) LC stimulation train in control animals ($n = 21$ cells) and in reserpine-treated animals ($n = 12$ cells). The LC-evoked excitation of PeFLH neurons was reduced after catecholaminergic depletion. The asterisk indicates significant statistical differences ($*p < 0.05$; $**p < 0.01$).

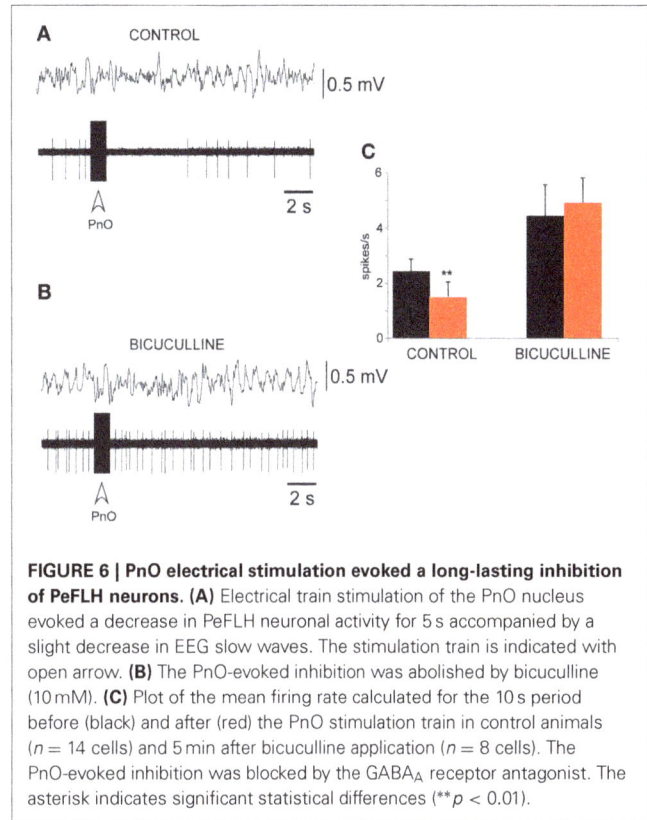

FIGURE 6 | PnO electrical stimulation evoked a long-lasting inhibition of PeFLH neurons. (A) Electrical train stimulation of the PnO nucleus evoked a decrease in PeFLH neuronal activity for 5 s accompanied by a slight decrease in EEG slow waves. The stimulation train is indicated with open arrow. **(B)** The PnO-evoked inhibition was abolished by bicuculline (10 mM). **(C)** Plot of the mean firing rate calculated for the 10 s period before (black) and after (red) the PnO stimulation train in control animals ($n = 14$ cells) and 5 min after bicuculline application ($n = 8$ cells). The PnO-evoked inhibition was blocked by the GABA$_A$ receptor antagonist. The asterisk indicates significant statistical differences ($**p < 0.01$).

DISCUSSION

The present results demonstrate using anatomical and electrophysiological methods the existence of a neuronal network involving the PeFLH area, LC, and PnO nuclei that would control the sleep-wake cycle. The Orx PeF neurons favor EEG activation by excitatory projections to the LC nucleus and simultaneously block REM sleep generation by inhibition of PnO neurons through GABAergic receptors. This study also reveals that the LC and PnO nuclei exerted a feedback control on neuronal activity of PeFLH area in order to maintain a normal succession of stages during the sleep-wakefulness cycle. Top-down and bottom-up regulatory mechanisms are engaged to control the succession of sleep-wakefulness stages.

Both Orx-1 and Orx-2 receptors are expressed in the rodent brainstem (Greco and Shiromani, 2001; Marcus et al., 2001). Whereas the distribution of both receptors is quite similar in the PnO nucleus (Greco and Shiromani, 2001; Cluderay et al., 2002; Brischoux et al., 2008), LC nucleus shows a much more prominent expression for Orx-1 receptor mRNA and protein (Trivedi et al., 1998; Greco and Shiromani, 2001); Orx-2 receptors appear to be virtually absent in noradrenergic neurons of the LC nucleus (Brischoux et al., 2008). In agreement with these results, our data show that application of the Orx-1 receptor antagonist SB-334867 into the LC nucleus prevents the excitatory effect evoked by PeFLH stimulation. The lesion of neurons expressing the Orx-2 receptor in the lateral hypothalamus, by using the toxin Orx 2-saporin, have already revealed the implication of this receptor in different narcoleptic signs (Gerashchenko et al., 2001, 2003).

The additional utilization of selective Orx-2 antagonists in the future could further help elucidate differential roles in regions expressing both receptors, such as the PnO.

The PeFLH area has been implicated in the regulation of behavioral arousal during wakefulness (Kilduff and Peyron, 2000; Siegel, 2004; Szymusiak and McGinty, 2008). This area contains Orx neurons mainly located in the PeF nucleus that are active during wakefulness and silent or with a low activity during non-REM and REM sleep (Alam et al., 2002; Koyama et al., 2003; Lee et al., 2005a,b; Suntsova et al., 2007). In a previous study we showed that Orx PeF neurons activate GABAergic receptors to inhibit PnO neurons, controlling the onset of REM sleep and thus, facilitating wakefulness (Nuñez et al., 2006a). In agreement with this observation, Lu and collaborators demonstrated that activation of PeF cells with bicuculline blocked the ability of pontine carbachol injections to elicit REM sleep (Lu et al., 2007). In the present study we show that there is a reciprocal connection between PnO and PeF nuclei. Both pathways have an inhibitory effect mediated by the activation of GABA$_A$ receptors because effects were blocked by local application of the GABA$_A$ receptor antagonist bicuculline. This experiment does not discard that other pathways could activated by PeFLH stimulation through other neurotransmitter actions. Consequently, when PeF neurons are active they block the possibility of REM sleep generation while PnO neurons activation during REM sleep inhibits PeF neurons and prevents wakefulness. Moreover, GABAergic sleep-active anterior hypothalamic neurons project to the PeF nucleus and GABA release is increased in this region during slow wave sleep (Nitz and Siegel, 1996; Saper et al., 2001, 2005; Uschakov et al., 2006). Thus, during slow wave and REM sleep PeF Orx neurons are inhibited. The absence of Orx is associated with narcolepsy, a disorder manifested by an uncontrollable occurrence of REM sleep (Chemelli et al., 1999; Lin et al., 1999; Thannickal et al., 2000). In agreement with this, Orx knock-out mice show an increase of slow wave and REM sleep during the darkness period, whereas wakefulness is decreased (Chemelli et al., 1999).

In this study we further demonstrated *in vivo* that PeF neurons facilitate wakefulness by direct excitation of LC neurons, which contribute to arousal by excitation of thalamic and cortical neurons (McCormick and Prince, 1988; McCormick, 1989; Aston-Jones, 2005). Previous studies in brain slices or neuronal cultures have demonstrated that Orx depolarizes LC neurons, increasing their firing rate (Soffin et al., 2002; Murai and Akaike, 2005). Also, the firing rates of LC neurons increased after microiontophoretic injection of Orx (Bourgin et al., 2000). LC neurons recorded in the present study showed similar spontaneous firing rate in control conditions from anesthetized rats that previous studies (Aston-Jones and Bloom, 1981; Bourgin et al., 2000) and also are consistent with these previous studies in demonstrating that Orx increases neuronal excitability in the LC nucleus through the activation of the Orx-1 receptor, since excitability is diminished by the Orx-1 receptor antagonist SB-334867 (Gompf and Aston-Jones, 2008). Orx innervation of LC neurons projecting to the cortex has been reported recently (Cid-Pellitero and Garzon, 2011). This Orx innervation probably supplies excitatory inputs to LC nucleus that are critical for cortical activation in transitions from sleep to wakefulness and during EEG activation.

The activity of LC neurons is involved in maintenance of wakefulness and EEG activation. These neurons are active during wakefulness, decrease their firing rate during slow wave sleep and are silent during REM sleep (Hobson and McCarley, 1975; Aston-Jones and Bloom, 1981). Unilateral lesions of the LC nucleus in cats enhance REM sleep (Caballero and De Andres, 1986). Carter and collaborators, using an optogenetic approach to stimulate or inhibit LC neurons found that silencing LC neurons blocked Orx-mediated sleep-to-wakefulness transitions while increasing the excitability of LC neurons enhanced these transitions (Carter et al., 2012, 2013).

Consequently with the above results, the LC nucleus plays a key role in regulating the sleep-wakefulness cycle. To favor the wakefulness stage, LC neurons activate PeF neurons by a direct pathway from LC nucleus to PeFLH area, as shown here. Moreover, electrical stimulation of LC nucleus induced an increase in the neuronal firing rate of PeF neurons by activation of catecholaminergic receptors. The lateral hypothalamus receives a moderately dense noradrenergic innervation (Baldo et al., 2003), most of which arises from outside the LC nucleus (Yoshida et al., 2006). Our study shows that neurons labeled after retrograde tracer injections in LC nucleus were located in the ventral sector of PeFLH area. Previous studies have described dense projections from PeFLH to the LC in the rat (Luppi et al., 1995; España et al., 2005; Lee et al., 2005b) and in the cat (Torterolo et al., 2013). The PeFLH neurons projecting to the LC distribute within the hypothalamic region containing the Orx cell group without any observed rostrocaudal or mediolateral topography, as occur in our experiments. However, retrogradely-labeled lateral hypothalamic neurons after

LC nucleus tracer injections have been reported to locate also in the dorsal half of the Orx-containing cell group (España et al., 2005). This difference may be due to the tracer infusion volume or the tracer uptake.

It is reasonable to believe that both effects, inhibition of REM sleep generation and facilitation of arousal, could be performed by the same PeF neuronal population. However, our anatomical results indicate there are two different neuronal populations sending separate projections to PnO and LC nuclei. In fact, injections of retrograde tracers in PnO nucleus resulted in labeled neurons in the PeF nucleus and in the medial sector of the PeFLH area, while neurons labeled after retrograde tracer injections in LC nucleus were located in the ventral sector of PeFLH area. Taken together, these results suggest the existence of a neuronal network between the lateral hypothalamus and brainstem structures that may control the appropriate succession of the stages during sleep-wakefulness cycle. Moreover, Orx neurons of the PeFLH area seem to be an important organizer of the wakefulness and sleep stages based on their anatomical projections and synaptic interactions with different brainstem "sleep generators." Thus, some sleep disorders such as narcolepsy or insomnia may be due to alterations of the Orx system.

AUTHOR CONTRIBUTIONS

Conceived and designed the experiments: Angel Núñez, Miguel Garzón, and Margarita L. Rodrigo-Angulo. Performed and analyzed electrophysiological experiments: Angel Núñez and Silvia Tortorella. Performed and analyzed anatomical experiments: Miguel Garzón and Margarita L. Rodrigo-Angulo. Wrote the paper: Angel Núñez, Miguel Garzón, and Margarita L. Rodrigo-Angulo.

ACKNOWLEDGMENTS

This work was supported by grant from Ministerio de Economia y Competitividad (BFU2009-06991). We thank G. de la Fuente and M. Callejo for technical assistance and C. F. Warren for revision of English language usage.

REFERENCES

Abrahamson, E. E., and Moore, R. Y. (2001). The posterior hypothalamic area: chemoarchitecture and afferent connections. *Brain Res.* 889, 1–22. doi: 10.1016/S0006-8993(00)03015-8

Alam, M. N., Gong, H., Alam, T., Jaganath, R., McGinty, D., and Szymusiak, R. (2002). Sleep-waking discharge patterns of neurons recorded in the rat perifornical lateral hypothalamic area. *J. Physiol. (Lond.)* 538, 619–631. doi: 10.1113/jphysiol.2001.012888

Aston-Jones, G. (2005). Brain structures and receptors involved in alertness. *Sleep Med.* 6(Suppl. 1), S3–S7. doi: 10.1016/S1389-9457(05)80002-4

Aston-Jones, G., and Bloom, F. E. (1981). Activity of norepinephrine-containing locus coeruleus neurons in behaving rats anticipates fluctuations in the sleep-waking cycle. *J. Neurosci.* 1, 876–886.

Baldo, B. A., Daniel, R. A., Berridge, C. W., and Kelley, A. E. (2003). Overlapping distributions of orexin/hypocretin- and dopamine-beta-hydroxylase immunoreactive fibers in rat brain regions mediating arousal, motivation, and stress. *J. Comp. Neurol.* 464, 220–237. doi: 10.1002/cne.10783

Bernard, R., Lydic, R., and Baghdoyan, H. A. (2003). Hypocretin-1 causes G protein activation and increases ACh release in rat pons. *Eur. J. Neurosci.* 18, 1775–1785. doi: 10.1046/j.1460-9568.2003.02905.x

Bernard, R., Lydic, R., and Baghdoyan, H. A. (2006). Hypocretin (orexin) receptor subtypes differentially enhance acetylcholine release and activate g protein subtypes in rat pontine reticular formation. *J. Pharmacol. Exp. Ther.* 317, 163–171. doi: 10.1124/jpet.105.097071

Beuckmann, C. T., Sinton, C. M., Williams, S. C., Richardson, J. A., Hammer, R. E., Sakurai, T., et al. (2004). Expression of a poly-glutamine-ataxin-3 transgene in orexin neurons induces narcolepsy-cataplexy in the rat. *J. Neurosci.* 24, 4469–4477. doi: 10.1523/JNEUROSCI.5560-03.2004

Bittencourt, J. C., Presse, F., Arias, C., Peto, C., Vaughan, J., Nahon, J. L., et al. (1992). The melanin-concentrating hormone system of the rat brain: an immuno- and hybridization histochemical characterization. *J. Comp. Neurol.* 319, 218–245. doi: 10.1002/cne.903190204

Bourgin, P., Huitron-Resendiz, S., Spier, A. D., Fabre, V., Morte, B., Criado, J. R., et al. (2000). Hypocretin-1 modulates rapid eye movement sleep through activation of locus coeruleus neurons. *J. Neurosci.* 20, 7760–7765.

Brischoux, F., Mainville, L., and Jones, B. E. (2008). Muscarinic-2 and orexin-2 receptors on GABAergic and other neurons in the rat mesopontine tegmentum and their potential role in sleep-wake state control. *J. Comp. Neurol.* 510, 607–630. doi: 10.1002/cne.21803

Burlet, S., Tyler, C. J., and Leonard, C. S. (2002). Direct and indirect excitation of laterodorsal tegmental neurons by hypocretin/orexin peptides: implications for wakefulness and narcolepsy. *J. Neurosci.* 22, 2862–2872.

Caballero, A., and De Andres, I. (1986). Unilateral lesions in locus coeruleus area enhance paradoxical sleep. *Electroencephalogr. Clin. Neurophysiol.* 64, 339–346. doi: 10.1016/0013-4694(86)90158-6

Camacho Evangelista, A., and Reinoso Suarez, F. (1964). Activating and synchronizing centers in cat brain: electroencephalograms after lesions. *Science* 146, 268–270. doi: 10.1126/science.146.3641.268

Carter, M. E., Brill, J., Bonnavion, P., Huguenard, J. R., Huerta, R., and de Lecea, L. (2012). Mechanism for hypocretin-mediated sleep-to-wake transitions. *Proc. Natl. Acad. Sci. U.S.A.* 109, E2635–E2644. doi: 10.1073/pnas.1202526109

Carter, M. E., de Lecea, L., and Adamantidis, A. (2013). Functional wiring of hypocretin and LC-NE neurons: implications for arousal. *Front. Behav. Neurosci.* 7:43. doi: 10.3389/fnbeh.2013.00043

Chemelli, R. M., Willie, J. T., Sinton, C. M., Elmquist, J. K., Scammell, T., Lee, C., et al. (1999). Narcolepsy in orexin knockout mice: molecular genetics of sleep regulation. *Cell* 98, 437–451. doi: 10.1016/S0092-8674(00)81973-X

Cid-Pellitero, E. D., and Garzon, M. (2011). Hypocretin1/OrexinA-containing axons innervate locus coeruleus neurons that project to the rat medial prefrontal cortex. Implication in the sleep-wakefulness cycle and cortical activation. *Synapse* 65, 843–857. doi: 10.1002/syn.20912

Cluderay, J. E., Harrison, D. C., and Hervieu, G. J. (2002). Protein distribution of the orexin-2 receptor in the rat central nervous system. *Regul. Pept.* 104, 131–144. doi: 10.1016/S0167-0115(01)00357-3

de Lecea, L., Kilduff, T. S., Peyron, C., Gao, X., Foye, P. E., Danielson, P. E., et al. (1998). The hypocretins: hypothalamus-specific peptides with neuroexcitatory activity. *Proc. Natl. Acad. Sci. U.S.A.* 95, 322–327. doi: 10.1073/pnas.95.1.322

Eggermann, E., Serafin, M., Bayer, L., Machard, D., Saint-Mleux, B., Jones, B. E., et al. (2001). Orexins/hypocretins excite basal forebrain cholinergic neurones. *Neuroscience* 108, 177–181. doi: 10.1016/S0306-4522(01)00512-7

Erami, E., Azhdari-Zarmehri, H., Ghasemi-Dashkhasan, E., Esmaeili, M. H., and Semnanian, S. (2012). Intra-paragigantocellularis lateralis injection of orexin-A has an antinociceptive effect on hot plate and formalin tests in rat. *Brain Res.* 1478, 16–23. doi: 10.1016/j.brainres.2012.08.013

España, R. A., Baldo, B. A., Kelley, A. E., and Berridge, C. W. (2001). Wake-promoting and sleep-suppressing actions of hypocretin (orexin): basal forebrain sites of action. *Neuroscience* 106, 699–715. doi: 10.1016/S0306-4522(01)00319-0

España, R. A., Reis, K. M., Valentino, R. J., and Berridge, C. W. (2005). Organization of hypocretin/orexin efferents to locus coeruleus and basal forebrain arousal-related structures. *J. Comp. Neurol.* 481, 160–178. doi: 10.1002/cne.20369

Garzón, M., De Andrés, I., and Reinoso-Suárez, F. (1998). Sleep patterns after carbachol delivery in the ventral oral pontine tegmentum of the cat. *Neuroscience* 83, 1137–1144. doi: 10.1016/S0306-4522(97)00494-6

Gerashchenko, D., Blanco-Centurion, C., Greco, M. A., and Shiromani, P. J. (2003). Effects of lateral hypothalamic lesion with the neurotoxin hypocretin-2-saporin on sleep in Long-Evans rats. *Neuroscience* 116, 223–235. doi: 10.1016/S0306-4522(02)00575-4

Gerashchenko, D., Kohls, M. D., Greco, M., Waleh, N. S., Salin-Pascual, R., Kilduff, T. S., et al. (2001). Hypocretin-2-saporin lesions of the lateral hypothalamus produce narcoleptic-like sleep behavior in the rat. *J. Neurosci.* 21, 7273–7283.

Gompf, H. S., and Aston-Jones, G. (2008). Role of orexin input in the diurnal rhythm of locus coeruleus impulse activity. *Brain Res.* 1224, 43–52. doi: 10.1016/j.brainres.2008.05.060

Greco, M. A., and Shiromani, P. J. (2001). Hypocretin receptor protein and mRNA expression in the dorsolateral pons of rats. *Mol. Brain Res.* 88, 176–182. doi: 10.1016/S0169-328X(01)00039-0

Guilleminault, C., and Fromherz, S. (2005). "Narcolepsy: diagnosis and management," in *Principles and Practice of Sleep Medicine*, eds M. H. Kryger, T. I. Roth, and W. C. Dement (Philadelphia, PA: Elsevier Saunders), 780–790. doi: 10.1016/B0-72-160797-7/50072-0

Hagan, J. J., Leslie, R. A., Patel, S., Evans, M. L., Wattam, T. A., Holmes, S., et al. (1999). Orexin A activates locus coeruleus cell firing and increases arousal in the rat. *Proc. Natl. Acad. Sci. U.S.A.* 96, 10911–10916. doi: 10.1073/pnas.96.19.10911

Hara, J., Beuckmann, C. T., Nambu, T., Willie, J. T., Chemelli, R. M., Sinton, C. M., et al. (2001). Genetic ablation of orexin neurons in mice results in narcolepsy, hypophagia, and obesity. *Neuron* 30, 345–354. doi: 10.1016/S0896-6273(01)00293-8

Hobson, J. A., and McCarley, R. W. (1975). Sleep cycle oscillation: reciprocal discharge by two brainstem neuronal groups. *Science* 189, 55–58. doi: 10.1126/science.1094539

Horner, R. L., and Kubin, L. (1999). Pontine carbachol elicits multiple rapid eye movement sleep-like neural events in urethane-anaesthetized rats. *Neuroscience* 93, 215–226. doi: 10.1016/S0306-4522(99)00126-8

Horvath, T. L., Peyron, C., Diano, S., Ivanov, A., Aston-Jones, G., Kilduff, T. S., et al. (1999). Hypocretin (orexin) activation and synaptic innervation of the locus coeruleus noradrenergic system. *J. Comp. Neurol.* 415, 145–159. doi: 10.1002/(SICI)1096-9861(19991213)415:2<145::AID-CNE1>3.0.CO;2-2

Ivanov, A., and Aston-Jones, G. (2000). Hypocretin/orexin depolarizes and decreases potassium conductance in locus coeruleus neurons. *Neuroreport* 11, 1755–1758. doi: 10.1097/00001756-200006050-00031

Jones, B. E. (2008). Modulation of cortical activation and behavioral arousal by cholinergic and orexinergic systems. *Ann. N.Y. Acad. Sci.* 1129, 26–34. doi: 10.1196/annals.1417.026

Kilduff, T. S., and Peyron, C. (2000). The hypocretin/orexin ligand-receptor system: implications for sleep and sleep disorders. *Trends Neurosci.* 23, 359–365. doi: 10.1016/S0166-2236(00)01594-0

Kohlmeier, K. A., Burns, J., Reiner, P. B., and Semba, K. (2002). Substance P in the descending cholinergic projection to REM sleep-induction regions of the rat pontine reticular formation: anatomical and electrophysiological analyses. *Eur. J. Neurosci.* 15, 176–196. doi: 10.1046/j.0953-816x.2001.01829.x

Koyama, Y., Takahashi, K., Kodama, T., and Kayama, Y. (2003). State-dependent activity of neurons in the perifornical hypothalamic area during sleep and waking. *Neuroscience* 119, 1209–1219. doi: 10.1016/S0306-4522(03)00173-8

Lee, M. G., Hassani, O. K., and Jones, B. E. (2005a). Discharge of identified orexin/hypocretin neurons across the sleep-waking cycle. *J. Neurosci.* 25, 6716–6720. doi: 10.1523/JNEUROSCI.1887-05.2005

Lee, H. S., Lee, B. Y., and Waterhouse, B. D. (2005b). Retrograde study of projections from the tuberomammillary nucleus to the dorsal raphe and the locus coeruleus in the rat. *Brain Res.* 1043, 65–75. doi: 10.1016/j.brainres.2005.02.050

Lin, L., Faraco, J., Li, R., Kadotani, H., Rogers, W., Lin, X., et al. (1999). The sleep disorder canine narcolepsy is caused by a mutation in the hypocretin (orexin) receptor 2 gene. *Cell* 98, 365–376. doi: 10.1016/S0092-8674(00)81965-0

Lu, J. W., Fenik, V. B., Branconi, J. L., Mann, G. L., Rukhadze, I., and Kubin, L. (2007). Disinhibition of perifornical hypothalamic neurones activates noradrenergic neurones and blocks pontine carbachol-induced REM sleep-like episodes in rats. *J. Physiol.* 582, 553–567. doi: 10.1113/jphysiol.2007.127613

Luppi, P. H., Aston-Jones, G., Akaoka, H., Chouvet, G., and Jouvet, M. (1995). Afferent projections to the rat locus coeruleus demonstrated by retrograde and anterograde tracing with cholera-toxin B subunit and *Phaseolus vulgaris* leucoagglutinin. *Neuroscience* 65, 119–160. doi: 10.1016/0306-4522(94)00481-J

Marcus, J. N., Aschkenasi, C. J., Lee, C. E., Chemelli, R. M., Saper, C. B., Yanagisawa, M., et al. (2001). Differential expression of orexin receptors 1 and 2 in the rat brain. *J. Comp. Neurol.* 435, 6–25. doi: 10.1002/cne.1190

McCormick, D. A. (1989). Cholinergic and noradrenergic modulation of thalamocortical processing. *Trends Neurosci.* 12, 215–221. doi: 10.1016/0166-2236(89)90125-2

McCormick, D. A., and Prince, D. A. (1988). Noradrenergic modulation of firing pattern in guinea pig and cat thalamic neurons, *in vitro*. *J. Neurophysiol.* 59, 978–996.

McGinty, D., and Szymusiak, R. (2003). Hypothalamic regulation of sleep and arousal. *Front. Biosci.* 8, s1074–s1083. doi: 10.2741/1159

Mileykovskiy, B. Y., Kiyashchenko, L. I., and Siegel, J. M. (2005). Behavioral correlates of activity in identified hypocretin/orexin neurons. *Neuron* 46, 787–798. doi: 10.1016/j.neuron.2005.04.035

Murai, Y., and Akaike, T. (2005). Orexins cause depolarization via nonselective cationic and K+ channels in isolated locus coeruleus neurons. *Neurosci. Res.* 51, 55–65. doi: 10.1016/j.neures.2004.09.005

Nishino, S., Ripley, B., Overeem, S., Lammers, G. J., and Mignot, E. (2000). Hypocretin (orexin) deficiency in human narcolepsy. *Lancet* 355, 39–40. doi: 10.1016/S0140-6736(99)05582-8

Nitz, D., and Siegel, J. M. (1996). GABA release in posterior hypothalamus across sleep-wake cycle. *Am. J. Physiol.* 271, R1707–R1712.

Nuñez, A., Moreno-Balandran, M. E., Rodrigo-Angulo, M. L., Garzon, M., and De Andres, I. (2006a). Relationship between the perifornical hypothalamic area and oral pontine reticular nucleus in the rat. Possible implication of the hypocretinergic projection in the control of rapid eye movement sleep. *Eur. J. Neurosci.* 24, 2834–2842. doi: 10.1111/j.1460-9568.2006.05159.x

Nuñez, A., Cervera-Ferri, A., Olucha-Bordonau, F., Ruiz-Torner, A., and Teruel, V. (2006b). Nucleus incertus contribution to hippocampal theta rhythm generation. *Eur. J. Neurosci.* 23, 2731–2738. doi: 10.1111/j.1460-9568.2006.04797.x

Nuñez, A., Rodrigo-Angulo, M. L., De Andres, I., and Reinoso-Suarez, F. (2002). Firing activity and postsynaptic properties of morphologically identified neurons of ventral oral pontine reticular nucleus. *Neuroscience* 115, 1165–1175. doi: 10.1016/S0306-4522(02)00478-5

Paxinos, G., and Watson, C. (2007). *The Rat Brain in Stereotaxic Coordinates*. San Diego, CA: Academic Press.

Peyron, C., Faraco, J., Rogers, W., Ripley, B., Overeem, S., Charnay, Y., et al. (2000). A mutation in a case of early onset narcolepsy and a generalized absence of hypocretin peptides in human narcoleptic brains. *Nat. Med.* 6, 991–997. doi: 10.1038/79690

Peyron, C., Tighe, D. K., van den Pol, A. N., de Lecea, L., Heller, H. C., Sutcliffe, J. G., et al. (1998). Neurons containing hypocretin (orexin) project to multiple neuronal systems. *J. Neurosci.* 18, 9996–10015.

Reinoso-Suárez, F., De Andrés, I., Rodrigo-Angulo, M. L., de la Roza, C., Nuñez, A., and Garzón, M. (1999). The anatomy of dreaming, and REM sleep. *Eur. J. Anat.* 3, 163–175.

Reinoso-Suarez, F., de Andres, I., Rodrigo-Angulo, M. L., and Garzon, M. (2001). Brain structures and mechanisms involved in the generation of REM sleep. *Sleep Med. Rev.* 5, 63–77. doi: 10.1053/smrv.2000.0136

Reinoso-Suárez, F., de Andrés, I., Rodrigo-Angulo, M. L., and Rodriguez-Veiga, E. (1994). Location and anatomical connections of a paradoxical sleep induction site in the brainstem of the cat. *Eur. J. Neurosci.* 6, 1829–1836. doi: 10.1111/j.1460-9568.1994.tb00575.x

Rodrigo-Angulo, M. L., Heredero, S., Rodriguez-Veiga, E., and Reinoso-Suarez, F. (2008). GABAergic and non-GABAergic thalamic, hypothalamic and basal forebrain projections to the ventral oral pontine reticular nucleus: their implication in REM sleep modulation. *Brain Res.* 1210, 116–125. doi: 10.1016/j.brainres.2008.02.095

Sakurai, T. (2005). Roles of orexin/hypocretin in regulation of sleep/wakefulness and energy homeostasis. *Sleep Med. Rev.* 9, 231–241. doi: 10.1016/j.smrv.2004.07.007

Sakurai, T., Amemiya, A., Ishii, M., Matsuzaki, I., Chemelli, R. M., Tanaka, H., et al. (1998). Orexins and orexins receptors: a family of hypothalamic neuropeptides and G protein-coupled receptors that regulate feeding behavior. *Cell* 92, 573–585. doi: 10.1016/S0092-8674(00)80949-6

Saper, C. B., Chou, T. C., and Scammell, T. E. (2001). The sleep switch: hypothalamic control of sleep and wakefulness. *Trends Neurosci.* 24, 726–731. doi: 10.1016/S0166-2236(00)02002-6

Saper, C. B., Lu, J., Chou, T. C., and Gooley, J. (2005). The hypothalamic integrator for circadian rhythms. *Trends Neurosci.* 28, 152–157. doi: 10.1016/j.tins.2004.12.009

Sasaki, K., Suzuki, M., Mieda, M., Tsujino, N., Roth, B., and Sakurai, T. (2011). Pharmacogenetic modulation of orexin neurons alters sleep/wakefulness states in mice. *PLoS ONE* 6:e20360. doi: 10.1371/journal.pone.0020360

Siegel, J. M. (2004). Hypocretin (orexin): role in normal behavior and neuropathology. *Annu. Rev. Psychol.* 55, 125–148. doi: 10.1146/annurev.psych.55.090902.141545

Soffin, E. M., Evans, M. L., Gill, C. H., Harries, M. H., Benham, C. D., and Davies, C. H. (2002). SB-334867-A antagonises orexin mediated excitation in the locus coeruleus. *Neuropharmacology* 42, 127–133. doi: 10.1016/S0028-3908(01)00156-3

Suntsova, N., Guzman-Marin, R., Kumar, S., Alam, M. N., Szymusiak, R., and McGinty, D. (2007). The median preoptic nucleus reciprocally modulates activity of arousal-related and sleep-related neurons in the perifornical lateral hypothalamus. *J. Neurosci.* 27, 1616–1630. doi: 10.1523/JNEUROSCI.3498-06.2007

Szymusiak, R., and McGinty, D. (2008). Hypothalamic regulation of sleep and arousal. *Ann. N.Y. Acad. Sci.* 1129, 275–286. doi: 10.1196/annals.1417.027

Takahashi, K., Wang, Q. P., Guan, J. L., Kayama, Y., Shioda, S., and Koyama, Y. (2005). State-dependent effects of orexins on the serotonergic dorsal raphe neurons in the rat. *Regul. Pept.* 126, 43–47. doi: 10.1016/j.regpep.2004.08.009

Teruel-Marti, V., Cervera-Ferri, A., Nuñez, A., Valverde-Navarro, A. A., Olucha-Bordonau, F. E., and Ruiz-Torner, A. (2008). Anatomical evidence for a pontoseptal pathway via the nucleus incertus in the rat. *Brain Res.* 1218, 87–96. doi: 10.1016/j.brainres.2008.04.022

Thakkar, M. M., Ramesh, V., Strecker, R. E., and McCarley, R. W. (2001). Microdialysis perfusion of orexin-A in the basal forebrain increases wakefulness in freely behaving rats. *Arch. Ital. Biol.* 139, 313–328.

Thannickal, T. C., Moore, R. Y., Nienhuis, R., Ramanathan, L., Gulyani, S., Aldrich, M., et al. (2000). Reduced number of hypocretin neurons in human narcolepsy. *Neuron* 27, 469–474. doi: 10.1016/S0896-6273(00)00058-1

Torterolo, P., Sampogna, S., and Chase, M. H. (2013). Hypocretinergic and non-hypocretinergic projections from the hypothalamus to the REM sleep executive area of the pons. *Brain Res.* 1491, 68–77. doi: 10.1016/j.brainres.2012.10.050

Trivedi, P., Yu, H., MacNeil, D. J., Van der Ploeg, L. H., and Guan, X. M. (1998). Distribution of orexin receptor mRNA in the rat brain. *FEBS Lett.* 438, 71–75. doi: 10.1016/S0014-5793(98)01266-6

Uschakov, A., Gong, H., McGinty, D., and Szymusiak, R. (2006). Sleep active neurons in the preoptic area project to hypothalamic paraventricular nucleus and perifornical lateral hypothalamus. *Eur. J. Neurosci.* 23, 3284–3296. doi: 10.1111/j.1460-9568.2006.04860.x

Vaughan, J. M., Fischer, W. H., Hoeger, C., Rivier, J., and Vale, W. (1989). Characterization of melanin-concentrating hormone from rat hypothalamus. *Endocrinology* 125, 1660–1665. doi: 10.1210/endo-125-3-1660

Willie, J. T., Chemelli, R. M., Sinton, C. M., Tokita, S., Williams, S. C., Kisanuki, Y. Y., et al. (2003). Distinct narcolepsy syndromes in orexin receptor-2 and orexin null mice: molecular genetic dissection of non-REM and REM sleep regulatory processes. *Neuron* 38, 715–730. doi: 10.1016/S0896-6273(03)00330-1

Xi, M. C., Morales, F. R., and Chase, M. H. (2001). Effects on sleep and wakefulness of the injection of hypocretin-1 (orexin-A) into the laterodorsal tegmental nucleus of the cat. *Brain Res.* 901, 259–264. doi: 10.1016/S0006-8993(01)02317-4

Yamanaka, A., Tsujino, N., Funahashi, H., Honda, K., Guan, J. L., Wang, Q. P., et al. (2002). Orexins activate histaminergic neurons via the orexin 2 receptor. *Biochem. Biophys. Res. Commun.* 290, 1237–1245. doi: 10.1006/bbrc.2001.6318

Yoshida, K., McCormack, S., Espana, R. A., Crocker, A., and Scammell, T. E. (2006). Afferents to the orexin neurons of the rat brain. *J. Comp. Neurol.* 494, 845–861. doi: 10.1002/cne.20859

Conflict of Interest Statement: The authors declare that the research was conducted in the absence of any commercial or financial relationships that could be construed as a potential conflict of interest.

Orexin-1 and orexin-2 receptor antagonists reduce ethanol self-administration in high-drinking rodent models

Rachel I. Anderson[1,2], Howard C. Becker[1,2,3], Benjamin L. Adams[4], Cynthia D. Jesudason[4] and Linda M. Rorick-Kehn[4]*

[1] Medical University of South Carolina, Charleston, SC, USA
[2] Charleston Alcohol Research Center, Charleston, SC, USA
[3] Ralph H. Johnson VA Medical Center, USA
[4] Lilly Research Laboratories, Eli Lilly and Company, Indianapolis, IN, USA

Edited by:
Michel A. Steiner, Actelion
Pharmaceuticals Ltd., Switzerland

Reviewed by:
Roberto Ciccocioppo, University of
Camerino, Italy
Valentina Vengeliene, Central
Institute of Mental Health, Germany

*Correspondence:
Linda M. Rorick-Kehn, Lilly Research
Laboratories, Neuroscience
Discovery Research, Lilly Corporate
Center, DC0510, Indianapolis, IN
46285, USA
e-mail: rorickkehnlm@lilly.com

To examine the role of orexin-1 and orexin-2 receptor activity on ethanol self-administration, compounds that differentially target orexin (OX) receptor subtypes were assessed in various self-administration paradigms using high-drinking rodent models. Effects of the OX_1 antagonist SB334867, the OX_2 antagonist LSN2424100, and the mixed $OX_{1/2}$ antagonist almorexant (ACT-078573) on home cage ethanol consumption were tested in ethanol-preferring (P) rats using a 2-bottle choice procedure. In separate experiments, effects of SB334867, LSN2424100, and almorexant on operant ethanol self-administration were assessed in P rats maintained on a progressive ratio operant schedule of reinforcement. In a third series of experiments, SB334867, LSN2424100, and almorexant were administered to ethanol-preferring C57BL/6J mice to examine effects of OX receptor blockade on ethanol intake in a binge-like drinking (drinking-in-the-dark) model. In P rats with chronic home cage free-choice ethanol access, SB334867 and almorexant significantly reduced ethanol intake, but almorexant also reduced water intake, suggesting non-specific effects on consummatory behavior. In the progressive ratio operant experiments, LSN2424100 and almorexant reduced breakpoints and ethanol consumption in P rats, whereas the almorexant inactive enantiomer and SB334867 did not significantly affect the motivation to consume ethanol. As expected, vehicle-injected mice exhibited binge-like drinking patterns in the drinking-in-the-dark model. All three OX antagonists reduced both ethanol intake and resulting blood ethanol concentrations relative to vehicle-injected controls, but SB334867 and LSN2424100 also reduced sucrose consumption in a different cohort of mice, suggesting non-specific effects. Collectively, these results contribute to a growing body of evidence indicating that OX_1 and OX_2 receptor activity influences ethanol self-administration, although the effects may not be selective for ethanol consumption.

Keywords: hypocretins/orexins, ethanol consumption, operant progressive ratio, P rat, C57BL/6J mouse

INTRODUCTION

Orexins A and B are neuropeptides synthesized in neurons originating in the lateral hypothalamus (LH) that project throughout the brain and bind to two widely expressed G-protein coupled receptors, orexin-1 (OX_1) and orexin-2 (OX_2). OX_1 receptors selectively bind orexin A, whereas OX_2 receptors bind orexin A and B with equal affinity (Sakurai et al., 1998). This neuropeptide system plays an established role in numerous behavioral and regulatory functions including sleep, arousal, and feeding behavior (Willie et al., 2001; Sakurai, 2002). While orexin neurons in the dorsomedial hypothalamus are believed to regulate arousal and stress responses, orexin neurons within the LH are hypothesized to play a role in regulating reward processing for natural rewards as well as drugs of abuse (Harris and Aston-Jones, 2006). This has led to the suggestion that the orexin system is involved in addiction (for review, see Sharf et al., 2010; Mahler et al., 2012). Although evidence previously supported functional

differences between the two receptors, with OX_2 receptor activity more closely related to arousal and OX_1 receptor activity more closely associated with reward (Aston-Jones et al., 2010), more recent research has revealed a role for OX_2 receptors in reward processes as well (Shoblock et al., 2011; Brown et al., 2013).

While a growing body of literature has shown that the orexin system interacts with drug-seeking behavior induced by numerous drugs of abuse such as cocaine, nicotine, and opiates (reviewed by Mahler et al., 2012), the orexin system also has been implicated in the motivational properties of ethanol. Administration of orexin A into the paraventricular nucleus within the LH resulted in elevated ethanol consumption in Sprague-Dawley rats (Schneider et al., 2007). Orexin antagonists that target both OX_1 and OX_2 receptors have been shown to influence ethanol consumption (Kim et al., 2012). For example, systemic administration of the OX_1 receptor antagonist SB334867 reduced ethanol intake and preference in Sprague-Dawley rats

(Moorman and Aston-Jones, 2009). This same antagonist has been shown to reduce relapse drinking, operant responding, and both cue- and stress-induced reinstatement in other rat strains (Richards et al., 2008; Dhaher et al., 2010; Jupp et al., 2011). The OX_2 receptor antagonist JNJ-10397049 also reduced ethanol self-administration and expression of ethanol conditioned place preference (Shoblock et al., 2011). Central administration of the OX_2 receptor antagonist TCS-OX2-29 reduced ethanol intake but did not alter cue-induced reinstatement of responding for ethanol (Brown et al., 2013). Although the dual $OX_{1/2}$ receptor antagonist almorexant has been shown to reduce operant ethanol self-administration when injected either systemically or directly into the ventral tegmental area (VTA; Srinivasan et al., 2012), effects of dual antagonism of both orexin receptors on ethanol consumption have not been as thoroughly explored.

There is some evidence to suggest that orexin antagonists may be particularly effective in subjects that show a high preference for ethanol. For example, an OX_1 receptor antagonist was more effective in reducing ethanol consumption among outbred Sprague-Dawley rats that demonstrated high vs. low ethanol preference (Moorman and Aston-Jones, 2009). Further, several studies that reported orexin antagonist-induced reductions in ethanol self-administration used rats selectively bred for high ethanol preference (Lawrence et al., 2006; Dhaher et al., 2010; Jupp et al., 2011; Brown et al., 2013). Taken together, these results suggest that blocking orexin activity in the brain may be particularly effective in reducing ethanol consumption under conditions in which subjects exhibit a high propensity for ethanol self-administration. The present study was designed to characterize the relative contributions of OX_1 and OX_2 receptor-mediated signaling in modulating ethanol consumption using three different self-administration paradigms in high-drinking rodents. The OX_1 receptor antagonist SB334867 (Smart et al., 2001) is >1000-fold selective for OX_1 over OX_2 receptors, whereas the novel OX_2 receptor antagonist N-((1H-imidazol-2-yl)methyl)-N-([1,1'-biphenyl]-2-yl)-4-fluorobenzenesulfonamide hydrochloride (LSN2424100) is >200-fold selective for OX_2 over OX_1 receptors (Fitch et al., 2014). The dual OX_1/OX_2 antagonist almorexant (ACT-078573; Brisbare-Roch et al., 2007), which is approximately 1.3-fold OX_2-preferring (Fitch et al., 2014), was also tested for comparison to the more selective compounds. Each of these compounds was tested in three different experiments: home cage free-choice drinking in female P rats, progressive ratio operant responding maintained by ethanol in female P rats, and ethanol consumption in a binge-drinking model (drinking-in-the-dark) in male C57BL/6J mice. Some of the P rat experiments included either the inactive enantiomer of almorexant as a negative control or naltrexone as a positive control.

MATERIALS AND METHODS
SUBJECTS
All experiments were conducted in compliance with the Guide for the Care and Use of Laboratory Animals under protocols approved by the local Institutional Animal Care and Use Committees. Rat experiments were conducted in adult female selectively bred Alcohol-Preferring (P) rats generously supplied by the Indiana University School of Medicine (maintained as a

private colony at Taconic Inc., Germantown, NY). For the home cage ethanol consumption studies, a total of 32 female P rats were individually housed with 24-h *ad libitum* access to 15% (v/v) ethanol, water, and food. All 32 P rats had chronic access to ethanol in the home cage for approximately 8–14 months before the current studies were conducted. P rats were divided into 3 groups. One group ($n = 10$) was used to test the effects of SB334867 and a second group ($n = 11$) was used to test the effects of LSN2424100 (one rat was excluded from the experiment due to low baseline drinking). A within-subjects experimental design was used to test the OX_1 and OX_2 receptor antagonists. These rats, along with another group of 11 (i.e., all 32 P rats) were tested in the almorexant study using a between-subjects design ($n = 8$/dose).

A separate cohort of female P rats ($n = 10$) used in operant experiments were pair-housed with food and water available *ad libitum* and maintained on a 12-h light/dark cycle (lights on at 6:00 AM). All operant procedures were conducted during the light phase (between 10 AM and 4 PM). In order to reduce the total number of animals used, within-subjects designs were employed for the operant and home cage consumption experiments. To avoid potential carryover effects, a 3–4 day washout period was imposed between different drug doses, and a 4–7 day washout period was included between the different drug experiments. Baseline performance of the rats (operant and home cage consumption) was monitored on non-dose days to confirm that ethanol intake returned to baseline levels prior to testing.

For the mouse experiments, a total of 166 adult male C57BL/6J mice (Jackson Laboratories, Bar Harbor, ME) were used in the binge drinking experiments, which were conducted using a between-subjects design. Mice were individually housed throughout experimentation under a 12-h reverse light/dark cycle (lights off at 8:00 AM). All testing occurred during the dark cycle.

DRUGS
N-((1H-imidazol-2-yl)methyl)-N-([1,1'-biphenyl]-2-yl)-4-fluorobenzenesulfonamide hydrochloride (LSN2424100), SB334867, (S)-almorexant (ACT-078573), and the inactive (R) enantiomer of almorexant were synthesized at Lilly Research Laboratories (Indianapolis, IN). Naltrexone hydrochloride was purchased from Sigma Aldrich (St. Louis, MO). For rat experiments, the OX_1 antagonist SB334867 was dissolved in a vehicle of 10% (2-hydroxypropyl)-β-cyclodextrin, 2% dimethyl sulfoxide, and 0.05% lactic acid in water, and administered by intraperitoneal (i.p.) injection in a dose volume of 1 ml/kg. The OX_2 antagonist LSN2424100 was suspended in 1% carboxymethyl cellulose, 0.25% polysorbate-80 and 0.05% Dow antifoam in water, and administered by i.p. injection in a dose volume of 1 ml/kg. The mixed $OX_{1/2}$ antagonist almorexant, and its inactive enantiomer, were dissolved in a 20% Captisol solution and administered orally (p.o.) in a dose volume of 1 ml/kg. Naltrexone was dissolved in water with the addition of 15 μl 85% lactic acid.

For mouse experiments, SB334867 was dissolved using 0.01% polysorbate-80 in saline. Almorexant was dissolved in 20% Captisol in water. LSN2424100 was suspended using 1% carboxymethyl cellulose and 0.25% polysorbate-80 in water. All compounds were administered by i.p. injection at a dose volume of 10 ml/kg.

PROCEDURE

Home cage 2-bottle choice drinking in P rats

P rats were housed individually in TSE LabMaster cages (TSE Systems, Bad Homburg, Germany) with food, water, and 15% ethanol (v/v) available at all times. Water and ethanol intake (in ml) were measured once every 5 min throughout the 12-h dark cycle and recorded for later analysis. In the first experiment, rats ($n = 10$) received vehicle, 3, 10, or 30 mg/kg SB334867 (i.p.), 60 min before onset of the 12-h dark phase of the light-dark cycle, using a within-subjects design. In the second experiment, rats ($n = 10$) received vehicle, naltrexone (10 mg/kg), or LSN2424100 at doses of 10 or 30 mg/kg (i.p.), 60 min before onset of the 12-h dark phase, using a within-subjects design (one rat was excluded from the experiment due to low baseline drinking). In the third experiment, rats ($n = 32$) received vehicle, naltrexone (10 mg/kg), or S-almorexant at doses of 60 or 100 mg/kg (p.o.), 60 min before onset of the dark cycle, using a between-subjects design. Naltrexone was included in the study design as a positive control, since this dose of naltrexone has been shown to effectively reduce ethanol consumption in P rats under these testing conditions. For all experiments, a 60-min pre-treatment period was chosen so that the onset of the dark cycle roughly coincided with the time at which maximal brain concentrations were achieved (data not reported). Consumption of water and ethanol was measured during the first 3 h of the dark cycle, based on the short half-lives and high metabolism of the compounds.

Operant progressive ratio responding in P rats

P rats were trained and tested 5 days per week in standard rat operant chambers (Med Associates, St. Albans, VT), housed within sound attenuating boxes. Operant chambers measured $30.5 \times 24.1 \times 21$ cm, with clear Plexiglas front and back walls, modular aluminum sidewalls, a metal bar floor and Plexiglas ceiling. A food cup was located in the center of one sidewall with retractable levers on either side of the food cup. A liquid dipper device allowed the delivery of 0.1 ml of 15% ethanol (v/v) into the food cup. A computer running the MED-IV software package (Med-Associates, St. Albans, VT) controlled stimulus presentations and recorded lever presses. Once subjects were trained to lever press for ethanol reinforcement on a fixed ratio-1 (FR1) schedule of reinforcement, the response requirement for each reinforcement was slowly increased to FR2 and then FR3 over 1–2 weeks. When rats demonstrated a stable level of responding on the FR3 schedule, progressive ratio testing began. The progressive ratio schedule involved increasing response requirements within each session. The response requirement increased from 1 to 2 after three ethanol presentations, and continued to increase by two after every three ethanol presentations (see Rodd et al., 2003). Experimental sessions terminated after 60 min. Total responses on the active and inactive levers, breakpoints [defined as the highest fixed ratio (FR) value reached during the session], and the amount of ethanol consumed (ml; converted to g/kg) were recorded for analysis.

Experiments were conducted using a within-subject design, with 3–4 days washout between administration of different doses, which were counterbalanced using a Latin square design. One group of $n = 10$ rats was used to test the effects of SB334867,

LSN2424100, and almorexant on operant responding maintained on a progressive ratio schedule, in separate experiments. Drugs were administered two days per week (Tues and Fri) to allow for washout between subsequent doses. Rats received vehicle, 3, 10, or 30 mg/kg SB334867 (i.p., 30 min prior to the session); vehicle, 3, 10, or 30 mg/kg LSN2424100 (i.p., 30 min prior to the session); or vehicle, 10, 30, or 60 mg/kg almorexant or 60 mg/kg of the inactive enantiomer of almorexant (p.o., 60 min prior to the session). On all other days, rats received progressive ratio operant testing without any drug treatments to maintain operant performance and confirm return to baseline behaviors. One rat was excluded from testing 60 mg/kg almorexant due to observation of a skin rash not related to the study drug.

Binge drinking in C57BL/6J mice

One week prior to ethanol intake testing, mice were given daily saline injections (i.p.) to acclimate them to handling and injection procedures. Ethanol consumption was assessed using a 4-day drinking-in-the-dark (DID) paradigm during which the water bottle in the home cage was replaced with a single bottle of ethanol (20% v/v) starting 3 h after the onset of the dark cycle. This procedure has been shown to produce high blood ethanol concentrations (BECs) resulting from high levels of ethanol consumption in a relatively short period of time (Rhodes et al., 2005). On the first three days, animals were injected with saline or vehicle 30 min prior to a 2-h period of access to ethanol. On the 4th day, drugs were administered via i.p. injection 30 min prior to the test session, which was extended to 4 h. One cohort of mice was administered vehicle, 3, 10, or 30 mg/kg SB334867 ($n = 10$/dose). A second cohort of mice was tested with vehicle, 15, 30, or 60 mg/kg LSN2424100 ($n = 9$–10/dose). A third cohort of animals was given vehicle, 25, 50, or 100 mg/kg almorexant ($n = 10$/dose). In order to assess resulting BECs, immediately upon removal of ethanol bottles, blood samples were collected from the retro-orbital sinus and centrifuged. The plasma was assayed using an Analox Instruments analyzer (Lunenburg, MA).

In order to assess the specificity of drug effects on ethanol consumption, an additional group of ethanol-naïve animals was tested with sucrose solution (1% w/v) in the same DID paradigm (Days 1–3: 2-h access with saline injections; Day 4: 4-h test session with drug pretreatment). On the 4th day, vehicle, 3, 10, or 30 mg/kg ($n = 6$–7/dose) SB334867 was administered prior to the 4-h access period. During a subsequent week of testing, these same mice were administered either vehicle or 100 mg/kg almorexant ($n = 14$/dose) before the 4-h intake session. In a separate cohort of mice, vehicle or 60 mg/kg LSN2424100 ($n = 9$–10/dose) was administered prior to the 4-h test.

Data analysis

For subjects treated with SB334867 and LSN2424100 in the home cage drinking studies, ethanol and water intake (g/kg and ml/kg, respectively) during the first 3 h of the dark cycle were calculated and analyzed separately using repeated measures analyses of variance (ANOVAs), with drug dose as a within-subjects factor (IBM SPSS Statistics, Armonk, NY). The positive control, naltrexone, was compared with vehicle using an independent samples t-test. For subjects treated with almorexant, ethanol and water intake were analyzed using ANOVAs with drug dose as a between-subjects factor. The positive control, naltrexone, was compared with vehicle using an independent samples t-test. All significant within-subject effects were further explored using paired-samples t-tests, except for the between-subjects almorexant study, for which Tukey's HSD test was used.

For subjects treated with SB334867 and LSN2424100 in the operant progressive ratio paradigm, total active lever responses, total ethanol consumption (g/kg), and breakpoints (highest FR value reached) were calculated and analyzed via repeated measures ANOVAs, with dose as a within-subjects factor. The negative control, R-almorexant, was compared with vehicle using a separate paired samples t-test. All significant within-subject effects were further explored using paired-samples t-tests. Total responding on the inactive levers was negligible, so those data were not analyzed.

For the mouse drinking studies, ethanol consumption during each 4-h test session was expressed in g/kg and subjected to a One-Way ANOVA with dose as a between-subjects factor. BEC data (mg/dl) were analyzed similarly. Sucrose data were expressed as ml/kg and subjected to independent samples t-tests. Because only the doses of LSN2424100 and almorexant that reduced ethanol consumption were tested with sucrose, the 3 and 10 mg/kg SB334867 data were excluded from the analysis for consistency across compounds.

RESULTS

HOME CAGE 2-BOTTLE CHOICE DRINKING IN P RATS
SB334867
In the first experiment, rats received vehicle, 3, 10, or 30 mg/kg SB334867. A significant main effect of dose was observed [$F_{(3, 27)} = 4.36$, $p < 0.05$]. Follow-up paired-samples t-tests indicated that the 10 and 30 mg/kg doses of SB334867 significantly reduced ethanol intake relative to vehicle ($ps < 0.05$ and 0.01, respectively; **Figure 1A**, filled bars). No significant effects emerged in the analysis of water consumption ($p > 0.05$; **Figure 1A**, open bars).

LSN2424100
In the second experiment, rats received vehicle, 10, or 30 mg/kg LSN2424100, or 10 mg/kg naltrexone. As shown in **Figure 1B**, LSN2424100 did not significantly affect ethanol intake ($p > 0.05$; filled bars). However, a paired-samples t-test revealed that naltrexone significantly attenuated ethanol intake [$t_{(9)} = 3.31$, $p < 0.015$]. Neither LSN2424100 nor naltrexone produced significant effects on water intake ($ps > 0.05$; **Figure 1B**, open bars).

Almorexant
In the third experiment, rats received vehicle, 60 or 100 mg/kg almorexant, or 10 mg/kg naltrexone in a between-subjects design. Almorexant significantly reduced ethanol intake [$F_{(2, 20)} = 3.12$, $p = 0.05$]. A *post-hoc* Tukey's HSD test revealed that only the 100 mg/kg dose of almorexant significantly affected ethanol intake, while effects at the 60 mg/kg dose were not statistically significant (**Figure 1C**, filled bars). An independent-samples t-test revealed that naltrexone also significantly reduced ethanol consumption [$t_{(13)} = 3.08$, $p < 0.01$; **Figure 1C**, filled

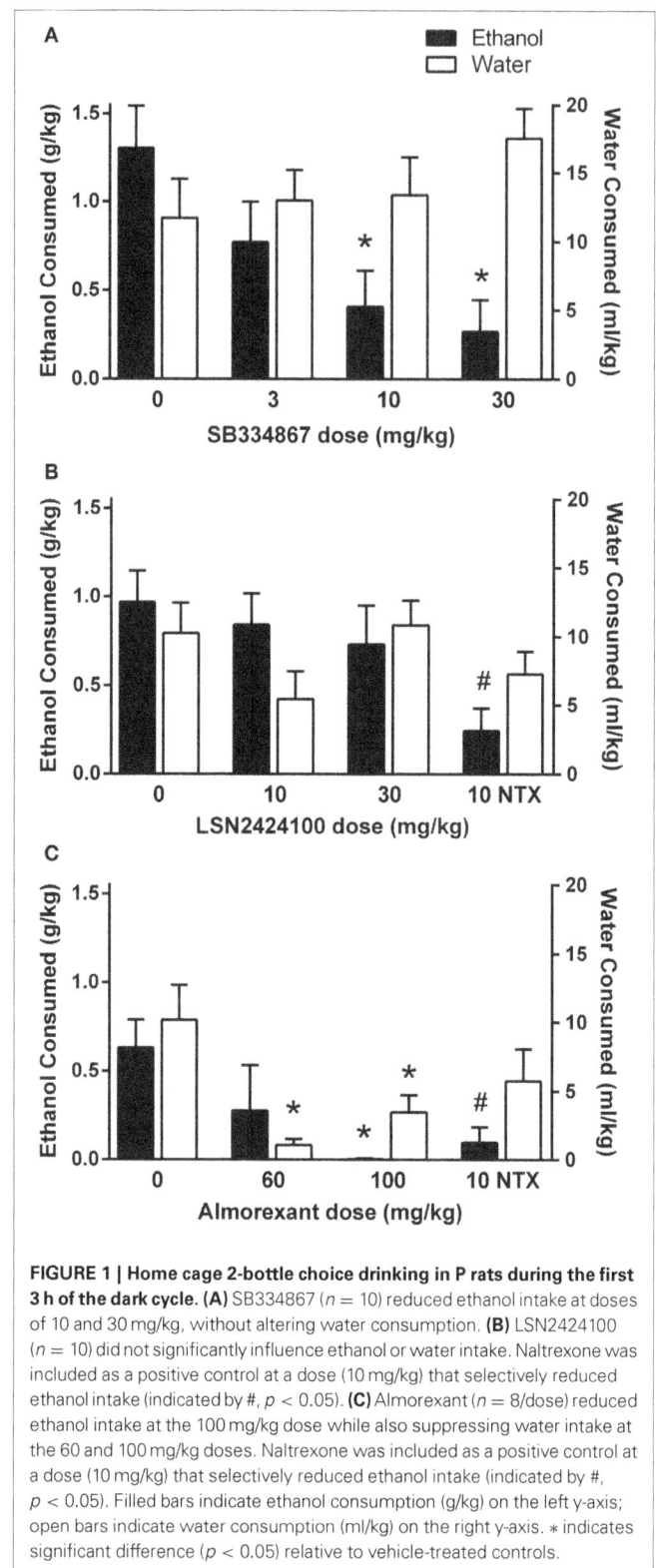

FIGURE 1 | Home cage 2-bottle choice drinking in P rats during the first 3 h of the dark cycle. (A) SB334867 ($n = 10$) reduced ethanol intake at doses of 10 and 30 mg/kg, without altering water consumption. (B) LSN2424100 ($n = 10$) did not significantly influence ethanol or water intake. Naltrexone was included as a positive control at a dose (10 mg/kg) that selectively reduced ethanol intake (indicated by #, $p < 0.05$). (C) Almorexant ($n = 8$/dose) reduced ethanol intake at the 100 mg/kg dose while also suppressing water intake at the 60 and 100 mg/kg doses. Naltrexone was included as a positive control at a dose (10 mg/kg) that selectively reduced ethanol intake (indicated by #, $p < 0.05$). Filled bars indicate ethanol consumption (g/kg) on the left y-axis; open bars indicate water consumption (ml/kg) on the right y-axis. * indicates significant difference ($p < 0.05$) relative to vehicle-treated controls.

bars]. Almorexant significantly reduced home cage water intake [$F_{(2, 21)} = 10.60$, $p < 0.01$; **Figure 1C**, open bars]. A *post-hoc* Tukey's HSD test revealed that both the 60 and 100 mg/kg doses of almorexant significantly reduced water consumption ($ps < 0.01$).

OPERANT PROGRESSIVE RATIO RESPONDING IN P RATS

SB334867

Although a trend toward efficacy was observed for SB334867 on progressive ratio responding for ethanol, statistical analysis revealed no significant effects of the drug on the number of active lever responses (data not shown), breakpoints (**Figure 2A**), or total ethanol consumption (**Figure 2B**; all $ps > 0.05$).

LSN2424100

The OX_2 antagonist LSN2424100 significantly reduced breakpoints [main effect of dose: $F_{(3, 36)} = 4.61$, $p < 0.01$] and resulting ethanol consumption [main effect of dose: $F_{(3, 36)} = 6.59$, $p < 0.01$]. *Post-hoc* tests indicated that the 30 mg/kg dose

was significantly different from vehicle (see **Figures 2C,D**). LSN2424100 also significantly reduced active lever presses [$F_{(3, 27)} = 3.67$, $p < 0.05$; data not shown].

Almorexant

Almorexant significantly reduced active lever presses [main effect of dose: $F_{(3, 24)} = 25.26$, $p < 0.001$]. Paired-samples t-tests indicated that doses of 10, 30, and 60 mg/kg significantly reduced active lever responding ($ps < 0.05$; data not shown). A paired-samples t-test indicated that the inactive enantiomer of almorexant did not significantly affect responses on the active lever ($p > 0.05$). Similarly, almorexant significantly reduced breakpoints [$F_{(3, 24)} = 32.32$, $p < 0.001$], with significant effects at doses of

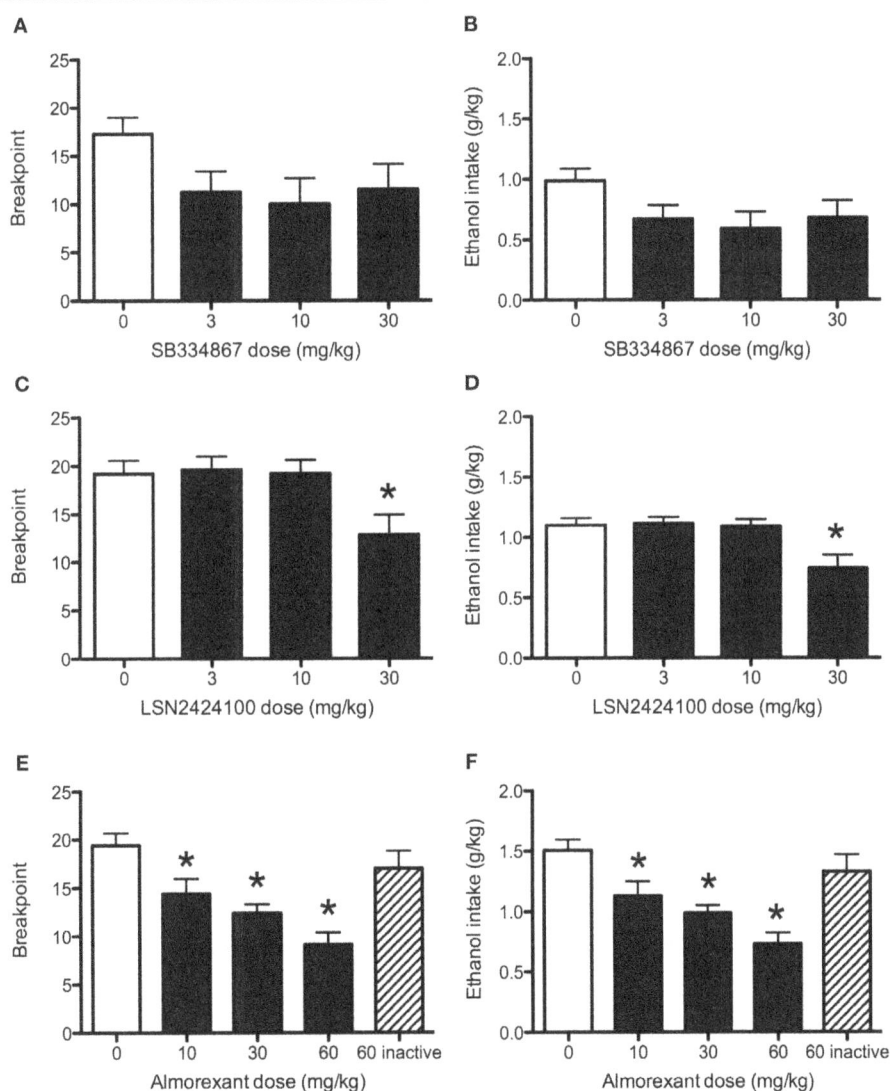

FIGURE 2 | Operant progressive ratio responding in P rats. SB334867 ($n = 8$) did not significantly reduce breakpoints **(A)** or ethanol consumption **(B)** maintained by a progressive ratio operant schedule of reinforcement. The 30 mg/kg dose of LSN2424100 ($n = 10$) reduced the motivation to consume ethanol as indicated by reductions in breakpoints **(C)** and corresponding ethanol consumption **(D)**. **(E,F)** Almorexant ($n = 10$) reduced breakpoints and

ethanol consumption at all doses tested (10, 30, and 60 mg/kg) doses. As expected, the inactive enantiomer (60 mg/kg) did not significantly affect progressive ratio operant responding for ethanol or ethanol consumption. Breakpoint was defined as the highest fixed ratio value reached by rats during the operant session. ∗ indicates significant difference ($p < 0.05$) relative to vehicle-treated controls.

10 ($p < 0.01$), 30 and 60 mg/kg ($ps < 0.001$; **Figure 2E**), while the inactive enantiomer did not ($p > 0.05$). Almorexant also significantly attenuated ethanol consumption [$F_{(3, 24)} = 32.29, p < 0.001$] at doses of 10 ($p < 0.01$), 30, and 60 mg/kg ($ps < 0.001$; **Figure 2F**). A paired-samples t-test indicated that the inactive R-enantiomer of almorexant did not significantly affect ethanol consumption ($p > 0.05$).

BINGE DRINKING IN C57BL/6J MICE
SB334867
Analysis revealed a main effect of dose [$F_{(3, 36)} = 3.6, p < 0.05$], with the 30 mg/kg SB334867 dose reducing ethanol intake relative to vehicle-injected controls (**Figure 3A**). BEC data indicated a similar pattern, with a main effect of dose emerging [$F_{(3, 36)} = 4.4, p < 0.05$]. While *post-hoc* tests revealed no significant differences between vehicle and any doses of SB334867, pairwise comparisons indicated that the 30 mg/kg dose resulted in lower BECs than both the 3 and 10 mg/kg doses (**Figure 3B**). Analysis of sucrose consumption (**Figure 3C**) revealed that 30 mg/kg SB334867 suppressed sucrose intake relative to vehicle [$t_{(11)} = 2.74, p < 0.05$].

LSN2424100
Analysis of ethanol intake on the test day revealed a main effect of dose [$F_{(3, 35)} = 4.3, p < 0.05$], with the 60 mg/kg dose reducing ethanol consumption relative to vehicle-injected control mice (**Figure 3D**). This reduction was mirrored in BEC data [main effect of dose: $F_{(3, 35)} = 6.1, p < 0.01$], with the 60 mg/kg dose resulting in lower BECs (**Figure 3E**). Analysis of sucrose consumption data (**Figure 3F**) revealed a significant suppression in mice administered the 60 mg/kg dose relative to vehicle [$t_{(17)} = 8.76, p < 0.001$].

Almorexant
Analysis revealed a main effect of dose [$F_{(3, 36)} = 5.0, p < 0.01$], with the 100 mg/kg dose reducing ethanol intake relative to vehicle-injected controls (**Figure 3G**). Analysis of BEC data also revealed a main effect of dose [$F_{(3, 36)} = 9.0, p < 0.001$], with both the 50 and 100 mg/kg doses of almorexant resulting in lower BECs than vehicle-treated control mice (**Figure 3H**). Analysis of sucrose consumption data revealed a trend ($p = 0.085$) for almorexant to reduce sucrose consumption, an effect that did not reach statistical significance (**Figure 3I**).

DISCUSSION
Data from the present series of experiments provide evidence that blockade of OX_1 and OX_2 receptors reduces ethanol self-administration in a variety of high-drinking rodent paradigms, although observed effects were dependent on the specific procedures used to evaluate ethanol-seeking behavior. The OX_1 receptor antagonist reduced home cage ethanol drinking in rats and binge-like drinking in mice, without influencing progressive ratio operant responding in rats. Blockade of OX_2 receptors did not alter home-cage ethanol intake in rats, but did lower breakpoints and reduce ethanol consumption in the progressive ratio procedure in P rats as well as reducing binge-like drinking in mice. Dual antagonism of OX_1 and OX_2 receptors resulted in reduced ethanol

consumption in rats and mice in addition to decreasing breakpoints and ethanol consumption in the operant progressive ratio model. Due to an established role for orexin in the regulation of feeding behavior, it was important to assess the specificity of these drug effects by measuring the ability of the these compounds to alter consumption of another caloric solution. Indeed, results from the present study indicated that some of the test compounds also reduced sucrose consumption in mice.

The majority of previous work exploring the role of orexin in ethanol reward has focused on blockade of OX_1 receptors with SB334867, with this compound typically reducing ethanol self-administration (Lawrence et al., 2006; Richards et al., 2008; Moorman and Aston-Jones, 2009; Jupp et al., 2011). In accordance with these findings, we demonstrate here that SB334867 reduced home cage ethanol intake in P rats with a long history of ethanol consumption. SB334867 has been previously shown to reduce breakpoints in an operant progressive ratio procedure in male iP rats (Jupp et al., 2011). In contrast, SB334867 did not significantly alter breakpoints or corresponding ethanol consumption in female P rats in the present study. It is unclear whether this discrepancy can be attributed to sex differences, experimental procedural differences, or differences between respective inbred lines. In the current study, we reported for the first time that SB334867 reduced binge-like ethanol intake in the drinking-in-the-dark procedure in mice. Oddly, the BEC values reported in the vehicle-injected mice were lower than expected given the high ethanol consumption. This apparent disparity may be a consequence of the long length of the testing period. Although not assessed in the current study, different patterns of ethanol consumption over the 4-h period may have resulted in different BEC values. The dose of SB334867 that effectively reduced ethanol intake also suppressed consumption of a 1% sucrose solution. However, previous reports indicate that SB334867 did not affect operant self-administration of a 5% sucrose solution (Richards et al., 2008). It is tempting to speculate that self-administration of the 1% sucrose solution used in the current experiments may be more susceptible to disruption by OX antagonists because it is less palatable to the mice than the 5% sucrose solution in other studies. Further experiments will be required to explore this possibility. Overall, the data reported herein complement and extend previous literature reports demonstrating that SB334867 attenuates ethanol self-administration.

Although previous work has examined OX_2 receptor involvement in operant ethanol self-administration and reinstatement procedures, the present study is the first to examine the effects of OX_2 antagonism on voluntary home cage ethanol consumption, breakpoints in an operant progressive ratio procedure, and binge-like ethanol drinking using the novel compound LSN2424100. This OX_2 antagonist did not alter ethanol consumption under voluntary continuous access conditions in P rats but did reduce breakpoints in the operant progressive ratio procedure, indicating reduced motivation to consume ethanol (Richardson and Roberts, 1996) in alcohol-preferring rats. Consistent with the reduction in operant breakpoints, LSN2424100 also decreased ethanol intake in the progressive ratio model. Our data are consistent with and complement earlier studies in which other selective OX_2 receptor antagonists (JNJ-10397049 and

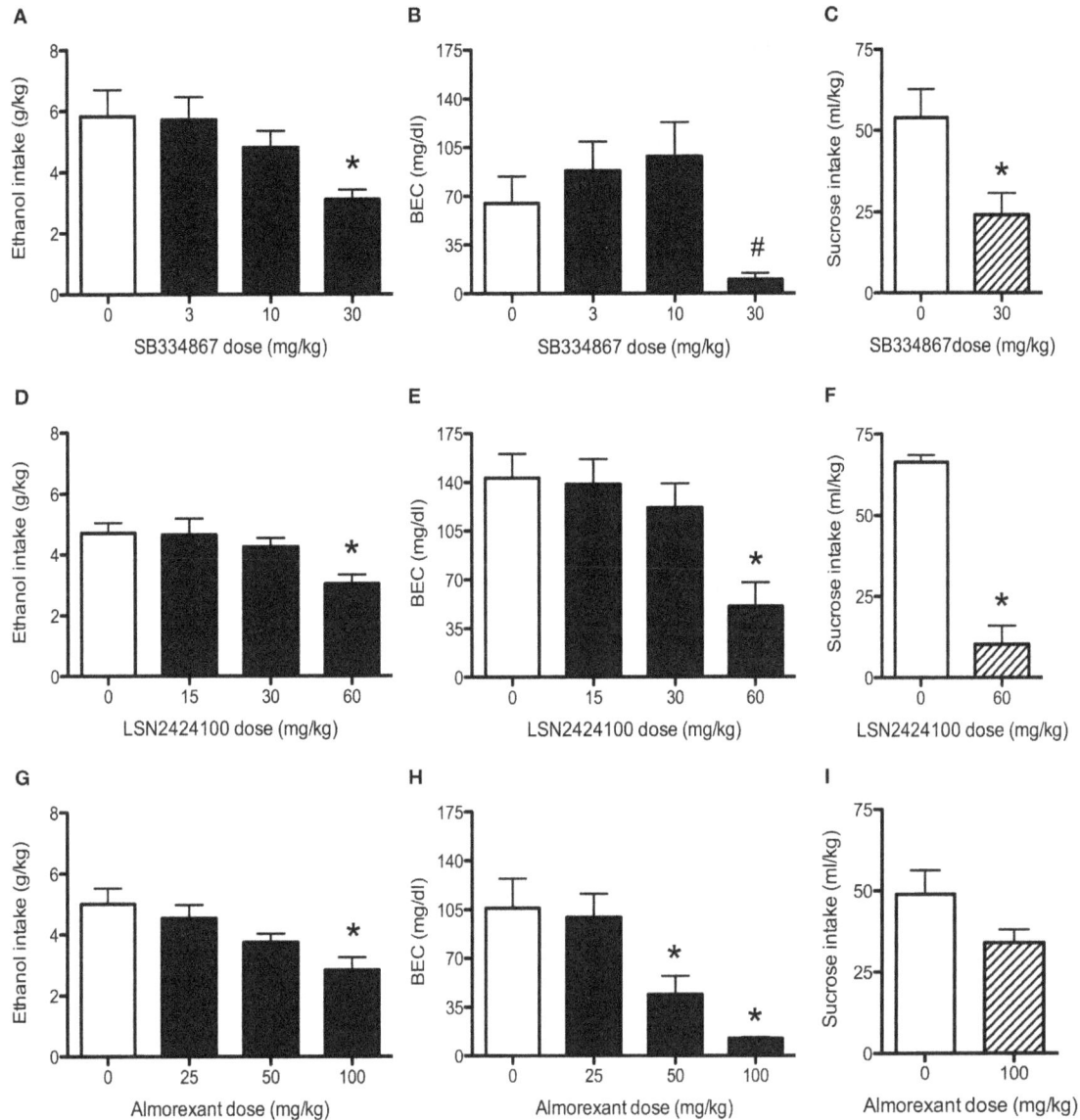

FIGURE 3 | Binge drinking in C57BL/6J mice. (A) SB334867 ($n = 10$) reduced ethanol consumption at the 30 mg/kg dose. **(B)** The 30 mg/kg dose of SB334867 resulted in lower BECs relative to both the 10 and 30 mg/kg doses (indicated by #, $p < 0.05$). **(C)** In a separate cohort of mice, SB334867 (30 mg/kg) also reduced consumption of a 1% sucrose solution ($n = 6$–7). **(D)** LSN2424100 ($n = 10$) reduced ethanol consumption at the 60 mg/kg dose. **(E)** The same dose resulted in lower BECs relative to vehicle-injected controls. **(F)** The 60 mg/kg dose of LSN2424100 significantly reduced consumption of a 1% sucrose solution ($n = 9$–10). **(G)** Almorexant ($n = 10$) reduced ethanol intake at the 100 mg/kg dose. **(H)** Both the 50 and 100 mg/kg doses of almorexant resulted in lower BECs. **(I)** In a separate cohort of mice, almorexant (100 mg/kg) did not significantly reduce consumption of a 1% sucrose solution ($n = 14$). ∗ indicates significant difference ($p < 0.05$) relative to vehicle-injected controls.

TCS-OX2-29) decreased ethanol self-administration using other operant paradigms in rats (Shoblock et al., 2011; Brown et al., 2013).

Because it is well-known that OX antagonists reduce wakefulness and suppress motor activity in general (e.g., Brisbare-Roch et al., 2007), one might argue that the breakpoint reduction seen in P rats is simply due to reduced locomotor activity. This is unlikely given that the same dose of LSN2424100 (30 mg/kg) did not alter ethanol or water consumption in the home cage drinking procedure reported here. Indeed, although OX receptor antagonists facilitate sleep, they do not produce overt motor impairment or sedative-like effects that are commonly associated with benzodiazepine receptor agonists, such as zolpidem (Steiner et al., 2011). To the contrary, rats receiving OX receptor antagonists, including those tested here, can perform operant and other motor tasks without any observable impairment (Steiner et al., 2011; Rorick-Kehn et al., unpublished observations). That LSN2424100 reduced ethanol self-administration in the operant progressive ratio assay, but not when ethanol was provided under unlimited access conditions, may suggest that OX_2

receptor-mediated signaling does not directly modulate ethanol reward. Rather, OX_2 receptors may be involved in modulating motivational circuits in the brain that underlie drug-seeking behavior. Indeed, it is not uncommon for drugs to differentially influence ethanol's appetitive/motivational effects vs. consummatory behavior (ethanol drinking *per se*) (e.g., Czachowski et al., 2001, 2002). Alternatively, the differential efficacy of LSN2424100 in these two procedures may reflect the varying ethanol histories of the rats tested in each model.

In mice, a high dose of LSN2424100 (60 mg/kg) reduced ethanol consumption in the binge-like drinking procedure; however, the same dose also suppressed sucrose consumption, suggesting that this dose was high enough to produce non-specific effects. Whether the suppression in sucrose intake reflects sleep-promoting effects or a general reduction in consummatory behaviors cannot be determined from the present series of studies. It is interesting that the reduction in sucrose intake (~85% reduction) was more dramatic than the reduction in ethanol intake (~36% reduction). The reasons for this difference are not clear. Further work will be necessary to better characterize the nature of these effects.

Antagonism of both OX_1 and OX_2 receptors by almorexant reduced ethanol drinking in rats with continuous home-cage access and in limited access binge-drinking in mice, and also attenuated breakpoints and ethanol consumption in the progressive ratio model in rats. The data presented here confirm and extend previous reports that almorexant suppressed operant self-administration of both ethanol and sucrose in Long-Evans rats (Srinivasan et al., 2012). Importantly, we demonstrate here that the inactive enantiomer of almorexant did not suppress breakpoints or ethanol self-administration in rats, indicating that the effect was specific to blockade of OX_1 and OX_2 receptors rather than unknown off-target pharmacological effects. Our data in regard to the specificity of almorexant effects were mixed. Specifically, almorexant reduced home-cage water drinking in rats, suggesting potential non-specific effects on fluid consumption, but it did not significantly attenuate sucrose intake in the mice. Almorexant has previously been shown to reduce operant responding for both ethanol and 5% sucrose when administered systemically; however, when administered directly into the VTA, effects were selective for ethanol (Srinivasan et al., 2012). In the current report, it is unclear whether the reduced water intake in rats, and the tendency for reduced sucrose intake in mice, reflects non-specific consummatory effects or transient sedative effects that may dissipate over the course of the extended drinking session. Additional examination of the selectivity of effects of the compounds tested in the present work, including assays of locomotor activity, is warranted.

The drinking paradigms employed in the present study involved different amounts of total ethanol exposure. Previous studies have reported alterations in the orexin system following long-term ethanol exposure. For example, chronic voluntary ethanol consumption (~5 g/kg/day for 70 days) has been reported to upregulate hypothalamic preproorexin mRNA in P rats (Lawrence et al., 2006) whereas a reduction in orexin mRNA has been reported after chronic ethanol consumption (~0.75–2.5 g/kg/day for 28 days) in Sprague-Dawley rats (Morganstern et al., 2010). Several methodological differences

between the two studies may account for the seemingly contradictory results, including differences in total daily ethanol exposure (~5 g/kg/day vs. ~0.75–2.5 g/kg/day), differences in genetic background (selectively bred P rats vs. Sprague-Dawley rats), and end-point measured (preproorexin vs. orexin A mRNA). Nonetheless, further studies will be required to determine the impact of long-term ethanol exposure on the brain orexin system, and whether adaptations in orexin signaling resulting from chronic ethanol exposure contribute to the development of addiction. Indeed, others have demonstrated that orexin-A stimulates dopamine cell firing in the VTA, increases dopamine release in the prefrontal cortex (PFC), and potentiates PFC-evoked excitation of VTA dopamine cells (Narita et al., 2006; Vittoz and Berridge, 2006; Moorman and Aston-Jones, 2010). Moreover, Borgland et al. (2006) demonstrated that orexin signaling in the VTA plays a critical role in synaptic plasticity associated with cocaine addiction. The relevance of orexin-mediated signaling in critical processes associated with addiction to drugs of abuse, including ethanol, is beginning to be understood, and will likely be further informed by the development and characterization of additional selective tool compounds from different chemical scaffolds, such as LSN2424100 reported here, that can be used to explore the relative roles of OX_1- and OX_2-receptor-mediated signaling. Future studies in models of ethanol dependence using selective pharmacological tools may provide valuable information about the therapeutic potential of orexin antagonists for the treatment of alcohol abuse and alcoholism.

ACKNOWLEDGMENTS

Financial support for P-rat studies was provided by Eli Lilly and Company. Mouse studies were supported by NIH/NIAAA grants to Howard C. Becker (P50 AA010761, U01 AA014095, and U01 AA020929) and the Department of Veterans Affairs. Rachel I. Anderson is supported by NIH/NIAAA grant T32 AA007474.

REFERENCES

Aston-Jones, G., Smith, R. J., Sartor, G. C., Moorman, D. E., Massi, L., Tahsili-Fahadan, P., et al. (2010). Lateral hypothalamic orexin/hypocretin neurons: a role in reward-seeking and addiction. *Brain Res.* 1314, 74–90. doi: 10.1016/j.brainres.2009.09.106

Borgland, S. L., Taha, S. A., Sarti, F., Fields, H. L., and Bonci, A. (2006). Orexin A in the VTA is critical for the induction of synaptic plasticity and behavioral sensitization to cocaine. *Neuron* 49, 589–601. doi: 10.1016/j.neuron.2006.01.016

Brisbare-Roch, C., Dingemanse, J., Koberstein, R., Hoever, P., Aissaoui, H., Flores, S., et al. (2007). Promotion of sleep by targeting the orexin system in rats, dogs and humans. *Nat. Med.* 13, 150–155. doi: 10.1038/nm1544

Brown, R. M., Khoo, S. Y., and Lawrence, A. J. (2013). Central orexin (hypocretin) 2 receptor antagonism reduces ethanol self-administration, but not cue-conditioned ethanol-seeking, in ethanol-preferring rats. *Int. J. Neuropsychopharmacol.* 16, 2067–2079. doi: 10.1017/S1461145713000333

Czachowski, C. L., Legg, B. H., and Samson, H. H. (2001). Effects of acamprosate on ethanol-seeking and self-administration in the rat. *Alcohol. Clin. Exp. Res.* 25, 344–350. doi: 10.1111/j.1530-0277.2001.tb02220.x

Czachowski, C. L., Santini, L. A., Legg, B. H., and Samson, H. H. (2002). Separate measures of ethanol seeking and drinking in the rat: effects of remoxipride. *Alcohol* 28, 39–46. doi: 10.1016/S0741-8329(02)00236-7

Dhaher, R., Hauser, S. R., Getachew, B., Bell, R. L., McBride, W. J., McKinzie, D. L., et al. (2010). The orexin-1 receptor antagonist SB-334867 reduces alcohol relapse drinking, but not alcohol-seeking, in alcohol-preferring (P) rats. *J. Addict. Med.* 4, 153–159. doi: 10.1097/ADM.0b013e3181bd893f

Fitch, T. E., Benvenga, M. J., Jesudason, C. D., Zink, C., Vandergriff, A. B., Menezes, M. M., et al. (2014). LSN2424100: a novel, potent orexin-2 receptor antagonist with selectivity over orexin-1 receptors and activity in an animal model predictive of antidepressant-like efficacy. *Front. Neurosci.* 8:5. doi: 10.3389/fnins.2014.00005

Harris, G. C., and Aston-Jones, G. (2006). Arousal and reward: a dichotomy in orexin function. *Trends Neurosci.* 29, 571–577. doi: 10.1016/j.tins.2006.08.002

Jupp, B., Krivdic, B., Krstew, E., and Lawrence, A. J. (2011). The orexin(1) receptor antagonist SB-334867 dissociates the motivational properties of alcohol and sucrose in rats. *Brain Res.* 1391, 54–59. doi: 10.1016/j.brainres.2011.03.045

Kim, A. K., Brown, R. M., and Lawrence, A. J. (2012). The role of orexins/hypocretins in alcohol use and abuse: an appetitive-reward relationship. *Front. Behav. Neurosci.* 6:78. doi: 10.3389/fnbeh.2012.00078

Lawrence, A. J., Cowen, M. S., Yang, H. J., Chen, F., and Oldfield, B. (2006). The orexin system regulates alcohol-seeking in rats. *Br. J. Pharmacol.* 148, 752–759. doi: 10.1038/sj.bjp.0706789

Mahler, S. V., Smith, R. J., Moorman, D. E., Sartor, G. C., and Aston-Jones, G. (2012). Multiple roles for orexin/hypocretin in addiction. *Prog. Brain Res.* 198, 79–121. doi: 10.1016/B978-0-444-59489-1.00007-0

Moorman, D. E., and Aston-Jones, G. (2009). Orexin-1 receptor antagonism decreases ethanol consumption and preference selectively in high-ethanol–preferring Sprague–Dawley rats. *Alcohol* 43, 379–386. doi: 10.1016/j.alcohol.2009.07.002

Moorman, D. E., and Aston-Jones, G. (2010). Orexin/hypocretin modulates response of ventral tegmental dopamine neurons to prefrontal activation: diurnal influences. *J. Neurosci.* 30, 15585–15599. doi: 10.1523/JNEUROSCI.2871-10.2010

Morganstern, I., Chang, G. Q., Barson, J. R., Ye, Z., Karatayev, O., and Leibowitz, S. F. (2010). Differential effects of acute and chronic ethanol exposure on orexin expression in the perifornical lateral hypothalamus. *Alcohol. Clin. Exp. Res.* 34, 886–896. doi: 10.1111/j.1530-0277.2010.01161.x

Narita, M., Nagumo, Y., Hashimoto, S., Narita, M., Khotib, J., Miyatake, M., et al. (2006). Direct involvement of orexinergic systems in the activation of the mesolimbic dopamine pathway and related behaviors induced by morphine. *J. Neurosci.* 26, 398–405. doi: 10.1523/JNEUROSCI.2761-05.2006

Rhodes, J. S., Best, K., Belknap, J. K., Finn, D. A., and Crabbe, J. C. (2005). Evaluation of a simple model of ethanol drinking to intoxication in C57BL/6J mice. *Physiol. Behav.* 84, 53–63. doi: 10.1016/j.physbeh.2004.10.007

Richards, J. K., Simms, J. A., Steensland, P., Taha, S. A., Borgland, S. L., Bonci, A., et al. (2008). Inhibition of orexin-1/hypocretin-1 receptors inhibits yohimbine-induced reinstatement of ethanol and sucrose seeking in Long-Evans rats. *Psychopharmacology (Berl.)* 199, 109–117. doi: 10.1007/s00213-008-1136-5

Richardson, N. R., and Roberts, D. C. S. (1996). Progressive ratio schedules in drug self-administration studies in rats: a method to evaluate reinforcing efficacy. *J. Neurosci. Methods* 66, 1–11. doi: 10.1016/0165-0270(95)00153-0

Rodd, Z. A., Bell, R. L., Kuc, K. A., Murphy, J. M., Lumeng, L., Li, T. K., et al. (2003). Effects of repeated alcohol deprivations on operant ethanol self-administration by alcohol-preferring (P) rats. *Neuropsychopharmacology* 28, 1614–1621. doi: 10.1038/sj.npp.1300214

Sakurai, T. (2002). Roles of orexins in the regulation of feeding and arousal. *Sleep Med.* 3(Suppl. 2), S3–S9. doi: 10.1016/S1389-9457(02)00156-9

Sakurai, T., Amemiya, A., Ishii, M., Matsuzaki, I., Chemelli, R. M., Tanaka, H., et al. (1998). Orexins and orexin receptors: a family of hypothalamic neuropeptides and G protein-coupled receptors that regulate feeding behavior. *Cell* 92, 573–585. doi: 10.1016/S0092-8674(00)80949-6

Schneider, E. R., Rada, P., Darby, R. D., Leibowitz, S. F., and Hoebel, B. G. (2007). Orexigenic peptides and alcohol intake: differential effects of orexin, galanin, and ghrelin. *Alcohol. Clin. Exp. Res.* 31, 1858–1865. doi: 10.1111/j.1530-0277.2007.00510.x

Sharf, R., Sarhan, M., and Dileone, R. J. (2010). Role of orexin/hypocretin in dependence and addiction. *Brain Res.* 1314, 130–138. doi: 10.1016/j.brainres.2009.08.028

Shoblock, J. R., Welty, N., Aluisio, L., Fraser, I., Motley, S. T., Morton, K., et al. (2011). Selective blockade of the orexin-2 receptor attenuates ethanol self-administration, place preference, and reinstatement. *Psychopharmacology (Berl.)* 215, 191–203. doi: 10.1007/s00213-010-2127-x

Smart, D., Sabido-David, C., Brough, S. J., Jewitt, F., Johns, A., Porter, R. A., et al. (2001). SB-334867-A: the first selective orexin-1 receptor antagonist. *Br. J. Pharmacol.* 132, 1179–1182. doi: 10.1038/sj.bjp.0703953

Srinivasan, S., Simms, J. A., Nielsen, C. K., Lieske, S. P., and Bito-Onon, J. J., Yi, H., et al. (2012). The dual orexin/hypocretin receptor antagonist, almorexant, in the ventral tegmental area attenuates ethanol self-administration. *PLoS ONE* 7:e44726. doi: 10.1371/journal.pone.0044726

Steiner, M. A., Lecourt, H., Strasser, D. S., Brisbare-Roch, C., and Jenck, F. (2011). Differential effects of the dual orexin receptor antagonist almorexant and the GABA(A)-alpha1 receptor modulator zolpidem, alone or combined with ethanol, on motor performance in the rat. *Neuropsychopharmacology* 36, 848–856. doi: 10.1038/npp.2010.224

Vittoz, N. M., and Berridge, C. W. (2006). Hypocretin/orexin selectively increases dopamine efflux within the prefrontal cortex: involvement of the ventral tegmental area. *Neuropsychopharmacology* 31, 384–395. doi: 10.1038/sj.npp.1300807

Willie, J. T., Chemelli, R. M., Sinton, C. M., and Yanagisawa, M. (2001). To eat or to sleep? Orexin in the regulation of feeding and wakefulness. *Annu. Rev. Neurosci.* 24, 429–458. doi: 10.1146/annurev.neuro.24.1.429

Conflict of Interest Statement: Financial support for P-rat studies was provided by Eli Lilly and Company. Benjamin L. Adams, Cynthia D. Jesudason, and Linda M. Rorick-Kehn are employees of, and stockholders in, Eli Lilly and Company.

Orexin antagonists for neuropsychiatric disease: progress and potential pitfalls

Jiann Wei Yeoh[†], Erin J. Campbell[†], Morgan H. James[†], Brett A. Graham and Christopher V. Dayas*

Neurobiology of Addiction Laboratory, The Centre for Translational Neuroscience and Mental Health Research, School of Biomedical Sciences and Pharmacy, University of Newcastle and the Hunter Medical Research Institute, Newcastle, NSW, Australia

Edited by:
Michel A. Steiner, Actelion Pharmaceuticals Ltd., Switzerland

Reviewed by:
Andrew Lawrence, Florey Neuroscience Institutes, Australia
Remi Martin-Fardon, The Scripps Research Institute, USA
Ronald See, Medical University of South Carolina, USA

*Correspondence:
Christopher V. Dayas, Neurobiology of Addiction Laboratory, The Centre for Translational Neuroscience and Mental Health Research, School of Biomedical Sciences and Pharmacy, University of Newcastle and the Hunter Medical Research Institute, Medical Sciences Building, Newcastle, NSW 2308, Australia
e-mail: christopher.dayas@newcastle.edu.au

[†]These authors have contributed equally to this work.

The tight regulation of sleep/wake states is critical for mental and physiological wellbeing. For example, dysregulation of sleep/wake systems predisposes individuals to metabolic disorders such as obesity and psychiatric problems, including depression. Contributing to this understanding, the last decade has seen significant advances in our appreciation of the complex interactions between brain systems that control the transition between sleep and wake states. Pivotal to our increased understanding of this pathway was the description of a group of neurons in the lateral hypothalamus (LH) that express the neuropeptides orexin A and B (hypocretin, Hcrt-1 and Hcrt-2). Orexin neurons were quickly placed at center stage with the demonstration that loss of normal orexin function is associated with the development of narcolepsy—a condition in which sufferers fail to maintain normal levels of daytime wakefulness. Since these initial seminal findings, much progress has been made in our understanding of the physiology and function of the orexin system. For example, the orexin system has been identified as a key modulator of autonomic and neuroendocrine function, arousal, reward and attention. Notably, studies in animals suggest that dysregulation of orexin function is associated with neuropsychiatric states such as addiction and mood disorders including depression and anxiety. This review discusses the progress associated with therapeutic attempts to restore orexin system function and treat neuropsychiatric conditions such as addiction, depression and anxiety. We also highlight potential pitfalls and challenges associated with targeting this system to treat these neuropsychiatric states.

Keywords: hypothalamus, orexin, stress, anxiety, depression, cocaine, reinstatement, reward seeking

OVERVIEW—THE OREXIN SYSTEM IN BRIEF

First described in 1996, the orexins are two neuropeptides expressed by a few thousand neurons within the perifornical area (PFA), the dorsomedial hypothalamus (DMH) and the lateral hypothalamus (LH) (de Lecea et al., 1998; Sakurai et al., 1998). The binding target of these ligands, termed orexin A and B, are two G-protein coupled receptors OxR1 and OxR2 (de Lecea et al., 1998; Sakurai et al., 1998). Orexin A is non-selective for both OxR1 and OxR2 whereas orexin B is more selective for OxR2 (Sakurai et al., 1998; Ammoun et al., 2003). A key feature of this relatively small population of neurons is their widespread projections throughout the brain, including other hypothalamic nuclei, the midline paraventricular thalamus (PVT), brain stem nuclei and a number of structures involved in reward behavior including the ventral tegmental area (VTA) and nucleus accumbens shell (NACs) (Peyron et al., 1998). In these projection areas, the expression of orexin receptor subtypes is partially overlapping, however, some regions preferentially express one receptor subtype, presumably providing some degree of selectivity (certainly in terms of potential pharmacological selectivity of different target regions). For example, the prefrontal cortex predominantly expresses OxR1, whereas the nucleus accumbens (NAC) mainly expresses OxR2 (Marcus et al., 2001).

Consistent with the widespread projections of these neurons, orexins have been implicated in a number of physiological functions, including regulation of sleep (Chemelli et al., 1999), energy metabolism (Burdakov et al., 2005), arousal (Sutcliffe and de Lecea, 2002; Taheri et al., 2002), behavioral and neuroendocrine responses to stress (Ida et al., 2000; Furlong et al., 2009) and reward-seeking behavior (Boutrel et al., 2005; Harris et al., 2005; Lawrence et al., 2006; Marchant et al., 2012). The role of orexin in this diverse range of functions has been reviewed extensively elsewhere (Boutrel and de Lecea, 2008; Aston-Jones et al., 2010; Boutrel et al., 2010; Lawrence, 2010; James et al., 2012; Mahler et al., 2012). In this review, we will highlight new research focused on changes in the intra-hypothalamic LH-orexin circuitry induced by drugs of abuse and stress. We will also outline recent data highlighting the clinical potential of single and dual orexin receptor antagonists (SORAs and DORAs) for neuropsychiatric conditions including addiction, anxiety and depression. However, we also discuss recent findings indicating that several challenges must be overcome for the therapeutic value of SORAs and DORAs to be fully realized.

CELLULAR AND MOLECULAR EVIDENCE FOR TARGETING THE LH-OREXIN SYSTEM IN DRUG ADDICTION

Until recently, work on the relationship between the orexin system and addiction has been heavily focused on the antagonism of orexin actions in downstream projection areas (James et al., 2011; Brown et al., 2013; Mahler et al., 2013). At the same time, the issue of how drugs of addiction might alter the properties of orexin neurons has been largely overlooked. Interestingly, gene expression analysis has shown that the LH is highly transcriptionally responsive to addictive drugs (Ahmed et al., 2005). Ahmed et al. (2005) found that rats given extended access to cocaine displayed a profound increase in both pre- and post-synaptic markers of plasticity in the LH. Further, studies from the feeding literature suggest that excitatory inputs onto orexin neurons can undergo significant rewiring in response to food-deprivation and re-feeding. These results suggest that the LH orexin circuitry is likely to undergo experience-dependent neuroplasticity in response to cocaine treatment.

Given the above evidence, our group has undertaken a series of studies to assess how drugs might remodel LH orexin circuits. In these experiments, rats were exposed to 7 days of cocaine injections or allowed to self-administer cocaine for 14 days before excitatory synaptic transmission was assessed in LH slices. This work showed that both experimenter- and self-administered cocaine significantly increased excitatory drive in the LH through pre-synaptic mechanisms, assessed using mEPSCs frequency, amplitude and paired pulse ratio (Yeoh et al., 2012). Consistent with our electrophysiological findings, the number of putative excitatory but not inhibitory inputs onto PFA/LH cells were significantly increased, as measured by immunolabeling for vesicular glutamate transporter 2 (VGLUT2) or vesicular GABA transporter (VGAT; Yeoh et al., 2012). Importantly, a population of recorded neurons that were recovered with neurobiotin labeling and immunolabeled for orexin confirmed that these increases in excitatory drive occurred in orexin neurons.

Somewhat surprisingly, a recent study by a different group failed to find evidence of pre-synaptic plasticity in orexin neurons after 3 days of cocaine exposure (Rao et al., 2013). However, this regimen of cocaine exposure did promote long-term potentiation (LTP) at glutamate synapses onto orexin neurons, which persisted for more than 5 days post-withdrawal (Rao et al., 2013). The differences in the Rao et al. (2013) study and our own may in part be explained by differences in experimental procedures. In our study, we carried out both intraperitoneal (i.p) injections and cocaine self-administration in rats as compared to the Rao study, which employed a conditioned place preference (CPP) model whereby mice received only experimenter-administered cocaine injections. Animals that underwent i.p injections in our study received a slightly higher dose of cocaine for a longer period of time as compared to Rao and colleagues (15 mg/kg/7 days vs. 10 mg/kg/3 days). Further, our animals which were trained to self-administer cocaine (14 days, 0.25 mg/0.1 ml/infusion) did not show signs of post-synaptic adaptations. Therefore, species differences are unlikely to have contributed to this disparity. Furthermore, preliminary experiments in our laboratory indicate similar presynaptic effects in mice. A more likely explanation might be that in our study, all experimental procedures were carried out during

the active (dark) phase while CPP procedures performed by Rao et al. (2013) occurred during the inactive (light) phase. Despite these differences in experimental procedures, both experiments indicate that cocaine induces synaptic plasticity in LH orexin circuitry (**Figures 1A, B**). These data, which indicate that addiction leads to an overstimulation of orexin neurons, may provide a mechanistic rationale for antagonizing the downstream actions of enhanced orexin signaling in addiction using SORAs and DORAs.

Furthermore, evidence exists that altered feeding behavior modifies LH orexin neuron circuitry at a cellular level. Specifically, work using an orexin-GFP mouse to selectively study the properties of orexin neurons showed an increase in miniature excitatory post-synaptic currents (mEPSCS), a measure of increased synaptic drive, in LH slices of mice that underwent mild food restriction for 24 h, as compared to normally-fed controls. Consistent with these electrophysiological findings, and similar to our LH addiction experiments, overnight food restriction promoted the formation of excitatory VGLUT2 synapses onto orexin neurons. These cellular effects of food restriction were rapidly reversed by re-feeding (Horvath and Gao, 2005), contrasting the addiction work where comparable cellular perturbations persisted beyond the removal of drug. Together, these behavioral and cellular studies highlight the potential impact for SORAs and DORAs on appetite and natural rewards.

Importantly, the source of the enhanced excitatory drive to orexin neurons remains to be determined. The LH receives significant glutamatergic inputs from other brain regions such as the prefrontal cortex, lateral septum and basolateral amygdala. For example, Morshedi and Meredith (2008) have shown that a sensitizing regimen of amphetamine upregulates Fos immunoreactivity in medial prefrontal cortex neurons projecting to the LH. Further, cocaine CPP has also been demonstrated to produce increased Fos immunoreactivity in the lateral septum, another area that projects to the LH (Sartor and Aston-Jones, 2012). It is also worth noting the possibility that local glutamatergic neurons may provide positive feedback to the orexin system in cocaine-exposed animals (Li et al., 2002; Jennings et al., 2013). Nonetheless, further studies are needed to confirm the likely source of these increased glutamatergic inputs onto orexin neurons in response to cocaine exposure and to determine how other classes of drugs might also rewire LH-orexin circuits. A final point that should be noted is that recent elegant work by Burdakov's group has demonstrated the existence of two subpopulations of orexin neurons in the LH (termed H-type and D-type), which can be distinguished electrophysiologically and anatomically (Schöne et al., 2011). It will be important for future studies to determine if drugs of abuse (or stress) differentially affect these orexin cell subtypes.

EFFECTS OF SORAs AND DORAs ON DRUG-SEEKING BEHAVIORS

A number of SORAs now exist, the most common being those that target the OxR1. These include SB-334867 (Porter et al., 2001; Smart et al., 2001), SB-674042 (Langmead et al., 2004), SB-408124 (Langmead et al., 2004), SB-410220 (Porter et al., 2001; Langmead et al., 2004), GSK1059865 (Gozzi et al., 2011) and, most recently, ACT-335827 (Steiner et al., 2013a) all of which have

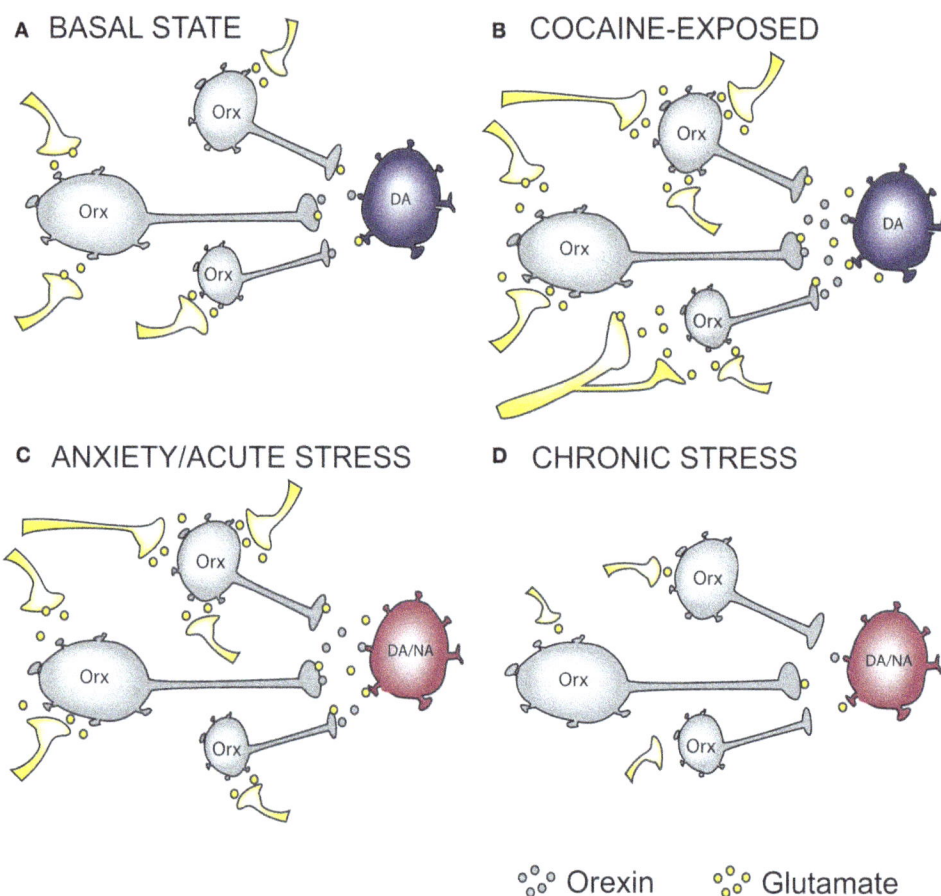

FIGURE 1 | The effect of cocaine and stress exposure on orexin neurons.
(A) Under basal conditions, orexin (Orx) neurons in the lateral hypothalamus receive excitatory inputs, thus providing "normal" glutamatergic and orexinergic (excitatory) tone onto downstream projection targets such as ventral tegmental area (VTA) dopamine (DA) neurons. **(B)** Based on recent studies, we propose that chronic cocaine-exposure rewires glutamatergic inputs onto Orx neurons resulting in increased excitatory drive onto DA neurons in the VTA. **(C)** Anxiety and acute stress are able to cause enhanced excitatory drive to DA neurons in the VTA and Noradrenergic (NA) neurons in the Locus Coeruleus (LC), an important projection target of orexin neurons. **(D)** Glutamatergic inputs onto Orx neurons in chronically stressed animals are impaired resulting in reduced excitatory drive onto DA and/or NA neurons. On the basis of this simplified hypothetical mechanistic rationale, orexin receptor antagonism represents a possible therapeutic intervention to treat anxiety and addictions. In the case of reduced orexin system activity, as may occur in some forms of depression or in response to chronic stress, mechanisms to augment orexin function may be required. Whether chronic modulation of these systems can be achieved without precipitating the expression of an alternate neuropsychiatric state warrants careful consideration.

at least 50-fold selectivity for OxR1 over OxR2 (Scammell and Winrow, 2011; Zhou et al., 2011). Amongst these compounds, SB-334867 has been most widely studied in terms of behavioral pharmacology, largely due to the high selectivity, potency and availability of this drug (Scammell and Winrow, 2011; Zhou et al., 2011).

A large number of studies have demonstrated that OxR1 antagonists are effective at blocking addiction-related behaviors across a range of drug classes. With respect to self-administration behavior, treatment with SB-334867 effectively attenuates ethanol and nicotine self-administration under both low-effort fixed ratio (FR) and higher-effort progressive ratio (PR) schedules (Lawrence et al., 2006; Schneider et al., 2007; Hollander et al., 2008; LeSage et al., 2010; Jupp et al., 2011; Martin-Fardon and Weiss, 2012). Interestingly, in the case of cocaine, SB-334867 has no effect on self-administration behavior under FR1 or FR3 conditions (Smith et al., 2009; Espana et al., 2010) but does attenuate self-administration under higher-effort schedules, including FR5 (Hollander et al., 2012) and PR (Borgland et al., 2009; Espana et al., 2010). These findings imply that in general, the orexin system has limited actions on the primary rewarding effects of cocaine, but is important to overcome increased motivational demands or effort to procure rewards. In contrast, SB-334867 effectively blocks the expression of CPP for amphetamine (Hutcheson et al., 2011) and morphine (Sharf et al., 2010), a widely used measure of the rewarding effects of drugs of abuse. Systemic SB-334867 treatment also attenuates reinstatement of cocaine-seeking behavior elicited by drug cues (Smith et al., 2009), contexts (Smith et al., 2010) and footshock stress (Boutrel et al., 2005), but not a cocaine prime (Mahler et al., 2013). Similarly, SB-334867 attenuates cue- and stress-induced reinstatement of alcohol seeking (Lawrence et al., 2006;

Richards et al., 2008; Jupp et al., 2011) as well as cue-induced, but not primed, heroin seeking (Smith and Aston-Jones, 2012). SB-334867 also attenuates cue- (Plaza-Zabala et al., 2013), but not footshock- (Plaza-Zabala et al., 2010) induced reinstatement of nicotine seeking—the latter result being a particularly surprising outcome. Thus, a wealth of preclinical studies support the premise that the use of OxR1 SORAs have the potential to decrease addiction-related behaviors, suggesting they may have clinical value in preventing relapse in abstinent patients.

In contrast to OxR1 antagonists, fewer studies have assessed the effects of selective OxR2 antagonists on addiction-related behaviors. This is likely due to the more recent development of these compounds and a predicted increase in the likelihood of sedation (Zhou et al., 2011). Selective OxR2 antagonists include JNJ-10397049 (McAtee et al., 2004; Dugovic et al., 2009), EMPA (Malherbe et al., 2009a), and TCS-OX2-29 (Hirose et al., 2003), all of which have at least a 250-fold selectivity for OxR2 (Scammell and Winrow, 2011; Zhou et al., 2011). Studies exploring the effects of these OxR2 SORAs have reported less consistent effects on drug-motivated behaviors compared to the OxR1 SORA SB-334867. For example, Shoblock et al. (2010) showed that JNJ-10397049 dose-dependently deceased ethanol self-administration, as well as the acquisition, expression and reinstatement of ethanol CPP. In contrast, Brown et al. (2013) showed that TCS-OX2-29 attenuated ethanol self-administration but had no effect on cue-induced reinstatement of extinguished ethanol seeking. Interestingly, these authors identified the nucleus accumbens core (NACc) as an important site for OxR2 signaling, as infusions of TCS-OX2-29 into the NACc, but not shell, reduced ethanol self-administration. In contrast, OxR2 SORAs have been shown to have no effect on cocaine self-administration or reinstatement (Smith et al., 2009) or the expression of nicotine withdrawal symptoms (Plaza-Zabala et al., 2012). Thus, regarding SORAs, the case for OxR1-based therapies in treating addiction is better developed than for antagonists targeting OxR2.

With respect to DORAs, a large number of these compounds have been developed, prompted largely by their potential as a novel treatment for insomnia. Indeed, at least three pharmaceutical companies (GSK, MERCK, Actelion) have initiated clinical trials investigating the utility of DORAs in modulating the sleep-wake cycle. These DORAs include almorexant (ACT-078573; Brisbare-Roch et al., 2007; Malherbe et al., 2009b); suvorexant (MK-4305; Cox et al., 2010), Merck DORA-1 (Bergman et al., 2008), Merck DORA-5 (Whitman et al., 2009), and SB-649868 (Renzulli et al., 2011). Only a limited number of studies have examined the effects of DORAs on addiction-related behaviors, with this work focusing almost exclusively on almorexant. For example, systemic and intra-VTA almorexant treatment was shown to attenuate ethanol self-administration (Srinivasan et al., 2012). Similarly, systemic almorexant blocked nicotine self-administration behavior (LeSage et al., 2010). Interestingly, whilst almorexant attenuated the expression of CPP to high doses of cocaine and amphetamine, it had no effect on morphine CPP (Steiner et al., 2013c). This study also showed that almorexant reduced the expression of behavioral sensitization to morphine but not to cocaine or amphetamine (Steiner et al., 2013c).

EFFECT OF SORAs AND DORAs ON FOOD AND NATURAL REWARD-SEEKING BEHAVIOR

An important consideration with respect to the potential clinical application of orexin receptor antagonists is the effect of these compounds on other appetitive behaviors, including food seeking. Indeed, studies carried out immediately following the discovery of the orexin peptides firmly implicated orexin in feeding behavior, with intracerebroventricular (i.c.v.) infusions of orexin shown to increase food consumption (Sakurai et al., 1998) whereas systemic treatment with SB-334867 was found to block feeding behavior (Haynes et al., 2000).

Since these initial demonstrations, subsequent studies have sought to investigate whether doses of orexin receptor antagonists that are required to block drug seeking also affect feeding behavior. For example, Martin-Fardon and colleagues recently showed that systemic administration of SB-334867 (1–10 mg/kg, i.p) attenuated reinstatement of cocaine seeking, but not sweetened-condensed milk seeking, elicited by discriminative cues (Martin-Fardon and Weiss, 2014). Similarly, Jupp et al. (2011) showed that systemic injections of SB-334867 (5 mg/kg) were sufficient to reduce responding for both ethanol and sucrose under an FR3 schedule of reinforcement. However, SB-334867 (5 mg/kg) attenuated responding for ethanol but not sucrose under a PR schedule. The authors suggested that the contribution of orexin A to motivation for alcohol is independent of non-specific effects on appetitive drive. Likewise, Hollander et al. (2012) showed that systemic injections of SB-334867 (2–4 mg/kg) reduced cocaine self-administration, but had no effect on responding for food rewards under an FR5 schedule. Comparable effects have also been shown with doses of SB-334867 that attenuate responding for nicotine (LeSage et al., 2010). Further, we have previously reported that intra-VTA infusions of SB-334867, at doses that suppress cue-induced cocaine seeking, had no effect on reinstatement for a natural reward (sweetened condensed milk; James et al., 2012). With respect to OxR2 antagonists, Brown et al. (2013) showed that central infusions of 100 μg TCS-OX2-29 reduced self-administration of ethanol, but had no effect on sucrose self-administration. In contrast however, LeSage et al. (2010) showed that systemic treatment with the DORA almorexant attenuated responding for both food pellets and nicotine. Similarly, systemic almorexant suppressed ethanol self-administration, and responding for sucrose (Srinivasan et al., 2012).

Taken together, these data indicate that a putative therapeutic window exists in which SORAs could be used to treat addiction-relevant behaviors, including 'relapse,' without producing 'off-target' effects on natural reward-seeking behavior. Conversely, it appears likely that the use of DORAs in the treatment of addiction may be associated with a risk of interfering with natural appetitive processes or promoting sedation. It is also important to acknowledge that there are very few studies that have assessed the effect of subchronic or chronic orexin receptor antagonism on drug or food-motivated behavior (discussed below).

RECENT PROGRESS IMPLICATING THE OREXIN SYSTEM IN STRESS-RELATED NEUROENDOCRINE RESPONSES

Activation of the hypothalamic-pituitary-adrenal (HPA) axis is an important component of the adaptive response to stress (Dayas et al., 2001; Day and Walker, 2007; Ulrich-Lai and Herman, 2009). In this regard it is noteworthy that the neuroendocrine paraventricular nucleus (PVN), the apex of the HPA axis, contains both OxR1 and OxR2 and that both receptor sub-types are expressed in the anterior and intermediate lobe of the pituitary gland (Trivedi et al., 1998; Date et al., 2000). Consistent with this anatomical evidence, several reports have suggested that orexins can modulate the HPA axis. For example, i.c.v. injections of orexin have been shown to increase Fos-protein expression in PVN corticotropin-releasing factor (CRF) neurons (Sakamoto et al., 2004), provoke adrenocorticotropin-releasing hormone (ACTH) release from the anterior pituitary, and increase the release of corticosterone from the adrenal glands (Jászberényi et al., 2000; Kuru et al., 2000; Russell et al., 2001; Moreno et al., 2005).

Importantly, researchers using systemic administration of orexin receptor antagonists have reported less consistent effects on HPA axis activity as would have been predicted from studies assessing HPA axis activity after orexin peptide infusions. For example, systemic injections of the OxR1 antagonist GSK-1059865 did not alter corticosterone responses to the pharmacological stressor yohimbine in rats (Gozzi et al., 2011, 2013). Further, oral treatment with almorexant had no effect on basal, social interaction, novelty or restraint stress-induced corticosterone release (Steiner et al., 2013b). Systemic SB-334867 administration also did not attenuate withdrawal-induced increases in plasma corticosterone release (Laorden et al., 2012) despite reducing the physical symptoms associated with morphine withdrawal in Wistar rats.

These equivocal effects of orexin on HPA axis function are somewhat surprising given the abundance of orexin receptors in the PVN and pituitary (Trivedi et al., 1998). Interestingly, i.c.v. administration of TCS-OX2-29, a selective OxR2 antagonist, attenuated swim stress-induced increases in plasma ACTH release (Chang et al., 2007) and, intra-PVT infusions of SB-334867 attenuated the ACTH response to restraint but only following repeated swim stress (Heydendael et al., 2011). Thus, any role of orexin in HPA axis control might depend on prior stress exposure, the category of stressor e.g., physical vs. psychological, its intensity and duration, or whether in repeated stress experiments, homotypic or heterotypic stressors are applied.

Despite the above data, exposure to psychological and physical stressors increase surrogate indices of orexin system function. For example, increased Fos-protein expression is observed in orexin neurons following exposure to acute footshock (Harris and Aston-Jones, 2006), fear-associated contexts and novel environments (Furlong et al., 2009). Interestingly, similar effects are not observed following acute immobilization stress (Furlong et al., 2009), however this form of stress does increase orexin mRNA levels in the LH (Ida et al., 2000). An explanation for these contrasting findings remains to be determined, however, one interpretation is that only sufficiently intense or salient stimuli recruit the orexin system and that prior arousal state strongly influences the likelihood of orexin system recruitment. With respect to pharmacological stressors, increased Fos-expression is observed in orexin neurons following systemic injections of the anxiogenic drug FG-7142 (Johnson et al., 2012), caffeine (Johnson et al., 2012) and intravenous administration of sodium

lactate (Johnson et al., 2010). Additionally, systemic administration of OxR1 antagonist GSK-1059865 has demonstrated functional inhibition in stress-relevant brain regions such as the NAC, dorsal thalamus, amygdala, and ventral hippocampus following the administration of yohimbine (Gozzi et al., 2013).

Acute stress also appears to have long lasting effects on orexin gene expression. For example, 2 weeks following a single session of footshock stress, increased prepro-orexin mRNA levels were observed in both the medial and lateral divisions of the hypothalamus (Chen et al., 2013). Elevated levels of orexin-A peptide in the cerebrospinal fluid (CSF) of Wistar rats have also been demonstrated following a short-term forced swimming paradigm (Martins et al., 2004). In addition, increased orexin mRNA was observed in rats immediately following morphine withdrawal (Zhou et al., 2006). Consistent with this Fos-activity mapping of orexin cell reactivity to stress, acute orexin peptide infusions evoke anxiety-like behavior. Specifically, i.c.v. administration of orexin-A produced anxiogenic-like effects i.e., increased the time spent in the closed arms of the elevated plus maze and the time spent in the dark compartment of the light-dark test (Suzuki et al., 2005). Orexins have also been shown to modulate the activity of extrahypothalamic CRF systems with i.c.v. injections of orexin-A found to increase the percentage of CRF cells that express Fos in the central amygdaloid nucleus (Sakamoto et al., 2004). Together, this evidence forms the basis for the hypothesis that manipulation of the orexin system using SORAs and DORAs will likely also impact on stress–induced anxiety-like behavior.

EFFECT OF SORAs AND DORAs ON ACUTE BEHAVIORAL STRESS REACTIVITY AND ANXIETY-LIKE BEHAVIOR

Several recent preclinical studies indicate that SORAs and DORAs have a limited effect on basal/non-stress evoked behavioral responses including anxiety-like behavior. For example, systemic treatment with SB-334867 in both rats and mice had no effect on activity in the elevated plus maze and social interaction task, two common tests of anxiety-like behavior (Johnson et al., 2010; Rodgers et al., 2013). However, intra-PVT SB-334867 infusions resulted in decreased anxiety-like behavior in the elevated plus maze (Heydendael et al., 2011). This could indicate an important role for orexin signaling in the PVT in regulating basal arousal or anxiety state.

Importantly, SORAs reliably attenuated anxiety-like behavior evoked by an acute psychological or physical stressor. For example, systemic SB-334867 administration reduced the expression of anxiety-like behavior induced by acute nicotine (Plaza-Zabala et al., 2010) and sodium lactate injections (Johnson et al., 2010) as well as cat odor (Staples and Cornish, 2014). Administration of SORAs also reduced physiological responses such as increased heart rate and body temperature produced by exposure to acute i.p injection stress (Rusyniak et al., 2012). With regards to OxR2 antagonists, intra-PVT infusions of TCS-OX2-29 reduce anxiety-like behavior elicited by footshock stress (Li et al., 2010) suggesting a role for orexin signaling through the OxR2 in stress-relevant behaviors.

There are also several recent animal studies that have explored the role for the orexin system in anxiety-like behavioral responses to conditioned cues that predict the presentation of a fearful stimulus, such as footshock. This approach has been used to explore brain mechanisms responsible for generating panic disorder and post-traumatic stress disorder in humans (Grillon, 2008). In male Sprague-Dawley rats, Sears et al. (2013) administered SB-334867 i.c.v. before fear conditioning and demonstrated an impairment in conditioned stimulus (CS)-induced freezing behavior 24 h after CS/unconditioned stimulus (US) presentation. Further, systemic injections of TCS-1102 decreased conditioned and generalized fear and anxiety-like behavior in an open field in rats previously exposed to footshock stress (Chen et al., 2013). Moreover, OxR1 knockout mice demonstrated a reduction in freezing behavior in both cued and contextual fear conditioning. Interestingly, OxR2 knockout mice also showed reduced freezing behavior to contextual but not conditioned fear (Soya et al., 2013). Consistent with a role for both receptor subtypes in aspects of conditioned fear responses, Steiner et al. (2012) reported that oral administration of almorexant reduced fear-potentiated startle in response to a CS but found no change in elevated plus maze behavior. Interestingly, human genetic studies have linked a polymorphism in Orx-2 receptor gene with panic disorder (Annerbrink et al., 2011).

Together these data indicate that exposure to acute stress and the expression of anxiety-like behavior is generally associated with increases in orexin system activity. Further, orexin antagonists appear to be potential candidates for the suppression of anxiety-like behavior and maladaptive stress-reactivity. Importantly, as is outlined below, recent evidence suggests that chronic suppression of the orexin system may be associated with the development of depression-like symptomology. These findings have significant implications for the potential use of orexin antagonists in the treatment of neuropsychiatric disorders.

EFFECT OF CHRONIC STRESS ON THE OREXIN SYSTEM AND IMPLICATIONS FOR DEPRESSION

In recent human studies, a polymorphism in Orx-1 receptor gene has been associated with major mood disorders and increased orexin peptide levels were correlated with positive emotions and social interaction (Rainero et al., 2011; Blouin et al., 2013). Non-genetic factors, such as chronic stress, have also implicated orexin in the etiology of depression (Katz et al., 1981; Kendler et al., 1999; Charney and Manji, 2004; Russo and Nestler, 2013). This link has been studied in animal models typically involving extended periods of psychological stress exposure (Lutter et al., 2008). Increasing evidence from these types of studies links chronic stress exposure to a downregulation of orexin system activity. For example, mice exposed to the well characterized social defeat model of chronic stress, which evokes symptoms thought to mimic depression in humans, display reduced orexin mRNA expression, lowered orexin cell number, and diminished levels of orexin A and orexin B peptide (Lutter et al., 2008; Nocjar et al., 2012). Similarly, Wistar-Kyoto (WKY) rats, which exhibit a depressive-like behavioral phenotype, express lower numbers of orexin neurons and a smaller orexin soma size compared to Wistar rats (Allard et al., 2004). The WKY rat strain also exhibits reduced prepro-orexin mRNA levels and orexin A immunoreactivity is reduced in the hypothalamus, thalamus, septum and amygdala (Taheri et al., 2001).

Early life stress (ELS) is a known risk factor for the development of stress-related mood disorders in adulthood (Graham et al., 1999). Surprisingly though, work has shown that ELS in fact increases frontal cortical OxR1 and hypothalamic orexin A levels in adulthood (Feng et al., 2007). Given these results, we recently investigated the effects of ELS on the reactivity of the orexin system to a second psychological stressor in adulthood. Both male and female rats exposed to neonatal maternal separation displayed a hypo-active orexin cell response to stress in adulthood. These animals also displayed reduced open field behavior but notably no overt anxiety-like behavior was observed on an elevated plus maze. Our interpretation of these data is that the ELS procedures evoked behaviors more akin to a depression-like profile after stress however further behavioral tests will be necessary to further explore this hypothesis (Campbell et al., 2013).

What effect a second stressor, such as restraint in adulthood, might have on LH-orexin circuits is unknown. This would seem important given the behavioral effects of this "two-hit" paradigm outlined above (Campbell et al., 2013). It is possible that increased drive to this system reflects an attempt to enhance orexin activity and prevent the expression of depression-like behavior. It may be that in response to a significant subsequent stressor, the reduced functional integrity at a synaptic and molecular level is unmasked, which may then develop into a depressive-like state. Regardless, taken together with the Fos data outlined above, our findings suggest that ELS can have long-term impacts on the normal functioning of orexin cells.

Consistent with a process where ELS can induce orexin cell dysfunction and depression-like behaviors, clinical evidence supports the possibility that decreased orexin signaling might promote depression-like behaviors. For example, reduced concentrations of orexin A were reported from CSF samples of adults with major depressive disorder and chronic, combat-related post-traumatic stress disorder (Brundin et al., 2007a,b, 2009; Strawn et al., 2010). Additionally, reduced orexin A mRNA has been correlated with increased scores on the Hamilton rating scale for depression (Rotter et al., 2011). Interestingly, infusions of orexin peptides into the ventricles of rats have been shown to have antidepressant-like effects. For example, i.c.v. administration of orexin reduces the duration of immobility in the forced swim test, and this effect is blocked by the administration of the OxR1 antagonist, SB-334867 (Ito et al., 2008). Thus, it is possible that in some forms of depression, increasing orexin system signaling may have therapeutic benefit. In line with this interpretation, we recently found that a period of exercise in adolescence prevented reductions in orexin system function and the expression of stress-related behavior in rats exposed to ELS (Campbell et al., 2013).

Despite the above work, it is important to acknowledge that there are both preclinical animal and human data that do not support a link between a hypoactive orexin system and depression. For example, Mikrouli et al. (2011) demonstrated that the Flinders Sensitive Line, considered a genetic rat model of depression, displayed elevated, not depressed, levels of orexin neurons compared to controls. Further, Nollet et al. (2011) demonstrated that mice subjected to unpredictable chronic mild stress displayed increased depressive-like behavior following the tail suspension test but presented with elevated orexin neuron activity in the DMH and PFA subregions of the hypothalamus. Interestingly, these authors were able to reverse this elevation in orexin cell activity with 6 weeks of fluoxetine treatment. Similarly, exposure to unpredictable chronic mild stress produced depressive-like behaviors in the tail suspension test, elevated plus maze and resident-intruder task; and 7 weeks exposure to the DORA almorexant produced an antidepressant-like behavioral effect in these tasks (Nollet et al., 2012). And, in a recent study, OxR1 mRNA expression in the amygdala was reported to be positively correlated with increased depressive-like behavior in the forced swim test (Arendt et al., 2013) - however it is possible that this effect might be caused by downregulated orexin system function. Finally, a recent study reported that decreased depressive-like behavior is observed in OxR1 knockout mice, whereas OxR2 knockout mice exhibit *increased* depressive-related behavior, possibly pointing to a differential role for OxR1 vs. OxR2 in the regulation of these behaviors (Scott et al., 2011). These authors highlight the fact that behavioral pharmacology studies typically use the non-selective OxR agonist orexin-A, along with SORAs at doses that are potentially non-selective *in vivo*, therefore making it difficult to differentiate roles for OxR1 vs. OxR2 in the regulation of depression-like behavior.

In human studies, Salomon et al. (2003) reported that orexin A CSF levels were higher in depressed patients and treatment with sertraline, an antidepressant drug, resulted in an attenuation of CSF orexin levels. Furthermore, a positive correlation between orexin plasma concentrations, depressive symptoms and global distress indices on the brief symptom inventory is seen following alcohol withdrawal (von der Goltz et al., 2011). Finally, Schmidt et al. (2011) failed to find any association between CSF orexin A levels and depression.

Taken together, these results suggest that acute stress may activate the orexin system in order to enhance an animal's ability to cope or adapt appropriately to a potential threat (**Figure 1C**). If these stressors persist, chronic or repeated exposure to stress may downregulate orexin system function (**Figure 1D**). Hypoactivity of the orexin system may impair an animal's ability to adapt to stress and lead to the expression of depressive-like behavior. Data from human and animal studies not supporting this link may reflect the heterogeneous nature of depression—i.e., depression presenting with and without anxiety or anxiety presenting with or without depression. Supporting this conclusion, Johnson et al. (2010) found that patients exhibiting panic anxiety displayed increased CSF orexin levels compared to patients exhibiting panic anxiety with comorbid major depressive disorder. It will be important for human and animal studies exploring the link between the orexin system dysfunction and neuropsychiatric conditions to consider the heterogeneous nature of these conditions.

POTENTIAL PITFALLS FOR APPROACHES TO TREAT NEUROPSYCHIATRIC DISORDERS USING OREXIN RECEPTOR ANTAGONISTS

As outlined above, significant progress has been made in our understanding of the contribution of the orexin system to normal and "pathological" behavior. In the case of addiction, there

seems sufficient evidence to conclude that the orexin system is important for drug-seeking behavior, particularly for relapse-like behavior provoked by drug-cues and stress but not by drug itself. Further, several studies indicate that orexin antagonists, and in particular selective OxR1 antagonists, can reduce drug-seeking at doses that have minimal effects on natural reward-seeking behavior (Jupp et al., 2011; Hollander et al., 2012; James et al., 2012; Brown et al., 2013). Comparison of orexin's role in drug taking vs. seeking behavior also highlights that orexin receptor antagonists have effects on rewarded self-administration, but importantly these effects generally emerge only under high effort schedules of reinforcement. These data combine to produce a compelling case that orexin receptors represent promising targets for the treatment of addiction. This is particularly true given the long-established interaction between addiction and maladaptation of natural reward seeking brain pathways. For example, increased excitatory drive to the orexin system is thought to heighten orexin signaling in key reward-seeking regions such as the VTA and may contribute to the persistent plasticity within dopamine neurons seen after long-term cocaine self-administration and increased relapse vulnerability (Chen et al., 2008; James et al., 2012)

It is important given the clinical promise of SORAs and DORAs for neuropsychiatric disorders that studies continue to assess the potential for off-target effects, tolerance to prolonged orexin receptor blockade and differential or counter-regulatory effects on OxR1 vs. 2, as well as any possible compensatory adaptations that may occur in other hypothalamic neuropeptide systems in response to chronic orexin receptor blockade. Studies to date indicate a limited profile of chronic SORA and DORA tolerance. For example, Steiner et al. (2013c) showed that 12 days of chronic almorexant treatment had no effect on the maintenance of CPP or locomotor sensitization in animals exposed to cocaine, morphine or amphetamine. However, as mentioned above, Nollet et al. (2012) exposed mice to chronic almorexant treatment (7 weeks), which produced an antidepressant-like effect in the tail suspension test, elevated plus maze and resident-intruder task following exposure to unpredictable chronic mild stress. Interestingly, chronic treatment with the OxR1 antagonist ACT-335827 (4 weeks) did not alter total energy intake in cafeteria diet fed rats compared to controls (Steiner et al., 2013b). In contrast, chronic SB-334867 treatment (14 days) had anti-obesity effects in a model of genetically obese mice by reducing food intake and body weight gain over the 14 day period (Haynes et al., 2002).

In one of the few examples where repeated doses of an orexin antagonist have been studied for addiction and relapse prevention, Zhou and colleagues demonstrated that chronic SB-334867 exposure resulted in a complex pattern of effects (Zhou et al., 2011). Specifically, they found that repeated SB-334867 exposure prior to extinction sessions resulted in reduced cocaine-seeking behavior in rats during extinction; however, repeated SB-334867 treatment during extinction increased cue-induced reinstatement and had no effect on cocaine primed reinstatement. Importantly, McNally and colleagues have also shown that cocaine and alcohol-seeking do not necessarily evoke a specific drug context-related activation of the orexin system, rather, recruitment of this pathway is necessary but not sufficient for drug-seeking behavior (Hamlin et al., 2007, 2008). It is also interesting to note that the OxR1 antagonist, SB-334867, has been shown to reduce cue-induced reinstatement of cocaine seeking behavior in male rodents yet no effect was seen in female rats (Zhou et al., 2012). Future work should focus on differentiating arousal vs. reward related function of the orexin neurons in the context of addiction. Sex-specific effects of stress and drug exposure on orexin circuitry also warrant further scrutiny.

With respect to the potential use of orexin receptor antagonists for anxiety and depression, recently, Johnson et al. (2010, 2012) proposed the use of OxR1 antagonists in the treatment of panic disorder. Certainly, the available data appears to support an important role for orexin signaling in ameliorating anxiety-like states in animal models. Studies employing chronic stress paradigms, however, suggests that a more complicated picture exists and that the effects of repeated SORA or DORA treatment may be unpredictable (Zhou et al., 2012). Emerging data indicates that ELS and chronic stress can downregulate the activity of the orexin system in response to chronic stress (Lutter et al., 2008; Nocjar et al., 2012; Campbell et al., 2013). There is also a developing clinical literature indicating that depression may be associated with decreased orexin system function (Brundin et al., 2007a,b, 2009). These studies raise potential concerns for the long-term use of orexin antagonists in the treatment of addiction and anxiety disorders, as long-term suppression of the orexin system may precipitate depressive-like symptoms. Similarly, the emergence of anxiety or depression under conditions of augmented orexin system function will need to be carefully considered. Therefore, a greater understanding of the changes to orexin receptor expression in relevant brain regions will be necessary to confidently predict the potential outcomes of therapeutic manipulation of orexin signaling under these conditions. Further we propose that a thorough evaluation of chronic and subchronic orexin receptor antagonism in preclinical animal models of anxiety and depression is necessary. Together, such approaches may be able to identify therapeutic dosing regimens with preferential effects on the different aspects for the orexin system that influence mood, as well as drug- and natural-reward behaviors. Finally, the evidence that drugs of abuse or stress can rewire inputs onto orexin neurons indicates that targeting these changes within the LH might offer an alternative strategy. This would negate the mixed downstream effects of SORAs and DORAs in mood, addiction and reward by reducing aberrant orexin cell activity at the site of dysfunction, rather than simply masking the downstream effects using antagonists. For example, our group is currently investigating the changes in LH-orexin circuits responsible for the increased excitatory drive observed after cocaine or ELS.

In conclusion, significant progress has been made toward an understanding of the role of the orexin system in normal and pathological behaviors. Unsurprisingly, given the widespread projections of the orexin system, the role for these neurons crosses many domains including basic physiological responses to more complex functions. Our view is that only a comprehensive dissection of the changes in LH-circuit function, both within the hypothalamus and in target regions of these neurons, will reveal

appropriate therapeutic avenues to augment or suppress dysregulated orexin function in neuropsychiatric and neurological disease states.

REFERENCES

Ahmed, S. H., Lutjens, R., van der Stap, L. D., Lekic, D., Romano-Spica, V., Morales, M., et al. (2005). Gene expression evidence for remodeling of lateral hypothalamic circuitry in cocaine addiction. *Proc. Natl. Acad. Sci. U.S.A.* 102, 11533–11538. doi: 10.1073/pnas.0504438102

Allard, J. S., Tizabi, Y., Shaffery, J. P., Trouth, C. O., and Manaye, K. (2004). Stereological analysis of the hypothalamic hypocretin/orexin neurons in an animal model of depression. *Neuropeptides* 38, 311–315. doi: 10.1016/j.npep.2004.06.004

Ammoun, S., Holmqvist, T., Shariatmadari, R., Oonk, H. B., Detheux, M., Parmentier, M., et al. (2003). Distinct recognition of OX1 and OX2 receptors by orexin peptides. *J. Pharmacol. Exp. Ther.* 305, 507–514. doi: 10.1124/jpet.102.048025

Annerbrink, K., Westberg, L., Olsson, M., Andersch, S., Sjödin, I., Holm, G., et al. (2011). Panic disorder is associated with the Val308Iso polymorphism in the hypocretin receptor gene. *Psychiatr. Genet.* 21, 85–89. doi: 10.1097/YPG.0b013e328341a3db

Arendt, D. H., Ronan, P. J., Oliver, K. D., Callahan, L. B., Summers, T. R., and Summers, C. H. (2013). Depressive behavior and activation of the orexin/hypocretin system. *Behav. Neurosci.* 127, 86–94. doi: 10.1037/a0031442

Aston-Jones, G., Smith, R. J., Sartor, G. C., Moorman, D. E., Massi, L., Tahsili-Fahadan, P., et al. (2010). Lateral hypothalamic orexin/hypocretin neurons: a role in reward-seeking and addiction. *Brain Res.* 1314, 74–90. doi: 10.1016/j.brainres.2009.09.106

Bergman, J. M., Roecker, A. J., Mercer, S. P., Bednar, R. A., Reiss, D. R., Ransom, R. W., et al. (2008). Proline bis-amides as potent dual orexin receptor antagonists. *Bioorg. Med. Chem. Lett.* 18, 1425–1430. doi: 10.1016/j.bmcl.2008.01.001

Blouin, A. M., Fried, I., Wilson, C. L., Staba, R. J., Behnke, E. J., Lam, H. A., et al. (2013). Human hypocretin and melanin-concentrating hormone levels are linked to emotion and social interaction. *Nat. Commun.* 4:1547. doi: 10.1038/ncomms2461

Borgland, S. L., Chang, S. J., Bowers, M. S., Thompson, J. L., Vittoz, N., Floresco, S. B., et al. (2009). Orexin A/hypocretin-1 selectively promotes motivation for positive reinforcers. *J. Neurosci.* 29, 11215–11225. doi: 10.1523/JNEUROSCI.6096-08.2009

Boutrel, B., Cannella, N., and de Lecea, L. (2010). The role of hypocretin in driving arousal and goal-oriented behaviors. *Brain Res.* 1314, 103–111. doi: 10.1016/j.brainres.2009.11.054

Boutrel, B., and de Lecea, L. (2008). Addiction and arousal: the hypocretin connection. *Physiol. Behav.* 93, 947–951. doi: 10.1016/j.physbeh.2007.11.022

Boutrel, B., Kenny, P. J., Specio, S. E., Martin-Fardon, R., Markou, A., Koob, G. F., et al. (2005). Role for hypocretin in mediating stress-induced reinstatement of cocaine-seeking behavior. *Proc. Natl. Acad. Sci. U.S.A.* 102, 19168–19173. doi: 10.1073/pnas.0507480102

Brisbare-Roch, C., Dingemanse, J., Koberstein, R., Hoever, P., Aissaoui, H., Flores, S., et al. (2007). Promotion of sleep by targeting the orexin system in rats, dogs and humans. *Nat. Med.* 13, 150–155. doi: 10.1038/nm1544

Brown, R. M., Khoo, S. Y.-S., and Lawrence, A. J. (2013). Central orexin (hypocretin) 2 receptor antagonism reduces ethanol self-administration, but not cue-conditioned ethanol-seeking, in ethanol-preferring rats. *Int. J. Neuropsychopharmacol.* 16, 2067–2079. doi: 10.1017/S1461145713000333

Brundin, L., Bjorkqvist, M., Petersen, A., and Traskman-Bendz, L. (2007a). Reduced orexin levels in the cerebrospinal fluid of suicidal patients with major depressive disorder. *Eur. Neuropsychopharmacol.* 17, 573–579. doi: 10.1016/j.euroneuro.2007.01.005

Brundin, L., Bjorkqvist, M., Traskman-Bendz, L., and Petersen, A. (2009). Increased orexin levels in the cerebrospinal fluid the first year after a suicide attempt. *J. Affect. Disord.* 113, 179–182. doi: 10.1016/j.jad.2008.04.011

Brundin, L., Petersen, A., Bjorkqvist, M., and Traskman-Bendz, L. (2007b). Orexin and psychiatric symptoms in suicide attempters. *J. Affect. Disord.* 100, 259–263. doi: 10.1016/j.jad.2006.10.019

Burdakov, D., Gerasimenko, O., and Verkhratsky, A. (2005). Physiological changes in glucose differentially modulate the excitability of hypothalamic melanin-concentrating hormones and orexin neurons *in situ. J. Neurosci.* 25, 2429–2433. doi: 10.1523/JNEUROSCI.4925-04.2005

Campbell, E. J., James, M. H., Richardson, H. N., Hodgson, D. M., and Dayas, C. V. (2013). *Orexin (Hypocretin) Neurons are Hyporesponsive to Stress in Adulthood Following Maternal Separation: Effects Reversed by Voluntary Exercise in Male but not Female Rats.* San Diego, CA: Paper presented at the Society for Neuroscience.

Chang, H., Saito, T., Ohiwa, N., Tateoka, M., Deocaris, C. C., Fujikawa, T., et al. (2007). Inhibitory effects of an orexin-2 receptor antagonist on orexin A- and stress-induced ACTH responses in conscious rats. *Neurosci. Res.* 57, 462–466. doi: 10.1016/j.neures.2006.11.009

Charney, D. S., and Manji, H. K. (2004). Life stress, genes, and depression: multiple pathways lead to increased risk and new opportunities for intervention. *Sci. STKE* 2004, 1–11. doi: 10.1126/stke.2252004re5

Chemelli, R. M., Willie, J. T., Sinton, C. M., Elmquist, J. K., Scammell, T., Lee, C., et al. (1999). Narcolepsy in orexin knockout mice: molecular genetics of sleep regulation. *Cell* 98, 437–451. doi: 10.1016/S0092-8674(00)81973-X

Chen, B. T., Bowers, M. S., Martin, M., Hopf, F. W., Guillory, A. M., Carelli, R. M., et al. (2008). Cocaine but not natural reward self-administration nor passive cocaine infusions produces persistent LTP in VTA. *Neuron* 59, 288–297. doi: 10.1016/j.neuron.2008.05.024

Chen, X., Wang, H., Lin, Z., Li, S., Li, Y., Bergen, H. T., et al. (2013). Orexins (hypocretins) contribute to fear and avoidance in rats exposed to a single episode of footshocks. *Brain Struct. Funct.* doi: 10.1007/s00429-013-0626-3. [Epub ahead of print].

Cox, C. D., Breslin, M. J., Whitman, D. B., Schreier, J. D., McGaughey, G. B., Bogusky, M. J., et al. (2010). Discovery of the dual orexin receptor antagonist [(7R)-4-(5-chloro-1,3-benzoxazol-2-yl)-7-methyl-1,4-diazepan-1-yl][5-methyl-2-(2H -1,2,3-triazol-2-yl)phenyl]methanone (MK-4305) for the treatment of insomnia. *J. Med. Chem.* 53, 5320–5332. doi: 10.1021/jm100541c

Date, Y., Mondal, M. S., Matsukura, S., Ueta, Y., Yamashita, H., Kaiya, H., et al. (2000). Distribution of orexin/hypocretin in the rat median eminence and pituitary. *Brain Res. Mol. Brain Res.* 76, 1–6. doi: 10.1016/S0169-328X(99)00317-4

Day, T. A., and Walker, F. R. (2007). More appraisal please: a commentary on Pfaff et al. (2007) "Relations between mechanisms of CNS arousal and mechanisms of stress." *Stress* 10, 311–313. doi: 10.1080/10253890701638204

Dayas, C. V., Buller, K. M., Crane, J. W., Xu, Y., and Day, T. A. (2001). Stressor categorization: acute physical and psychological stressors elicit distinctive recruitment patterns in the amygdala and in medullary noradrenergic cell groups. *Eur. J. Neurosci.* 14, 1143–1152. doi: 10.1046/j.0953-816x.2001. 01733.x

de Lecea, L., Kilduff, T. S., Peyron, C., Gao, X., Foye, P. E., Danielson, P. E., et al. (1998). The hypocretins: hypothalamus-specific peptides with neuroexcitatory activity. *Proc. Natl. Acad. Sci. U.S.A.* 95, 322–327. doi: 10.1073/pnas.95.1.322

Dugovic, C., Shelton, J. E., Aluisio, L. E., Fraser, I. C., Jiang, X., Sutton, S. W., et al. (2009). Blockade of orexin-1 receptors attenuates orexin-2 receptor antagonism-induced sleep promotion in the rat. *J. Pharmacol. Exp. Ther.* 330, 142–151. doi: 10.1124/jpet.109.152009

Espana, R. A., Oleson, E. B., Locke, J. L., Brookshire, B. R., Roberts, D. C., and Jones, S. R. (2010). The hypocretin-orexin system regulates cocaine self-administration via actions on the mesolimbic dopamine system. *Eur. J. Neurosci.* 31, 336–348. doi: 10.1111/j.1460-9568.2009.07065.x

Feng, P., Vurbic, D., Wu, Z., and Strohl, K. P. (2007). Brain orexins and wake regulation in rats exposed to maternal deprivation. *Brain Res.* 1154, 163–172. doi: 10.1016/j.brainres.2007.03.077

Furlong, T. M., Vianna, D. M. L., Liu, L., and Carrive, P. (2009). Hypocretin/orexin contributes to the expression of some but not all forms of stress and arousal. *Eur. J. Neurosci.* 30, 1603–1614. doi: 10.1111/j.1460-9568.2009.06952.x

Gozzi, A., Lepore, S., Vicentini, E., Merlo-Pich, E., and Bifone, A. (2013). Differential effect of orexin-1 and CRF-1 antagonism on stress circuits: a fMRI study in the rat with the pharmacological stressor Yohimbine. *Neuropsychopharmacology* 38, 2120–2130. doi: 10.1038/npp.2013.109

Gozzi, A., Turrini, G., Piccoli, L., Massagrande, M., Amantini, D., Antolini, M., et al. (2011). Functional magnetic resonance imaging reveals different neural substrates for the effects of orexin-1 and orexin-2 receptor antagonists. *PLoS ONE* 6:e16406. doi: 10.1371/journal.pone.0016406

Graham, Y. P., Heim, C., Goodman, S. H., Miller, A. H., and Nemeroff, C. B. (1999). The effects of neonatal stress on brain development:

implications for psychopathology. *Dev. Psychopathol.* 11, 545–565. doi: 10.1017/S0954579499002205

Grillon, C. (2008). Models and mechanisms of anxiety: evidence from startle studies. *Psychopharmacology (Berl.)* 199, 421–437. doi: 10.1007/s00213-007-1019-1

Hamlin, A. S., Clemens, K. J., and McNally, G. P. (2008). Renewal of extinguished cocaine-seeking. *Neuroscience* 151, 659–670. doi: 10.1016/j.neuroscience.2007. 11.018

Hamlin, A. S., Newby, J., and McNally, G. P. (2007). The neural correlates and role of D1 dopamine receptors in renewal of extinguished alcohol-seeking. *Neuroscience* 146, 525–536. doi: 10.1016/j.neuroscience.2007.01.063

Harris, G. C., and Aston-Jones, G. (2006). Arousal and reward: a dichotomy in orexin function. *Trends Neurosci.* 29, 571–577. doi: 10.1016/j.tins.2006. 08.002

Harris, G. C., Wimmer, M., and Aston-Jones, G. (2005). A role for lateral hypothalamic orexin neurons in reward seeking. *Nature* 437, 556–559. doi: 10.1038/nature04071

Haynes, A. C., Chapman, H., Taylor, C., Moore, G. B., Cawthorne, M. A., Tadayyon, M., et al. (2002). Anorectic, thermogenic and anti-obesity activity of a selective orexin-1 receptor antagonist in ob/ob mice. *Regul. Pept.* 104, 153–159. doi: 10.1016/S0167-0115(01)00358-5

Haynes, A. C., Jackson, B., Chapman, H., Tadayyon, M., Johns, A., Porter, R. A., et al. (2000). A selective orexin-1 receptor antagonist reduces food consumption in male and female rats. *Regul. Pept.* 96, 45–51. doi: 10.1016/S0167-0115(00)00199-3

Heydendael, W., Sharma, K., Iyer, V., Luz, S., Piel, D., Beck, S., et al. (2011). Orexins/hypocretins act in the posterior paraventricular thalamic nucleus during repeated stress to regulate facilitation to novel stress. *Endocrinology* 152, 4738–4752. doi: 10.1210/en.2011-1652

Hirose, M., Egashira, S., Goto, Y., Hashihayata, T., Ohtake, N., Iwaasa, H., et al. (2003). N-acyl 6,7-dimethoxy-1,2,3,4-tetrahydroisoquinoline: the first orexin-2 receptor selective non-peptidic antagonist. *Bioorg. Med. Chem. Lett.* 13, 4497–4499. doi: 10.1016/j.bmcl.2003.08.038

Hollander, J. A., Lu, Q., Cameron, M. D., Kamenecka, T. M., and Kenny, P. J. (2008). Insular hypocretin transmission regulates nicotine reward. *Proc. Natl. Acad. Sci. U.S.A.* 105, 19480–19485. doi: 10.1073/pnas.0808023105

Hollander, J. A., Pham, D., Fowler, C. D., and Kenny, P. J. (2012). Hypocretin-1 receptors regulate the reinforcing and reward-enhancing effects of cocaine: pharmacological and behavioral genetics evidence. *Front. Behav. Neurosci.* 6:47. doi: 10.3389/fnbeh.2012.00047

Horvath, T. L., and Gao, X. B. (2005). Input organization and plasticity of hypocretin neurons: possible clues to obesity's association with insomnia. *Cell Metab.* 1, 279–286. doi: 10.1016/j.cmet.2005.03.003

Hutcheson, D. M., Quarta, D., Halbout, B., Rigal, A., Valerio, E., and Heidbreder, C. (2011). Orexin-1 receptor antagonist SB-334867 reduces the acquisition and expression of cocaine-conditioned reinforcement and the expression of amphetamine-conditioned reward. *Behav. Pharmacol.* 22, 173–181. doi: 10.1097/FBP.0b013e328343d761

Ida, T., Nakahara, K., Murakami, T., Hanada, R., Nakazato, M., and Murakami, N. (2000). Possible involvement of orexin in the stress reaction in rats. *Biochem. Biophys. Res. Commun.* 270, 318–323. doi: 10.1006/bbrc.2000.2412

Ito, N., Yabe, T., Gamo, Y., Nagai, T., Oikawa, T., Yamada, H., et al. (2008). I.c.v. administration of orexin-A induces an antidepressive-like effect through hippocampal cell proliferation. *Neuroscience* 157, 720–732. doi: 10.1016/j.neuroscience.2008.09.042

James, M. H., Charnley, J. L., Levi, E. M., Jones, E., Yeoh, J. W., Smith, D. W., et al. (2011). Orexin-1 receptor signalling within the ventral tegmental area, but not the paraventricular thalamus, is critical to regulating cue-induced reinstatement of cocaine-seeking. *Int. J. Neuropsychopharmacol.* 14, 684–690. doi: 10.1017/S1461145711000423

James, M. H., Yeoh, J. W., Graham, B. A., and Dayas, C. V. (2012). Insights for developing pharmacological treatments for psychostimulant relapse targeting hypothalamic peptide systems. *Addict. Res. Ther.* s4, 1–13. doi: 10.4172/2155-6105. S4-008

Jászberényi, M., Bujdosó, E., Pataki, I., and Telegdy, G. (2000). Effects of orexins on the hypothalamic-pituitary-adrenal system. *J. Neuroendocrinol.* 12, 1174–1178. doi: 10.1046/j.1365-2826.2000.00572.x

Jennings, J. H., Rizzi, G., Stamatakis, A. M., Ung, R. L., and Stuber, G. D. (2013). The inhibitory circuit architecture of the lateral hypothalamus orchestrates feeding. *Science* 341, 1517–1521. doi: 10.1126/science.1241812

Johnson, P. L., Samuels, B. C., Fitz, S. D., Federici, L. M., Hammes, N., Early, M. C., et al. (2012). Orexin 1 receptors are a novel target to modulate panic responses and the panic brain network. *Physiol. Behav.* 107, 733–742. doi: 10.1016/j.physbeh.2012.04.016

Johnson, P. L., Truitt, W., Fitz, S. D., Minick, P. E., Dietrich, A., Sanghani, S., et al. (2010). A key role for orexin in panic anxiety. *Nat. Med.* 16, 111–115. doi: 10.1038/nm.2075

Jupp, B., Krivdic, B., Krstew, E., and Lawrence, A. J. (2011). The orexin(1) receptor antagonist SB-334867 dissociates the motivational properties of alcohol and sucrose in rats. *Brain Res.* 1391, 54–59. doi: 10.1016/j.brainres.2011.03.045

Katz, R. J., Roth, K. A., and Carroll, B. J. (1981). Acute and chronic stress effects on open field activity in the rat: implications for a model of depression. *Neurosci. Biobehav. Rev.* 5, 247–251. doi: 10.1016/0149-7634(81)90005-1

Kendler, K. S., Karkowski, L. M., and Prescott, C. A. (1999). Causal relationship between stressful life events and the onset of major depression. *Am. J. Psychiatry* 156, 837–841.

Kuru, M., Ueta, Y., Serino, R., Nakazato, M., Yamamoto, Y., Shibuya, I., et al. (2000). Centrally administered orexin/hypocretin activates HPA axis in rats. *Neuroreport* 11, 1977–1980. doi: 10.1097/00001756-200006260-00034

Langmead, C. J., Jerman, J. C., Brough, S. J., Scott, C., Porter, R. A., and Herdon, H. J. (2004). Characterisation of the binding of [3H]-SB-674042, a novel nonpeptide antagonist, to the human orexin-1 receptor. *Br. J. Pharmacol.* 141, 340–346. doi: 10.1038/sj.bjp.0705610

Laorden, M. L., Ferenczi, S., Pinter-Kubler, B., Gonzalez-Martin, L. L., Lasheras, M. C., Kovacs, K. J., et al. (2012). Hypothalamic orexin–a neurons are involved in the response of the brain stress system to morphine withdrawal. *PLoS ONE* 7:e36871. doi: 10.1371/journal.pone.0036871

Lawrence, A. J. (2010). Regulation of alcohol-seeking by orexin (hypocretin) neurons. *Brain Res.* 1314, 124–129. doi: 10.1016/j.brainres.2009.07.072

Lawrence, A. J., Cowen, M. S., Yang, H. J., Chen, F., and Oldfield, B. (2006). The orexin system regulates alcohol-seeking in rats. *Br. J. Pharmacol.* 148, 752–759. doi: 10.1038/sj.bjp.0706789

LeSage, M. G., Perry, J. L., Kotz, C. M., Shelley, D., and Corrigall, W. A. (2010). Nicotine self-administration in the rat: effects of hypocretin antagonists and changes in hypocretin mRNA. *Psychopharmacology (Berl.)* 209, 203–212. doi: 10.1007/s00213-010-1792-0

Li, Y., Gao, X.-B., Sakurai, T., and Van den Pol, A. N. (2002). Hypocretin/orexin excites hypocretin neurons via a local glutamate neuron - A potential mechanism for orchestrating the hypothalamic arousal system. *Neuron* 36, 1169–1181. doi: 10.1016/S0896-6273(02)01132-7

Li, Y., Li, S., Wei, C., Wang, H., Sui, N., and Kirouac, G. J. (2010). Orexins in the paraventricular nucleus of the thalamus mediate anxiety-like responses in rats. *Psychopharmacology (Berl.)* 212, 251–265. doi: 10.1007/s00213-010-1948-y

Lutter, M., Krishnan, V., Russo, S. J., Jung, S., McClung, C. A., and Nestler, E. J. (2008). Orexin signaling mediates the antidepressant-like effect of calorie restriction. *J. Neurosci.* 28, 3071–3075. doi: 10.1523/JNEUROSCI.5584-07.2008

Mahler, S., Smith, R., and Aston-Jones, G. (2013). Interactions between VTA orexin and glutamate in cue-induced reinstatement of cocaine seeking in rats. *Psychopharmacology (Berl.)* 226, 687–698. doi: 10.1007/s00213-012-2681-5

Mahler, S. V., Smith, R. J., Moorman, D. E., Sartor, G. C., and Aston-Jones, G. (2012). Multiple roles for orexin/hypocretin in addiction. *Prog. Brain Res.* 198, 79–121. doi: 10.1016/B978-0-444-59489-1.00007-0

Malherbe, P., Borroni, E., Gobbi, L., Knust, H., Nettekoven, M., Pinard, E., et al. (2009a). Biochemical and behavioural characterization of EMPA, a novel high-affinity, selective antagonist for the OX(2) receptor. *Br. J. Pharmacol.* 156, 1326–1341. doi: 10.1111/j.1476-5381.2009.00127.x

Malherbe, P., Borroni, E., Pinard, E., Wettstein, J. G., and Knoflach, F. (2009b). Biochemical and electrophysiological characterization of almorexant, a dual orexin 1 receptor (OX1)/orexin 2 receptor (OX2) antagonist: comparison with selective OX1 and OX2 antagonists. *Mol. Pharmacol.* 76, 618–631. doi: 10.1124/mol.109.055152

Marchant, N. J., Millan, E. Z., and McNally, G. P. (2012). The hypothalamus and the neurobiology of drug seeking. *Cell. Mol. Life Sci.* 69, 581–597. doi: 10.1007/s00018-011-0817-0

Marcus, J. N., Aschkenasi, C. J., Lee, C. E., Chemelli, R. M., Saper, C. B., Yanagisawa, M., et al. (2001). Differential expression of orexin receptors 1 and 2 in the rat brain. *J. Comp. Neurol.* 435, 6–25. doi: 10.1002/cne.1190

Martin-Fardon, R., and Weiss, F. (2012). *N*-(2-Methyl-6-benzoxazolyl)-*N′*-1,5-n aphthyridin-4-yl urea (SB334867), a hypocretin receptor-1 antagonist, preferentially prevents ethanol seeking: comparison with natural reward seeking. *Addict. Biol.* doi: 10.1111/j.1369-1600.2012.00480.x. [Epub ahead of print].

Martin-Fardon, R., and Weiss, F. (2014). Blockade of hypocretin receptor-1 preferentially prevents cocaine seeking: comparison with natural reward seeking. *Neuroreport.* doi: 10.1097/WNR.0000000000000120. [Epub ahead of print].

Martins, P. J., D'Almeida, V., Pedrazzoli, M., Lin, L., Mignot, E., and Tufik, S. (2004). Increased hypocretin-1 (orexin-a) levels in cerebrospinal fluid of rats after short-term forced activity. *Regul. Pept.* 117, 155–158. doi: 10.1016/j.regpep.2003.10.003

McAtee, L. C., Sutton, S. W., Rudolph, D. A., Li, X., Aluisio, L. E., Phuong, V. K., et al. (2004). Novel substituted 4-phenyl-[1,3]dioxanes: potent and selective orexin receptor 2 (OX(2)R) antagonists. *Bioorg. Med. Chem. Lett.* 14, 4225–4229. doi: 10.1016/j.bmcl.2004.06.032

Mikrouli, E., Wortwein, G., Soylu, R., Mathe, A. A., and Petersen, A. (2011). Increased numbers of orexin/hypocretin neurons in a genetic rat depression model. *Neuropeptides* 45, 401–406. doi: 10.1016/j.npep.2011.07.010

Moreno, G., Perelló, M., Gaillard, R., and Spinedi, E. (2005). Orexin a stimulates hypothalamic-pituitary-adrenal (HPA) axis function, but not food intake, in the absence of full hypothalamic NPY-ergic activity. *Endocrine* 26, 99–106. doi: 10.1385/endo:26:2:099

Morshedi, M. M., and Meredith, G. E. (2008). Repeated amphetamine administration induces Fos in prefrontal cortical neurons that project to the lateral hypothalamus but not the nucleus accumbens or basolateral amygdala. *Psychopharmacology (Berl.)* 197, 179–189. doi: 10.1007/s00213-007-1021-7

Nocjar, C., Zhang, J., Feng, P., and Panksepp, J. (2012). The social defeat animal model of depression shows diminished levels of orexin in mesocortical regions of the dopamine system, and of dynorphin and orexin in the hypothalamus. *Neuroscience* 218, 138–153. doi: 10.1016/j.neuroscience.2012.05.033

Nollet, M., Gaillard, P., Minier, F., Tanti, A., Belzung, C., and Leman, S. (2011). Activation of orexin neurons in dorsomedial/perifornical hypothalamus and antidepressant reversal in a rodent model of depression. *Neuropharmacology* 61, 336–346. doi: 10.1016/j.neuropharm.2011.04.022

Nollet, M., Gaillard, P., Tanti, A., Girault, V., Belzung, C., and Leman, S. (2012). Neurogenesis-independent antidepressant-like effects on behavior and stress axis response of a dual orexin receptor antagonist in a rodent model of depression. *Neuropsychopharmacology* 37, 2210–2221. doi: 10.1007/s00213-007-1021-7

Peyron, C., Tighe, D. K., van den Pol, A. N., de Lecea, L., Heller, H. C., Sutcliffe, J. G., et al. (1998). Neurons containing hypocretin (orexin) project to multiple neuronal systems. *J. Neurosci.* 18, 9996–10015.

Plaza-Zabala, A., Flores, Á., Maldonado, R., and Berrendero, F. (2012). Hypocretin/orexin signaling in the hypothalamic paraventricular nucleus is essential for the expression of nicotine withdrawal. *Biol. Psychiatry* 71, 214–223. doi: 10.1016/j.biopsych.2011.06.025

Plaza-Zabala, A., Flores, A., Martin-Garcia, E., Saravia, R., Maldonado, R., and Berrendero, F. (2013). A role for hypocretin/orexin receptor-1 in cue-induced reinstatement of nicotine-seeking behavior. *Neuropsychopharmacology* 38, 1724–1736. doi: 10.1038/npp.2013.72

Plaza-Zabala, A., Martin-Garcia, E., de Lecea, L., Maldonado, R., and Berrendero, F. (2010). Hypocretins regulate the anxiogenic-like effects of nicotine and induce reinstatement of nicotine-seeking behavior. *J. Neurosci.* 30, 2300–2310. doi: 10.1523/JNEUROSCI.5724-09.2010

Porter, R. A., Chan, W. N., Coulton, S., Johns, A., Hadley, M. S., Widdowson, K., et al. (2001). 1,3-Biarylureas as selective non-peptide antagonists of the orexin-1 receptor. *Bioorg. Med. Chem. Lett.* 11, 1907–1910. doi: 10.1016/S0960-894X(01)00343-2

Rainero, I., Ostacoli, L., Rubino, E., Gallone, S., Picci, L. R., Fenoglio, P., et al. (2011). Association between major mood disorders and the hypocretin receptor 1 gene. *J. Affect. Disord.* 130, 487–491. doi: 10.1016/j.jad.2010.10.033

Rao, Y., Mineur, Y. S., Gan, G., Wang, A. H., Liu, Z. W., Wu, X., et al. (2013). Repeated *in vivo* exposure of cocaine induces long-lasting synaptic plasticity in hypocretin/orexin-producing neurons in the lateral hypothalamus in mice. *J. Physiol.* 591(Pt 7), 1951–1966. doi: 10.1113/jphysiol.2012.246983

Renzulli, C., Nash, M., Wright, M., Thomas, S., Zamuner, S., Pellegatti, M., et al. (2011). Disposition and metabolism of [14C]SB-649868, an orexin 1 and 2 receptor antagonist, in humans. *Drug Metab. Dispos.* 39, 215–227. doi: 10.1124/dmd.110.035386

Richards, J. K., Simms, J. A., Steensland, P., Taha, S. A., Borgland, S. L., Bonci, A., et al. (2008). Inhibition of orexin-1/hypocretin-1 receptors inhibits yohimbine-induced reinstatement of ethanol and sucrose seeking in Long-Evans rats. *Psychopharmacology (Berl.)* 199, 109–117. doi: 10.1007/s00213-008-1136-5

Rodgers, R. J., Wright, F. L., Snow, N. F., and Taylor, L. J. (2013). Orexin-1 receptor antagonism fails to reduce anxiety-like behaviour in either plus-maze-naïve or plus-maze-experienced mice. *Behav. Brain Res.* 243, 213–219. doi: 10.1016/j.bbr.2012.12.064

Rotter, A., Asemann, R., Decker, A., Kornhuber, J., and Biermann, T. (2011). Orexin expression and promoter-methylation in peripheral blood of patients suffering from major depressive disorder. *J. Affect. Disord.* 131, 186–192. doi: 10.1016/j.jad.2010.12.004

Russell, S. H., Small, C. J., Dakin, C. L., Abbott, C. R., Morgan, D. G., Ghatei, M. A., et al. (2001). The central effects of orexin-A in the hypothalamic-pituitary-adrenal axis *in vivo* and *in vitro* in male rats. *J. Neuroendocrinol.* 13, 561–566. doi: 10.1046/j.1365-2826.2001.00672.x

Russo, S. J., and Nestler, E. J. (2013). The brain reward circuitry in mood disorders. *Nat. Rev. Neurosci.* 14, 609–625. doi: 10.1038/nrn3381

Rusyniak, D. E., Zaretsky, D. V., Zaretskaia, M. V., Durant, P. J., and DiMicco, J. A. (2012). The orexin-1 receptor antagonist SB-334867 decreases sympathetic responses to a moderate dose of methamphetamine and stress. *Physiol. Behav.* 107, 743–750. doi: 10.1016/j.physbeh.2012.02.010

Sakamoto, F., Yamada, S., and Ueta, Y. (2004). Centrally administered orexin-A activates corticotropin-releasing factor-containing neurons in the hypothalamic paraventricular nucleus and central amygdaloid nucleus of rats: possible involvement of central orexins on stress-activated central CRF neurons. *Regul. Pept.* 118, 183–191. doi: 10.1016/j.regpep.2003.12.014

Sakurai, T., Amemiya, A., Ishii, M., Matsuzaki, I., Chemelli, R. M., Tanaka, H., et al. (1998). Orexins and orexin receptors: a family of hypothalamic neuropeptides and G protein-coupled receptors that regulate feeding behavior. *Cell* 92, 573–585. doi: 10.1016/S0092-8674(00)80949-6

Salomon, R. M., Ripley, B., Kennedy, J. S., Johnson, B., Schmidt, D., Zeitzer, J. M., et al. (2003). Diurnal variation of cerebrospinal fluid hypocretin-1 (Orexin-A) levels in control and depressed subjects. *Biol. Psychiatry* 54, 96–104. doi: 10.1016/S0006-3223(02)01740-7

Sartor, G. C., and Aston-Jones, G. (2012). A septal-hypothalamic pathway drives orexin neurons, which is necessary for conditioned cocaine preference. *J. Neurosci.* 32, 4623–4631. doi: 10.1523/JNEUROSCI.4561-11.2012

Scammell, T. E., and Winrow, C. J. (2011). Orexin receptors: pharmacology and therapeutic opportunities. *Annu. Rev. Pharmacol. Toxicol.* 51, 243–266. doi: 10.1146/annurev-pharmtox-010510-100528

Schmidt, F. M., Arendt, E., Steinmetzer, A., Bruegel, M., Kratzsch, J., Strauss, M., et al. (2011). CSF-hypocretin-1 levels in patients with major depressive disorder compared to healthy controls. *Psychiatry Res.* 190, 240–243. doi: 10.1016/j.psychres.2011.06.004

Schneider, E. R., Rada, P., Darby, R. D., Leibowitz, S. F., and Hoebel, B. G. (2007). Orexigenic peptides and alcohol intake: differential effects of orexin, galanin, and ghrelin. *Alcohol. Clin. Exp. Res.* 31, 1858–1865. doi: 10.1111/j.1530-0277.2007.00510.x

Schöne, C., Venner, A., Knowles, D., Karnani, M. M., and Burdakov, D. (2011). Dichotomous cellular properties of mouse orexin/hypocretin neurons. *J. Physiol.* 589, 2767–2779. doi: 10.1113/jphysiol.2011.208637

Scott, M. M., Marcus, J. N., Pettersen, A., Birnbaum, S. G., Mochizuki, T., Scammell, T. E., et al. (2011). Hcrtr1 and 2 signaling differentially regulates depression-like behaviors. *Behav. Brain Res.* 222, 289–294. doi: 10.1016/j.bbr.2011.02.044

Sears, R. M., Fink, A. E., Wigestrand, M. B., Farb, C. R., de Lecea, L., and LeDoux, J. E. (2013). Orexin/hypocretin system modulates amygdala-dependent threat learning through the locus coeruleus. *Proc. Natl. Acad. Sci. U.S.A.* 110, 20260–20265. doi: 10.1073/pnas.1320325110

Sharf, R., Guarnieri, D. J., Taylor, J. R., and DiLeone, R. J. (2010). Orexin mediates morphine place preference, but not morphine-induced hyperactivity or sensitization. *Brain Res.* 1317, 24–32. doi: 10.1016/j.brainres.2009.12.035

Shoblock, J. R., Welty, N., Aluisio, L., Fraser, I., Motley, S. T., Morton, K., et al. (2010). Selective blockade of the orexin-2 receptor attenuates ethanol

self-administration, place preference, and reinstatement. *Psychopharmacology (Berl.)* 215, 191–203. doi: 10.1007/s00213-010-2127-x

Smart, D., Sabido-David, C., Brough, S. J., Jewitt, F., Johns, A., Porter, R. A., et al. (2001). SB-334867-A: the first selective orexin-1 receptor antagonist. *Br. J. Pharmacol.* 132, 1179–1182. doi: 10.1038/sj.bjp.0703953

Smith, R. J., and Aston-Jones, G. (2012). Orexin/hypocretin 1 receptor antagonist reduces heroin self-administration and cue-induced heroin seeking. *Eur. J. Neurosci.* 35, 798–804. doi: 10.1111/j.1460-9568.2012.08013.x

Smith, R. J., See, R. E., and Aston-Jones, G. (2009). Orexin/hypocretin signaling at the orexin 1 receptor regulates cue-elicited cocaine-seeking. *Eur. J. Neurosci.* 30, 493–503. doi: 10.1111/j.1460-9568.2009.06844.x

Smith, R. J., Tahsili-Fahadan, P., and Aston-Jones, G. (2010). Orexin/hypocretin is necessary for context-driven cocaine-seeking. *Neuropharmacology* 58, 179–184. doi: 10.1016/j.neuropharm.2009.06.042

Soya, S., Shoji, H., Hasegawa, E., Hondo, M., Miyakawa, T., Yanagisawa, M., et al. (2013). Orexin receptor-1 in the locus coeruleus plays an important role in cue-dependent fear memory consolidation. *J. Neurosci.* 33, 14549–14557. doi: 10.1523/JNEUROSCI.1130-13.2013

Srinivasan, S., Simms, J. A., Nielsen, C. K., Lieske, S. P., Bito-Onon, J. J., Yi, H., et al. (2012). The dual orexin/hypocretin receptor antagonist, almorexant, in the ventral tegmental area attenuates ethanol self-administration. *PLoS ONE* 7:e44726. doi: 10.1371/journal.pone.0044726

Staples, L. G., and Cornish, J. L. (2014). The orexin-1 receptor antagonist SB-334867 attenuates anxiety in rats exposed to cat odor but not the elevated plus maze: An investigation of Trial 1 and Trial 2 effects. *Horm. Behav.* doi: 10.1016/j.yhbeh.2013.12.014. [Epub ahead of print].

Steiner, M. A., Gatfield, J., Brisbare-Roch, C., Dietrich, H., Treiber, A., Jenck, F., et al. (2013a). Discovery and characterization of ACT-335827, an orally available, brain penetrant orexin receptor type 1 selective antagonist. *ChemMedChem* 8, 898–903. doi: 10.1002/cmdc.201300003

Steiner, M. A., Lecourt, H., and Jenck, F. (2012). The brain orexin system and almorexant in fear-conditioned startle reactions in the rat. *Psychopharmacology* 223, 465–475. doi: 10.1007/s00213-012-2736-7

Steiner, M. A., Lecourt, H., and Jenck, F. (2013c). The dual orexin receptor antagonist almorexant, alone and in combination with morphine, cocaine and amphetamine, on conditioned place preference and locomotor sensitization in the rat. *Int. J. Neuropsychopharmacol.* 16, 417–432. doi: 10.1017/S1461145712000193

Steiner, M. A., Sciarretta, C., Brisbare-Roch, C., Strasser, D. S., Studer, R., and Jenck, F. (2013b). Examining the role of endogenous orexins in hypothalamus–pituitary–adrenal axis endocrine function using transient dual orexin receptor antagonism in the rat. *Psychoneuroendocrinology* 38, 560–571. doi: 10.1016/j.psyneuen.2012.07.016

Strawn, J. R., Pyne-Geithman, G. J., Ekhator, N. N., Horn, P. S., Uhde, T. W., Shutter, L. A., et al. (2010). Low cerebrospinal fluid and plasma orexin-A (hypocretin-1) concentrations in combat-related posttraumatic stress disorder. *Psychoneuroendocrinology* 35, 1001–1007. doi: 10.1016/j.psyneuen.2010.01.001

Sutcliffe, J. G., and de Lecea, L. (2002). The hypocretins: setting the arousal threshold. *Nat. Rev. Neurosci.* 3, 339–349. doi: 10.1038/nrn808

Suzuki, M., Beuckmann, C. T., Shikata, K., Ogura, H., and Sawai, T. (2005). Orexin-A (hypocretin-1) is possibly involved in generation of anxiety-like behavior. *Brain Res.* 1044, 116–121. doi: 10.1016/j.brainres.2005.03.002

Taheri, S., Gardiner, J., Hafizi, S., Murphy, K., Dakin, C., Seal, L., et al. (2001). Orexin A immunoreactivity and preproorexin mRNA in the brain of Zucker and WKY rats. *Neuroreport* 12, 459–464. doi: 10.1097/00001756-200103050-00008

Taheri, S., Zeitzer, J. M., and Mignot, E. (2002). The role of hypocretins (orexins) in sleep regulation and narcolepsy. *Annu. Rev. Neurosci.* 25, 283–313. doi: 10.1146/annurev.neuro.25.112701.142826

Trivedi, P., Yu, H., MacNeil, D. J., Van der Ploeg, L. H., and Guan, X. M. (1998). Distribution of orexin receptor mRNA in the rat brain. *FEBS Lett.* 438, 71–75. doi: 10.1016/S0014-5793(98)01266-6

Ulrich-Lai, Y. M., and Herman, J P. (2009). Neural regulation of endocrine and autonimic stress responses. *Nat. Rev. Neurosci.* 10, 397–409. doi: 10.1038/nrn2647

von der Goltz, C., Koopmann, A., Dinter, C., Richter, A., Grosshans, M., Fink, T., et al. (2011). Involvement of orexin in the regulation of stress, depression and reward in alcohol dependence. *Horm. Behav.* 60, 644–650. doi: 10.1016/j.yhbeh.2011.08.017

Whitman, D. B., Cox, C. D., Breslin, M. J., Brashear, K. M., Schreier, J. D., Bogusky, M. J., et al. (2009). Discovery of a potent, CNS-penetrant orexin receptor antagonist based on an n,n-disubstituted-1,4-diazepane scaffold that promotes sleep in rats. *ChemMedChem* 4, 1069–1074. doi: 10.1002/cmdc.200900069

Yeoh, J. W., James, M. H., Jobling, P., Bains, J. S., Graham, B. A., and Dayas, C. V. (2012). Cocaine potentiates excitatory drive in the perifornical/lateral hypothalamus. *J. Physiol.* 590(Pt 16), 3677–3689. doi: 10.1113/jphysiol.2012.230268

Zhou, L., Smith, R. J., Do, P. H., Aston-Jones, G., and See, R. E. (2012). Repeated orexin 1 receptor antagonism effects on cocaine seeking in rats. *Neuropharmacology* 63, 1201–1207. doi: 10.1016/j.neuropharm.2012.07.044

Zhou, L., Sun, W. L., and See, R. E. (2011). Orexin receptor targets for anti-relapse medication development in drug addiction. *Pharmaceuticals (Basel)* 4, 804–821. doi: 10.3390/ph4060804

Zhou, Y., Bendor, J., Hofmann, L., Randesi, M., Ho, A., and Kreek, M. J. (2006). Mu opioid receptor and orexin/hypocretin mRNA levels in the lateral hypothalamus and striatum are enhanced by morphine withdrawal. *J. Endocrinol.* 191, 137–145. doi: 10.1677/joe.1.06960

Conflict of Interest Statement: The authors declare that the research was conducted in the absence of any commercial or financial relationships that could be construed as a potential conflict of interest.

Orexin-1 receptor blockade dysregulates REM sleep in the presence of orexin-2 receptor antagonism

Christine Dugovic*, Jonathan E. Shelton, Sujin Yun, Pascal Bonaventure, Brock T. Shireman and Timothy W. Lovenberg

Neuroscience, Janssen Research & Development, L.L.C., San Diego, CA, USA

Edited by:
Michel A. Steiner, Actelion Pharmaceuticals Ltd., Switzerland

Reviewed by:
Michihiro Mieda, Kanazawa University, Japan
Markus Fendt, Otto-von-Guericke University Magdeburg, Germany
Claudia Betschart, Novartis, Switzerland

*Correspondence:
Christine Dugovic, Neuroscience, Janssen Research & Development, L.L.C., 3210 Merryfield Row, San Diego, CA 92121, USA
e-mail: cdugovic@its.jnj.com

In accordance with the prominent role of orexins in the maintenance of wakefulness via activation of orexin-1 (OX1R) and orexin-2 (OX2R) receptors, various dual OX1/2R antagonists have been shown to promote sleep in animals and humans. While selective blockade of OX2R seems to be sufficient to initiate and prolong sleep, the beneficial effect of additional inhibition of OX1R remains controversial. The relative contribution of OX1R and OX2R to the sleep effects induced by a dual OX1/2R antagonist was further investigated in the rat, and specifically on rapid eye movement (REM) sleep since a deficiency of the orexin system is associated with narcolepsy/cataplexy based on clinical and pre-clinical data. As expected, the dual OX1/2R antagonist SB-649868 was effective in promoting non-REM (NREM) and REM sleep following oral dosing (10 and 30 mg/kg) at the onset of the dark phase. However, a disruption of REM sleep was evidenced by a more pronounced reduction in the onset of REM as compared to NREM sleep, a marked enhancement of the REM/total sleep ratio, and the occurrence of a few episodes of direct wake to REM sleep transitions (REM intrusion). When administered subcutaneously, the OX2R antagonist JNJ-10397049 (10 mg/kg) increased NREM duration whereas the OX1R antagonist GSK-1059865 (10 mg/kg) did not alter sleep. REM sleep was not affected either by OX2R or OX1R blockade alone, but administration of the OX1R antagonist in combination with the OX2R antagonist induced a significant reduction in REM sleep latency and an increase in REM sleep duration at the expense of the time spent in NREM sleep. These results indicate that additional blockade of OX1R to OX2R antagonism elicits a dysregulation of REM sleep by shifting the balance in favor of REM sleep at the expense of NREM sleep that may increase the risk of adverse events. Translation of this hypothesis remains to be tested in the clinic.

Keywords: orexin-1, orexin-2, receptor antagonist, REM sleep, rat

INTRODUCTION

The orexin neuropeptides produced by lateral hypothalamic neurons play a critical role in the maintenance of wakefulness by activating two distinct receptors, the orexin-1 (OX1R) and the orexin-2 (OX2R) receptor that are widely distributed throughout the brain (De Lecea et al., 1998; Peyron et al., 1998; Sakurai et al., 1998). The orexin system is believed to stabilize the wake-sleep flip-flop switch in wake-active structures consisting of histaminergic, monoaminergic, and cholinergic neurons (Saper et al., 2001), and also to regulate the onset of rapid eye movement (REM) sleep and associated muscular atonia in the brainstem (Lu et al., 2006). In accordance with the prominent function of orexins in sustaining wakefulness, pharmacological blockade of both OX1R and OX2R (OX1/2R) has been shown to promote sleep in various species, and the dual OX1/2R antagonists almorexant, SB-649868 and suvorexant have been clinically validated for the treatment of insomnia (Winrow and Renger, 2014). Further investigations conducted in rodent models on the specific role of OX1R and OX2R in sleep modulation indicate that while selective blockade of OX2R seems to be sufficient to initiate and prolong sleep (Dugovic et al., 2009; Mang et al., 2012), the beneficial effect

of additional inhibition of OX1R remains controversial (Morairty et al., 2012).

OX1R and OX2R are differentially distributed in structures regulating sleep and wake, with OX1R exclusively expressed in the locus coeruleus, OX2R selectively expressed in the tubero-mammillary nucleus, and both receptors co-expressed in the dorsal raphe (Sakurai et al., 1998; Marcus et al., 2001), suggesting a distinct function between the two orexin receptors. It has been proposed that OX2R signaling is essential for the promotion of wakefulness and the transition to non-REM (NREM) sleep and that both OX1R and OX2R contribute to REM sleep suppression (Willie et al., 2003; Mieda et al., 2011; Mochizuki et al., 2011). Loss or disruption of orexin signaling in human and animal narcolepsy is associated with reduced activity of the wake-promoting system, frequent transitions into NREM sleep, and abnormal intrusions of REM sleep into wake accompanied by loss of muscular tone and cataplexy (Nishino, 2007). During their dark/active phase, mice lacking the orexin peptide as well as mice lacking both OX1R and OX2R spend more time in REM sleep, whereas NREM sleep duration is unaffected as compared to their corresponding wild type (Willie et al., 2003; Sakurai,

2007; Mang et al., 2012). Previous work in our lab has indicated that simultaneous blockade of OX1R attenuates the NREM sleep-promoting effects evoked by a selective OX2R antagonist but not the REM sleep promotion when assessed for a 2-h period during the light/rest phase in rats (Dugovic et al., 2009).

In the present study, we further explored the respective contributions of OX1R and OX2R on the sleep-promoting effects elicited by pharmacological blockade of both receptors, and specifically on REM sleep since a deficiency of the orexin system is associated with narcolepsy/cataplexy based on clinical and pre-clinical data. In order to detect possible events reminiscent of narcoleptic-like symptoms such as REM intrusion into wakefulness, the investigation was conducted during the active phase of the animals. The effects of the dual OX1/2R antagonist SB-649868 (Di Fabio et al., 2011) were compared to those obtained by co-administration of the selective OX1R antagonist GSK-1059865 (Gozzi et al., 2011) and the selective OX2R antagonist JNJ-10397049 (McAtee et al., 2004) during the dark phase in rats.

MATERIALS AND METHODS
ANIMALS
Studies were performed in male Sprague–Dawley rats (Harlan Laboratories, weighing 350–450 g). Animals were approximately 4 months of age at the start of the study and were housed individually in cages under controlled conditions with lights on at 6 AM (12:12 light/dark schedule) while temperature was maintained at $22 \pm 2°C$. During the course of the study, animals had *ad libitum* access to food and water. All procedures detailed in this investigation were implemented in accordance with policies established by the Guide for the Care and Use of Laboratory Animals as adopted by the United States National Institutes of Health.

DRUGS AND EXPERIMENTAL DESIGN
SB-649868 is a dual OX1/2R antagonist with similar potency at both receptor subtypes (pKi OX1R = 9.5, pKi OX2R = 9.4) and the doses tested were selected in accordance with the pharmacokinetic profile and hypnotic activity in rats described for this compound (Di Fabio et al., 2011). GSK-1059865 is a selective OX1R antagonist that shows a 80 fold higher selectivity vs. OX2R (Gozzi et al., 2011). We confirmed the high selectivity of GSK-1059865 (pKi OX1R = 8.3, pKi OX2R = 6.4; unpublished data). GSK-1059865 (10 mg/kg) achieved about 90% OX1R occupancy 15 min after subcutaneous (sc) administration which was maintained for 4 h, as determined by *ex vivo* autoradiography in the rat brain (manuscript in preparation). JNJ-10397049 is a selective OX2R antagonist (pKi OX2R = 8.2, pKi OX1R = 5.7). JNJ-10397049 (30 mg/kg) achieved about 80% of OX2R occupancy 15 min after sc administration which was maintained for 6 h, as determined by *ex vivo* autoradiography in rat cortex (Dugovic et al., 2009). SB-649868, JNJ-10397049, and GSK-1059865 were synthesized at Janssen Research & Development, L.L.C. SB-649868 (10 and 30 mg/kg) was dosed orally as a suspension of 0.5% methylcellulose in a volume of 1 ml/kg. JNJ-10397049 (10 mg/kg) and GSK-1059865 (10 mg/kg) were administered via the subcutaneous (sc) route. GSK-1059865 and JNJ-10397049 were formulated in 5% pharmasolve, 20%

solutol, 75% hydroxypropyl-β-cyclodextrin (20% w/v), and were injected as a free base form of the compound in a volume of 1 ml/kg.

The dose-response experiment with SB-649868 was carried out in a group of animals ($n = 8$) assigned to three treatment conditions (vehicle, $n = 8$; 10 mg/kg, $n = 7$; 30 mg/kg, $n = 7$). The experiment with the simultaneous coadministration of GSK-1059865 and JNJ-10397049 was carried out on a separate group of rats ($n = 7$) assigned to four treatment conditions (vehicle + vehicle, GSK-1059865 + vehicle, vehicle + JNJ-10397049, and GSK-1059865 + JNJ-10397049). Both experiments were conducted in a randomized cross-over design and a minimum of 3 days washout period were allowed between two treatments.

SLEEP RECORDING AND ANALYSIS
Animals were implanted with telemetric devices for polysomnographic recording of sleep-wake patterns as previously described (Dugovic et al., 2009). To determine states of vigilance, polysomnographic waveforms were acquired from two stainless steel screw electrodes that were implanted under isofluorane anesthesia in the frontal and parietal cortex for the electroencephalogram (EEG) and in dorsal nuchal muscles for the electromyogram (EMG). Electrodes were coupled to a sterile two-channel telemetric device (PhysioTel F40-EET; Data Sciences International, St. Paul, MN) that had been implanted in the intraperitoneal cavity in order to acquire measurements of body temperature and locomotor activity. After a 2-week period of recovery from surgery, animals were transferred to their designated housing/procedure room to allow for adaptation to the recording chamber and environment.

EEG and EMG signals were recorded for up to 12 h post-drug administration and were digitized at a sampling rate of 100 Hz on an IBM PC-compatible computer using Dataquest A.R.T software (Data Sciences International). Using the computer software program SleepSign (Kissei Comtec, Nagano, Japan), consecutive EEG/EMG recordings were divided into individual 10 sepochs that were then visually assigned vigilance states based upon conventional criteria for wake, NREM sleep and REM sleep as described previously. EEG activity within specific vigilance states was determined by power spectral analysis using the Fast Fourier Transform performed within a frequency range of 1–30 Hz. Values for power spectra were divided into four frequency bands: delta (1–4 Hz), theta (4–10 Hz), sigma (10–15 Hz), and beta (15–30 Hz).

Analysis of sleep-wake parameters included latency (onset) to NREM sleep (defined as the time interval to the first six consecutive NREM epochs) and REM sleep (the first two consecutive REM epochs post-injection), the duration of wake, NREM and REM sleep and bout analysis (number and duration) for each vigilance state. In addition, episodes of direct wake to REM sleep (DREM) transitions were assessed. A DREM transition was defined as an abrupt episode of nuchal atonia and EEG dominance of theta activity lasting at least a 10 s epoch with at least six consecutive 10 s epochs of wake (60 s) preceding the episode. As a comparison, a criteria of at least 40 s of wakefulness preceding an episode of cataplexy has been defined in mouse models of narcolepsy (Scammell et al., 2009).

Results were averaged and expressed as mean ±s.e.m. in defined time intervals. To determine whether differences were significant at a given interval, either a One-Way analysis of variance (ANOVA) with Newman–Keuls or Dunnett's multiple comparison *post-hoc* analysis, or Two-Way repeated measures ANOVA followed by a Bonferroni *post-hoc* test was performed.

RESULTS

DIFFERENTIAL NREM AND REM SLEEP-PROMOTING EFFECTS OF THE DUAL OX1/2R ANTAGONIST SB-649868

When administered at the onset of the dark phase, the dual OX1/2R antagonist SB-649868 significantly reduced the latencies for NREM and REM sleep, and significantly prolonged the time spent in each of these sleep states at the two doses tested, 10 and 30 mg/kg (**Figure 1**). However, REM sleep was predominantly affected relative to NREM sleep in regard to its onset and total duration. The latency for NREM sleep was reduced by half (**Figure 1A**), whereas the latency for REM sleep was

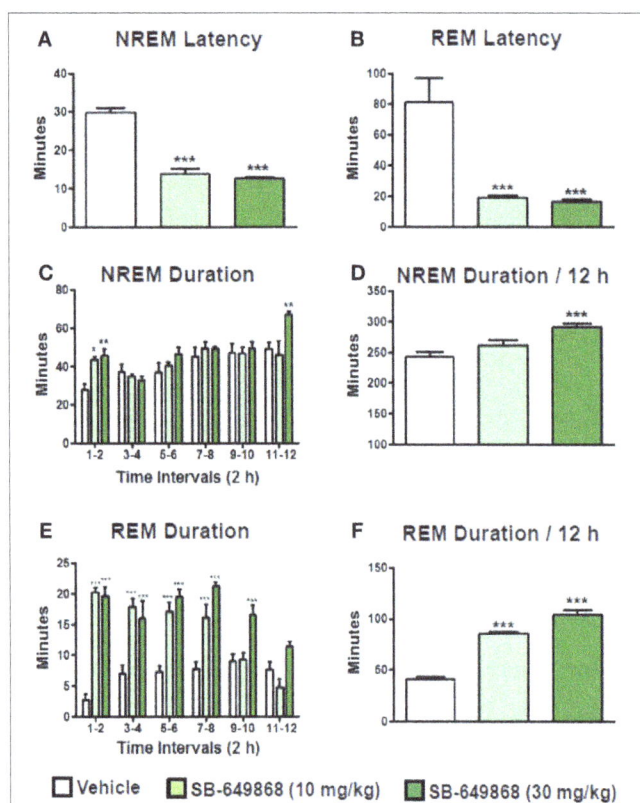

FIGURE 1 | Sleep-promoting effects of the dual OX1/2R antagonist SB-649868 in rats. Latency to NREM **(A)** and REM **(B)** sleep and duration of NREM **(C,D)** and REM **(E,F)** sleep during the 12-h dark phase after oral dosing (10 and 30 mg/kg) are expressed in minutes and are represented as means ± s.e.m. (n = 7–8 animals per condition). $*P < 0.05$, $**P < 0.01$, and $***P < 0.001$ vs. vehicle, based on One-Way ANOVA followed by Dunnett's multiple comparison *post-hoc* test **(A)** [$F_{(2, 19)}$ = 70.60, $p < 0.001$], **(B)** [$F_{(2, 19)}$ = 14.05, $p < 0.001$], **(D)** [$F_{(2, 19)}$ = 9.57, $p = 0.001$], and **(F)** [$F_{(2, 19)}$ = 127.50, $p < 0.001$] or two-way ANOVA (interaction Time × Treatment) followed by Bonferroni *post-hoc* test **(C)** [$F_{(10, 144)}$ = 2.45, $p = 0.011$] and **(E)** [$F_{(10, 114)}$ = 8.07, $p < 0.001$].

diminished by about 75% (**Figure 1B**) as compared to the vehicle condition, leading to an almost similar onset for both states. Similarly, the time course of the effects on REM sleep differed from the effects on NREM sleep. The increase in NREM sleep duration occurred mostly during the first 2 h after the treatment (**Figure 1C**), whereas the increase in REM duration lasted for 8 h at the 10 mg/kg dose and for the entire 12-h dark phase following the dose of 30 mg/kg (**Figure 1E**). In the total 12-h period, the increase in NREM sleep duration was significant at the high dose only (**Figure 1D**) whereas REM sleep was significantly increased at both doses tested (**Figure 1F**). Further analysis of the sleep macrostructure showed that while the numbers of both NREM and REM bouts were dose-dependently enhanced, the NREM bout duration was reduced but the REM bout duration was prolonged (**Table 1**). Therefore, the net increase in the time spent in NREM sleep might be attenuated due to a decrease in NREM sleep continuity in spite of the increase in its frequency. In contrast, both the frequency and continuity in REM sleep were increased, leading to a larger increment in the total REM sleep duration. In addition, a careful visual analysis of the EEG and EMG signals revealed scarce episodes of direct transitions from wake to REM sleep (DREM). DREM episodes occurred in 3 out of 7 rats treated with the highest dose of 30 mg/kg, and in one animal which received the dose of 10 mg/kg as illustrated in the hypnogram and the EEG/EMG traces corresponding to this event (**Figure 2**). Power spectral analysis indicates that the averaged EEG relative power in the theta frequency band (4–10 Hz) during this DREM episode (45% of the total power) was comparable to the relative theta power during a normal episode of REM sleep (49%) shown in **Figure 2** for this animal. The averaged EEG theta activity contributed to 26% of the total power during the 40 s wake episode preceding DREM and to 31% during the 50 s wake episode following DREM, indicating a distinct range of power density values compared to the theta activity during DREM.

DISINHIBITION OF REM SLEEP BY ADDITIONAL PHARMACOLOGICAL BLOCKADE OF OX1R TO OX2R ANTAGONISM

To further investigate the differential actions of the dual OX1/2R antagonist on NREM and REM sleep, rats were administered either with the selective OX1R antagonist GSK-1059865

Table 1 | NREM and REM bout analysis after oral administration of the dual OX1/2R antagonist SB-649868 in rats.

	NREM bout number	NREM bout duration (min)	REM bout number	REM bout duration (min)
Vehicle	154.4 ± 4.8	1.57 ± 0.04	31.9 ± 2.5	1.32 ± 0.07
10 mg/kg	211.1 ± 9.1***	1.22 ± 0.07***	46.7 ± 2.8**	1.85 ± 0.09**
30 mg/kg	248.4 ± 7.6***	1.15 ± 0.04***	52.0 ± 3.2***	2.02 ± 0.13***

Values (means ± s.e.m. n = 7–8 animals per condition) are calculated for the 12-h dark phase after compound administration

$**P < 0.01$ *and* $***P < 0.001$ *vs. Vehicle based on one-way ANOVA followed by Dunnett's multiple comparison post-hoc test.*

NREM Bout Number [$F_{(2,19)}$ = 44.58, $p < 0.001$]; NREM Bout Duration [$F_{(2,19)}$ = 19.38, $p < 0.001$]; REM Bout Number [$F_{(2,19)}$ = 14.10, $p < 0.001$]; REM Bout Duration [$F_{(2,19)}$ = 13.94, $p < 0.001$].

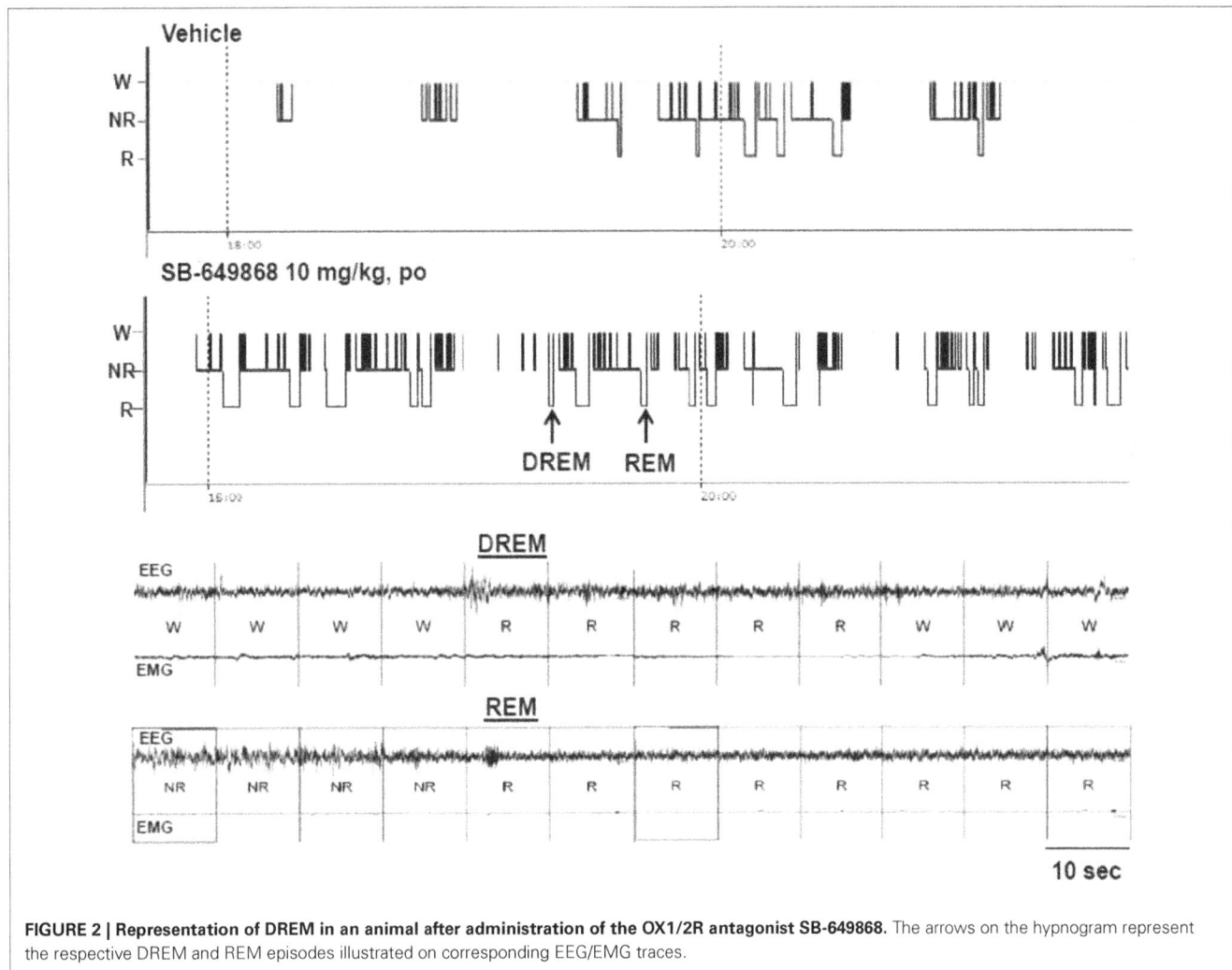

FIGURE 2 | Representation of DREM in an animal after administration of the OX1/2R antagonist SB-649868. The arrows on the hypnogram represent the respective DREM and REM episodes illustrated on corresponding EEG/EMG traces.

(10 mg /kg) or the selective OX2R antagonist JNJ-10397049 (10 mg/kg) alone, or in combination at the onset of the dark phase. The results were presented in **Figure 3** for the first 6-h period after dosing, based on the shorter duration of both the sleep-promoting effect of JNJ-10397049 and the sleep response elicited by simultaneous injection of GSK-1059865 at the respective doses tested. Sleep-wake parameters were not affected during the second 6-h period (data not shown). Administration of the OX2R antagonist alone induced a significant reduction in NREM sleep latency (**Figure 3A**) and an increase in NREM sleep duration (**Figures 3C,D**) relative to vehicle treatment. While the OX1R antagonist had no effect on NREM sleep by itself, its administration significantly attenuated the NREM sleep prolongation evoked by the OX2R antagonist (**Figures 3C,D**). Indeed, in the combined treatment condition the NREM bout duration was significantly reduced relative to all other conditions (**Table 2**), accounting for the less pronounced increment in total NREM sleep duration. The time course analysis shows that the reduced effect on NREM sleep occurred 2 h after the additional administration of GSK-1059865 (**Figure 3C**), and consequently the NREM sleep latency was not affected (**Figure 3A**). REM sleep

onset (**Figure 3B**) and REM sleep duration (**Figures 3E,F**) were not altered by either OX1R or OX2R pharmacological blockade. In contrast, when receiving the combined treatment the animals displayed a reduced REM sleep latency (**Figure 3B**) and the time spent in REM sleep was significantly increased as compared to treatment with vehicle, OX1R or OX2R antagonist alone (**Figures 3E,F**). This REM sleep-promoting effect was observed mainly during the first 4 h following the treatment (**Figure 3E**) and was due to a significant prolongation of the REM bout duration as well as a tendency to enhanced REM bout numbers (**Table 2**). Ultimately, the results showed that additional pharmacological blockade of OX1R attenuated the NREM sleep-promoting effects of an OX2R antagonist by increasing REM sleep duration and concomitantly decreasing NREM sleep duration, leading to a significant enhancement of the REM/total sleep ratio (% REM/TS) as illustrated in **Figure 3G**. Similarly, a markedly elevated % REM/TS was found following the administration of the dual OX1/2R antagonist SB-649868 at the doses of 10 mg/kg (24.6%) and 30 mg/kg (26.4%) as compared to vehicle treatment (14.6%) over the 12-h dark phase. Therefore, both experimental approaches produced a disinhibition of REM

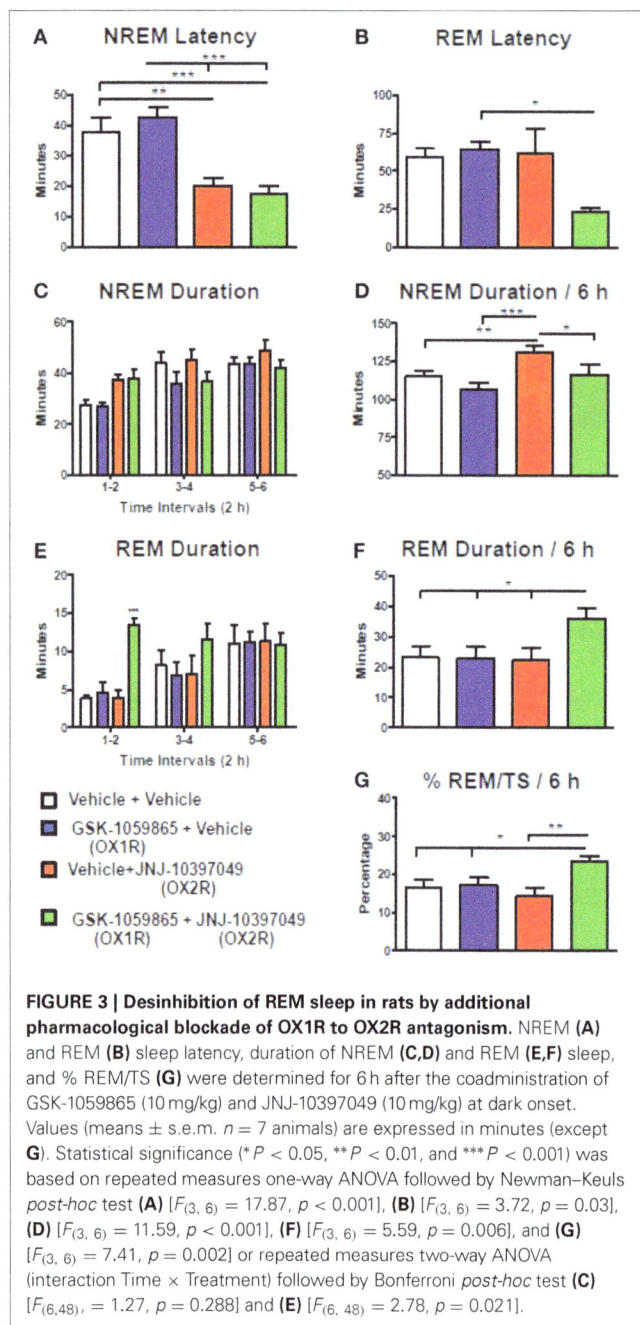

FIGURE 3 | Desinhibition of REM sleep in rats by additional pharmacological blockade of OX1R to OX2R antagonism. NREM **(A)** and REM **(B)** sleep latency, duration of NREM **(C,D)** and REM **(E,F)** sleep, and % REM/TS **(G)** were determined for 6 h after the coadministration of GSK-1059865 (10 mg/kg) and JNJ-10397049 (10 mg/kg) at dark onset. Values (means ± s.e.m. $n = 7$ animals) are expressed in minutes (except **G**). Statistical significance (*$P < 0.05$, **$P < 0.01$, and ***$P < 0.001$) was based on repeated measures one-way ANOVA followed by Newman–Keuls post-hoc test **(A)** [$F_{(3, 6)} = 17.87$, $p < 0.001$], **(B)** [$F_{(3, 6)} = 3.72$, $p = 0.03$], **(D)** [$F_{(3, 6)} = 11.59$, $p < 0.001$], **(F)** [$F_{(3, 6)} = 5.59$, $p = 0.006$], and **(G)** [$F_{(3, 6)} = 7.41$, $p = 0.002$] or repeated measures two-way ANOVA (interaction Time × Treatment) followed by Bonferroni post-hoc test **(C)** [$F_{(6,48)}, = 1.27$, $p = 0.288$] and **(E)** [$F_{(6, 48)} = 2.78$, $p = 0.021$].

Table 2 | NREM and REM bout analysis after co-administration of the OX1R antagonist GSK-1059865 (10 mg/kg) and the OX2R antagonist JNJ-10397049 (10 mg/kg) in rats.

	NREM bout number	NREM bout duration (min)	REM bout number	REM bout duration (min)
Vehicle + Vehicle	82.7 ± 2.6	1.39 ± 0.07	19.6 ± 2.0	1.13 ± 0.13
GSK-1059865 + Vehicle	70.7 ± 3.7*[a]	1.51 ± 0.10[c]	18.1 ± 1.7	1.21 ± 0.17
Vehicle + JNJ-10397049	101.0 ± 4.2**	1.30 ± 0.07	17.7 ± 3.6	1.37 ± 0.18
GSK-1059865 + JNJ-10397049	97.9 ± 3.0*	1.17 ± 0.07*,[b]	23.0 ± 2.1	1.55 ± 0.11**,[b]

Values (means ± s.e.m. $n = 7$ animals) are calculated for the 6-h period following the treatment.
*$P < 0.05$ and **$P < 0.01$ vs. Vehicle + Vehicle
[a]$P < 0.001$ vs. Vehicle + JNJ-10397049 and GSK-1059865 + JNJ-10397049
[b]$P < 0.01$ vs. GSK-1059865 + Vehicle
[c]$P < 0.05$ vs. Vehicle + JNJ-10397049
As determined by repeated measures One-Way ANOVA followed by Newman–Keuls post-hoc test.
NREM Bout Number [$F_{(3, 6)} = 13.69$, $p < 0.001$]; NREM Bout Duration [$F_{(3, 6)} = 7.79$, $p = 0.001$];
REM Bout Number [$F_{(3, 6)} = 1.28$, $p = 0.313$]; REM Bout Duration [$F_{(3, 6)} = 6.76$, $p = 0.003$].

pronounced NREM sleep-promoting effect. Similarly, administration of a selective OX1R antagonist in combination with a selective OX2R antagonist exclusively enhanced REM sleep by counteracting the NREM sleep-promoting effects evoked by the OX2R blockade. Therefore, transient pharmacological inhibition of the two receptors, either by a dual OX1/2R antagonist or by simultaneous blockade of OX1R to OX2R antagonism, disrupted sleep architecture by shifting the balance in favor of REM sleep at the expense of NREM sleep.

Selective pharmacological blockade of OX2R by JNJ-10397049 promotes sleep by inhibiting the output of wake active neurons, mainly by suppressing histamine release in the hypothalamus (Dugovic et al., 2009). Conversely, orexin-A administration increased cortical histamine release without affecting the norepinephrine or serotonin release in mice (Hong et al., 2005). The robust hypnotic properties of several selective OX2R antagonists after systemic administration in rats and mice have been confirmed by other groups (Gozzi et al., 2011; Morairty et al., 2012; Betschart et al., 2013). In these dose-response studies, results showed that NREM sleep was firstly increased at low dosage and that REM sleep was progressively enhanced at higher doses, with no obvious change in the REM/TS ratio indicating a preservation of the sleep architecture. By contrast to selective OX2R antagonists, pharmacological (using various OX1R antagonists with distinct chemical structures) or genetic selective inhibition of OX1R in rodent models has been reported to minimally affect sleep-wake states in baseline conditions (Smith et al., 2003; Sakurai, 2007; Dugovic et al., 2009; Gozzi et al., 2011). Controversial data has been reported in one study with the OX1R antagonist SB-334867 (Morairty et al., 2012) which is less selective and less potent than GSK-1059865 and exhibits off target activities (Gotter et al., 2012). Our results confirm the absence of sleep-promoting

sleep by shifting the balance in favor of REM sleep at the expense of NREM sleep. However, unlike with SB-649868, no DREM episodes were detected with the coadministration of GSK-1059865 and JNJ-10397049.

DISCUSSION

The present investigation demonstrated that pharmacological blockade of both OX1R and OX2R is effective in promoting both NREM and REM sleep but produced an alteration of the sleep stages distribution due to a striking impact on REM sleep. The dual OX1/2R antagonist SB-649868 primarily reduced REM sleep latency and prolonged REM sleep time in comparison to a less effects of GSK-1059865 previously reported by Gozzi et al. (2011), and a more recent study showed that the new selective OX1R antagonist ACT-335827 did not alter sleep in rats (Steiner et al., 2013). However, due to the paucity of publically available selective orexin compounds, SB-334867 remains so far the most studied OX1R antagonist and has been found to reverse the arousal and REM sleep suppression induced by pharmacological (orexin-A injection) or optogenetic activation of orexin neurons through OX1R in the locus coeruleus (Bourgin et al., 2000; Smith et al., 2003; Carter et al., 2012).

Within the last decade, dual OX1/2R antagonists have been developed as therapeutics for insomnia and their hypnotic properties have been demonstrated in animals, human volunteers, and insomnia patients. The development of the former compounds almorexant and SB-649868 has been stopped for undisclosed adverse effects; suvorexant is in the latest stage of clinical development and is followed by its back up compound filorexant (Winrow and Renger, 2014). In the present study, rats treated with SB-649868 at the onset of their active/dark phase displayed a markedly reduced REM sleep latency and the first episode of REM sleep was observed shortly after NREM sleep onset (**Figure 1**). While both sleep stages were enhanced, the predominant increase in REM sleep was reflected by the abnormally elevated REM/TS ratio compared to vehicle treatment. These data are in agreement with those previously found in rats when SB-649868 was dosed in the middle of the dark phase (Di Fabio et al., 2011). A similar increase in the proportion of REM vs. NREM sleep has been reported in mice dosed with almorexant or suvorexant (Mang et al., 2012; Betschart et al., 2013; Black et al., 2013), although not in rats (Brisbare-Roch et al., 2007; Winrow et al., 2011).

Our visual examination of EEG/EMG recordings revealed the occurrence of at least one episode of REM intrusion into wake (DREM) in 4 out of 7 animals dosed with SB-649868 (**Figure 2**). Simultaneous video recordings were not performed, therefore the behaviors associated with this activity during this unusual state transition in these rats are unclear. However, we did not observe any DREM event with the coadministration of the OX1R antagonist GSK-1059865 and the OX2R antagonist JNJ-10397049. While both compounds exhibit efficient brain-penetrating properties (see *ex vivo* receptor occupancy in methods), the REM sleep promotion produced by SB-649868 was much more pronounced and long-lasting as compared to the combined treatment, that might increase the possibility to trigger DREM transitions. In a murine model of narcolepsy, the orexin/ataxin-3 transgenic mouse, almorexant exacerbated spontaneous cataplexy, and possibly elicited cataplexy-like events in some wild type mice after wheel running activity (Black et al., 2013). In a preliminary investigation conducted in mice deficient for the OX2R, we also observed episodes of DREM following the treatment with another dual OX1/2R antagonist (Dugovic et al., 2012). Mice lacking both orexin receptors or the orexin peptide exhibit some cataplexy spontaneously (Sakurai, 2007) that can be substantially increased by pleasurable activity such as wheel running or eating highly palatable foods (Espana et al., 2007; Clark et al., 2009; Oishi et al., 2013). Cataplexy, a pathological intrusion of REM sleep atonia into wakefulness, has not been reported with almorexant or suvorexant in clinical or preclinical studies in situations where cataplexy is not provoked (Brisbare-Roch et al., 2007; Winrow and Renger, 2014). However, there are no disclosed clinical trials with an OX1/2R antagonist under conditions of positive emotional stimuli that are known to trigger cataplexy in narcolepsy with cataplexy patients.

Narcoleptic patients also exhibit sleep onset REM (SOREM) episodes usually defined as REM sleep latency shorter than 15 min (Nishino and Mignot, 1997). After SB-649868 administration, SOREM episodes were observed in Phase I studies (Bettica et al., 2012a), in a model of situational insomnia in healthy volunteers (Bettica et al., 2012b), as well as in patients with primary insomnia (Bettica et al., 2012c). Although SOREM episodes were not detected after administration of almorexant or suvorexant in primary insomnia patients, it is noteworthy that the latency for REM sleep was significantly reduced at half the dose required to shorten the latency to persistent sleep for both compounds (Herring et al., 2012; Hoever et al., 2012). In patients with primary insomnia treated with suvorexant or SB-649868, the increase in total sleep time resulted from a higher percentage of time spent in REM sleep and to a lesser degree in stage-2 sleep (Bettica et al., 2012c; Herring et al., 2012). Therefore, the preferential sleep-promoting action of dual OX1/2R antagonists on REM sleep relative to NREM sleep in animal studies seems to be predictive of the alterations in sleep architecture observed in humans.

The results of the experiment conducted in rats receiving the selective OX1R antagonist GSK-1059865 and the selective OX2R antagonist JNJ-10397049 in combination were consistent with the data obtained with the dual OX1/2R antagonist SB-649868. While REM sleep was not affected either by the OX2R antagonist or the OX1R antagonist alone, their coadministration reduced REM sleep latency and prolonged REM sleep time. Concurrently, the magnitude of the NREM sleep promoting effect elicited by the OX2R blockade was attenuated, demonstrating a shift in the balance between NREM and REM sleep. In a previous investigation carried out during the light/rest phase of the rat using the same selective OX2R antagonist, but with the OX1R antagonist SB-408124 which displayed less brain penetration (Gotter et al., 2012), we mainly observed a diminution in NREM sleep with the combined treatment vs. the OX2R antagonism alone (Dugovic et al., 2009). Together, these data indicate that additional OX1R blockade attenuated the NREM sleep promoting effect of an OX2R antagonist by disinhibiting REM sleep likely through OX1R.

In summary, we demonstrated that OX1R blockade dysregulates REM sleep in the presence of OX2R antagonism. These findings reinforce the consensus based on various animal models that wake to NREM sleep transitions depend on OX2R signaling and that REM sleep dysregulation occurs by the loss of both OX1R and OX2R function (Willie et al., 2003; Mieda et al., 2011; Mochizuki et al., 2011), thereby confirming the distinct contribution of OX1R and OX2R in the control of sleep-wake states. Key insights recently gained from the above clinical studies suggest that transient blockade of orexin receptors by dual OX1/2R antagonists induce a preferential disinhibition of REM sleep relative to NREM sleep, and may cause a dysregulation of REM sleep. Since the blockade of OX2R is sufficient to initiate and promote sleep in animals, future clinical studies with selective

OX2R antagonists should answer the question of whether this hypothesis is translatable to humans.

AUTHOR CONTRIBUTIONS

Christine Dugovic designed research, analyzed data, and wrote manuscript; Jonathan E. Shelton analyzed data and edited manuscript; Sujin Yun conducted research and analyzed data; Pascal Bonaventure participated in research design and edited manuscript; Brock T. Shireman provided compounds; Timothy W. Lovenberg participated in research design.

ACKNOWLEDGMENTS

We gratefully acknowledge the contribution of Dr. Kevin Sharp and the vivarium staff.

REFERENCES

Betschart, C., Hintermann, S., Behnke, D., Cotesta, S., Fendt, M., Gee, C. E., et al. (2013). Identification of a novel series of orexin receptor antagonists with a distinct effect on sleep architecture for the treatment of insomnia. *J. Med. Chem.* 56, 7590–7607. doi: 10.1021/jm4007627

Bettica, P., Nucci, G., Pyke, C., Squassante, L., Zamuner, S., Ratti, E., et al. (2012a). Phase I studies on the safety, tolerability, pharmacokinetics and pharmacodynamics of SB-649868, a novel dual orexin receptor antagonist. *J. Psychopharmacol.* 26, 1058–1070. doi: 10.1177/0269881111408954

Bettica, P., Squassante, L., Groeger, J. A., Gennery, B., Winsky-Sommerer, R., and Dijk, D. J. (2012b). Differential effects of a dual orexin receptor antagonist (SB-649868) and zolpidem on sleep initiation and consolidation, SWS, REM sleep, and EEG power spectra in a model of situational insomnia. *Neuropsychopharmacology* 37, 1224–1233. doi: 10.1038/npp.2011.310

Bettica, P., Squassante, L., Zamuner, S., Nucci, G., Danker-Hopfe, H., and Ratti, E. (2012c). The orexin antagonist SB-649868 promotes and maintains sleep in men with primary insomnia. *Sleep* 35, 1097–1104. doi: 10.5665/sleep.1996

Black, S. W., Morairty, S. R., Fisher, S. P., Chen, T. M., Warrier, D. R., and Kilduff, T. S. (2013). Almorexant promotes sleep and exacerbates cataplexy in a murine model of narcolepsy. *Sleep* 36, 325–336. doi: 10.5665/sleep.2442

Bourgin, P., Huitron-Resendiz, S., Spier, A. D., Fabre, V., Morte, B., Criado, J. R., et al. (2000). Hypocretin-1 modulates rapid eye movement sleep through activation of locus coeruleus neurons. *J. Neurosci.* 20, 7760–7765.

Brisbare-Roch, C., Dingemanse, J., Koberstein, R., Hoever, P., Aissaoui, H., Flores, S., et al. (2007). Promotion of sleep by targeting the orexin system in rats, dogs and humans. *Nat. Med.* 13, 150–155. doi: 10.1038/nm1544

Carter, M. E., Brill, J., Bonnavion, P., Huguenard, J. R., Huerta, R., and De Lecea, L. (2012). Mechanism for Hypocretin-mediated sleep-to-wake transitions. *Proc. Natl. Acad. Sci. U.S.A.* 109, E2635–E2644. doi: 10.1073/pnas.1202526109

Clark, E. L., Baumann, C. R., Cano, G., Scammell, T. E., and Mochizuki, T. (2009). Feeding-elicited cataplexy in orexin knockout mice. *Neuroscience* 161, 970–977. doi: 10.1016/j.neuroscience.2009.04.007

De Lecea, L., Kilduff, T. S., Peyron, C., Gao, X., Foye, P. E., Danielson, P. E., et al. (1998). The hypocretins: hypothalamus-specific peptides with neuroexcitatory activity. *Proc. Natl. Acad. Sci. U.S.A.* 95, 322–327. doi: 10.1073/pnas.95.1.322

Di Fabio, R., Pellacani, A., Faedo, S., Roth, A., Piccoli, L., Gerrard, P., et al. (2011). Discovery process and pharmacological characterization of a novel dual orexin 1 and orexin 2 receptor antagonist useful for treatment of sleep disorders. *Bioorg. Med. Chem. Lett.* 21, 5562–5567. doi: 10.1016/j.bmcl.2011.06.086

Dugovic, C., Shelton, J. E., Aluisio, L. E., Fraser, I. C., Jiang, X., Sutton, S. W., et al. (2009). Blockade of orexin-1 receptors attenuates orexin-2 receptor antagonism-induced sleep promotion in the rat. *J. Pharmacol. Exp. Ther.* 330, 142–151. doi: 10.1124/jpet.109.152009

Dugovic, C., Yun, S., Shelton, J., Bonaventure, P., Shireman, B., and Lovenberg, T. (2012). Respective role of orexin-1 and orexin-2 receptors in the effects of a dual ox1/2r antagonist on sleep. *Sleep* 35, A32.

Espana, R. A., McCormack, S. L., Mochizuki, T., and Scammell, T. E. (2007). Running promotes wakefulness and increases cataplexy in orexin knockout mice. *Sleep* 30, 1417–1425.

Gotter, A. L., Webber, A. L., Coleman, P. J., Renger, J. J., and Winrow, C. J. (2012). international union of basic and clinical pharmacology. LXXXVI. orexin receptor function, nomenclature and pharmacology. *Pharmacol. Rev.* 64, 389–420. doi: 10.1124/pr.111.005546

Gozzi, A., Turrini, G., Piccoli, L., Massagrande, M., Amantini, D., Antolini, M., et al. (2011). Functional magnetic resonance imaging reveals different neural substrates for the effects of orexin-1 and orexin-2 receptor antagonists. *PLoS ONE* 6:e16406. doi: 10.1371/journal.pone.0016406

Herring, W. J., Snyder, E., Budd, K., Hutzelmann, J., Snavely, D., Liu, K., et al. (2012). Orexin receptor antagonism for treatment of insomnia: a randomized clinical trial of suvorexant. *Neurology* 79, 2265–2274. doi: 10.1212/WNL.0b013e31827688ee

Hoever, P., Dorffner, G., Benes, H., Penzel, T., Danker-Hopfe, H., Barbanoj, M. J., et al. (2012). Orexin receptor antagonism, a new sleep-enabling paradigm: a proof-of-concept clinical trial. *Clin. Pharmacol. Ther.* 91, 975–985. doi: 10.1038/clpt.2011.370

Hong, Z. Y., Huang, Z. L., Qu, W. M., and Eguchi, N. (2005). Orexin A promotes histamine, but not norepinephrine or serotonin, release in frontal cortex of mice. *Acta Pharmacol. Sin.* 26, 155–159. doi: 10.1111/j.1745-7254.2005.00523.x

Lu, J., Sherman, D., Devor, M., and Saper, C. B. (2006). A putative flip-flop switch for control of REM sleep. *Nature* 441, 589–594. doi: 10.1038/nature04767

Mang, G. M., Durst, T., Burki, H., Imobersteg, S., Abramowski, D., Schuepbach, E., et al. (2012). The dual orexin receptor antagonist almorexant induces sleep and decreases orexin-induced locomotion by blocking orexin 2 receptors. *Sleep* 35, 1625–1635. doi: 10.5665/sleep.2232

Marcus, J. N., Aschkenasi, C. J., Lee, C. E., Chemelli, R. M., Saper, C. B., Yanagisawa, M., et al. (2001). Differential expression of orexin receptors 1 and 2 in the rat brain. *J. Comp. Neurol.* 435, 6–25. doi: 10.1002/cne.1190

McAtee, L. C., Sutton, S. W., Rudolph, D. A., Li, X., Aluisio, L. E., Phuong, V. K., et al. (2004). Novel substituted 4-phenyl-[1,3]dioxanes: potent and selective orexin receptor 2 (OX(2)R) antagonists. *Bioorg. Med. Chem. Lett.* 14, 4225–4229. doi: 10.1016/j.bmcl.2004.06.032

Mieda, M., Hasegawa, E., Kisanuki, Y. Y., Sinton, C. M., Yanagisawa, M., and Sakurai, T. (2011). Differential roles of orexin receptor-1 and -2 in the regulation of non-REM and REM sleep. *J. Neurosci.* 31, 6518–6526. doi: 10.1523/JNEUROSCI.6506-10.2011

Mochizuki, T., Arrigoni, E., Marcus, J. N., Clark, E. L., Yamamoto, M., Honer, M., et al. (2011). Orexin receptor 2 expression in the posterior hypothalamus rescues sleepiness in narcoleptic mice. *Proc. Natl. Acad. Sci. U.S.A.* 108, 4471–4476. doi: 10.1073/pnas.1012456108

Morairty, S. R., Revel, F. G., Malherbe, P., Moreau, J. L., Valladao, D., Wettstein, J. G., et al. (2012). Dual hypocretin receptor antagonism is more effective for sleep promotion than antagonism of either receptor alone. *PLoS ONE* 7:e39131. doi: 10.1371/journal.pone.0039131

Nishino, S. (2007). Clinical and neurobiological aspects of narcolepsy. *Sleep Med.* 8, 373–399. doi: 10.1016/j.sleep.2007.03.008

Nishino, S., and Mignot, E. (1997). Pharmacological aspects of human and canine narcolepsy. *Prog. Neurobiol.* 52, 27–78. doi: 10.1016/S0301-0082(96)00070-6

Oishi, Y., Williams, R. H., Agostinelli, L., Arrigoni, E., Fuller, P. M., Mochizuki, T., et al. (2013). Role of the medial prefrontal cortex in cataplexy. *J. Neurosci.* 33, 9743–9751. doi: 10.1523/JNEUROSCI.0499-13.2013

Peyron, C., Tighe, D. K., Van Den Pol, A. N., De Lecea, L., Heller, H. C., Sutcliffe, J. G., et al. (1998). Neurons containing hypocretin (orexin) project to multiple neuronal systems. *J. Neurosci.* 18, 9996–10015.

Sakurai, T. (2007). The neural circuit of orexin (hypocretin): maintaining sleep and wakefulness. *Nat. Rev. Neurosci.* 8, 171–181. doi: 10.1038/nrn2092

Sakurai, T., Amemiya, A., Ishii, M., Matsuzaki, I., Chemelli, R. M., Tanaka, H., et al. (1998). Orexins and orexin receptors: a family of hypothalamic neuropeptides and G protein-coupled receptors that regulate feeding behavior. *Cell* 92, 573–585. doi: 10.1016/S0092-8674(00)80949-6

Saper, C. B., Chou, T. C., and Scammell, T. E. (2001). The sleep switch: hypothalamic control of sleep and wakefulness. *Trends Neurosci.* 24, 726–731. doi: 10.1016/S0166-2236(00)02002-6

Scammell, T. E., Willie, J. T., Guilleminault, C., and Siegel, J. M. (2009). A consensus definition of cataplexy in mouse models of narcolepsy. *Sleep* 32, 111–116.

Smith, M. I., Piper, D. C., Duxon, M. S., and Upton, N. (2003). Evidence implicating a role for orexin-1 receptor modulation of paradoxical sleep in the rat. *Neurosci. Lett.* 341, 256–258. doi: 10.1016/S0304-3940(03)00066-1

Steiner, M. A., Gatfield, J., Brisbare-Roch, C., Dietrich, H., Treiber, A., Jenck, F., et al. (2013). Discovery and characterization of ACT-335827, an orally available, brain penetrant orexin receptor type 1 selective antagonist. *ChemMedChem* 8, 898–903. doi: 10.1002/cmdc.201300003

Willie, J. T., Chemelli, R. M., Sinton, C. M., Tokita, S., Williams, S. C., Kisanuki, Y. Y., et al. (2003). Distinct narcolepsy syndromes in Orexin receptor-2 and Orexin null mice: molecular genetic dissection of Non-REM and REM sleep regulatory processes. *Neuron* 38, 715–730. doi: 10.1016/S0896-6273(03) 00330-1

Winrow, C. J., Gotter, A. L., Cox, C. D., Doran, S. M., Tannenbaum, P. L., Breslin, M. J., et al. (2011). Promotion of sleep by suvorexant-a novel dual orexin receptor antagonist. *J. Neurogenet.* 25, 52–61. doi: 10.3109/01677063.2011. 566953

Winrow, C. J., and Renger, J. J. (2014). Discovery and development of orexin receptor antagonists as therapeutics for insomnia. *Br. J. Pharmacol.* 17, 283–293. doi: 10.1111/bph.12261

Conflict of Interest Statement: All the authors are full-time employees of Janssen Research & Development, L.L.C.

The hypocretin/orexin antagonist almorexant promotes sleep without impairment of performance in rats

Stephen R. Morairty[1]*, Alan J. Wilk[1], Webster U. Lincoln[1], Thomas C. Neylan[2] and Thomas S. Kilduff[1]

[1] SRI International, Center for Neuroscience, Biosciences Division, Menlo Park, CA, USA
[2] Department of Psychiatry, SF VA Medical Center/NCIRE/University of California, San Francisco, CA, USA

Edited by:
Christopher J. Winrow, Merck, USA

Reviewed by:
Collin Park, University of South
Florida, USA
Michihiro Mieda, Kanazawa
University, Japan

*Correspondence:
Stephen R. Morairty, SRI
International, 333 Ravenswood Ave.,
Menlo Park, CA, USA
e-mail: stephen.morairty@sri.com

The hypocretin receptor (HcrtR) antagonist almorexant (ALM) has potent hypnotic actions but little is known about neurocognitive performance in the presence of ALM. HcrtR antagonists are hypothesized to induce sleep by disfacilitation of wake-promoting systems whereas GABA$_A$ receptor modulators such as zolpidem (ZOL) induce sleep through general inhibition of neural activity. To test the hypothesis that less functional impairment results from HcrtR antagonist-induced sleep, we evaluated the performance of rats in the Morris Water Maze in the presence of ALM vs. ZOL. Performance in spatial reference memory (SRM) and spatial working memory (SWM) tasks were assessed during the dark period after equipotent sleep-promoting doses (100 mg/kg, po) following undisturbed and sleep deprivation (SD) conditions. ALM-treated rats were indistinguishable from vehicle (VEH)-treated rats for all SRM performance measures (distance traveled, latency to enter, time within, and number of entries into, the target quadrant) after both the undisturbed and 6 h SD conditions. In contrast, rats administered ZOL showed impairments in all parameters measured compared to VEH or ALM in the undisturbed conditions. Following SD, ZOL-treated rats also showed impairments in all measures. ALM-treated rats were similar to VEH-treated rats for all SWM measures (velocity, time to locate the platform and success rate at finding the platform within 60 s) after both the undisturbed and SD conditions. In contrast, ZOL-treated rats showed impairments in velocity and in the time to locate the platform. Importantly, ZOL rats only completed the task 23–50% of the time while ALM and VEH rats completed the task 79–100% of the time. Thus, following equipotent sleep-promoting doses, ZOL impaired rats in both memory tasks while ALM rats performed at levels comparable to VEH rats. These results are consistent with the hypothesis that less impairment results from HcrtR antagonism than from GABA$_A$-induced inhibition.

Keywords: hypocretins/orexins, cognitive impairment, memory impairment, hypnotics, water maze, spatial reference memory, spatial working memory, EEG

INTRODUCTION

Insomnia is a highly prevalent condition affecting 10–30% of the general population; (NIH, 2005; Roth, 2007; Mai and Buysse, 2008). Sleep loss and sleep disruption can lead to a degradation of neurocognitive performance as assessed by objective and subjective measures (Wesensten et al., 1999; Belenky et al., 2003; Lamond et al., 2007). Prescription sleep medications are often used to treat insomnia and obtain desired amounts of sleep. Presently, nonbenzodiazepine, positive allosteric modulators of the GABA$_A$ receptor such as zolpidem (ZOL) are the most widely prescribed hypnotic medications. Although known to induce sleep, these compounds have been shown to significantly impair psychomotor and memory functions in rodents (Huang et al., 2010; Uslaner et al., 2013; Zanin et al., 2013), non-human primates (Makaron et al., 2013; Soto et al., 2013; Uslaner et al., 2013) and humans (Balkin et al., 1992; Wesensten et al., 1996, 2005; Mattila et al., 1998; Mintzer and Griffiths, 1999; Verster et al., 2002; Storm et al., 2007; Otmani et al., 2008; Gunja, 2013). Such impairment can be particularly troubling when there is an urgent need for highly functional performance in the presence of drug such as with first responders, military personnel, and caregivers. Further, complex behaviors during the sleep period (e.g., eating, cooking, driving, conversations, sex) have been associated with these medications (Dolder and Nelson, 2008). Therefore, more effective hypnotics are needed that facilitate sleep that is easily reversible in the event of an unexpected awakening that demands unimpaired cognitive and psychomotor performance.

Recently, antagonism of the hypocretin (Hcrt; also called orexin) receptors has been identified as a target mechanism for the next generation of sleep medications (Brisbare-Roch et al., 2007; Dugovic et al., 2009; Whitman et al., 2009; Hoever et al., 2010, 2012a,b; Coleman et al., 2012; Herring et al., 2012; Winrow et al., 2012; Betschart et al., 2013). The Hcrt system is well known to play an important role in the maintenance of wakefulness (de Lecea, 2012; Inutsuka and Yamanaka, 2013; Mieda and Sakurai, 2013; Saper, 2013). Hcrt fibers project throughout the central nervous system (CNS), with particularly dense projections and receptor expression found in arousal centers including the locus coeruleus, the tuberomammilary nucleus, dorsal raphe nuclei, laterodorsal tegmentum, pedunculopontine tegmentum, and the basal forebrain (Peyron et al., 1998; Marcus et al., 2001). The excitatory effects of the Hcrt peptides on these arousal centers is hypothesized to stabilize and maintain wakefulness. Therefore, blockade of the Hcrt system should disfacilitate these arousal centers, creating conditions that are permissive for sleep to occur.

The current study tests the hypothesis that the dual Hcrt receptor antagonist almorexant (ALM) produces less functional impairment than ZOL. The rationale that underlies this hypothesis is that ZOL causes a general inhibition of neural activity whereas ALM specifically disfacilitates wake-promoting systems. We tested this hypothesis using tests of spatial reference memory (SRM) and spatial working memory (SWM) in the Morris Water Maze. Although the concentrations of ALM and ZOL administered prior to these tests were equipotent in hypnotic efficacy, the performance of rats treated with ALM were superior to that of rats treated with ZOL.

MATERIALS AND METHODS
ANIMALS
One hundred fifty three male Sprague Dawley rats (300 g at time of purchase; Charles River, Wilmington, MA) were distributed among the 12 groups as described in **Table 1**. All animals were individually housed in temperature-controlled recording chambers (22 $\pm$ 2°C, 50 $\pm$ 25% relative humidity) under a 12:12 light/dark cycle with food and water available *ad libitum*. All experimental procedures were approved by SRI International's Institutional Animal Care and Use Committee and were in accordance with National Institute of Health (NIH) guidelines.

SURGICAL PROCEDURES
Rats were instrumented with sterile telemetry transmitters (F40-EET, Data Sciences Inc., St Paul, MN) as previously described (Morairty et al., 2008, 2012; Revel et al., 2012, 2013). Briefly, under isoflurane anesthesia, transmitters were placed intraperitoneally and biopotential leads were routed subcutaneously to the head and neck. Holes were drilled into the skull at 1.5 mm anterior to bregma and 1.5 mm lateral to midline, and 6 mm posterior to bregma and 4 mm lateral to midline on the right hemisphere. Two biopotential leads used as EEG electrodes were inserted into the holes and affixed to the skull with dental acrylic. Two biopotential leads used as EMG electrodes were positioned bilaterally through the nuchal muscles.

IDENTIFICATION OF SLEEP/WAKE STATES
After at least 3 weeks post-surgical recovery, EEG, and EMG were recorded via telemetry using DQ ART 4.1 software (Data Sciences Inc., St Paul, MN). Following completion of data collection, the EEG, and EMG recordings were scored in 10 s epochs as waking (W), rapid eye movement sleep (REM), or non-rapid eye movement sleep (NREM) by expert scorers blinded to the treatments using NeuroScore software (Data Sciences Inc., St Paul, MN). Sleep latency was defined as the first 60 s of continuous sleep following drug administration. Recordings were started at Zeitgeber time (ZT) 12 (lights off) and continued until animals performed the water maze tests.

SLEEP DEPRIVATION PROCEDURES
Animals were sleep deprived (SD) from ZT12-18 by progressive manual stimulation concurrent with EEG and EMG recording. The rats were continuously observed and, when they appeared to attempt to sleep, progressive interventions were employed to keep them awake: removal of cage tops, tapping on cages, placement of brushes inside the cage, or stroking of vibrissae or fur with an artist's brush.

DRUGS
Almorexant (ALM; ACT-078573), was synthesized at SRI International (Menlo Park, CA. USA) according to the patent literature. Zolpidem (ZOL) was a gift from Actelion Pharmaceuticals Ltd. For the SWM task, rats were dosed with ALM (100 mg/kg, p.o.), ZOL (100 mg/kg, p.o.) or vehicle (VEH; 1.25% hydroxypropyl methyl cellulose, 0.1% dioctyl sodium sulfosuccinate, and 0.25% methyl cellulose in water) at ZT18 and left undisturbed until time to perform memory tasks (see below). For the SRM task, most rats were also administered ALM, ZOL, and VEH p.o. at the concentrations above. However, one cohort of rats was administered drugs i.p. For these rats, ALM was administered at 100 mg/kg ($N = 6$), ZOL at 30 mg/kg ($N = 8$) and VEH ($N = 7$). ZOL is approximately 3X more potent i.p. than p.o. (Vanover et al., 1999) while ALM is equipotent through both routes of administration. Analysis of the sleep/wake data confirmed the equipotent effects of both drugs through both routes of administration at the concentrations tested.

WATER MAZE
All water maze (WM) tasks occurred in a pool 68″ in diameter and 25″ in depth, containing water at 24 $\pm$ 2°C made opaque by the addition of non-toxic, water soluble black paint and milk powder. Since all tests took place during the dark period, distinctive spatial cues were made of small "rice" lights colored blue, yellow, and green. Patterns of lights in distinct shapes (circle, square, diamond, "T" shape) were clearly visible from within the pool. Preliminary studies determined the minimum number of lights that were needed for learning to occur. A 10 cm diameter platform was submerged approximately 1 cm below the surface of the water in one of 6 locations (**Figure 1**). The platform location determined the orientation of the 4 quadrants used for analysis. Both WM tasks were similar to previous reports (Wenk, 2004; Ward et al., 2009).

TEST OF SPATIAL REFERENCE MEMORY
The acquisition phase occurred in one session consisting of 12–15 consecutive trials with a 60 s inter-trial interval. For each trial,

Table 1 | The number of rats tested for each of the 12 experimental groups.

Test	No SD			6 h SD		
	VEH	ALM	ZOL	VEH	ALM	ZOL
Reference memory	14	13	17	16	16	8
Working memory	11	12	12	12	11	11

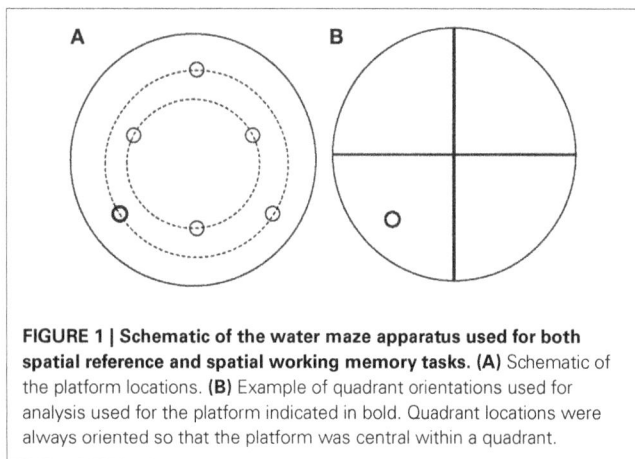

FIGURE 1 | Schematic of the water maze apparatus used for both spatial reference and spatial working memory tasks. (A) Schematic of the platform locations. **(B)** Example of quadrant orientations used for analysis used for the platform indicated in bold. Quadrant locations were always oriented so that the platform was central within a quadrant.

rats were placed in the WM facing the wall in one of three quadrants that did not contain the hidden platform. The location of the hidden platform remained constant across all trials. Rats were given 60 s to locate the platform. If the rats did not locate the platform within this period, they were guided to the platform location. When the rats reached the platform, they were allowed to remain on the platform for approximately 15 s before being placed in a dry holding cage for the next 60 s. This training sequence continued until the rats learned the task, typically 12–15 trials.

On the following day, rats were dosed with ALM, ZOL or VEH at ZT18 and a retention probe trial was performed 90 min later in which the rats were returned to the WM but the platform had been removed. A total of 40 rats were subjected to SD for 6 h prior to drug administration, and 42 were left undisturbed during this period (**Table 1**). Rats were started in the quadrant opposite the target quadrant and allowed to swim for 30 s. All trials were recorded by video camera and analyzed with Ethovision XT software (Noldus, Leesburg, VA). Test measures for the retention probe were time spent in target quadrant, latency to target quadrant, frequency of entrance into target quadrant, and total distance traveled. Swim speed was calculated to control for nonspecific effects.

TEST OF SPATIAL WORKING MEMORY

The SWM task consisted of 6 pairs of trials, one for each platform location (**Figure 1A**). In the first trial, a cued platform marked with a flag was placed in one of 6 positions in the WM. Rats were released facing the wall from one of the 3 quadrants not containing the platform and were allowed 120 s to locate the cued platform before the researcher guided the rats to the platform. This procedure provided all rats the opportunity to learn the platform location even if they did not find it on their own. After 15 s on the platform, the rats were removed from the WM and placed in a holding cage. The flag was then removed but the platform remained in the same location as in the first trial. Following a delay of 1, 5, or 10 min in the holding cage, the rats were placed back in the WM into one of the 2 quadrants that did not contain the platform and was not the starting quadrant during the first trial. Once the rats found the platform, they were removed after approximately 5 s and placed back in a holding cage for 10 min

before a new pair of trials with a novel platform location was given. The order of delays was counterbalanced so that each rat was tested twice at 1, 5, or 10 min delays between the cued and hidden platforms. All trials were recorded by video camera and analyzed with Ethovision XT software (Noldus, Leesburg, VA). Test measures were time to locate the platform and the swim velocity during all tests.

STATISTICAL ANALYSIS

Statistical analyses were performed using SigmaPlot 12.3 (Systat Software Inc., San Jose, CA). Sleep/wake data (W, NREM, and REM time) were analyzed in 30 min bins and compared between drug groups using Two-Way mixed-model ANOVA on factors "drug group" (between subjects) and "time" (within subjects). SRM performance parameters (latency, duration and frequency in target quadrant, total distance traveled) were analyzed using a One-Way ANOVA. SWM performance measures (velocity, time to platform, percent found) by delay time were analyzed using Two-Way mixed-model ANOVA on factors "drug group" (between subjects) and "time" (within subjects). Significance levels were set at $\alpha = 0.05$. When ANOVA indicated significance, Bonferroni t-tests were used for *post hoc* analyses.

RESULTS

Drug concentrations were chosen to be equipotent at sleep promotion based on our previous experience (Morairty et al., 2012). Although ZOL produced a more rapid onset to sleep under both SD and undisturbed conditions (No SD: ZOL = 6.6 min, VEH = 32.2 min, ALM = 25.4 min; SD: ZOL = 5.9 min, VEH = 20.0 min, ALM = 15.5 min), ALM- and ZOL-treated rats slept equivalent amounts during the last hour before the WM test (**Figure 2**; No SD: ZOL = 69.4%, ALM = 62.3%, VEH = 37.6%; SD: ZOL = 69.6%, ALM = 71.5%, VEH = 52.0%).

TEST OF SPATIAL REFERENCE MEMORY

For all performance measures analyzed, rats treated with ZOL showed significant impairments while ALM- and VEH-treated rats were indistinguishable (**Figure 3**). Following ZOL, the latency to the target zone increased (No SD: ZOL = 14.1 s, VEH = 5.7 s, ALM = 5.8 s; SD: ZOL = 18.4 s, VEH = 4.2 s, ALM = 3.6 s) and the duration in the target zone (No SD: ZOL = 5.5 s, VEH = 8.4 s, ALM = 7.9 s; SD: ZOL = 4.8 s, VEH = 7.7 s, ALM = 7.8 s), frequency entering the target zone (No SD: ZOL = 1.2, VEH = 2.7, ALM = 2.5; SD: ZOL = 0.9, VEH = 2.8, ALM = 2.9) and the distance traveled (No SD: ZOL = 472 cm, VEH = 666 cm, ALM = 725 cm; SD: ZOL = 343 cm, VEH = 709 cm, ALM = 775 cm) all decreased compared to VEH and ALM-treated rats. ALM-treated rats did not differ from VEH-treated rats on any of these four measures. Performance in the SRM task was not significantly affected by 6 h SD for any measure within any group.

Swim patterns in the WM were different for ZOL-treated rats compared to VEH- and ALM-treated rats (**Figure 4**). Both VEH and ALM rats repeatedly swam across the WM and typically swam through the area where the hidden platform was present on the previous day (**Figure 4A**). In contrast, ZOL-treated rats primarily swam around the perimeter of the WM, a pattern typical of a rat during its first exposure to the WM.

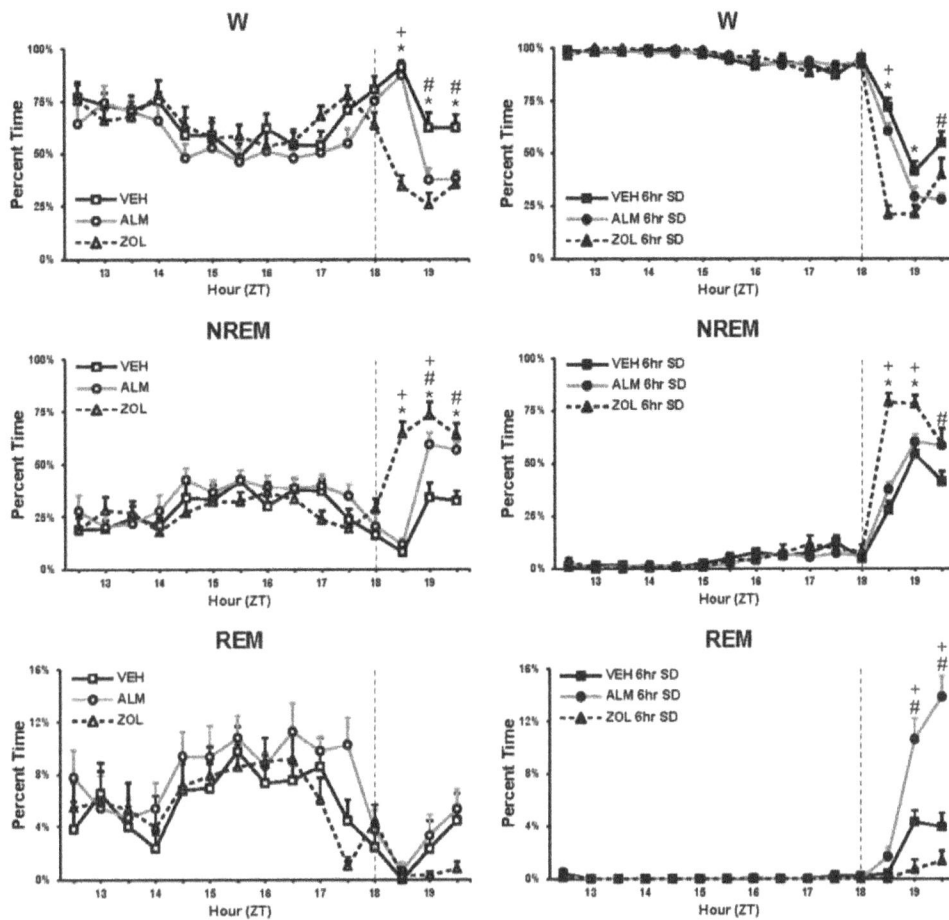

FIGURE 2 | Percent time spent in W, NREM, and REM during baseline (left panels) and during 6 h SD (right panels). The vertical line in each panel at ZT18 depicts the time of drug administration. At the end of the recording time displayed in these panels, rats were tested in the water maze. Note that, for the 60 min prior to testing (ZT19.5), the ALM and ZOL groups slept similar amounts. *, ZOL different from VEH; +, ZOL different ALM; #, ALM different from VEH; $p < 0.05$.

TEST OF SPATIAL WORKING MEMORY

ZOL-treated rats performed poorly in the SWM task compared to either VEH- or ALM-treated rats (**Figures 5, 6**). ZOL-treated rats took longer to find the platform (No SD: ZOL = 43.4–47.3 s, VEH = 20.6–30.0 s, ALM = 22.5–30.7 s; SD: ZOL = 48.0–55.5 s, VEH = 26.9–31.0 s, ALM = 25.6–28.2 s) and swam more slowly (No SD: ZOL = 14.0–14.2 cm/s, VEH = 18.0–19.6 cm/s, ALM = 18.9–20.4 cm/s; SD: ZOL = 9.9–10.9 cm/s, VEH = 15.7–16.8 cm/s, ALM = 17.5–18.1 cm/s) than the VEH or ALM rats (**Figure 5**). These measures were not affected by increasing the delay from 1 to 5 min or 10 min for any of the 6 groups of rats.

The goal for the SWM task was to locate the platform. VEH- and ALM-treated rats found the platform the majority of the time in both SD and undisturbed conditions (83.3–100% for VEH and 79.2–87.5% for ALM; **Figure 6**). Conversely, ZOL-treated rats failed to find the platform most of the time (22.7 50.0% success rate). Interestingly, ZOL-treated rats also often failed to find the cued platform during the training phase of each pair of trials (**Figure 7**). The ZOL-treated rats in the baseline group found

the cued platform 54.4% of the time while the SD ZOL-treated group were successful 53.8% of the time as compared to 98.6% for ALM-treated rats in the baseline group and 100% following SD and 100% of the time for all VEH-treated rats. A trend toward improved performance was observed with progressive trials in the ZOL-treated rats.

DISCUSSION

Though differing in the latency to induce sleep at the doses tested, ALM, and ZOL were equally effective at promoting sleep during the 90 min period prior to performance testing and both compounds significantly increased sleep compared to VEH. ALM-treated rats were indistinguishable from VEH-treated rats in their performance of both the SRM and SWM tasks. In contrast, ZOL caused significant impairments in both tasks. Specifically, in the SRM task, ZOL increased the latency to, the duration in, and the frequency of entering the target zone. In the SWM task, ZOL increased the time to find the platform, decreased the swim velocity and decreased the success rate in finding the platform. These results support the hypothesis that dual Hcrt receptor antagonism

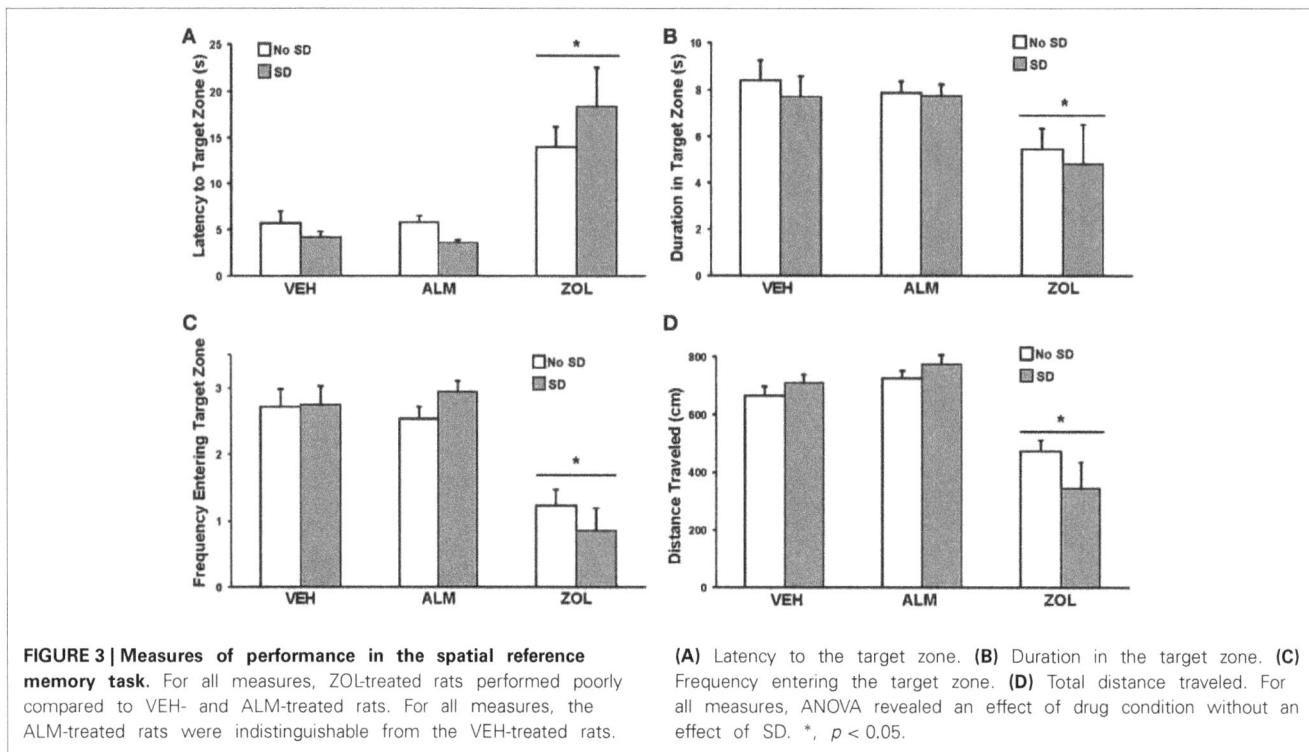

FIGURE 3 | Measures of performance in the spatial reference memory task. For all measures, ZOL-treated rats performed poorly compared to VEH- and ALM-treated rats. For all measures, the ALM-treated rats were indistinguishable from the VEH-treated rats.

(A) Latency to the target zone. **(B)** Duration in the target zone. **(C)** Frequency entering the target zone. **(D)** Total distance traveled. For all measures, ANOVA revealed an effect of drug condition without an effect of SD. *, $p < 0.05$.

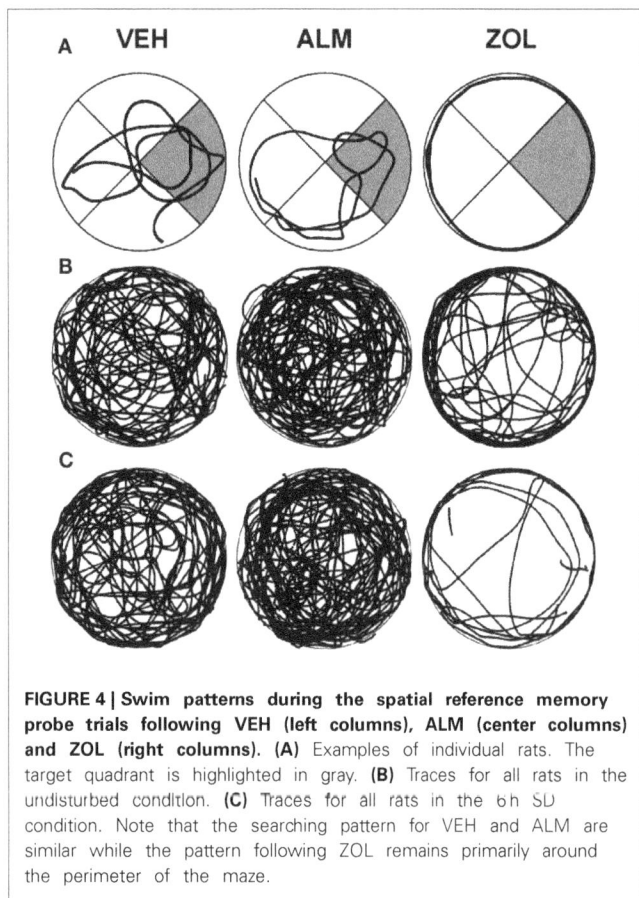

FIGURE 4 | Swim patterns during the spatial reference memory probe trials following VEH (left columns), ALM (center columns) and ZOL (right columns). (A) Examples of individual rats. The target quadrant is highlighted in gray. **(B)** Traces for all rats in the undisturbed condition. **(C)** Traces for all rats in the 6 h SD condition. Note that the searching pattern for VEH and ALM are similar while the pattern following ZOL remains primarily around the perimeter of the maze.

effectively promotes sleep without the functional impairments observed following GABA$_A$ receptor modulation.

An alternative explanation of the results obtained is that ZOL-treated rats were not motivated to perform the tasks rather than having memory/cognitive deficits. ZOL-treated rats had decreased distance traveled during the SRM task and decreased velocity during the SWM task, which could indicate a lack of motivation to escape the WM. Further, the lower success rate in finding the cued platform during the training trials for the SWM task could be interpreted as an absence of motivation to escape. However, ZOL rats did not simply float in the WM; they swam continuously, primarily circling the perimeter of the WM. As mentioned above, this swim pattern is typical of an untrained rat during its first exposure to the WM. Although not measured in this study, it is possible that the decreased distance traveled during the SRM task and decreased velocity during the SWM task are due to motor deficits produced by ZOL. This hypothesis is supported by previous studies that found prominent motor effects following ZOL administration (Depoortere et al., 1986; Steiner et al., 2011; Milic et al., 2012).

The SD protocol in these studies was included to assess whether moderate increases in sleep drive would exacerbate any cognitive deficits found following ALM or ZOL administration and also produce deficits in VEH-treated rats. While the primary active period of nocturnal rodents such as the rat is during the dark phase, rats still sleep approximately 30% of the time during this period and increasing wake duration during the dark period should create a mild sleep deficit (see **Figure 2**). Therefore, a portion of our experimental protocol involved SD during the 6 h of the dark period just prior to drug administration at ZT18.

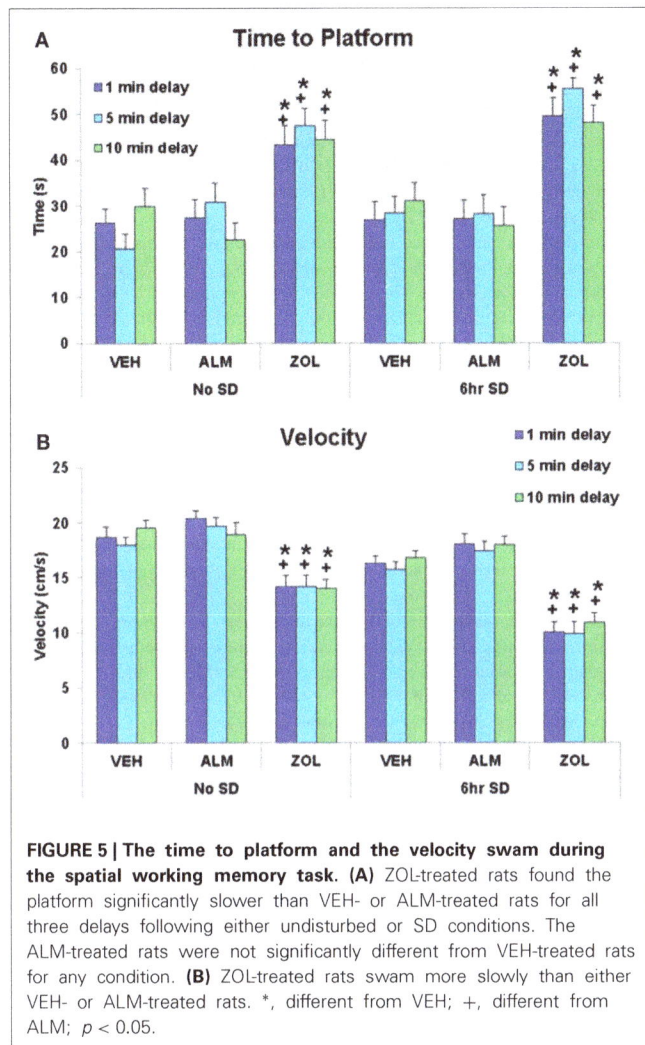

FIGURE 5 | The time to platform and the velocity swam during the spatial working memory task. (A) ZOL-treated rats found the platform significantly slower than VEH- or ALM-treated rats for all three delays following either undisturbed or SD conditions. The ALM-treated rats were not significantly different from VEH-treated rats for any condition. (B) ZOL-treated rats swam more slowly than either VEH- or ALM-treated rats. *, different from VEH; +, different from ALM; $p < 0.05$.

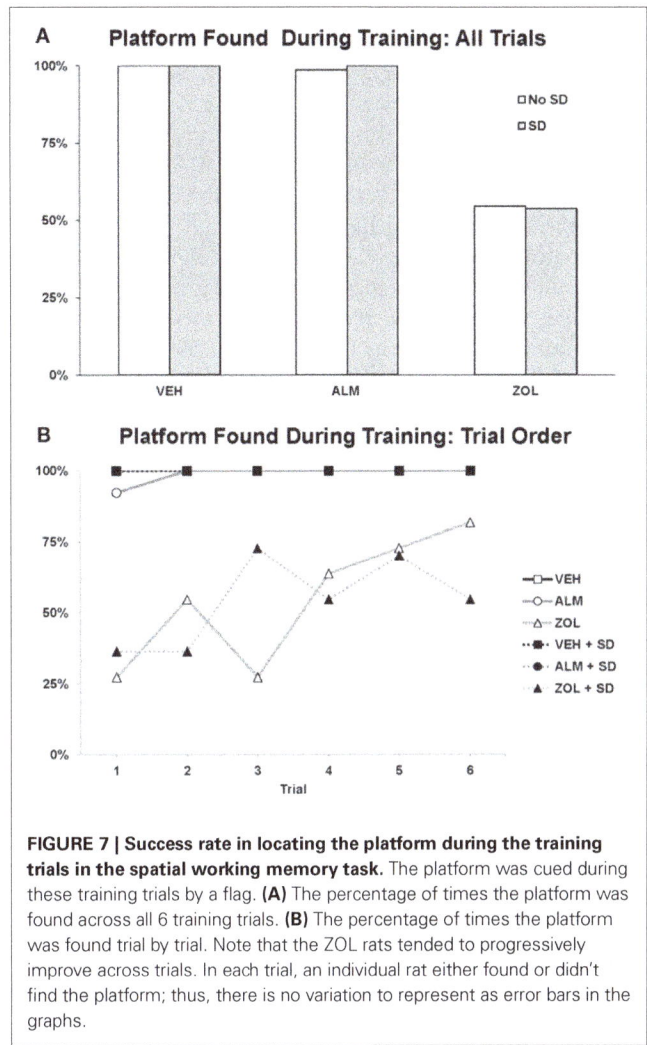

FIGURE 7 | Success rate in locating the platform during the training trials in the spatial working memory task. The platform was cued during these training trials by a flag. (A) The percentage of times the platform was found across all 6 training trials. (B) The percentage of times the platform was found trial by trial. Note that the ZOL rats tended to progressively improve across trials. In each trial, an individual rat either found or didn't find the platform; thus, there is no variation to represent as error bars in the graphs.

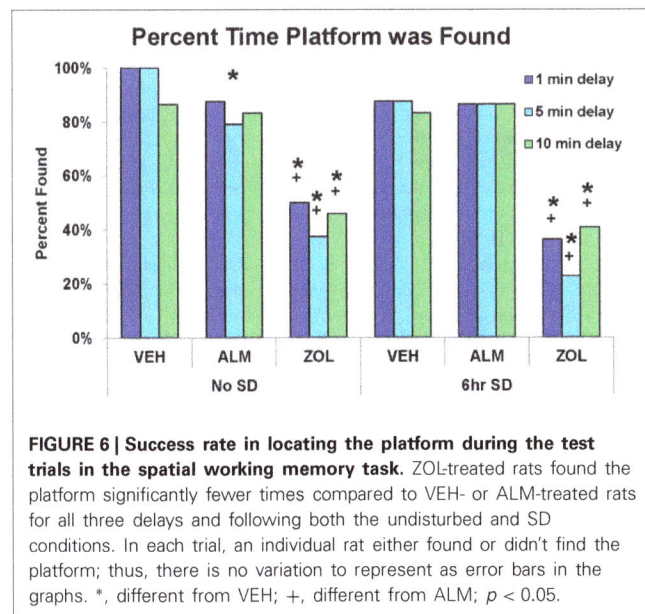

FIGURE 6 | Success rate in locating the platform during the test trials in the spatial working memory task. ZOL-treated rats found the platform significantly fewer times compared to VEH- or ALM-treated rats for all three delays and following both the undisturbed and SD conditions. In each trial, an individual rat either found or didn't find the platform; thus, there is no variation to represent as error bars in the graphs. *, different from VEH; +, different from ALM; $p < 0.05$.

Although we did not find significant effects of SD vs. non-SD within any of the 3 dosing conditions, these results are likely due to the fact that we allowed the rats to sleep after drug administration until water maze testing began. This undisturbed period lasted only 60–90 min but provided an opportunity for the experimental subjects to recover from this mild sleep deprivation. If the SD were continued until testing, increased memory deficits might have been observed. Further studies are needed to determine whether this is indeed to case.

ZOL is a widely prescribed hypnotic medication that can be well-tolerated when taken as directed (Greenblatt and Roth, 2012). However, numerous adverse effects associated with ZOL usage have been reported including driving impairment (Verster et al., 2006; Gunja, 2013), effects on balance and postural tone (Zammit et al., 2008), interference with memory consolidation (Balkin et al., 1992; Wesensten et al., 1996, 2005; Mintzer and Griffiths, 1999; Morgan et al., 2010) and increased incidence of complex behaviors during sleep (Hoever et al., 2010). Some studies investigated the effects of daytime administration of ZOL and tested psychomotor function upon arousal from naps (Wesensten et al., 2005; Storm et al., 2007), a protocol which our experiments closely mimic. In these studies, ZOL or melatonin was administered at either 10:00 or 13:00. Following a 1.5–2 h nap opportunity, subjects were awakened and required to perform a series of psychomotor and cognitive tests. Significant performance decrements were observed following ZOL in cognitive, vigilance and memory tasks while little to no decrements were found following melatonin. The results of ZOL administration on rat cognitive performance in the current study correlate well with these deficits found in humans.

In contrast, the high level of performance following ALM in both of our memory tasks suggests a high degree of safety at concentrations with hypnotic efficacy. Indeed, a recent study found no performance decrements in a variant of the WM SRM task at three-fold the concentration of ALM that we used (Dietrich and Jenck, 2010). Furthermore, another recent study found no effect of ALM at 300 mg/kg on motor function (Steiner et al., 2011). In humans, however, psychometric test battery assessment of the effect of ALM administered in the daytime found reductions in vigilance, alertness, and visuomotor and motor coordination at dose concentrations of 400–1000 mg (Hoever et al., 2010, 2012a). Notably, 400 mg ALM is within the therapeutic dose range required to improve sleep in patients with primary insomnia (Hoever et al., 2012b). Therefore, performance deficits following ALM occur within the range of hypnotic efficacy in humans. In one report, pharmacokinetic/pharmacodynamic modeling suggests that doses of 500 mg ALM and 10 mg ZOL are equivalent with respect to subjectively assessed alertness (Hoever et al., 2010). Since we find hypnotic efficacy to be achieved at roughly similar dose concentrations, there may be species differences in pharmacokinetic/pharmacodynamics of ALM and/or ZOL. While not uncommon, this makes direct translational interpretations of the present data more difficult. Regardless, in both rodents and humans, ALM appears to have a significantly better safety profile than ZOL with regards to cognitive/memory domains.

CONCLUSION

ALM and ZOL are effective hypnotics in multiple mammalian species (Brisbare-Roch et al., 2007; Hoever et al., 2010, 2012a,b; Morairty et al., 2012). They act through entirely different mechanisms of action, and their effects on cognition, psychomotor vigilance and memory are in stark contrast to one another. We found that at equipotent hypnotic concentrations, ZOL impaired SRM and SWM but ALM did not. These results support the hypothesis that antagonism of the Hcrt system can provide hypnotic efficacy without the impairments found by inducing sleep through GABA$_A$ modulation.

ACKNOWLEDGMENTS

We thank Sarah Black, Jacqueline DeRose, Sinom Fisher, Gregory Parks, Michael Schwartz, Alexia Thomas and Rhiannan Williams for feedback on the manuscript. Supported by USAMRMC grant W81XWH-09-2-0081.

REFERENCES

Balkin, T. J., O'Donnell, V. M., Wesensten, N., McCann, U., and Belenky, G. (1992). Comparison of the daytime sleep and performance effects of zolpidem versus triazolam. *Psychopharmacology* 107, 83–88. doi: 10.1007/BF02244970

Belenky, G., Wesensten, N. J., Thorne, D. R., Thomas, M. L., Sing, H. C., Redmond, D. P., et al. (2003). Patterns of performance degradation and restoration during sleep restriction and subsequent recovery: a sleep dose-response study. *J. Sleep Res.* 12, 1–12. doi: 10.1046/j.1365-2869.2003.00337.x

Betschart, C., Hintermann, S., Behnke, D., Cotesta, S., Fendt, M., Gee, C. E., et al. (2013). Identification of a novel series of orexin receptor antagonists with a distinct effect on sleep architecture for the treatment of insomnia. *J. Med. Chem.* 56, 7590–7607. doi: 10.1021/jm4007627

Brisbare-Roch, C., Dingemanse, J., Koberstein, R., Hoever, P., Aissaoui, H., Flores, S., et al. (2007). Promotion of sleep by targeting the orexin system in rats, dogs and humans. *Nat. Med.* 13, 150–155. doi: 10.1038/nm1544

Coleman, P. J., Schreier, J. D., Cox, C. D., Breslin, M. J., Whitman, D. B., Bogusky, M. J., et al. (2012). Discovery of [(2R,5R)-5-{[(5-fluoro pyridin-2-yl)oxy]methyl}-2-methylpiperidin-1-yl][5-methyl-2 -(pyrimidin-2-yl)phenyl]methanone (MK-6096): a dual orexin receptor antagonist with potent sleep-promoting properties. *ChemMedChem* 7, 415–424, 337. doi: 10.1002/cmdc.201200025

de Lecea, L. (2012). Hypocretins and the neurobiology of sleep-wake mechanisms. *Prog. Brain Res.* 198, 15–24. doi: 10.1016/B978-0-444-59489-1.00003-3

Depoortere, H., Zivkovic, B., Lloyd, K. G., Sanger, D. J., Perrault, G., Langer, S. Z., and Bartholini, G. (1986). Zolpidem, a novel nonbenzodiazepine hypnotic. I. Neuropharmacological and behavioral effects. *J. Pharmacol. Exp. Ther.* 237, 649–658.

Dietrich, H., and Jenck, F. (2010). Intact learning and memory in rats following treatment with the dual orexin receptor antagonist almorexant. *Psychopharmacology* 212, 145–154. doi: 10.1007/s00213-010-1933-5

Dolder, C. R., and Nelson, M. H. (2008). Hypnosedative-induced complex behaviours: incidence, mechanisms and management. *CNS Drugs* 22, 1021–1036. doi: 10.2165/0023210-200822120-00005

Dugovic, C., Shelton, J. E., Aluisio, L. E., Fraser, I. C., Jiang, X., Sutton, S. W., et al. (2009). Blockade of orexin-1 receptors attenuates orexin-2 receptor antagonism-induced sleep promotion in the rat. *J. Pharmacol. Exp. Ther.* 330, 142–151. doi: 10.1124/jpet.109.152009

Greenblatt, D. J., and Roth, T. (2012). Zolpidem for insomnia. *Expert Opin. Pharmacother.* 13, 879–893. doi: 10.1517/14656566.2012.667074

Gunja, N. (2013). In the Zzz zone: the effects of z-drugs on human performance and driving. *J. Med. Toxicol.* 9, 163–171. doi: 10.1007/s13181-013-0294-y

Herring, W. J., Snyder, E., Budd, K., Hutzelmann, J., Snavely, D., Liu, K., et al. (2012). Orexin receptor antagonism for treatment of insomnia: a randomized clinical trial of suvorexant. *Neurology* 79, 2265–2274. doi: 10.1212/WNL.0b013e31827688ee

Hoever, P., de Haas, S., Winkler, J., Schoemaker, R. C., Chiossi, E., van Gerven, J., and Dingemanse, J. (2010). Orexin receptor antagonism, a new sleep-promoting paradigm: an ascending single-dose study with almorexant. *Clin. Pharmacol. Ther.* 87, 593–600. doi: 10.1038/clpt.2010.19

Hoever, P., de Haas, S. L., Dorffner, G., Chiossi, E., van Gerven, J. M., and Dingemanse, J. (2012a). Orexin receptor antagonism: an ascending multiple-dose study with almorexant. *J. Psychopharmacol.* 26, 1071–1080. doi: 10.1177/0269881112448946

Hoever, P., Dorffner, G., Benes, H., Penzel, T., Danker-Hopfe, H., Barbanoj, M. J., et al. (2012b). Orexin receptor antagonism, a new sleep-enabling paradigm: a proof-of-concept clinical trial. *Clin. Pharmacol. Ther.* 91, 975–985. doi: 10.1038/clpt.2011.370

Huang, M. P., Radadia, K., Macone, B. W., Auerbach, S. H., and Datta, S. (2010). Effects of eszopiclone and zolpidem on sleep-wake behavior, anxiety-like behavior and contextual memory in rats. *Behav. Brain Res.* 210, 54–66. doi: 10.1016/j.bbr.2010.02.018

Inutsuka, A., and Yamanaka, A. (2013). The regulation of sleep and wakefulness by the hypothalamic neuropeptide orexin/hypocretin. *Nagoya J. Med. Sci.* 75, 29–36.

Lamond, N., Jay, S. M., Dorrian, J., Ferguson, S. A., Jones, C., and Dawson, D. (2007). The dynamics of neurobehavioural recovery following sleep loss. *J. Sleep Res.* 16, 33–41. doi: 10.1111/j.1365-2869.2007.00574.x

Mai, E., and Buysse, D. J. (2008). Insomnia: prevalence, impact, pathogenesis, differential diagnosis, and evaluation. *Sleep Med. Clin.* 3, 167–174. doi: 10.1016/j.jsmc.2008.02.001

Makaron, L., Moran, C. A., Namjoshi, O., Rallapalli, S., Cook, J. M., and Rowlett, J. K. (2013). Cognition-impairing effects of benzodiazepine-type drugs: role of

GABAA receptor subtypes in an executive function task in rhesus monkeys. *Pharmacol. Biochem. Behav.* 104, 62–68. doi: 10.1016/j.pbb.2012.12.018

Marcus, J. N., Aschkenasi, C. J., Lee, C. E., Chemelli, R. M., Saper, C. B., Yanagisawa, M., et al. (2001). Differential expression of orexin receptors 1 and 2 in the rat brain. *J. Comp. Neurol.* 435, 6–25. doi: 10.1002/cne.1190

Mattila, M. J., Vanakoski, J., Kalska, H., and Seppala, T. (1998). Effects of alcohol, zolpidem, and some other sedatives and hypnotics on human performance and memory. *Pharmacol. Biochem. Behav.* 59, 917–923. doi: 10.1016/S0091-3057(97)00506-6

Mieda, M., and Sakurai, T. (2013). Orexin (hypocretin) receptor agonists and antagonists for treatment of sleep disorders. Rationale for development and current status. *CNS Drugs* 27, 83–90. doi: 10.1007/s40263-012-0036-8

Milic, M., Divljakovic, J., Rallapalli, S., van Linn, M. L., Timic, T., Cook, J. M., et al. (2012). The role of alpha1 and alpha5 subunit-containing GABAA receptors in motor impairment induced by benzodiazepines in rats. *Behav. Pharmacol.* 23, 191–197. doi: 10.1097/FBP.0b013e3283512c85

Mintzer, M. Z., and Griffiths, R. R. (1999). Selective effects of zolpidem on human memory functions. *J. Psychopharmacol.* 13, 18–131. doi: 10.1177/026988119901300103

Morairty, S. R., Hedley, L., Flores, J., Martin, R., and Kilduff, T. S. (2008). Selective 5HT2A and 5HT6 receptor antagonists promote sleep in rats. *Sleep* 31, 34–44.

Morairty, S. R., Revel, F. G., Malherbe, P., Moreau, J. L., Valladao, D., Wettstein, J. G., et al. (2012). Dual hypocretin receptor antagonism is more effective for sleep promotion than antagonism of either receptor alone. *PLoS ONE* 7:e39131. doi: 10.1371/journal.pone.0039131

Morgan, P. T., Kehne, J. H., Sprenger, K. J. and Malison, R. T. (2010). Retrograde effects of triazolam and zolpidem on sleep-dependent motor learning in humans. *J. Sleep Res.* 19, 157–164. doi: 10.1111/j.1365-2869.2009.00757.x

NIH. (2005). National Institutes of Health State of the Science Conference statement on Manifestations and Management of Chronic Insomnia in Adults. *Sleep* 28, 1049–57.

Otmani, S., Demazieres, A., Staner, C., Jacob, N., Nir, T., Zisapel, N., et al. (2008). Effects of prolonged-release melatonin, zolpidem, and their combination on psychomotor functions, memory recall, and driving skills in healthy middle aged and elderly volunteers. *Hum. Psychopharmacol.* 23, 693–705. doi: 10.1002/hup.980

Peyron, C., Tighe, D. K., van den Pol, A. N., de Lecea, L., Heller, H. C., Sutcliffe, J. G., et al. (1998). Neurons containing hypocretin (orexin) project to multiple neuronal systems. *J. Neurosci.* 18, 9996–10015.

Revel, F. G., Moreau, J. L., Gainetdinov, R. R., Ferragud, A., Velazquez-Sanchez, C., Sotnikova, T. D., et al. (2012). Trace amine-associated receptor 1 partial agonism reveals novel paradigm for neuropsychiatric therapeutics. *Biol. Psychiatry* 72, 934–942. doi: 10.1016/j.biopsych.2012.05.014

Revel, F. G., Moreau, J. L., Pouzet, B., Mory, R., Bradaia, A., Buchy, D., et al. (2013). A new perspective for schizophrenia: TAAR1 agonists reveal antipsychotic- and antidepressant-like activity, improve cognition and control body weight. *Mol. Psychiatry* 18, 543–556. doi: 10.1038/mp.2012.57

Roth, T. (2007). Insomnia: definition, prevalence, etiology, and consequences. *J. Clin. Sleep Med.* 3, S7–S10.

Saper, C. B. (2013). The neurobiology of sleep. *Continuum (Minneap Minn)* 19, 19–31. doi: 10.1212/01.CON.0000427215.07715.73

Soto, P. L., Ator, N. A., Rallapalli, S. K., Biawat, P., Clayton, T., Cook, J. M., et al. (2013). Allosteric modulation of GABAA receptor subtypes: effects on visual recognition and visuospatial working memory in rhesus monkeys. *Neuropsychopharmacology* 38, 2315–2325. doi: 10.1038/npp.2013.137

Steiner, M. A., Lecourt, H., Strasser, D. S., Brisbare-Roch, C. and Jenck, F. (2011). Differential effects of the dual orexin receptor antagonist almorexant and the GABA(A)-alpha1 receptor modulator zolpidem, alone or combined with ethanol, on motor performance in the rat. *Neuropsychopharmacology* 36, 848–856. doi: 10.1038/npp.2010.224

Storm, W. F., Eddy, D. R., Welch, C. B., Hickey, P. A., Fischer, J., and Cardenas, R. (2007). Cognitive performance following premature awakening from zolpidem or melatonin induced daytime sleep. *Aviat. Space Environ. Med.* 78, 10–20.

Uslaner, J. M., Tye, S. J., Eddins, D. M., Wang, X., Fox, S. V., Savitz, A. T., et al. (2013). Orexin receptor antagonists differ from standard sleep drugs by promoting sleep at doses that do not disrupt cognition. *Sci. Transl. Med.* 5, 179ra44. doi: 10.1126/scitranslmed.3005213

Vanover, K. E., Edgar, D. M., Seidel, W. F., Hogenkamp, D. J., Fick, D. B., Lan, N. C., et al. (1999). Response-rate suppression in operant paradigm as predictor of soporific potency in rats and identification of three novel sedative-hypnotic neuroactive steroids. *J. Pharmacol. Exp. Ther.* 291, 1317–1323.

Verster, J. C., Veldhuijzen, D. S., Patat, A., Olivier, B., and Volkerts, E. R. (2006). Hypnotics and driving safety: meta-analyses of randomized controlled trials applying the on-the-road driving test. *Curr. Drug Saf.* 1, 63–71. doi: 10.2174/157488606775252674

Verster, J. C., Volkerts, E. R., Schreuder, A. H., Eijken, E. J., van Heuckelum, J. H., Veldhuijzen, D. S., et al. (2002). Residual effects of middle-of-the-night administration of zaleplon and zolpidem on driving ability, memory functions, and psychomotor performance. *J. Clin. Psychopharmacol.* 22, 576–583. doi: 10.1097/00004714-200212000-00007

Ward, C. P., McCarley, R. W., and Strecker, R. E. (2009). Experimental sleep fragmentation impairs spatial reference but not working memory in Fischer/Brown Norway rats. *J. Sleep Res.* 18, 238–244. doi: 10.1111/j.1365-2869.2008.00714.x

Wenk, G. L. (2004). Assessment of spatial memory using the radial arm maze and Morris water maze. *Curr. Protoc. Neurosci. Chapter 8, Unit 8.5A.* doi: 10.1002/0471142301.ns0805as26

Wesensten, N. J., Balkin, T. J., and Belenky, G. (1999). Does sleep fragmentation impact recuperation? A review and reanalysis. *J. Sleep Res.* 8, 237–245. doi: 10.1046/j.1365-2869.1999.00161.x

Wesensten, N. J., Balkin, T. J., and Belenky, G. L. (1996). Effects of daytime administration of zolpidem and triazolam on performance. *Aviat. Space Environ. Med.* 67, 115–120.

Wesensten, N. J., Balkin, T. J., Reichardt, R. M., Kautz, M. A., Saviolakis, G. A., and Belenky, G. (2005). Daytime sleep and performance following a zolpidem and melatonin cocktail. *Sleep* 28, 93–103.

Whitman, D. B., Cox, C. D., Breslin, M. J., Brashear, K. M., Schreier, J. D., Bogusky, M. J., et al. (2009). Discovery of a potent, CNS-penetrant orexin receptor antagonist based on an n,n-disubstituted-1,4-diazepane scaffold that promotes sleep in rats. *ChemMedChem* 4, 1069–1074. doi: 10.1002/cmdc.200900069

Winrow, C. J., Gotter, A. L., Cox, C. D., Tannenbaum, P. L., Garson, S. L., Doran, S. M., et al. (2012). Pharmacological characterization of MK-6096 - a dual orexin receptor antagonist for insomnia. *Neuropharmacology* 62, 978–987. doi: 10.1016/j.neuropharm.2011.10.003

Zammit, G., Wang-Weigand, S., and Peng, X. (2008). Use of computerized dynamic posturography to assess balance in older adults after nighttime awakenings using zolpidem as a reference. *BMC Geriatr.* 8:15. doi: 10.1186/1471-2318-8-15

Zanin, K. A., Patti, C. L., Sanday, L., Fernandes-Santos, L., Oliveira, L. C., Poyares, D., et al. (2013). Effects of zolpidem on sedation, anxiety, and memory in the plus-maze discriminative avoidance task. *Psychopharmacology* 226, 459–474. doi: 10.1007/s00213-012-2756-3

Conflict of Interest Statement: The authors declare that the research was conducted in the absence of any commercial or financial relationships that could be construed as a potential conflict of interest.

The selective orexin receptor 1 antagonist ACT-335827 in a rat model of diet-induced obesity associated with metabolic syndrome

Michel A. Steiner[1]*, Carla Sciarretta[2†], Anne Pasquali[3†] and Francois Jenck[1]

[1] CNS Pharmacology Neurobiology, Actelion Pharmaceuticals Ltd., Allschwil, Switzerland
[2] Immunology, Actelion Pharmaceuticals Ltd., Allschwil, Switzerland
[3] Cardiology, Actelion Pharmaceuticals Ltd., Allschwil, Switzerland

Edited by:
Christopher J. Winrow, Merck, USA

Reviewed by:
Ciaran J. Faherty, Cadence
Pharmaceuticals, USA
Arshad M. Khan, University of Texas
at El Paso, USA

*Correspondence:
Michel A. Steiner, Actelion
Pharmaceuticals Ltd.,
Gewerbestrasse 16, 4123 Allschwil,
Switzerland
e-mail: michel.steiner@actelion.com

[†] These authors have contributed
equally to this work.

The orexin system regulates feeding, nutrient metabolism and energy homeostasis. Acute pharmacological blockade of orexin receptor 1 (OXR-1) in rodents induces satiety and reduces normal and palatable food intake. Genetic OXR-1 deletion in mice improves hyperglycemia under high-fat (HF) diet conditions. Here we investigated the effects of chronic treatment with the novel selective OXR-1 antagonist ACT-335827 in a rat model of diet-induced obesity (DIO) associated with metabolic syndrome (MetS). Rats were fed either standard chow (SC) or a cafeteria (CAF) diet comprised of intermittent human snacks and a constant free choice between a HF/sweet (HF/S) diet and SC for 13 weeks. Thereafter the SC group was treated with vehicle (for 4 weeks) and the CAF group was divided into a vehicle and an ACT-335827 treatment group. Energy and water intake, food preference, and indicators of MetS (abdominal obesity, glucose homeostasis, plasma lipids, and blood pressure) were monitored. Hippocampus-dependent memory, which can be impaired by DIO, was assessed. CAF diet fed rats treated with ACT-335827 consumed less of the HF/S diet and more of the SC, but did not change their snack or total kcal intake compared to vehicle-treated rats. ACT-335827 increased water intake and the high-density lipoprotein associated cholesterol proportion of total circulating cholesterol. ACT-335827 slightly increased body weight gain (4% vs. controls) and feed efficiency in the absence of hyperphagia. These effects were not associated with significant changes in the elevated fasting glucose and triglyceride (TG) plasma levels, glucose intolerance, elevated blood pressure, and adiposity due to CAF diet consumption. Neither CAF diet consumption alone nor ACT-335827 affected memory. In conclusion, the main metabolic characteristics associated with DIO and MetS in rats remained unaffected by chronic ACT-335827 treatment, suggesting that pharmacological OXR-1 blockade has minimal impact in this model.

Keywords: diet-induced obesity, metabolic syndrome, food intake, orexin, orexin receptor antagonist, ACT-335827, food preference, lipid metabolism

INTRODUCTION

Metabolic syndrome (MetS) represents a group of risk factors for diabetes and cardiovascular disease; it is characterized by abdominal obesity plus two of four factors including: elevated circulating triglyceride (TG) levels, reduced circulating high density lipoprotein-associated cholesterol (HDLc) levels, elevated blood pressure, and elevated fasting plasma glucose levels (International Diabetes Federation; http://www.idf.org). Diet-induced obesity (DIO), which is a major causative factor of MetS, can also result in cognitive impairments and in poorer hippocampus-dependent memory function (Eskelinen et al., 2008; Francis and Stevenson, 2011). The current primary intervention for MetS is to lower body weight through reduced energy consumption, a change of diet composition, and increased physical activity (De Flines and Scheen, 2010). Pharmacological treatments are expected to additionally help

patients to restrict over-eating by reducing systemic and brain signals responsible for driving high caloric palatable food intake (Adamo and Tesson, 2008).

Orexin neuropeptides A and B modulate energy balance and metabolic homeostasis (Sakurai, 2006) but also palatable food and sweet reward perception (Di Sebastiano and Coolen, 2012). Orexins are expressed by a discrete number of neurons in the lateral hypothalamus (De Lecea et al., 1998; Sakurai et al., 1998) and their effects are mediated by the G-protein-coupled orexin receptors type 1 and 2. OXRs are expressed widely in orexinergic projection areas throughout the brain including the mesolimbic system, implicated in reward/aversion, and including several mid- and hindbrain regions, implicated in regulating energy homeostasis and food intake (Trivedi et al., 1998; Marcus et al., 2001). For instance, some orexin neurons project to the ventral tegmental area (VTA), where they synapse with dopaminergic and GABAergic neurons (Balcita-Pedicino and Sesack, 2007); other orexin neurons innervate neuropeptide Y and pro-opiomelanocortin expressing neurons of the arcuate nucleus (Niimi et al., 2001; Tsuneki et al., 2010). Orexin neurons also receive multiple afferent input (Yoshida et al., 2006) from cortico-limbic regions, involved in either positive or negative emotional processing, as well as from local hypothalamic areas, involved in defense reactions, in autonomic and in circadian regulation (Furudono et al., 2006); in addition, orexin neuron activation is modulated by the anorectic adipokine leptin, by the orectic peptide ghrelin, by circulating non-essential amino acids, and by falling glucose levels (Yamanaka et al., 2003; Williams et al., 2008; Louis et al., 2010; Karnani and Burdakov, 2011). OXR mRNA or protein is also found in the periphery including enteric neurons, stomach, pancreas, adrenal gland, and white and brown adipose tissue (Kirchgessner and Liu, 1999; Blanco et al., 2002; Digby et al., 2006; Adeghate et al., 2010; Skrzypski et al., 2011). The relative functional significance of orexins in controlling energy homeostasis and food intake by acting both in the brain and periphery (Heinonen et al., 2008) has remained elusive but orexin peptide or OXR levels appear to be regulated under a variety of nutritional conditions such as food deprivation, sweetener-induced overconsumption and genetic obesity (Mondal et al., 1999; Karteris et al., 2005; Furudono et al., 2006).

The preferential OXR-1 antagonist SB-334867 has been described to reduce normal food intake in rats during the dark phase (Haynes et al., 2000) by decreasing meal size (Parise et al., 2011) and enhancing satiety onset (Ishii et al., 2005). In addition to impacting quantitative natural feeding the OXR-1 may play a key role in mediating the hedonic component of nutrient intake. SB-334867 centrally injected in the VTA of rats inhibited feeding stimulated by intra-nucleus accumbens injections of a mu-opioid receptor agonist (Zheng et al., 2007). The systemic administration of SB-334867 reduced the overconsumption of a HF diet in satiated rats (Choi et al., 2010), and another OXR-1 antagonist, GSK1059865, reduced the binge-like intake of a HF/S diet (Piccoli et al., 2012). Chronic administration of a high dose of SB-334867 to ob/ob female mice lacking leptin reduced food intake and weight gain (Haynes et al., 2002), and this effect was associated with improvements in glucose homeostasis. Contrarily, OXR-1 deficient mice became similarly obese to wild-type mice when challenged with a HF diet (Funato et al., 2009). However, consistent with the reported effects of chronic SB-334867 treatment, fasting blood glucose and serum insulin levels were improved in obese OXR-1 deficient mice (Funato et al., 2009). Finally, a series of studies exploring SB-334867 in operant responding models also suggest that blocking OXR-1 signaling can reduce the motivation to consume HF/S foods (Borgland et al., 2009; Choi et al., 2010; Cason and Aston-Jones, 2013). Central infusion of the OXR-2 specific agonist [Ala11,D-Leu15]Orexin-B over a period of 14 days decreased consumption of a HF diet and reduced DIO (Funato et al., 2009). Genetically elevating brain levels of orexins also prevented DIO by decreasing food intake and stimulating energy expenditure through a mechanism requiring OXR-2. Therefore, either blocking OXR-1 or activating OXR-2 signaling may provide benefits under conditions of prolonged access to high palatable food that will lead to DIO.

The purpose of our study was to test the effects of the novel OXR-1 antagonist ACT-335827 (Steiner et al., 2013) in a rat model of DIO associated with MetS. In comparison to the frequently used OXR-1 antagonist SB-334867, which may also bind to other neuronal receptors (Gotter et al., 2012; Morairty et al., 2012), ACT-335827 shows greater selectivity among a panel of more than 100 neuronal targets [it only binds to the melatonin MT_1 receptor with greater than 50% (i.e., 58%) inhibition at $10 \mu M$; (Steiner et al., 2013)]. Affinity of ACT-335827, measured by an intracellular calcium release assay, at the recombinant rat OXR-1 was between 7 and 25 nM (depending on incubation time) and between 630 and 1030 nM at the OXR-2. The calculated free brain concentration in Wistar rats after oral gavage of 300 mg/kg was between 97 nM at 1 h and 166 nM at 6 h following administration. Accordingly, the oral dose of 300 mg/kg was effective in reducing a number of anxiety and stress-related measures in the rat including autonomic activation, schedule-induced polydipsia, and fear-potentiated startle; similar to dual OXR antagonists (Steiner et al., 2012). However, in contrast to dual OXR antagonists, ACT-335827 did not simultaneously induce sleep or hypolocomotion at 300 mg/kg, likely because it did not block OXR-2 at his dose (Steiner et al., 2013).

In the present study MetS was induced in rats exposed to a CAF diet with constant access and free choice between HF/S diet or SC. In addition, highly caloric human snacks were provided 4 times weekly. Once metabolic disturbances were established (13 weeks), rats were treated daily before the onset of the dark phase with 300 mg/kg of ACT-335827 or vehicle for 4 weeks. The effects of chronic ACT-335827 treatment were monitored on energy and water intake, food preference, abdominal obesity, glucose homeostasis, plasma lipid levels, and blood pressure. Hippocampus-dependent cognitive function, which has been shown to be impaired in rodents exposed to DIO (Hwang et al., 2010; Davidson et al., 2012), was also assessed in parallel using a contextual fear-conditioning paradigm.

MATERIALS AND METHODS
ANIMALS
Thirty male Wistar rats (Harlan, Horst, NL) weighing 160–180 g (6–7 weeks old) were single-housed upon arrival and acclimated to the Actelion animal facility under a regular 12 h light/dark cycle (lights on at 6:00) for 2 weeks. During this time they were fed SC [Diet 2018S: 18% kcal fat, 24% kcal protein, 58% kcal carbohydrate (CHO) and 3.1 kcal/g; Harlan Teklad Diets, Madison, WI, USA] ad libitum. All experimental procedures were performed in strict accordance with the relevant licenses issued by the Basel-Land Veterinary office and adhered to Swiss federal regulations on animal experimentation.

DIETS
After acclimatization, rats were randomly divided into two groups. One group of 10 rats (250–325 g; 8–9 weeks old) continued to receive SC ad libitum and served as the control group for the effects of CAF diet feeding. A second group of 20 rats (275–320 g) was given a CAF diet comprised of a free choice

between SC and a HF/S diet (Diet 2126: 47% kcal fat, 19.5% kcal protein, 33.5% kcal CHO and 4.6 kcal/g; Provimi Kliba, Kaiseraugst, Switzerland), both provided *ad libitum*. The CAF diet group also received a human snack food 4 days per week of 15 kcal (weeks 1–5 of diet exposure), 30 kcal (weeks 6–13 of diet exposure), or *ad libitum* for 1 h at the beginning of the dark phase (weeks 14 to 18 of diet exposure). Seven types of snacks were provided (see Supplementary Table 1). One snack type was given per day and they were alternated between sweet and savory. The inclusion of human snacks, which are both highly caloric and high in sugar, fat, and salt, can be an important addition to rodent models of DIO, since voluntary over-snacking by humans may potentiate obesity, as well as glycemic and cardiovascular abnormalities (Kimokoti and Brown, 2011; Sampey et al., 2011).

EXPERIMENTAL DESIGN

Please see **Figure 1** for a schematic outline of the experimental design.

Both groups of animals (SC or CAF fed) were maintained on their respective diets for 13 weeks and their body weights were monitored once weekly. Blood glucose and plasma lipids levels were determined at the end of week 11, after a 16 h fast, and at the beginning of week 13, after a 6–8 h fast, respectively.

Chronic ACT-335827 or vehicle treatment began in week 14 of diet exposure. The CAF-diet fed rats were evenly assigned to a vehicle (CAF-Veh, $n = 11$) or an ACT-335827 (CAF-ACT, $n = 9$) treatment group based on their fasting blood glucose levels obtained in week 11. All SC fed rats received vehicle treatment only (SC-Veh, $n = 10$). ACT-335827 or vehicle was orally administered daily, 2 h before the onset of the dark phase. Body weights were recorded in the afternoon before the start of treatment and once weekly thereafter. Food and water intake in the home cages were continuously measured by an automated system (Phenomaster, TSE systems, Bad Hamburg, Germany).

In week 3 of treatment (week 16 of diet exposure), rats were tested in a contextual fear conditioning (CFC) paradigm. At the beginning of week 4 of treatment (week 17 of diet exposure),

blood pressure of the rats was measured in the morning. At the end of the same week, the rats were food deprived (16 h) before an oral glucose tolerance test (oGTT) in the morning. At the beginning of week 18 of diet exposure, the rats were sacrificed by decapitation 24 h after the last ACT-335827 administration and following a mild food deprivation (4–6 h).

DRUGS

ACT-335827 hydrobromide (Actelion Pharmaceuticals Ltd., Switzerland) was freshly prepared in 10% polyethylene glycol 400/0.5% methylcellulose in water, which served as vehicle (Veh). It was administered orally at 300 mg/kg based on the weight of the free base, in a volume of 5 mL/kg, and administered daily 2 h before the onset of the dark phase.

The 300 mg/kg dose was chosen based on the pharmacokinetics of this compound, which were outlined in the Introduction. At this dose, calculated free brain concentrations (>97 nM) were sufficient to allow a significant blockade of OXR-1 (affinity at the rat receptor: 7–25 nM, depending on the assay), without yet blocking the OXR-2 (affinity: 630–1030 nM). This was confirmed by the pharmacological actions of this compound, i.e., reducing stress-related outcomes without inducing sleep at this dose. Following oral administration of ACT-335827 at 300 mg/kg, calculated free brain concentrations were rising from 1 h (97 nM) to 6 h (166 nM), and declined thereafter (1 nM at 24 h). Rats consumed the majority of their food during the active, dark phase, and they increased their eating pattern just before the switch of the light-dark cycle. Thus, the rats were treated 2 h before onset of the dark phase, and also the snacks (the most caloric type of food used in this experiment) were provided at the beginning of the dark phase, in order to assure that the large majority of food intake during this chronic study would take place under full blockade of the OXR-1.

FASTING BLOOD GLUCOSE AND PLASMA LIPID ANALYSIS BEFORE CHRONIC DRUG TREATMENT

In week 11 of diet exposure, rats were fasted overnight (16 h). Using gentle restraint, a tail blood sample was obtained and

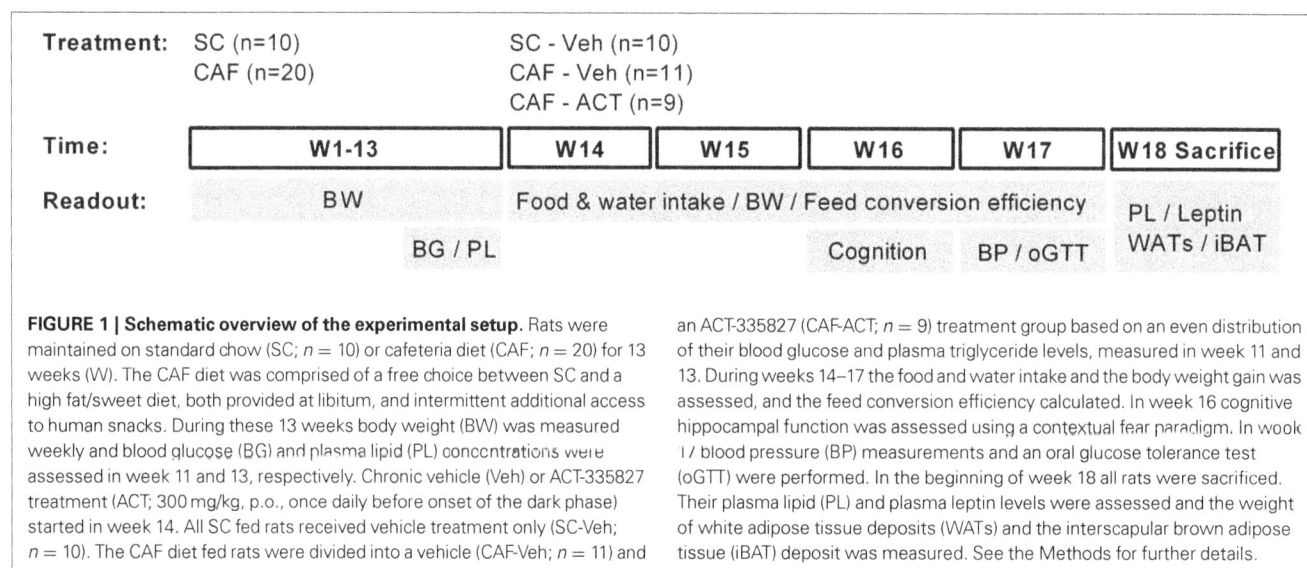

Treatment:	SC (n=10) CAF (n=20)	SC - Veh (n=10) CAF - Veh (n=11) CAF - ACT (n=9)				
Time:	W1-13	W14	W15	W16	W17	W18 Sacrifice
Readout:	BW	Food & water intake / BW / Feed conversion efficiency				PL / Leptin
	BG / PL			Cognition	BP / oGTT	WATs / iBAT

FIGURE 1 | Schematic overview of the experimental setup. Rats were maintained on standard chow (SC; $n = 10$) or cafeteria diet (CAF; $n = 20$) for 13 weeks (W). The CAF diet was comprised of a free choice between SC and a high fat/sweet diet, both provided at libitum, and intermittent additional access to human snacks. During these 13 weeks body weight (BW) was measured weekly and blood glucose (BG) and plasma lipid (PL) concentrations were assessed in week 11 and 13, respectively. Chronic vehicle (Veh) or ACT-335827 treatment (ACT; 300 mg/kg, p.o., once daily before onset of the dark phase) started in week 14. All SC fed rats received vehicle treatment only (SC-Veh; $n = 10$). The CAF diet fed rats were divided into a vehicle (CAF-Veh; $n = 11$) and

an ACT-335827 (CAF-ACT; $n = 9$) treatment group based on an even distribution of their blood glucose and plasma triglyceride levels, measured in week 11 and 13. During weeks 14–17 the food and water intake and the body weight gain was assessed, and the feed conversion efficiency calculated. In week 16 cognitive hippocampal function was assessed using a contextual fear paradigm. In week 17 blood pressure (BP) measurements and an oral glucose tolerance test (oGTT) were performed. In the beginning of week 18 all rats were sacrificed. Their plasma lipid (PL) and plasma leptin levels were assessed and the weight of white adipose tissue deposits (WATs) and the interscapular brown adipose tissue (iBAT) deposit was measured. See the Methods for further details.

glucose levels were determined using a Glucometer (ACCU-CHEK, Roche Diagnostics, Germany). For plasma lipid analysis in week 13, rats were mildly fasted (6–8 h) and blood samples were obtained by sublingual vein puncture under isoflurane anesthesia, divided between EDTA or heparin containing microtainer tubes, and kept on ice. Plasma was collected by centrifugation (2400 × g for 10 min at 4°C), placed in pre-chilled tubes and stored at −20°C. Levels of non-esterified fatty acid (NEFA), total cholesterol, and TG were assayed in plasma from EDTA-mixed blood, whereas HDL-cholesterol (HDLc) was quantified in plasma from heparinized blood. All lipids were measured using commercial enzyme assay kits and a fully automated analyzer (Beckman Coulter AU480, Nyon, Switzerland).

CONTEXTUAL FEAR CONDITIONING (CFC)

A single-training trial CFC paradigm was used to assess the effects of the CAF diet in combination with ACT-335827 treatment on hippocampus-dependent learning addressing simple contextual memory. For the training of conditioned fear, rats were singly placed in lit transparent plastic boxes (27 × 27 × 40 cm) equipped with stainless steel grid shock floors within an enclosed cubicle (Ugo Basile, Comerio, Italy) for 5 min. A 1 mA footshook was then delivered for 2 s. After 2 min the rats were returned to their home cages. 24 h later, rats were re-exposed to the same box for a 10 min testing phase. Freezing behavior (defined as absence of all movements except breathing) was measured using an automated video-tracking system (Anymaze; Stoelting Co., Wood Dale, IL, USA).

BLOOD PRESSURE

Blood pressure was indirectly measured by blood volume pressure recording (VPR) from the tail using the CODA 8-channel high throughput non-invasive blood pressure system (EMKA Technologies, Paris, France). Animals were pre-warmed at 37°C. They were then placed in restraining tubes and body temperature was maintained using a heating pad. An occlusion tail-cuff was inserted at the base of the tail and a transducer was placed 1 cm below. Rats underwent 7 cycles of measurements, lasting ~5 min, before they were returned to their home cage. Following manual reviewing, at least 3 of the 7 measurements derived from clearly defined and smooth VPRs were selected for further analysis. Based on this criteria, two CAF diet fed rats treated with ACT-335827, and one CAF diet fed rat treated with vehicle, were excluded from analyses. The systolic and diastolic blood pressures were derived by taking the mean of the 3 selected values. The mean blood pressure was calculated using the following formula: (systolic pressure - diastolic pressure)/3 + diastolic pressure.

ORAL GLUCOSE TOLERANCE TEST (oGTT)

An oGTT was performed between 8:00 and 12:00 at the end of the fourth week of treatment (week 17 of diet exposure) on overnight fasted rats (16 h). In the morning, tail vein blood was collected from rats of all treatment groups in random order for determination of fasting glucose levels (as described above). Approximately 30 min later, a freshly prepared solution of glucose (2 g/kg/5 mL in water) was orally administered to the rats in a staggered manner, and blood was again collected for glucose quantification 30, 60, 120, and 180 min following oral glucose administration.

TISSUE AND BLOOD COLLECTION AT SACRIFICE

Eighteen to Twenty hours after the last ACT-335827 or vehicle administration, rats were mildly fasted for 4–6 h before sacrifice by decapitation. Trunk blood was collected, divided between EDTA- and heparin- containing tubes, and kept on ice for ~2 h before centrifugation. Plasma was collected into pre-chilled tubes and stored at −20°C for lipid quantification (as described above) or at −80°C for leptin analysis by a commercially available leptin detection assay (Mesoscale, Gaithersburg, USA). Epididymal, abdominopelvic, and mesenteric white adipose tissues (WATs), as well as intrascapular brown adipose tissue (iBAT) were then rapidly isolated and weighed.

STATISTICAL ANALYSIS

For each rat, food intake in grams was converted to energy intake in kcal. For the time course analysis of energy and water intake and diet preference, kcal values or water volumes (mL) were cumulated over either 48 h or weekly. Body weight gain was expressed as the percentage change from baseline weight at the start of diet exposure or from the beginning of chronic treatment. The area under the curve (AUC) of the time course of blood glucose changes for each rat during the oGTT was calculated using the trapezoid rule. The weekly feed efficiency of each rat was determined by normalizing body weight gain to the total kcal intake of a given week.

For all measures, mean values and standard errors of the mean (s.e.m.) were calculated per treatment/diet group. Before the beginning of chronic treatment, the blood glucose and plasma TG levels of the CAF diet groups were compared to each other and to those of the SC fed group using unpaired two-tailed t-tests, except for diet preference and weight gain, which was analyzed using a Two-Way analysis of variance (ANOVA). Following the start of chronic vehicle or ACT-335827 treatment, for all readouts the effects of CAF diet feeding *per se* were determined by comparing CAF diet fed vehicle treated rats with SC fed vehicle treated rats using unpaired t-tests or Two-Way ANOVAs. The effects of ACT-335827 were also determined for all readouts by comparing vehicle-treated and ACT-335827-treated CAF fed rats using unpaired t-tests, and Two-Way or Three-Way ANOVAs where appropriate. CAF fed ACT-335827-treated rats were not compared to SC-fed vehicle-treated rats. *Post-hoc* mean comparisons were made using Tukey or Bonferroni tests. All statistical analyses were performed using GraphPad Prism 5.03 or Statistica (version 9) software, and statistical significance was accepted at $p < 0.05$.

RESULTS

PROFILE OF DIET GROUPS BEFORE TREATMENT ONSET

Over the 13 weeks of diet exposure, the body weight gain of CAF diet fed rats was significantly greater than that of SC fed rats [*Diet*: $F_{(1, 28)} = 12.20$, $p < 0.05$; *Time × Diet*: $F_{(12, 336)} = 3.42$, $p < 0.05$; **Figure 2A**]. *Post-hoc* analyses revealed significant group differences in weeks 8, 12, and 13 of diet exposure (**Figure 2A**).

Fasting glucose levels of CAF diet fed rats were significantly elevated at week 11 when compared to SC fed rats [$t_{(30)} = 2.3$, $p < 0.05$]. This parameter was used to divide CAF diet fed rats in two subgroups with a similar mean and distribution of glucose

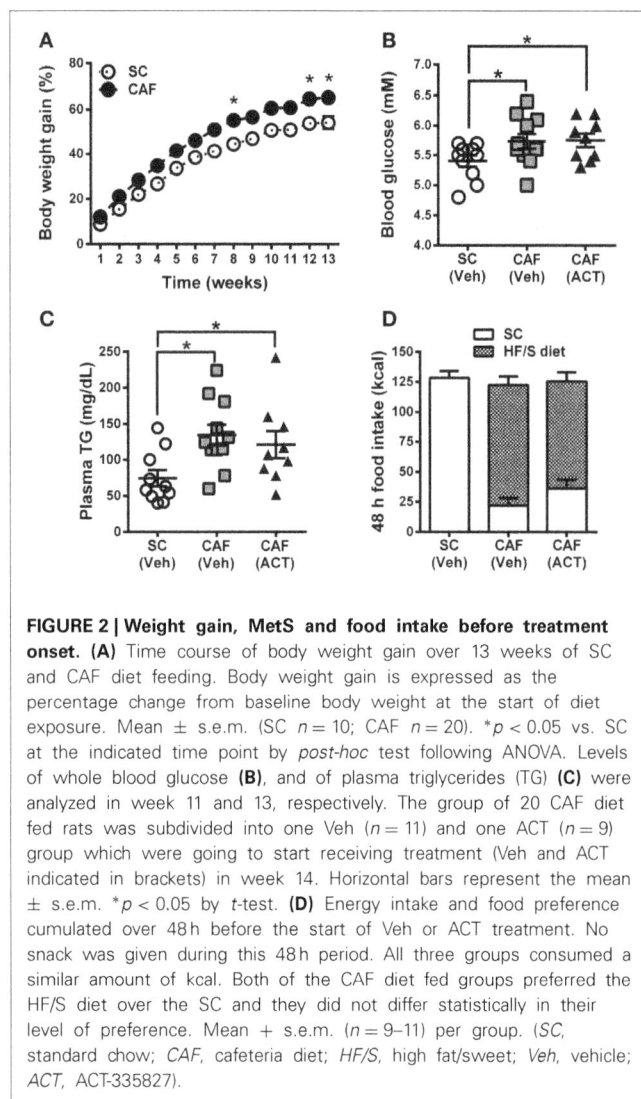

FIGURE 2 | **Weight gain, MetS and food intake before treatment onset.** **(A)** Time course of body weight gain over 13 weeks of SC and CAF diet feeding. Body weight gain is expressed as the percentage change from baseline body weight at the start of diet exposure. Mean ± s.e.m. (SC $n = 10$; CAF $n = 20$). *$p < 0.05$ vs. SC at the indicated time point by *post-hoc* test following ANOVA. Levels of whole blood glucose **(B)**, and of plasma triglycerides (TG) **(C)** were analyzed in week 11 and 13, respectively. The group of 20 CAF diet fed rats was subdivided into one Veh ($n = 11$) and one ACT ($n = 9$) group which were going to start receiving treatment (Veh and ACT indicated in brackets) in week 14. Horizontal bars represent the mean ± s.e.m. *$p < 0.05$ by *t*-test. **(D)** Energy intake and food preference cumulated over 48 h before the start of Veh or ACT treatment. No snack was given during this 48 h period. All three groups consumed a similar amount of kcal. Both of the CAF diet fed groups preferred the HF/S diet over the SC and they did not differ statistically in their level of preference. Mean + s.e.m. ($n = 9$–11) per group. (*SC*, standard chow; *CAF*, cafeteria diet; *HF/S*, high fat/sweet; *Veh*, vehicle; *ACT*, ACT-335827).

levels (**Figure 2B**) that were then assigned to receive either vehicle or ACT-335827 upon the start of treatment in week 14. Both subgroups showed similar significantly elevated fasting glucose levels compared to SC fed rats [CAF(Veh) vs. SC: $t_{(19)} = 2.14$, $p < 0.05$; CAF(ACT) vs. SC: $t_{(17)} = 2.39$, $p < 0.05$; CAF(Veh) vs. CAF(ACT): $t_{(18)} = 0.11$, $p = 0.91$].

At week 13 of diet exposure plasma TG levels were also found elevated in both groups fed a CAF diet as compared to SC [CAF(Veh) vs. SC: $t_{(19)} = 3.18$, $p < 0.01$; CAF(ACT) vs. SC: $t_{(17)} = 2.18$, $p < 0.05$] (**Figure 2C**). TG levels did not differ between the CAF diet fed groups [$t_{(18)} = 0.57$, $p = 0.56$]. Plasma levels of NEFA, total cholesterol, HDLc, or the proportion of HDLc in total cholesterol were not elevated in CAF diet fed rats compared to SC diet fed rats (data not shown).

Finally, before the start of chronic drug treatment in week 14, a 48 h assessment of the total energy intake of the HF/S diet and SC on days when no snacks were presented (**Figure 2D**) was performed. The two groups of rats exposed to the CAF diet and the rats fed SC did not differ in their total kcal intake. With respect

to food choice, both of the CAF diet fed groups consumed significantly more of the HF/S diet (77.3% of total calories) than SC (22.7% of total calories) [*Food*: $F_{(1, 18)} = 53.11$, $p < 0.05$], but they did not differ in their level of preference [*CAF diet* treatment *Group* × *Food*: $F_{(1, 18)} = 1.97$, $p = 0.18$]. With respect to water intake, the three groups of rats did not significantly differ (Supplementary Figure 1A).

In summary, rats fed the CAF diet gained more weight and showed elevated fasting blood glucose and plasma TG levels compared to rats fed SC. Forty-eight hours before the onset of chronic ACT-335827 or vehicle administration, the two CAF diet fed groups did not differ from each other in their total kcal and water intake and in their preference of the HF/S diet over SC.

ACT-335827 REDUCES THE PREFERENCE FOR A HF/S DIET WITHOUT AFFECTING WEEKLY TOTAL ENERGY INTAKE, AND INCREASES BODY WEIGHT GAIN AND FEED CONVERSION EFFICIENCY

In general, all three experimental groups slightly reduced their total energy intake over the 4 weeks of vehicle or ACT-335827 treatment [SC-Veh vs. CAF-Veh: *Time*: $F_{(3, 57)} = 17.2$, $p < 0.05$; CAF-Veh vs. CAF-ACT: *Time*: $F_{(3, 34)} = 21.57$, $p < 0.05$; **Figure 3A**]. Vehicle treated rats fed a CAF diet did not differ in their weekly total kcal intake compared to vehicle treated rats fed SC [*Diet*: $F_{(1, 19)} = 3.13$, $p = 0.09$; *Diet* × *Time*: $F_{(3, 57)} = 0.26$, $p = 0.85$]. Chronic administration of ACT-335827 did not affect the total kcal intake of the CAF diet compared to vehicle treatment [*Treatment*: $F_{(1, 18)} = 0.001$, $p = 0.98$; *Treatment* × *Time*: $F_{(3, 54)} = 0.92$, $p = 0.44$]. Both vehicle and ACT-335827 treated rats fed the CAF diet consumed significantly more of the HF/S diet than SC or snack [*Food*: $F_{(2, 36)} = 157.4$, $p < 0.05$]. Analysis of the contribution of each food type to the total kcal intake averaged over 4 weeks of vehicle treatment revealed that the rats obtained in average 74% of their total kcal from the HF/S diet, 18% from SC, and 8% from snacks. Rats chronically treated with ACT-335827 reduced their preference for the HF/S diet over SC [*Treatment* × *Food*: $F_{(2, 36)} = 8.22$, $p < 0.05$], irrespective of week of treatment [*Treatment* × *Food* × *Time*: $F_{(6, 108)} = 0.13$, $p = 1.28$].

More detailed analyses of the weekly energy intake of each food type separately over the 4 weeks of treatment revealed that ACT-335827 significantly increased the intake of SC as compared to vehicle [*Treatment*: $F_{(1, 18)} = 11.24$, $p < 0.05$], and this effect became stronger over time [*Treatment* × *Time*: $F_{(3, 54)} = 3.08$, $p < 0.05$; **Figure 3B**]. Indeed, *post-hoc* comparisons showed that ACT-335827 treatment significantly increased SC intake in weeks 3 and 4. Conversely, ACT-335827 treatment significantly decreased the intake of the HF/S diet as compared to vehicle [*Treatment*: $F_{(1, 18)} = 7.47$, $p < 0.05$], irrespective of week of treatment [*Treatment* × *Time*: $F_{(3, 54)} = 0.742$, $p = 0.53$; **Figure 3C**]. Finally, both the vehicle and ACT-335827 treated rats consumed a similar amount of the snack food over the 4 weeks of treatment [*Treatment*: $F_{(3, 54)} = 1.38$, $p = 0.26$; *Time*: $F_{(3, 54)} = 2.66$, $p = 0.06$; *Treatment* × *Time*: $F_{(3, 54)} = 1.38$, $p = 0.25$; **Figure 3D**].

Vehicle treated CAF diet fed rats and SC fed rats did not differ in their weight gain over the 4 weeks of treatment [*Time*: $F_{(4, 19)} = 14.91$, $p < 0.05$; *Diet* × *Time*: $F_{(1, 76)} = 0.48$, $p = 0.74$;

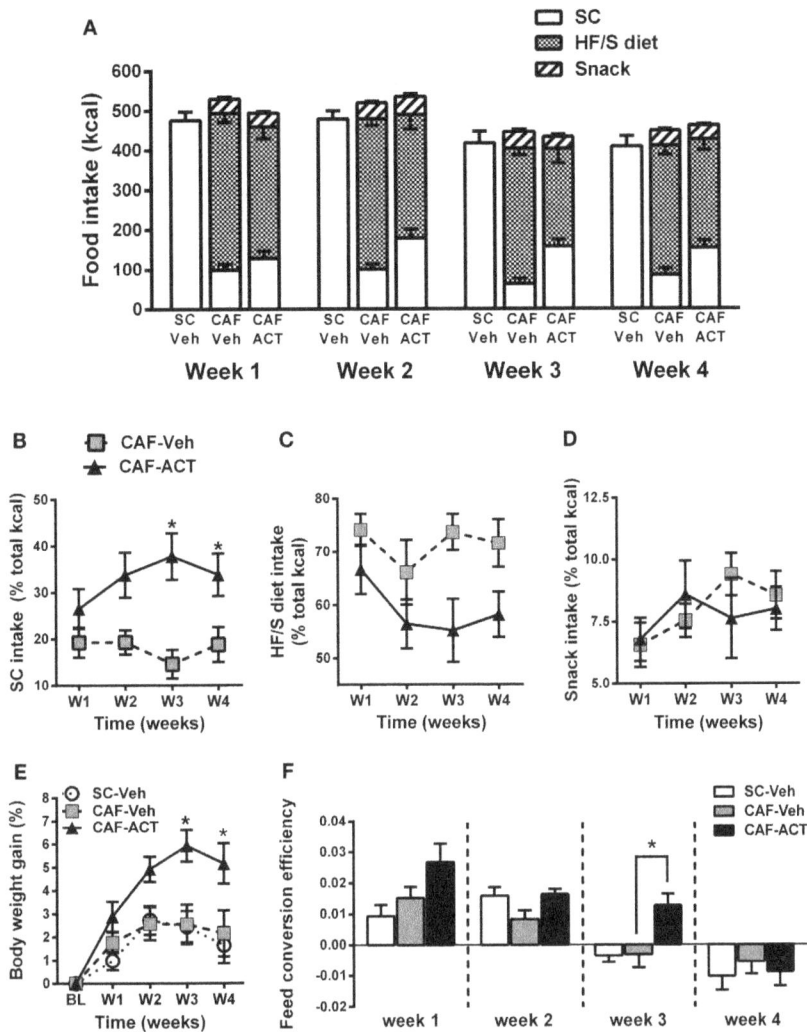

FIGURE 3 | Effect of diet and chronic ACT-335827 treatment on feeding behavior, body weight, and feed efficiency. (A) Total energy intake divided into SC, HF/S diet, and snack intake cumulated weekly. CAF-diet fed Rats chronically treated with ACT-335827 reduced their preference for the HF/S diet over SC. Snack intake was not affected by ACT-335827. For further statistical analyses see Results. **(B–D)** Energy intake of SC, HF/S diet, and snack expressed as the percentage of the total energy intake and cumulated in 1 week time bins over the 4 weeks (weeks 14–17) of Veh or ACT treatment. Significant differences between groups were revealed only for the SC intake, not for the HF/S diet or snack intake. $*p < 0.05$ vs. CAF-Veh at the indicated time points by post-hoc test following ANOVA. **(E)** Body weight gain expressed as a percentage change from baseline (BL) weight (i.e., at start of chronic treatment). CAF-Veh and SC-Veh groups did not statistically differ from each other. $*p < 0.05$ vs. CAF-Veh at the indicated time points by post-hoc test following ANOVA. **(F)** Weekly efficiency of conversion of total kcal intake into body weight gain. No significant differences were revealed between the SC-Veh and CAF-Veh groups. Mean ± s.e.m. ($n = 9$–11) per group. $*p < 0.05$ vs. CAF-Veh at the indicated time points by post-hoc test following ANOVA. Note that throughout this manuscript SC-Veh is always compared to CAF-Veh, and CAF-ACT is always compared to CAF-Veh. No comparisons between CAF-ACT and SC-Veh were made. (SC, standard chow; CAF, cafeteria diet; Veh, vehicle; ACT, ACT-335827; HF/S, high fat/sweet).

Figure 3E]. In the CAF diet fed groups, chronic ACT-335827 treatment significantly increased weight gain over 4 weeks compared to vehicle treatment [Treatment: $F_{(1, 18)} = 6.29$, $p < 0.05$; Treatment × Time: $F_{(4, 72)} = 5.42$, $p < 0.05$]. Post-hoc analysis revealed that this increase was due to significantly greater weight gains by the ACT-335827 treated rats in weeks 3 and 4.

Normalization of weekly energy intake to absolute body weight revealed that CAF diet fed rats treated with vehicle were not hyperphagic compared to SC fed rats or to ACT-335827 treated rats over the 4 weeks of treatment (data not shown). However, examination of the efficiency of feed conversion into body weight

gain of vehicle treated CAF diet fed and SC fed rats revealed a significant reduction for both groups over 4 weeks of treatment from a positive efficiency to a negative efficiency [Time: $F_{(3, 19)} = 21.9$, $p < 0.05$], but no effect of diet and no diet × time interaction [Diet: $F_{(1, 19)} = 0.07$, $p = 0.80$; Diet × Time: $F_{(3, 57)} = 1.88$, $p = 0.14$; **Figure 3F**]. Similarly, both groups of CAF fed rats showed decreasing feed efficiency over the 4 weeks of treatment [Time: $F_{(3, 19)} = 22.4$, $p < 0.05$]. However, ACT-335827 treatment inhibited this decrease compared to vehicle treatment [Treatment: $F_{(1, 19)} = 5.00$, $p < 0.05$], which was more pronounced during the first 3 weeks [Treatment × Time: $F_{(3, 54)} =$

2.65, $p = 0.06$] and reached significance in week 3 ($p < 0.05$; *post-hoc* test).

In summary, rats consuming a CAF diet and chronically treated with ACT-335827 slightly decreased their preference for a HF/S diet over SC without changing their weekly total kcal intake and snack consumption. CAF diet fed rats treated with ACT-335827 gained significantly more weight over 4 weeks compared to vehicle treatment, likely due to increased feed conversion efficiency.

ACT-335827 INCREASES WATER INTAKE IN CAF DIET FED RATS

Similar to the total food intake, overall water intake slightly decreased over the 4 weeks of treatment with vehicle or ACT-335827 independent of diet [SC-Veh vs. CAF-Veh: *Time*: $F_{(3, 57)} = 18.91$, $p < 0.05$; CAF-Veh vs. CAF-ACT: *Time*: $F_{(3, 54)} = 11.3$, $p < 0.05$; Supplementary Figure 1B]. Furthermore, vehicle treated rats fed CAF diet drank significantly less water than vehicle treated rats fed only SC, independent of week of treatment [*Diet*: $F_{(1, 19)} = 10.95$, $p < 0.05$; *Diet* × *Time*: $F_{(3, 57)} = 0.03$, $p = 0.93$]. In CAF fed rats, ACT-335827 treatment significantly increased water intake compared to vehicle treatment, largely irrespective of the week of administration [*Treatment*: $F_{(1, 18)} = 12.39$, $p < 0.05$; *Treatment* × *Time*: $F_{(3, 54)} = 2.38$, $p = 0.08$]. The effect reached statistical significance in the second and third week of treatment ($p < 0.05$; *post-hoc* test).

NO DETECTABLE EMOTIONAL OR COGNITIVE IMPAIRMENTS DUE TO CAF DIET EXPOSURE ALONE OR IN COMBINATION WITH CHRONIC ACT-335827 TREATMENT

Consumption of energy rich diets high in fat and/or sugar has been shown to impair learning and memory, particularly through their effects on hippocampal function. A CFC task was performed after 3 weeks of chronic ACT-335827 or vehicle treatment (17 weeks following the onset of CAF diet exposure).

During the fear conditioning training the rats of all groups responded with a similar amount of freezing over the 2 min following the presentation of a 1 mA foot shock (data not shown). When returned to the aversive conditioned context 24 h later, vehicle treated CAF-fed rats displayed a high level of freezing (~70%) over the entire 10 min of testing that was similar to that of both the vehicle treated rats fed SC [$t_{(19)} = 0.37, p = 0.72$] and the ACT335827 treated rats fed a CAF diet [$t_{(18)} = 0.61, p = 0.55$; **Figure 4**].

CAF DIET-INDUCED GLUCOSE INTOLERANCE IS NOT AFFECTED BY ACT-335827 TREATMENT

The effect of CAF diet exposure alone and in combination with ACT-335827 treatment on glucose homeostasis and tolerance were assessed. Following a 16 h fast, the blood glucose levels of vehicle-treated CAF fed rats were slightly elevated from those of SC fed vehicle treated rats, but the difference was not significant [$t_{(18)} = 0.77$, $p = 0.45$; **Figure 5A**]. In addition, ACT-335827 treatment of rats fed a CAF diet did not alter fasting glucose levels compared to vehicle treatment [$t_{(18)} = 1.91, p = 0.07$].

Upon oral glucose challenge, blood glucose levels were significantly elevated in vehicle treated CAF fed rats compared to

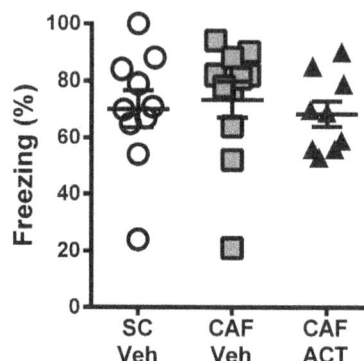

FIGURE 4 | Effect of CAF diet and ACT-335827 on cognition in week 16. Percentage of time spent freezing over a 10 min test of contextual conditioned fear. Mean ± s.e.m. ($n = 9$–11 per group). No statistical difference between groups was revealed. (*SC*, standard chow; *CAF*, cafeteria diet; *Veh*, vehicle; *ACT*, ACT-335827).

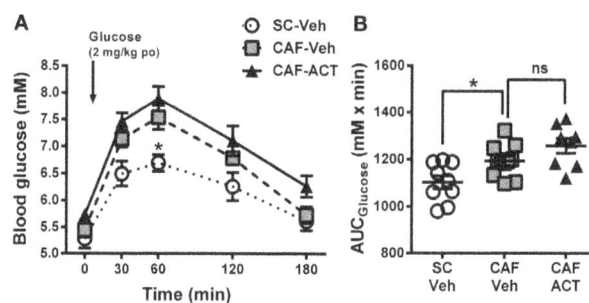

FIGURE 5 | Glucose homeostasis in week 17. (A) Oral glucose tolerance test (oGTT) performed on overnight fasted SC and CAF fed rats treated with Veh or ACT. Whole blood glucose was measured before (0 min) and at the indicated time points after the oral (po) administration of 2 mg/kg glucose (arrow). *$p < 0.05$ vs. CAF-Veh at the indicated time point by *post-hoc* test following ANOVA. Mean ± s.e.m. ($n = 8$–11) per group. Due to an incomplete blood sample set, data from one SC-Veh and one CAF-Veh rat had to be omitted because of repeated measures within subjects analyses. **(B)** AUC calculated individually for each rat. *$p < 0.05$ by *t*-test. The CAF-ACT group was statistically not different from the CAF-Veh group. (*SC*, standard chow; *CAF*, cafeteria diet; *Veh*, vehicle; *ACT*, ACT-335827; *po*, per os; *AUC*, area under the curve; *ns*, not significant).

SC fed rats [*Diet*: $F_{(2, 25)} = 9.85$, $p < 0.05$; **Figure 5A**], but the shape of the time course up to 180 min after challenge was not affected [*Diet* × *Time*: $F_{(8, 100)} = 1.33$, $p = 0.24$]. *Post-hoc* analyses revealed that the effect was most pronounced at the glucose peak (60 min after challenge), which was significantly higher in CAF fed rats than in SC fed rats. Analysis of the $AUC_{glucose}$ confirmed the glucose intolerance of the CAF-fed rats compared to SC-fed rats [$t_{(18)} = 2.72$, $p < 0.05$]. Chronic ACT-335827 treatment in combination with CAF diet feeding showed a trend to impair glucose tolerance but did not significantly alter the levels or time course of blood glucose elevations upon challenge [*Treatment*: $F_{(1, 17)} = 4.28$, $p = 0.054$; *Treatment* × *Time*: $F_{(4, 68)} = 0.23$, $p = 0.92$; **Figure 5B**], or the $AUC_{glucose}$ [$t_{(17)} = 1.80, p = 0.09$].

CAF DIET-INDUCED ELEVATION IN BLOOD PRESSURE IS NOT ALTERED BY CHRONIC ACT-335827 TREATMENT

Hypertension is correlated with central obesity and is an aspect of MetS. Compared to vehicle treated rats fed a SC diet, vehicle treated rats consuming a CAF diet for 17 weeks had significantly elevated diastolic [$t_{(18)} = 2.16, p < 0.05$], systolic [$t_{(18)} = 2.53, p < 0.05$], and mean blood pressure [$t_{(18)} = 2.37, p < 0.05$; Figure 6]. Chronic ACT-335827 treatment did not affect the elevation in blood pressure due to CAF diet feeding.

ACT-335827 DOES NOT AFFECT ELEVATIONS IN WAT AND iBAT MASS DUE TO A CAF DIET

Elevations in visceral white adipose tissue mass are associated with central obesity and are an indicator of MetS. The main visceral fat deposits in male rodents are the epididymal depot, the adominopelvic depot, and the mesenteric depot. At the time of sacrifice, following 4 weeks of chronic vehicle treatment, CAF diet fed rats had significantly heavier epididymal [$t_{(19)} = 2.43, p < 0.05$; Figure 7A] and adominopelvic [$t_{(19)} = 2.13, p < 0.05$; Figure 7B], but not mesenteric (Figure 7C) fat deposits, than SC fed rats. Moreover, the proportion of body weight represented by the combined mass of all three visceral fat deposits was significantly higher in vehicle treated rats fed a CAF diet compared to those fed SC [$t_{(19)} = 2.36, p < 0.05$; Figure 7D]. In addition to WAT, the CAF diet fed rats treated with vehicle also had significantly larger deposits of iBAT compared to vehicle treated SC fed rats [$t_{(19)} = 3.0, p < 0.05$; Figure 7E]. Chronic treatment with ACT-335827 did not significantly alter the elevations in visceral WAT depots and iBAT mass resulting from CAF diet feeding as compared to vehicle treatment.

ACT-335827 INCREASES THE PROPORTION OF PLASMA HDLc LEVELS, BUT DOES NOT ALTER ELEVATED PLASMA TG LEVELS DUE TO A CAF DIET

Plasma markers of MetS include reduced levels of HDLc and elevated TG levels. At the time of sacrifice following 4 weeks of vehicle or ACT-335827 treatment (and 18 weeks of diet exposure), plasma levels of HDLc (Figure 8A), total cholesterol

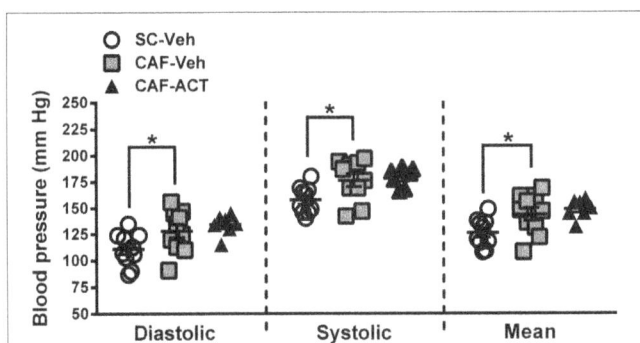

FIGURE 6 | Blood pressure in week 17. Diastolic, systolic, and mean blood pressures of SC or CAF diet fed rats treated with Veh or ACT. Horizontal bars represent the mean ± s.e.m. (n = 7–10) per group. Reliable data was not attainable from 1 CAF-Veh rat and from 2 CAF-ACT rats, and were therefore omitted from analyses. *p < 0.05 by t-test. No statistical difference was revealed between the CAF-ACT and the CAF-Veh group. (SC, standard chow; CAF, cafeteria diet; Veh, vehicle; ACT, ACT-335827).

(Figure 8B), or the proportion of HDLc relative to total cholesterol (Figure 8C) were not different between vehicle treated rats fed CAF diet or SC. However, plasma TG levels were significantly higher in vehicle treated CAF diet fed rats compared to SC fed rats [$t_{(18)} = 2.70, p < 0.05$; Figure 8D]. As expected from elevations in WAT and iBAT mass due to CAF diet feeding reported above, plasma levels of leptin were significantly elevated in these rats compared to SC fed rats [$t_{(18)} = 2.72, p < 0.05$; Figure 8E]. Finally, plasma levels of NEFA did not differ significantly between vehicle treated rats fed SC or CAF (Figure 8F).

ACT-335827 treatment of CAF diet fed rats did not significantly affect plasma levels of TG [$t_{(18)} = 0.61, p = 0.55$], cholesterol, NEFA, Plasma HDLc or leptin compared to vehicle treatment. However, the proportion of HDLc in the total plasma cholesterol was found significantly elevated [$t_{(18)} = 3.84, p < 0.05$; Figure 8C].

DISCUSSION

CAF DIET FEEDING AS A MODEL OF MetS

In humans, over-consumption of palatable food rich in fat, sugar, and salt facilitates MetS development. Under a CAF diet comprised of a choice between a HF/S diet and SC and an additional snack 4 times weekly, rats developed major signs of human MetS, including abdominal adiposity, elevated TG and fasting blood glucose levels, glucose intolerance, and elevated blood pressure when compared to rats fed only SC. Conversely, plasma levels of NEFA, total cholesterol, HDLc, and the ratio between the latter two, were not altered. These findings are in agreement with those of other DIO studies in rodents reporting a similar induction of partial abnormalities associated with MetS in man [e.g., (Sampey et al., 2011)]. An impairment of hippocampus-dependent memory function induced by DIO, which might be a consequence of altered blood-brain barrier integrity (Davidson et al., 2012) and/or a reduction of growth factors and proteins responsible for synaptic plasticity (Woo et al., 2013), has been demonstrated both in human and rodents (Kanoski and Davidson, 2011). Still, hippocampus memory function, which was assessed in the present study by employing a CFC paradigm, was not altered in rats fed a CAF diet compared to rats fed SC. Using a one-trial conditioning protocol and a shock intensity similar to ours, Hwang et al. showed that male mice fed a normal diet responded with ~50% freezing during the 6 min test of conditioned fear, whereas this was reduced to ~20% in mice fed a HF diet for 1 year (Hwang et al., 2010). A CAF diet exposure of only 4 months as in our study may have been insufficient to cause learning impairments in this test.

EFFECT OF CHRONIC ACT-335827 TREATMENT IN THE MetS MODEL

ACT-335827 treatment began in week 14 of CAF diet exposure, a time point when rats displayed elevated fasting blood glucose and plasma TG levels. Our results indicate that 4 weeks of ACT-335827 treatment did not significantly alter metabolic abnormalities and adiposity generated by CAF diet exposure alone, despite the animals showing an improved diet composition due to a slight but significant reduction in preference for the HF/S diet over SC. This reduction in HF/S diet intake upon OXR-1 blockade is

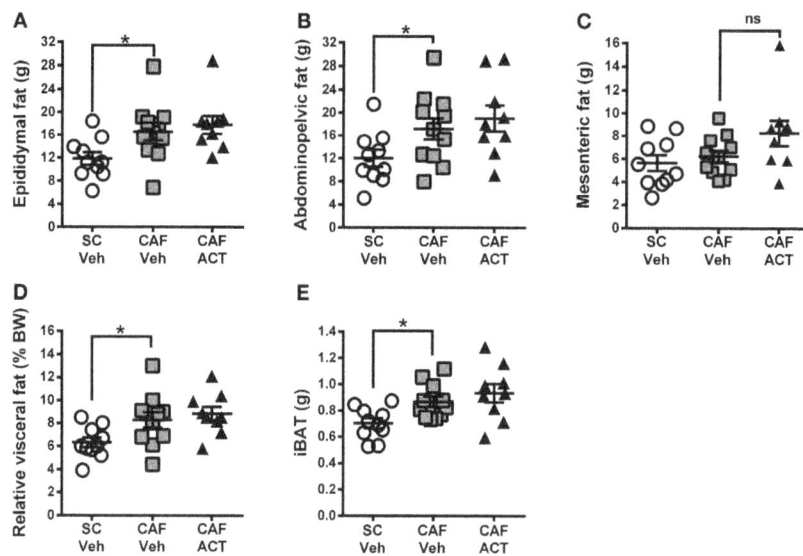

FIGURE 7 | Fat mass at sacrifice. The effect of SC or CAF diet exposure on the mass of epididymal **(A)**, abdominopelvic **(B)**, and mesenteric **(C)** visceral fat deposits in rats treated with Veh or ACT. **(D)** Normalization of cumulated visceral fat mass (in **A–C**) to body weight (BW) per rat and expressed as a percentage. **(E)** Mass of intrascapular brown adipose tissue (iBAT). Mean ± s.e.m. ($n = 9$–11 per group). *$p < 0.05$ by t-test. No statistical difference was revealed between the CAF-ACT and the CAF-Veh group. (*SC*, standard chow; *CAF*, cafeteria diet; *Veh*, vehicle; *ACT*, ACT-335827; *ns*, not significant).

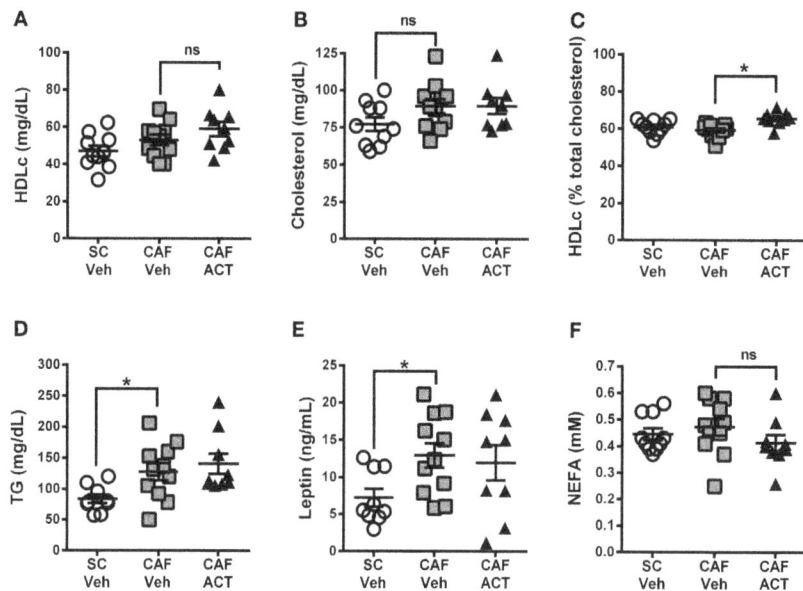

FIGURE 8 | Plasma lipids and leptin at sacrifice. Plasma levels of HDL-cholesterol (HDLc) **(A)**, total cholesterol **(B)**, HDL-c levels (in **A**) expressed as a percentage of total plasma cholesterol (in **B**) **(C)**, triglyceride (TG) levels **(D)**, leptin **(E)**, and non-esterified fatty acids (NEFA) **(F)**, in rats fed SC or a CAF diet and treated with Veh or ACT. Horizontal bars represent the mean ± s.e.m. ($n = 9$–11 per group). *$p < 0.05$ by t-test. (*SC*, standard chow; *CAF*, cafeteria diet; *Veh*, vehicle; *ACT*, ACT-335827; *HDL*, high density lipoprotein; *ns*, not significant).

consistent with other studies in rats suggesting a role for OXR-1 activation in positively regulating the motivation to consume palatable foods (Zheng et al., 2007; Choi et al., 2010). A decrease in reward perception under ACT-335827 treatment might also be expected to decrease intake of highly palatable snacks. However, consumption of the human snacks (presented for 1 h, 4 times weekly), was not affected by the drug. ACT-335827 administration may thus, be ineffective at reducing the binge-like intake of highly palatable foods under conditions, where either another type of palatable food (the HF/S diet) is freely available, or where no additional intermittent periods of stress or food-restriction occur. Using the OXR-1 antagonist GSK1059865, Piccoli et al.

showed that OXR-1 signaling is only involved in the binge-like intake of highly palatable food if an additional specific stressor component (e.g., smelling but no access to the palatable food) is present (Piccoli et al., 2012).

The reduced overall food intake among all experimental groups during weeks 3 and 4 of vehicle or ACT-335827 treatment may be due to the performance of the CFC test to assess cognition (in week 3), and a blood pressure analysis and an overnight period of fasting before the oGTT (in week 4). These procedures were likely a source of stress on the rats, which may have affected their energy consumption and led to a slight decline of body weight gain in week 4. It is unlikely that those procedures confounded the overall conclusions of the current study with regard to OXR-1 blockade because all experimental groups (SC-Veh, CAF-Veh, and CAF-ACT) were simultaneously affected. Moreover, the overall pattern of the different diet consumption, which was displayed by the different groups already in week 2 of chronic treatment (until when no additional potentially stressful experimental procedures had been performed) was actually maintained in weeks 3 and 4 as well (see **Figure 3A**). Whether the additional exposure to environmental stressors during weeks 3 and 4 actually intensified the preference of the CAF-ACT treated rats for consuming more of the SC as compared to the CAF diet, cannot be excluded.

Despite affecting HF/S food preference vs. SC, ACT-335827 had no impact on total calorie intake because the decrease in HF/S food intake was entirely compensated for by an increase in SC intake. As a result, given that chronic ACT-335827 treatment also increased body weight gain, feed efficiency was enhanced. Although not directly tested, these results suggest that ACT-335827 administration may reduce energy expenditure. Funato et al. (2009) showed that energy expenditure is reduced in OXR-1 deficient mice under low fat, but not high fat, feeding conditions. Conversely, ob/ob female mice showed even increased energy expenditure under chronic treatment with SB-334867 administered at 30 mg/kg (Haynes et al., 2002). The reason for these discrepancies remains unclear, but biological compensation, phenotypically expressed in knockout animals, and sex or species differences are likely explanations that can be considered. Moreover, the OXR-1 preferential antagonist SB-334867 has recently been tested by two independent groups for selectivity (Gotter et al., 2012; Morairty et al., 2012): these studies suggest that at high doses as applied by Haynes et al. (2002), SB-334867 could additionally interact with a number of other brain targets.

Orexins also stimulate BAT thermogenesis, but the individual role played by the OXR-1 in modulating BAT function is unclear (Haynes et al., 2002; Sellayah et al., 2011; Tupone et al., 2011). BAT is important for plasma TG clearance, which improves insulin resistance due to DIO (Bartelt et al., 2011). In the current study the elevated weight gain and feed efficiency seen with ACT-335827 treatment under CAF diet feeding was not associated with an altered elevation in iBAT mass or a change in plasma TG levels compared to vehicle treatment. This might suggest that BAT was functioning normally in ACT-335827 treated rats challenged with a CAF diet. However, UCP-1 levels, which serves as a marker of BAT thermogenesis (Haynes et al., 2002; Sellayah et al., 2011), were not analyzed to confirm this conclusion. An alternative possibility for the reduced energy expenditure is that ACT-335827

had an inhibitory effect on non-exercise activity thermogenesis, which can be generated by orexin A (Novak et al., 2006; Novak and Levine, 2009).

Interestingly, the elevated body weight gain and increased feed efficiency seen over 4 weeks of ACT-335827 treatment were not associated with an increase in visceral fat mass compared to vehicle treatment. Thus, the weight gained by ACT-335827 - treated-rats must have occurred in fat deposits not analyzed (e.g., subcutaneous) and/or in non-fat tissues. Blood pressure of CAF diet fed rats also remained unchanged by treatment.

Rats exposed to a CAF diet for 13 weeks marginally consumed less water than rats fed SC in the 48 h before vehicle or ACT-33527 treatment onset; this decrease became significant over the subsequent 4 weeks of vehicle administration. ACT-335827 treatment, however, countered this decrease, even though acute administration of ACT-335827 to rats under normal feeding conditions does not affect water intake during their active phase (Steiner et al., 2013).

The mechanisms by which orexins modulate water balance or glucose metabolism through OXR-1 and OXR-2 binding have not been extensively investigated. Existing evidence suggests that orexins induce glucose production in the liver (Yi et al., 2009) and facilitate glucose uptake in skeletal muscle (Shiuchi et al., 2009). In addition, orexins A and B have been shown to differentially modulate glucagon release from pancreas (Goncz et al., 2008; Adeghate and Hameed, 2011). The unaltered glucose homeostasis observed with chronic ACT-335827 treatment in CAF diet fed rats with existing glucose imbalance contrasts with the improved fasting glucose levels seen in obese OXR-1 deficient mice (Funato et al., 2009) and in ob/ob female mice chronically treated with a high dose of the preferential OXR-1 antagonist SB-334867 before obesity onset (Haynes et al., 2002). Again, developmental compensation, species differences or non OXR-1 related effects may be responsible for these discrepancies.

A final observation of our study was that CAF diet fed rats chronically treated with ACT-335827 had elevated HDLc to total cholesterol ratios. HDLc is cardioprotective due to its antioxidant, anti-inflammatory, and scavenging properties (Mooradian et al., 2008). HDLc has a complex metabolism, and elevated levels must be interpreted in context with the overall lipid profile (Mooradian et al., 2008). To our knowledge there has been no reported involvement of the orexin system in HDLc processing; the mechanism by which ACT-335827 affects HDLc metabolism warrants further examination.

It is difficult to directly compare the results that we obtained using ACT-335827 with previous investigations using other OXR-1 antagonists, because this is the first study exploring chronic pharmacological OXR-1 blockade in a rat model of DIO associated with MetS. It also has to be mentioned that most of our knowledge concerning the effects of OXR-1 inhibition on food intake in rodents derives from using the OXR-1 antagonist SB-334867, which at high dose is likely to affect additional neuronal targets (Gotter et al., 2012; Morairty et al., 2012). Another newer generation OXR-1 selective compound, GSK1059865, for instance did not confirm previous findings using SB-334867 (Choi et al., 2010) in the sense that GSK did not affect high palatable food intake *per se* under no-stress and no food restriction conditions

(Piccoli et al., 2012). Thus, it is desirable that future studies exploring the role of OXR-1 signaling in feeding further will employ not only SB-334867 but also other OXR-1 antagonists from different chemical classes.

Taken together, utilizing a free choice nutrient regime with additional human snacks as a model of DIO, this study was successful in inducing most aspects of human metabolic syndrome in Wistar rats. Chronic ACT-335827 treatment for 4 weeks reduced the preference for a high-fat/high-sweet diet compared to standard laboratory food pellets but had no effect on snack intake or absolute energy intake. ACT-335827 even slightly increased body weight gain. The main characteristics of human metabolic syndrome, including abdominal obesity, decreased glucose tolerance, enhanced blood pressure, and increased TGs remained unaffected by ACT-335827 treatment, at doses otherwise active in reducing environmental stress-induced outcomes (Steiner et al., 2013). It is concluded that continuous selective pharmacological blockade of OXR-1, in brain and periphery, under the applied experimental conditions has minimal impact on rat net energy balance resulting from food reward, nutrient metabolism, and physical homeostasis.

AUTHOR CONTRIBUTIONS

Michel A. Steiner conceived, designed and supervised the study and wrote part of the manuscript. Carla Sciarretta and Anne Pasquali designed and planned the study, performed the experiments, and collected and analyzed the data. Carla Sciarretta also wrote a large part of the manuscript, and Anne Pasquali performed the statistical analyses. Francois Jenck facilitated and supported the study and critically reviewed the manuscript.

ACKNOWLEDGMENTS

We thank Daniel Wanner for analyzing the plasma lipid contents and Céline Bortolamiol for help in performing the blood pressure measurements. We thank Christophe Cattaneo, Magali Vercauteren and Daniele Viviani for their technical advice.

SUPPLEMENTARY MATERIAL

The Supplementary Material for this article can be found online at: http://www.frontiersin.org/journal/10.3389/fphar.2013. 00165/abstract

REFERENCES

Adamo, K. B., and Tesson, F. (2008). Gene-environment interaction and the metabolic syndrome. *Novartis Found. Symp.* 293, 103–119. discussion: 119–127. doi: 10.1002/9780470696781.ch8

Adeghate, E., Fernandez-Cabezudo, M., Hameed, R., El-Hasasna, H., El Wasila, M., Abbas, T., et al. (2010). Orexin-1 receptor co-localizes with pancreatic hormones in islet cells and modulates the outcome of streptozotocin-induced diabetes mellitus. *PLoS ONE* 5:e8587. doi: 10.1371/journal.pone.0008587

Adeghate, E., and Hameed, R. (2011). Mechanism of orexin B-stimulated insulin and glucagon release from the pancreas of normal and diabetic rats. *Pancreas* 40, 131–136. doi: 10.1097/MPA.0b013e3181f74b4b

Balcita-Pedicino, J. J., and Sesack, S. R. (2007). Orexin axons in the rat ventral tegmental area synapse infrequently onto dopamine and gamma-aminobutyric acid neurons. *J. Comp. Neurol.* 503, 668–684. doi: 10.1002/cne.21420

Bartelt, A., Bruns, O. T., Reimer, R., Hohenberg, H., Ittrich, H., Peldschus, K., et al. (2011). Brown adipose tissue activity controls triglyceride clearance. *Nat. Med.* 17, 200–205. doi: 10.1038/nm.2297

Blanco, M., Garcia-Caballero, T., Fraga, M., Gallego, R., Cuevas, J., Forteza, J., et al. (2002). Cellular localization of orexin receptors in human adrenal gland, adrenocortical adenomas and pheochromocytomas. *Regul. Pept.* 104, 161–165. doi: 10.1016/S0167-0115(01)00359-7

Borgland, S. L., Chang, S. J., Bowers, M. S., Thompson, J. L., Vittoz, N., Floresco, S. B., et al. (2009). Orexin A/hypocretin-1 selectively promotes motivation for positive reinforcers. *J. Neurosci.* 29, 11215–11225. doi: 10.1523/JNEUROSCI.6096-08.2009

Cason, A. M., and Aston-Jones, G. (2013). Role of orexin/hypocretin in conditioned sucrose-seeking in rats. *Psychopharmacology (Berl)* 226, 155–165. doi: 10.1007/s00213-012-2902-y

Choi, D. L., Davis, J. F., Fitzgerald, M. E., and Benoit, S. C. (2010). The role of orexin-A in food motivation, reward-based feeding behavior and food-induced neuronal activation in rats. *Neuroscience* 167, 11–20. doi: 10.1016/j.neuroscience.2010.02.002

Davidson, T. L., Monnot, A., Neal, A. U., Martin, A. A., Horton, J. J., and Zheng, W. (2012). The effects of a high-energy diet on hippocampal-dependent discrimination performance and blood-brain barrier integrity differ for diet-induced obese and diet-resistant rats. *Physiol. Behav.* 107, 26–33. doi: 10.1016/j.physbeh.2012.05.015

De Flines, J., and Scheen, A. J. (2010). Management of metabolic syndrome and associated cardiovascular risk factors. *Acta Gastroenterol. Belg.* 73, 261–266.

De Lecea, L., Kilduff, T. S., Peyron, C., Gao, X., Foye, P. E., Danielson, P. E., et al. (1998). The hypocretins: hypothalamus-specific peptides with neuroexcitatory activity. *Proc. Natl. Acad. Sci. U.S.A.* 95, 322–327. doi: 10.1073/pnas.95.1.322

Digby, J. E., Chen, J., Tang, J. Y., Lehnert, H., Matthews, R. N., and Randeva, H. S. (2006). Orexin receptor expression in human adipose tissue: effects of orexin-A and orexin-B. *J. Endocrinol.* 191, 129–136. doi: 10.1677/joe.1.06886

Di Sebastiano, A. R., and Coolen, L. M. (2012). Orexin and natural reward: feeding, maternal, and male sexual behavior. *Prog. Brain Res.* 198, 65–77. doi: 10.1016/B978-0-444-59489-1.00006-9

Eskelinen, M. H., Ngandu, T., Helkala, E. L., Tuomilehto, J., Nissinen, A., Soininen, H., et al. (2008). Fat intake at midlife and cognitive impairment later in life: a population-based CAIDE study. *Int. J. Geriatr. Psychiatry* 23, 741–747. doi: 10.1002/gps.1969

Francis, H. M., and Stevenson, R. J. (2011). Higher reported saturated fat and refined sugar intake is associated with reduced hippocampal-dependent memory and sensitivity to interoceptive signals. *Behav. Neurosci.* 125, 943–955. doi: 10.1037/a0025998

Funato, H., Tsai, A. L., Willie, J. T., Kisanuki, Y., Williams, S. C., Sakurai, T., et al. (2009). Enhanced orexin receptor-2 signaling prevents diet-induced obesity and improves leptin sensitivity. *Cell Metab.* 9, 64–76. doi: 10.1016/j.cmet.2008.10.010

Furudono, Y., Ando, C., Yamamoto, C., Kobashi, M., and Yamamoto, T. (2006). Involvement of specific orexigenic neuropeptides in sweetener-induced overconsumption in rats. *Behav. Brain Res.* 175, 241–248. doi: 10.1016/j.bbr.2006.08.031

Goncz, E., Strowski, M. Z., Grotzinger, C., Nowak, K. W., Kaczmarek, P., Sassek, M., et al. (2008). Orexin-A inhibits glucagon secretion and gene expression through a Foxo1-dependent pathway. *Endocrinology* 149, 1618–1626. doi: 10.1210/en.2007-1257

Gotter, A. L., Webber, A. L., Coleman, P. J., Renger, J. J., and Winrow, C. J. (2012). International Union of basic and clinical pharmacology. LXXXVI. Orexin receptor function, nomenclature and pharmacology. *Pharmacol. Rev.* 64, 389–420. doi: 10.1124/pr.111.005546

Haynes, A. C., Chapman, H., Taylor, C., Moore, G. B., Cawthorne, M. A., Tadayyon, M., et al. (2002). Anorectic, thermogenic and anti-obesity activity of a selective orexin-1 receptor antagonist in ob/ob mice. *Regul. Pept.* 104, 153–159. doi: 10.1016/S0167-0115(01)00358-5

Haynes, A. C., Jackson, B., Chapman, H., Tadayyon, M., Johns, A., Porter, R. A., et al. (2000). A selective orexin-1 receptor antagonist reduces food consumption in male and female rats. *Regul. Pept.* 96, 45–51. doi: 10.1016/S0167-0115(00)00199-3

Heinonen, M. V., Purhonen, A. K., Makela, K. A., and Herzig, K. H. (2008). Functions of orexins in peripheral tissues. *Acta Physiol. (Oxf)* 192, 471–485. doi: 10.1111/j.1748-1716.2008.01836.x

Hwang, L. L., Wang, C. H., Li, T. L., Chang, S. D., Lin, L. C., Chen, C. P., et al. (2010). Sex differences in high-fat diet-induced obesity, metabolic alterations and learning, and synaptic plasticity deficits in mice. *Obesity (Silver Spring)* 18, 463–469. doi: 10.1038/oby.2009.273

Ishii, Y., Blundell, J. E., Halford, J. C., Upton, N., Porter, R., Johns, A., et al. (2005). Satiety enhancement by selective orexin-1 receptor antagonist SB-334867: influence of test context and profile comparison with CCK-8S. *Behav. Brain Res.* 160, 11–24. doi: 10.1016/j.bbr.2004.11.011

Kanoski, S. E., and Davidson, T. L. (2011). Western diet consumption and cognitive impairment: links to hippocampal dysfunction and obesity. *Physiol. Behav.* 103, 59–68. doi: 10.1016/j.physbeh.2010.12.003

Karnani, M., and Burdakov, D. (2011). Multiple hypothalamic circuits sense and regulate glucose levels. *Am. J. Physiol. Regul. Integr. Comp. Physiol.* 300, R47–R55. doi: 10.1152/ajpregu.00527.2010

Karteris, E., Machado, R. J., Chen, J., Zervou, S., Hillhouse, E. W., and Randeva, H. S. (2005). Food deprivation differentially modulates orexin receptor expression and signaling in rat hypothalamus and adrenal cortex. *Am. J. Physiol. Endocrinol. Metab.* 288, E1089–E1100. doi: 10.1152/ajpendo.00351.2004

Kimokoti, R. W., and Brown, L. S. (2011). Dietary management of the metabolic syndrome. *Clin. Pharmacol. Ther.* 90, 184–187. doi: 10.1038/clpt.2011.92

Kirchgessner, A. L., and Liu, M. (1999). Orexin synthesis and response in the gut. *Neuron* 24, 941–951. doi: 10.1016/S0896-6273(00)81041-7

Louis, G. W., Leininger, G. M., Rhodes, C. J., and Myers, M. G. Jr. (2010). Direct innervation and modulation of orexin neurons by lateral hypothalamic LepRb neurons. *J. Neurosci.* 30, 11278–11287. doi: 10.1523/JNEUROSCI.1340-10.2010

Marcus, J. N., Aschkenasi, C. J., Lee, C. E., Chemelli, R. M., Saper, C. B., Yanagisawa, M., et al. (2001). Differential expression of orexin receptors 1 and 2 in the rat brain. *J. Comp. Neurol.* 435, 6–25. doi: 10.1002/cne.1190

Mondal, M. S., Nakazato, M., Date, Y., Murakami, N., Hanada, R., Sakata, T., et al. (1999). Characterization of orexin-A and orexin-B in the microdissected rat brain nuclei and their contents in two obese rat models. *Neurosci. Lett.* 273, 45–48. doi: 10.1016/S0304-3940(99)00624-2

Mooradian, A. D., Haas, M. J., Wehmeier, K. R., and Wong, N. C. (2008). Obesity-related changes in high-density lipoprotein metabolism. *Obesity (Silver Spring)* 16, 1152–1160. doi: 10.1038/oby.2008.202

Morairty, S. R., Revel, F. G., Malherbe, P., Moreau, J. L., Valladao, D., Wettstein, J. G., et al. (2012). Dual hypocretin receptor antagonism is more effective for sleep promotion than antagonism of either receptor alone. *PLoS ONE* 7:e39131. doi: 10.1371/journal.pone.0039131

Niimi, M., Sato, M., and Taminato, T. (2001). Neuropeptide Y in central control of feeding and interactions with orexin and leptin. *Endocrine* 14, 269–273. doi: 10.1385/ENDO:14:2:269

Novak, C. M., Kotz, C. M., and Levine, J. A. (2006). Central orexin sensitivity, physical activity, and obesity in diet-induced obese and diet-resistant rats. *Am. J. Physiol. Endocrinol. Metab.* 290, E396–E403. doi: 10.1152/ajpendo.00293.2005

Novak, C. M., and Levine, J. A. (2009). Daily intraparaventricular orexin-A treatment induces weight loss in rats. *Obesity (Silver Spring)* 17, 1493–1498. doi: 10.1038/oby.2009.91

Parise, E. M., Lilly, N., Kay, K., Dossat, A. M., Seth, R., Overton, J. M., et al. (2011). Evidence for the role of hindbrain orexin-1 receptors in the control of meal size. *Am. J. Physiol. Regul. Integr. Comp. Physiol.* 301, R1692–R1699. doi: 10.1152/ajpregu.00044.2011

Piccoli, L., Micioni Di Bonaventura, M. V., Cifani, C., Costantini, V. J., Massagrande, M., Montanari, D., et al. (2012). Role of orexin-1 receptor mechanisms on compulsive food consumption in a model of binge eating in female rats. *Neuropsychopharmacology* 37, 1999–2011. doi: 10.1038/npp.2012.48

Sakurai, T. (2006). Roles of orexins and orexin receptors in central regulation of feeding behavior and energy homeostasis. *CNS Neurol. Disord. Drug Targets* 5, 313–325. doi: 10.2174/187152706777452218

Sakurai, T., Amemiya, A., Ishii, M., Matsuzaki, I., Chemelli, R. M., Tanaka, H., et al. (1998). Orexins and orexin receptors: a family of hypothalamic neuropeptides and G protein-coupled receptors that regulate feeding behavior. *Cell* 92, 573–585. doi: 10.1016/S0092-8674(00)80949-6

Sampey, B. P., Vanhoose, A. M., Winfield, H. M., Freemerman, A. J., Muehlbauer, M. J., Fueger, P. T., et al. (2011). Cafeteria diet is a robust model of human metabolic syndrome with liver and adipose inflammation: comparison to high-fat diet. *Obesity (Silver Spring)* 19, 1109–1117. doi: 10.1038/oby.2011.18

Sellayah, D., Bharaj, P., and Sikder, D. (2011). Orexin is required for brown adipose tissue development, differentiation, and function. *Cell Metab.* 14, 478–490. doi: 10.1016/j.cmet.2011.08.010

Shiuchi, T., Haque, M. S., Okamoto, S., Inoue, T., Kageyama, H., Lee, S., et al. (2009). Hypothalamic orexin stimulates feeding-associated glucose utilization in skeletal muscle via sympathetic nervous system. *Cell Metab.* 10, 466–480. doi: 10.1016/j.cmet.2009.09.013

Skrzypski, M., T Le, T., Kaczmarek, P., Pruszynska-Oszmalek, E., Pietrzak, P., Szczepankiewicz, D., et al. (2011). Orexin A stimulates glucose uptake, lipid accumulation and adiponectin secretion from 3T3-L1 adipocytes and isolated primary rat adipocytes. *Diabetologia* 54, 1841–1852. doi: 10.1007/s00125-011-2152-2

Steiner, M. A., Gatfield, J., Brisbare-Roch, C., Dietrich, H., Treiber, A., Jenck, F., et al. (2013). Discovery and characterization of ACT-335827, an orally available, brain penetrant orexin receptor type 1 selective antagonist. *ChemMedChem* 8, 898–903. doi: 10.1002/cmdc.201300003

Steiner, M. A., Lecourt, H., and Jenck, F. (2012). The brain orexin system and almorexant in fear-conditioned startle reactions in the rat. *Psychopharmacology (Berl)* 223, 465–475. doi: 10.1007/s00213-012-2736-7

Trivedi, P., Yu, H., Macneil, D. J., Van Der Ploeg, L. H., and Guan, X. M. (1998). Distribution of orexin receptor mRNA in the rat brain. *FEBS Lett.* 438, 71–75. doi: 10.1016/S0014-5793(98)01266-6

Tsuneki, H., Wada, T., and Sasaoka, T. (2010). Role of orexin in the regulation of glucose homeostasis. *Acta Physiol. (Oxf)* 198, 335–348. doi: 10.1111/j.1748-1716.2009.02008.x

Tupone, D., Madden, C. J., Cano, G., and Morrison, S. F. (2011). An orexinergic projection from perifornical hypothalamus to raphe pallidus increases rat brown adipose tissue thermogenesis. *J. Neurosci.* 31, 15944–15955. doi: 10.1523/JNEUROSCI.3909-11.2011

Williams, R. H., Alexopoulos, H., Jensen, L. T., Fugger, L., and Burdakov, D. (2008). Adaptive sugar sensors in hypothalamic feeding circuits. *Proc. Natl. Acad. Sci. U.S.A.* 105, 11975–11980. doi: 10.1073/pnas.0802687105

Woo, J., Shin, K. O., Park, S. Y., Jang, K. S., and Kang, S. (2013). Effects of exercise and diet change on cognition function and synaptic plasticity in high fat diet induced obese rats. *Lipids Health Dis.* 12, 144. doi: 10.1186/1476-511X-12-144

Yamanaka, A., Beuckmann, C. T., Willie, J. T., Hara, J., Tsujino, N., Mieda, M., et al. (2003). Hypothalamic orexin neurons regulate arousal according to energy balance in mice. *Neuron* 38, 701–713. doi: 10.1016/S0896-6273(03)00331-3

Yi, C. X., Serlie, M. J., Ackermans, M. T., Foppen, E., Buijs, R. M., Sauerwein, H. P., et al. (2009). A major role for perifornical orexin neurons in the control of glucose metabolism in rats. *Diabetes* 58, 1998–2005. doi: 10.2337/db09-0385

Yoshida, K., McCormack, S., Espana, R. A., Crocker, A., and Scammell, T. E. (2006). Afferents to the orexin neurons of the rat brain. *J. Comp. Neurol.* 494, 845–861. doi: 10.1002/cne.20859

Zheng, H., Patterson, L. M., and Berthoud, H. R. (2007). Orexin signaling in the ventral tegmental area is required for high-fat appetite induced by opioid stimulation of the nucleus accumbens. *J. Neurosci.* 27, 11075–11082. doi: 10.1523/JNEUROSCI.3542-07.2007

Conflict of Interest Statement: All authors are employees of Actelion Pharmaceuticals Ltd.

Kinetic properties of "dual" orexin receptor antagonists at OX$_1$R and OX$_2$R orexin receptors

Gabrielle E. Callander[1,2], Morenike Olorunda[3], Dominique Monna[3], Edi Schuepbach[3], Daniel Langenegger[3], Claudia Betschart[4], Samuel Hintermann[4], Dirk Behnke[4], Simona Cotesta[4], Markus Fendt[3†], Grit Laue[5], Silvio Ofner[4], Emmanuelle Briard[4], Christine E. Gee[3,6], Laura H. Jacobson[3†] and Daniel Hoyer[1,2,3]*

[1] *Department of Pharmacology and Therapeutics, Faculty of Medicine, Dentistry and Health Sciences, School of Medicine, The University of Melbourne, Parkville, VIC, Australia*
[2] *The Florey Institute of Neuroscience and Mental Health, The University of Melbourne, Parkville, VIC, Australia*
[3] *Department of Neuroscience, Novartis Institutes for Biomedical Research, Basel, Switzerland*
[4] *Global Discovery Chemistry, Novartis Institutes for Biomedical Research, Basel, Switzerland*
[5] *Metabolism and Pharmacokinetics, Novartis Institutes for Biomedical Research, Basel, Switzerland*
[6] *Centre for Neurobiology Hamburg, Institute for Synaptic Physiology, Hamburg, Germany*

Edited by:
Christopher J. Winrow, Merck, USA

Reviewed by:
Anthony J. Hannan, University of Melbourne, Australia
Zoë Bichler, National Neuroscience Institute, Singapore

***Correspondence:**
Daniel Hoyer, Department of Pharmacology and Therapeutics, Faculty of Medicine, Dentistry and Health Sciences, School of Medicine, The University of Melbourne, Parkville, VIC 3010, Australia
e-mail: d.hoyer@unimelb.edu.au

†Present address:
Markus Fendt, Institute for Pharmacology and Toxicology, Otto-von-Guericke University Magdeburg, Magdeburg, Germany; Laura H. Jacobson, The Florey Institute of Neuroscience and Mental Health, The University of Melbourne, Parkville, Australia

Orexin receptor antagonists represent attractive targets for the development of drugs for the treatment of insomnia. Both efficacy and safety are crucial in clinical settings and thorough investigations of pharmacokinetics and pharmacodynamics can predict contributing factors such as duration of action and undesirable effects. To this end, we studied the interactions between various "dual" orexin receptor antagonists and the orexin receptors, OX$_1$R and OX$_2$R, over time using saturation and competition radioligand binding with [^{3}H]-BBAC ((S)-N-([1,1'-biphenyl]-2-yl)-1-(2-((1-methyl-1H-benzo[d]imidazol-2-yl)thio)acetyl)pyrrolidine-2-carboxamide). In addition, the kinetics of these compounds were investigated in cells expressing human, mouse and rat OX$_1$R and OX$_2$R using FLIPR® assays for calcium accumulation. We demonstrate that almorexant reaches equilibrium very slowly at OX$_2$R, whereas SB-649868, suvorexant, and filorexant may take hours to reach steady state at both orexin receptors. By contrast, compounds such as BBAC or the selective OX$_2$R antagonist IPSU ((2-((1H-Indol-3-yl)methyl)-9-(4-methoxypyrimidin-2-yl)-2,9-diazaspiro[5.5]undecan-1-one) bind rapidly and reach equilibrium very quickly in binding and/or functional assays. Overall, the "dual" antagonists tested here tend to be rather unselective under non-equilibrium conditions and reach equilibrium very slowly. Once equilibrium is reached, each ligand demonstrates a selectivity profile that is however, distinct from the non-equilibrium condition. The slow kinetics of the "dual" antagonists tested suggest that *in vitro* receptor occupancy may be longer lasting than would be predicted. This raises questions as to whether pharmacokinetic studies measuring plasma or brain levels of these antagonists are accurate reflections of receptor occupancy *in vivo*.

Keywords: orexin receptor antagonists, dual orexin receptor antagonists, kinetics, radioligands

INTRODUCTION

The orexin receptors, OX$_1$R and OX$_2$R, were deorphanised in 1998, when two independent teams identified the peptides orexin A and orexin B (de Lecea et al., 1998; Sakurai et al., 1998). OX$_1$R and OX$_2$R are G protein-coupled receptors that share 64% amino acid sequence identity in humans and are highly conserved between species (de Lecea et al., 1998; Sakurai et al., 1998). Both

receptors can couple to G$_q$ and mobilize intracellular Ca^{2+} via activation of phospholipase C (Sakurai et al., 1998), whilst OX$_2$R can also couple G$_i$/G$_o$ and inhibit cAMP production via inhibition of adenylate cyclase (Zhu et al., 2003). In non-neuronal cells OX$_2$R is capable of extracellular signal-regulated kinase activation via G$_s$, G$_q$, and G$_i$ (Tang et al., 2008). In competition radioligand binding OX$_1$R has a 10–100 fold higher affinity for orexin A (20 nM) than for orexin B (250 nM), whereas OX$_2$R binds both orexin peptides with similar affinity (Sakurai et al., 1998).

Orexin is exclusively expressed by orexin producing neurons within the perifornical nucleus, the dorsomedial hypothalamic nucleus, and the dorsal and lateral hypothalamic areas (Peyron et al., 1998). Orexin producing neurons are limited to a few thousand in rodents, whereas in humans there are approximately 30,000–70,000. These neurons have both ascending and descending projections with dense projections to key

Abbreviations: 5-HT, serotonin; BBAC, (S)-N-([1,1'-biphenyl]-2-yl)-1-(2-((1-methyl-1H-benzo[d]imidazol-2-yl)thio)acetyl)pyrrolidine-2-carboxamide; BSA, Bovine Serum Albumin; cAMP, cyclic AMP; CHO, Chinese Hamster Ovary; DMEM, Dulbecco's Modified Eagle's Medium; F12, Ham's F12 nutrients mixture; FDA, Federal Drug Administration of the United States Department of Health and Human Services; FLIPR®, FLuorescent Imaging Plate Reader; GABA, γ-aminobutyric acid; HEK, Human Embryonic Kidney; IPSU, 2-((1H-Indol-3-yl)methyl)-9-(4-methoxypyrimidin-2-yl)-2,9-diazaspiro[5.5]undecan-1-one; KO, Knock Out; NSB, Non-specific Binding; OX$_1$R, orexin receptor 1; OX$_2$R, orexin receptor 2; REM, Rapid Eye Movement (sleep state).

nuclei of the ascending arousal system such as the adrenergic locus coeruleus, the serotonergic dorsal raphe, and the histaminergic tuberomammillary nucleus. These same regions also receive inhibitory projections from the ventrolateral preoptic area, which promote sleep (Sherin et al., 1998).

The orexin receptors are widely distributed in the brain in a pattern consistent with orexin neuron projections (Trivedi et al., 1998; Marcus et al., 2001). Although the expression patterns of the receptors are largely overlapping, OX_1R is selectively expressed in the locus coeruleus and OX_2R is expressed in the tuberomammillary nucleus. The broad distribution of the orexin system throughout the cortex, hippocampus, thalamic, and hypothalamic nuclei suggests it may modulate a variety of functions including arousal, appetite, metabolism, reward, stress, and autonomic function (Scammell and Winrow, 2011; Gotter et al., 2012).

Although orexin was originally named for its role in feeding behavior (Sakurai et al., 1998), the link between energy homeostasis and sleep/wakefulness is increasingly recognized (Yamanaka et al., 2003) and it is clear that the orexin system is crucial for the stability of wake and sleep states (Sakurai, 2007). The orexin system was first linked to the sleep disorder narcolepsy: a mutation in the OX_2R gene was found to cause canine narcolepsy (Lin et al., 1999) and the knockout (KO) of orexin peptides in mice also resulted in narcolepsy with cataplexy (Chemelli et al., 1999). Indeed, several orexin system KO and transgenic models exhibit sleep abnormalities reminiscent of narcolepsy (Chemelli et al., 1999; Hara et al., 2001a,b; Willie et al., 2003; Beuckmann et al., 2004). The absence of orexin neurons or peptides and the double receptor KO mouse models recapitulate the human narcoleptic symptoms, with narcoleptic and cataplectic phenotypes, whereas single orexin receptor KO mice have only a moderate (OX_2R) or no sleep phenotype (OX_1R) (Chemelli et al., 1999; Scammell et al., 2000; Hara et al., 2001a,b; Beuckmann et al., 2002; Willie et al., 2003; Kalogiannis et al., 2011).

Narcolepsy with cataplexy is associated with severe daytime sleepiness (Tafti et al., 2005) due to the complete disorganization of the sleep/wake cycle, with sudden onset of Rapid Eye Movement (REM) sleep and cataplexy (loss of skeletal muscle tone without the loss of consciousness triggered by emotions). Patients with narcolepsy have undetectable levels of orexin in cerebral spinal fluid (Nishino et al., 2000) and a marked decrease in orexin producing cells in the hypothalamus (Thannickal et al., 2000). The cause of human narcolepsy is neurodegeneration of orexin-containing neurons, possibly due to an autoimmune disease (Tafti, 2007), although the precise mechanism is not established.

Not surprisingly, the orexin system has attracted substantial attention for the development of drugs for the treatment of insomnia. Dual orexin receptor antagonists or possibly selective OX_2R antagonists are likely to be effective without some of the undesirable side effects of currently available treatments. Benzodiazepines and sedative hypnotics are commonly prescribed and inhibit arousal through activation or positive allosteric modulation of the $GABA_A$ receptor. However, reported side effects include morning sedation, anxiety, anterograde

amnesia, impaired balance and sleep behaviors such as sleep walking and eating (Buysse, 2013).

A number of orexin receptor antagonists have been developed that are expected to have advantages over classic sleep promoting drugs (see Uslaner et al., 2013). These have been reported as "dual" antagonists as they have apparently similar affinities for both OX_1R and OX_2R (Roecker and Coleman, 2008; Scammell and Winrow, 2011). Almorexant was the first compound for which clinical data was reported in volunteers and patients (Brisbare-Roch et al., 2007; Malherbe et al., 2009; Owen et al., 2009) followed closely by SB-649868 (also known as GW 649868) (Bettica et al., 2009a,b, 2012a,b,c), suvorexant, the most advanced antagonist that has successfully completed phase III clinical trials (Cox et al., 2010; Winrow et al., 2011; Connor et al., 2012; Herring et al., 2012b; Ivgy-May et al., 2012) and filorexant (Coleman et al., 2012; Winrow et al., 2012). Also in this issue, we present our characterization of IPSU (Hoyer et al., 2013), an orally bioavailable, brain penetrant OX_2R antagonist, on sleep architecture in mice.

During the characterization of orexin receptor antagonists, we and others (Malherbe et al., 2010; Mang et al., 2012; Morairty et al., 2012) have noticed that almorexant has peculiar kinetic features, in particular a very slow dissociation rate constant especially at OX_2R. Such features may be clinically relevant as they influence duration of action and potential for side effects. Therefore, we performed kinetic studies on the dual orexin receptor antagonists listed above in comparison with BBAC (**Figure 1**) and/or IPSU in radioligand binding and signaling studies at both OX_1R and OX_2R.

MATERIALS AND METHODS
CHEMICALS AND REAGENTS
[^{3}H]-BBAC ((S)-N-([1,1′-biphenyl]-2-yl)-1-(2-((1-methyl-1H-benzo[d]imidazol-2-yl)thio)acetyl)pyrrolidine-2-carboxamide, Specific activity 73.76Ci/mmol) was synthesized at Novartis Pharma AG Basel (Isotope Laboratories). BBAC, SB-649868, suvorexant, filorexant, and IPSU (2-((1H-Indol-3-yl)methyl)-9-(4-methoxypyrimidin-2-yl)-2,9-diazaspiro[5.5]undecan-1-one) were synthesized at Novartis Pharma AG. Almorexant was synthesized by Anthem Biosciences (Bangalore, India).

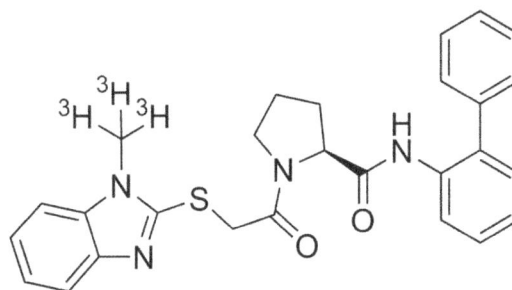

FIGURE 1 | Chemical structure of BBAC ((S)-N-([1,1′-biphenyl]-2-yl)-1-(2-((1-methyl-1H-benzo[d]imidazol-2-yl)thio)acetyl)pyrrolidine-2-carboxamide).

CELL CULTURE AND CELL MEMBRANE PREPARATION

Chinese Hamster Ovary (CHO) cells stably transfected with the cDNA encoding the human OX_1R (CHO-hOX_1) or OX_2R (CHO-hOX_2) were used (kindly provided by T. Cremer and Dr. S. Geisse, NIBR Basel, Switzerland). For measurements of calcium accumulation using FLIPR® (Fluorescent Imaging Plate Reader) assay, CHO or Human Embryonic Kidney (HEK) cells stably expressing mouse, rat or human OX_1R or OX_2R (kindly provided by Dr. A. Chen, GNF, San Diego, CA, USA) were used. All cells were cultured in 1:1 Dulbecco's Modified Eagle's Medium (DMEM)/Ham's F12 Nutrients Mixture (F12) supplemented with 10% (v/v) fetal bovine serum (FBS), $100\,\mu/ml$ ($100\,g/ml$)/streptomycin ($100\,\mu g/ml$), Fungizone ($250\,\mu g/ml$), and Geneticin (G418, $50\,mg/ml$). Cells were maintained in a humidified incubator at 37°C in 5% CO_2. For crude cell membrane preparations, cells were washed and harvested in $10\,mM$ HEPES (pH 7.5), and centrifuged at 4°C for 5 min at 2500 g. The cell pellet was either stored at $-80°C$ or used directly.

RADIOLIGAND BINDING ASSAYS

Cell membranes were resuspended in binding assay buffer at 4°C ($10\,mM$ HEPES, pH 7.5, 0.5% (w/v) bovine serum albumin (BSA), $5\,mM$ $MgCl_2$, $1\,mM$ $CaCl_2$, and 0.05% Tween 20) and homogenized with a Polytron homogenizer at 50 Hz for 20 s. Cells were incubated with [^3H]-BBAC in binding assay buffer in 96-deep well plates (Fisher Scientific). Aliquots of [^3H]-BBAC were measured using liquid scintillation spectrometry on a LS 6500 scintillation counter (Beckman Coulter) to determine the amount radioactivity added to each well. Non-specific Binding (NSB) was determined in the presence of $1\,\mu M$ almorexant. After the indicated incubation time, bound and free radioligand were separated by vacuum filtration using a Filtermate™ Cell Harvester (Perkin Elmer) and filtered onto 96-well deep GF/b filter plates (Millipore) which had been pre-treated with 0.5% (w/v) polyethyleneimine. Filter plates were rapidly washed three times with wash buffer ($10\,mM$ Tris-HCl, $154\,mM$ NaCl, pH 7.4) at 4°C, dried and $25\,\mu l$ of Microscint™ (Perkin Elmer) was added to each well. Radioactivity was quantified using a TopCount™ microplate counter (Perkin Elmer).

SATURATION BINDING

Binding was performed with eight concentrations of [^3H]-BBAC ($50\,\mu l$, 1–20 nM) to construct saturation curves. CHO-hOX_1 or CHO-hOX_2 cell membranes ($150\,\mu l$/well) were incubated for 60 min in 96-deep well plates at room temperature with radioligand in binding assay buffer ($50\,\mu l$) in the presence or absence of almorexant ($1\,\mu M$, $50\,\mu l$), in a final volume of $250\,\mu l$. [^3H]-BBAC binding was measured in triplicate in at least three independent experiments. Data in the figures is representative of the mean $\pm$ s.e.m. of a single experiment.

COMPETITION BINDING

Competition experiments were performed with a single concentration of radioligand and six concentrations of competitor (unlabeled ligands; BBAC, almorexant, SB-649868, suvorexant, filorexant or IPSU). 4.6 nM [^3H]-BBAC (chosen from saturation experiments to provide 80–90% specific binding, $50\,\mu l$) was added simultaneously with various concentrations of unlabeled ligand (0.1 nM–10 μM) to membranes ($150\,\mu l$/well) in $50\,\mu l$/well of assay buffer with a total volume of $250\,\mu l$/well. The amount of [^3H]-BBAC bound to receptors was determined at room temperature at different time points (ranging from 15 min to 4 h) and terminated by rapid vacuum filtration and liquid scintillation counting. Binding at a given concentration of competitor at a given time was measured in triplicate in at least three independent experiments. Data in figures is representative of the mean $\pm$ s.e.m. of a single experiment.

DATA ANALYSIS

All data was analyzed using GraphPad Prism 4.0 (GraphPad, San Diego, USA). The saturation data was fit to a non-linear regression model for saturation binding with consideration for one site binding. In addition, saturation binding data was also analyzed according to Scatchard (Scatchard, 1949; plots not shown). Competition binding data was fit to a non-linear regression model for competition binding with consideration for variable one site binding with a non-fixed Hill slope. The method of Cheng and Prusoff (1973) was used to convert IC_{50} values from competition binding curves to Ki (equilibrium dissociation constant) values.

FUNCTIONAL ANALYSIS OF DUAL ANTAGONISTS ON HUMAN OREXIN RECEPTORS

Determination of orexin A-stimulated calcium accumulation was performed over 2 days using FLIPR® (Fluorescent imaging plate reader from Molecular Devices-FLIPR384). Cells expressing either human, rat or mouse OX_1R or OX_2R were seeded at 8,000 cells/well in black 384 well clear bottom plates and incubated overnight at 37°C. The following day, medium was discarded and cells loaded with $50\,\mu l$ of $1\,mM$ Fluo-4 AM (Invitrogen F14202) in dimethyl sulfoxide in working buffer (Hanks' balanced salt solution, $10\,mM$ HEPES) and incubated for 60 min at 37°C. The loading buffer was removed and cells were washed with $100\,\mu l$ working buffer containing $200\,mM$ $CaCl_2$, 0.1% BSA, and $2.5\,mM$ Probenecid (pH 7.4) to remove the excess Fluo-4 AM. Working buffer was added and plates were incubated 10–15 min at room temperature. The assay plate was then transferred to the Molecular Devices-FLIPR384. The baseline calcium signal was recorded for 10 s, then the antagonist of interest was injected ($10\,\mu l$ at 3 times the final concentration) and the calcium signal recorded every second for 1 min, then every 2 s 40 times. Plates were then incubated at room temperature for 30 min, 1, 2, or 4 h. Calcium signals were again measured as above, this time orexin A ($15\,\mu l$) was injected at 3 times the final concentration. For each experiment, full orexin A concentration response curves were generated on each plate: they served to calculate the EC_{50} for that plate and to adapt the EC_{80} values in the subsequent experiments, which vary according to cell line and passage number.

The concentration response curves were analyzed according to the law of mass action, for both orexin A (EC_{50}), and antagonists (IC_{50}) with slope factors and maximal/minimal effects; the antagonist data was transformed according to Cheng and Prusoff (1973) ($K_i = IC_{50}/1 = (L/EC_{50})$) where L is the agonist concentration used in the assay and EC_{50} its concentration for half maximal activation and the antagonist data was finally expressed as K_i (nM) and pK_i values ($-\log$ M).

RESULTS

TIME-DEPENDENT CHANGES IN APPARENT AFFINITY AS DETERMINED IN RADIOLIGAND BINDING

[³H]-BBAC bound both OX_1R and OX_2R with high affinity and K_D values of about 7 nM and 1 nM, respectively (**Figure 2**). Binding reached equilibrium very quickly, as 15–30 min incubation time was sufficient to reach B_{max} and K_D values comparable to those measured after 4 h (data not shown).

Competition experiments were performed with the various antagonists at 15, 30, 45 min, 1, 2, or 4 h and the graphs illustrate the competition curves at the different times. As expected from the saturation experiments described above, as well as in further kinetic experiments to be reported elsewhere, BBAC reached equilibrium quickly at both OX_1R and OX_2R (15–30 min), and there was no significant difference in IC_{50} values measured between 30 min and 4 h, as illustrated by superimposable competition curves at both orexin receptors (**Figure 3**).

In contrast to BBAC, the competition curves for almorexant shifted to the left with time moderately at OX_1R and substantially at OX_2R (**Figure 4**). In other words, almorexant showed similar apparent affinity at OX_1R between 30 min and 4 h, whereas

the apparent affinity at OX_2R increased up to 4 h of incubation. The data suggests that equilibrium at OX_2R can only be reached after prolonged incubation, which also means that under short term conditions, almorexant is a dual orexin receptor antagonist, whereas after several hours of exposure, the compound becomes somewhat OX_2R selective.

The SB-649868 competition curves on OX_1R shifted to the left over time up to 4 h, whereas at OX_2R binding appeared to be rather stable (**Figure 5**), suggesting that the compound equilibrated very rapidly at OX_2R whereas it took hours to equilibrate at OX_1R. This means that although acting as a dual antagonist acutely, given sufficient time to equilibrate, SB-649868 will show some OX_1R selectivity.

Similarly, the suvorexant competition curves for both OX_1R and OX_2R shifted to the left over time, although the effect on OX_2R was somewhat less pronounced (**Figure 6**). Thus, suvorexant equilibrates slowly at both orexin receptors and since equilibrium is generally driven by the dissociation rate constant, this means that once steady state binding is reached, receptor occupancy will be long lasting.

The filorexant competition curves at OX_1R were rather insensitive to incubation time, whereas OX_2R curves shifted to the left over time, even up to 4 h (**Figure 7**). Thus, similar to the other dual orexin receptor antagonists tested here, filorexant reaches equilibrium only after several hours of incubation, especially at OX_2R.

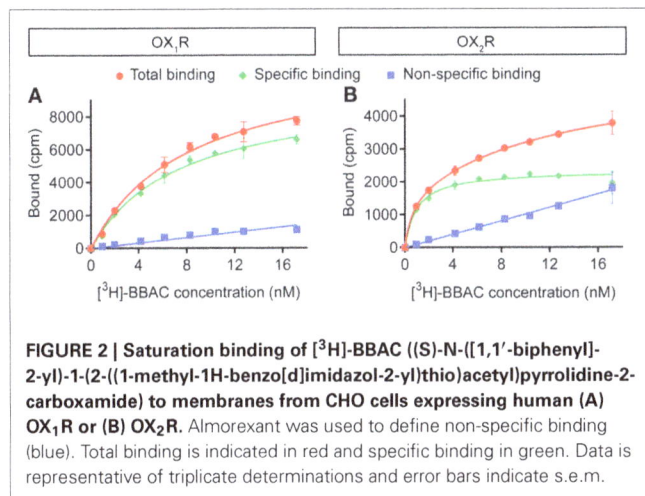

FIGURE 2 | Saturation binding of [³H]-BBAC ((S)-N-([1,1'-biphenyl]-2-yl)-1-(2-((1-methyl-1H-benzo[d]imidazol-2-yl)thio)acetyl)pyrrolidine-2-carboxamide) to membranes from CHO cells expressing human (A) OX₁R or (B) OX₂R. Almorexant was used to define non-specific binding (blue). Total binding is indicated in red and specific binding in green. Data is representative of triplicate determinations and error bars indicate s.e.m.

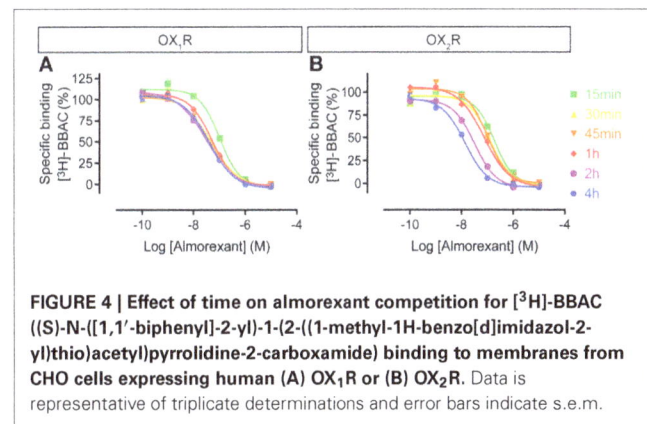

FIGURE 4 | Effect of time on almorexant competition for [³H]-BBAC ((S)-N-([1,1'-biphenyl]-2-yl)-1-(2-((1-methyl-1H-benzo[d]imidazol-2-yl)thio)acetyl)pyrrolidine-2-carboxamide) binding to membranes from CHO cells expressing human (A) OX₁R or (B) OX₂R. Data is representative of triplicate determinations and error bars indicate s.e.m.

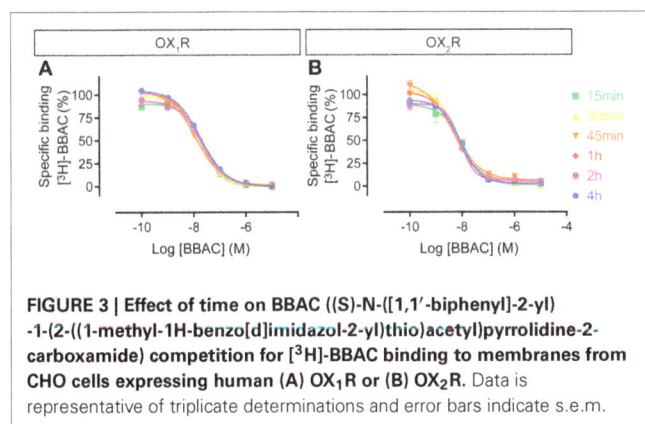

FIGURE 3 | Effect of time on BBAC ((S)-N-([1,1'-biphenyl]-2-yl)-1-(2-((1-methyl-1H-benzo[d]imidazol-2-yl)thio)acetyl)pyrrolidine-2-carboxamide) competition for [³H]-BBAC binding to membranes from CHO cells expressing human (A) OX₁R or (B) OX₂R. Data is representative of triplicate determinations and error bars indicate s.e.m.

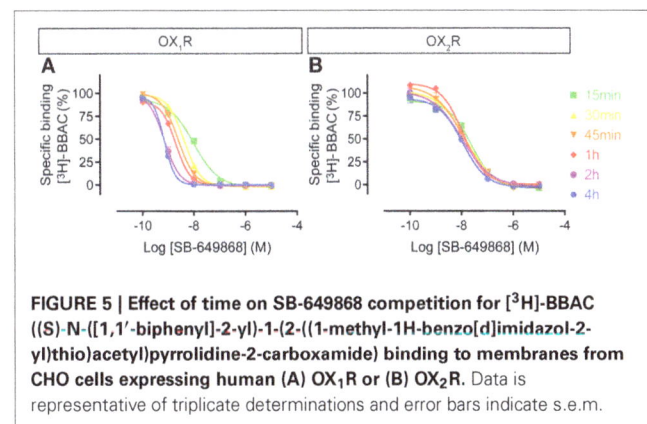

FIGURE 5 | Effect of time on SB-649868 competition for [³H]-BBAC ((S)-N-([1,1'-biphenyl]-2-yl)-1-(2-((1-methyl-1H-benzo[d]imidazol-2-yl)thio)acetyl)pyrrolidine-2-carboxamide) binding to membranes from CHO cells expressing human (A) OX₁R or (B) OX₂R. Data is representative of triplicate determinations and error bars indicate s.e.m.

The IPSU competition curves at OX_1R and OX_2R do not show time-dependency (**Figure 8**), since maximal inhibition was already achieved following 15 min of incubation. This suggests a very rapid binding and equilibrium and a tendency to a rightward shift, suggesting faster kinetics than for the radioligand.

TIME-DEPENDENT CHANGES IN APPARENT AFFINITY AS DETERMINED IN CALCIUM ASSAYS

In the calcium accumulation assays performed at mouse, rat and human OX_1R and OX_2R, we first confirmed that orexin A produces stable results and that the apparent potency is largely

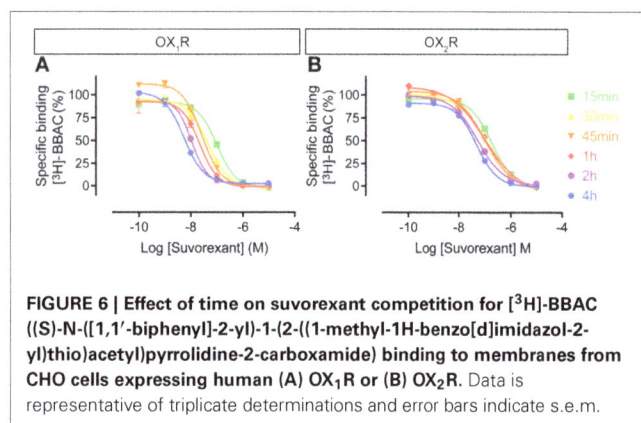

FIGURE 6 | Effect of time on suvorexant competition for [3H]-BBAC ((S)-N-([1,1′-biphenyl]-2-yl)-1-(2-((1-methyl-1H-benzo[d]imidazol-2-yl)thio)acetyl)pyrrolidine-2-carboxamide) binding to membranes from CHO cells expressing human (A) OX_1R or (B) OX_2R. Data is representative of triplicate determinations and error bars indicate s.e.m.

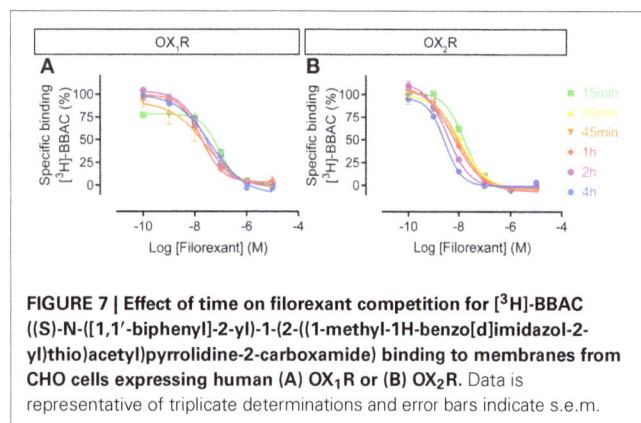

FIGURE 7 | Effect of time on filorexant competition for [3H]-BBAC ((S)-N-([1,1′-biphenyl]-2-yl)-1-(2-((1-methyl-1H-benzo[d]imidazol-2-yl)thio)acetyl)pyrrolidine-2-carboxamide) binding to membranes from CHO cells expressing human (A) OX_1R or (B) OX_2R. Data is representative of triplicate determinations and error bars indicate s.e.m.

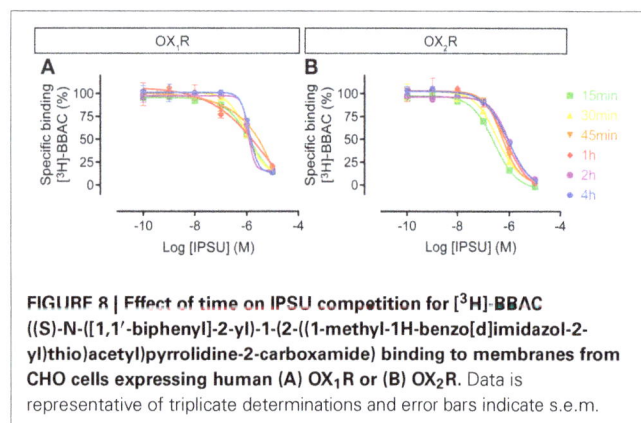

FIGURE 8 | Effect of time on IPSU competition for [3H]-BBAC ((S)-N-([1,1′-biphenyl]-2-yl)-1-(2-((1-methyl-1H-benzo[d]imidazol-2-yl)thio)acetyl)pyrrolidine-2-carboxamide) binding to membranes from CHO cells expressing human (A) OX_1R or (B) OX_2R. Data is representative of triplicate determinations and error bars indicate s.e.m.

comparable when the effects of antagonists are measured following incubation times of between 30 min and 4 h. Indeed, pEC_{50} values for orexin were largely time-independent at both OX_1R and OX_2R. This suggests the cells and receptors used were stable and would allow incubation times of up to 4 h in the subsequent experiments (**Tables 1**, **2**). At OX_1R, almorexant had an apparent antagonist potency which was constant, irrespective of the incubation time (30 min–4 h, **Table 1**). By contrast, at OX_2R, the apparent potency kept increasing with incubation time (**Table 2**), as suggested by the radioligand binding experiments. These results indicate that across the three species studied here there is an apparent OX_2R selectivity after longer incubation times. Filorexant showed time-independent potencies at OX_1R, whereas at OX_2R the apparent potencies increased with time. Suvorexant showed a time-dependent shift toward higher potency as time increased at both receptors, although the effects were more pronounced at OX_2R. For SB-649868, antagonism at both receptors tended to increase with time, although the increase was greater at OX_1R.

DISCUSSION

A thorough exploration of the pharmacokinetics and pharmacodynamics of drug candidates is important in drug development. Ideal sleep-enabling compounds have distinct profiles: rapid absorption and induction of sleep, low blood drug concentrations 8 h after dosing and efficacy in the absence of side effects (Wilson et al., 2010). Understanding the nuances of the kinetics of binding, such as the time taken to reach binding equilibrium, can provide valuable predictive information on duration of action and explain efficacy in patients.

With this in mind we sought to characterize the kinetic features of various "dual" orexin receptor antagonists at OX_1R and OX_2R. We selected antagonists that have either been used clinically or are currently under development for the treatment of insomnia and sleep disorders, including almorexant, SB-649868, suvorexant, and filorexant. We compared the kinetic features of these compounds with those of BBAC (a fast binding dual orexin receptor antagonist that was also used as a radioligand in the present studies) and IPSU, an OX_2R antagonist (see Betschart et al., 2013; Hoyer et al., 2013). Our results show clearly that each of the ligands tested has different properties at both OX_1R and OX_2R, especially with respect to kinetics and suggest that at steady state each of these compounds has a pharmacological profile different from that measured under non-equilibrium conditions.

We observed that the radioligand [3H]-BBAC binds with high affinity, rapidly and reversibly to both OX_1R and OX_2R. In competition assays, unlabeled BBAC was a fast dual receptor binder, as illustrated by competition curves which are virtually superimposable irrespective of receptor type or incubation time. The slight shift to the right as time increased indicates the concentration dependence of the association rate, since the concentrations of unlabeled ligand used in the competition experiments (**Figure 3**; up to 10 μM) are higher than those used for the radioligand (low nM). This suggests unlabeled BBAC reaches apparent equilibrium faster than [3H]-BBAC.

For the dual orexin receptor antagonists tested, time-dependent changes in the apparent affinities for the receptors

Table 1 | Ca^{2+} signaling in cells stably transfected with human (CHO), rat (HEK) or mouse (HEK) OX$_1$R in the presence of the endogenous agonist (orexin A) or putative dual orexin receptor antagonists (almorexant, filorexant, suvorexant, SB-649868, and IPSU).

| | OX$_1$R | | | | | | | | | | | |
| | 30 min | | | 1 h | | | 2 h | | | 4 h | | |
	pKi	s.e.m.	n	pKi	s.e.m.	n	pKi	s.e.m.	n	pKi	s.e.m.	n
HUMAN												
Orexin A	9.52	0.10	3	9.48	0.01	541	9.51	0.07	3	9.63	0.10	3
Almorexant	7.84	0.05	6	7.73	0.06	26	7.75	0.07	6	7.75	0.07	6
Filorexant	8.65	0.09	6	8.79	0.08	12	8.78	0.11	6	8.55	0.06	6
Suvorexant	8.39	0.09	6	8.74	0.10	8	8.75	0.12	6	8.73	0.15	6
SB-649868	9.03	0.05	6	8.87	0.09	12	9.29	0.08	6	9.38	0.10	6
IPSU	6.32	0.08	6	6.29	0.05	6	6.28	0.09	6	6.14	0.08	6
RAT												
Orexin A	8.92	0.08	3	9.01	0.09	3	9.01	0.05	3	8.86	0.09	3
Almorexant	7.90	0.06	6	7.90	0.07	6	7.95	0.08	6	7.76	0.08	6
Filorexant	9.12	0.13	6	9.21	0.18	6	9.30	0.17	6	8.92	0.18	6
Suvorexant	8.82	0.20	6	9.40	0.36	6	9.37	0.19	6	9.24	0.17	6
SB-649868	9.59	0.11	6	9.90	0.19	6	10.17	0.10	6	10.14	0.06	6
IPSU	6.65	0.05	6	6.62	0.06	6	6.56	0.13	6	6.25	0.06	6
MOUSE												
Orexin A	9.17	0.14	3	9.18	0.04	31	9.36	0.15	3	9.25	0.14	3
Almorexant	7.73	0.05	6	7.63	0.10	10	7.47	0.07	6	7.41	0.11	4
Filorexant	8.28	0.10	6	8.39	0.14	9	8.18	0.08	6	8.23	0.08	6
Suvorexant	8.90	0.14	6	8.98	0.18	4	9.03	0.08	6	8.99	0.08	6
SB-649868	9.80	0.12	6	9.37	0.14	7	10.39	0.16	6	10.33	0.17	6
IPSU	6.48	0.04	6	6.31	0.12	4	6.54	0.06	6	6.49	0.06	6

were found. The affinity of SB-649868 at hOX$_1$R increased markedly between 15 min and 4 h, whilst time had little effect on the affinity at hOX$_2$R (**Figure 5**). The opposite is true for almorexant, which displayed a leftward shift at hOX$_1$R and a very pronounced increase in affinity at hOX$_2$R as incubation time increased (**Figure 4**). Thus, SB-649868 and almorexant are slowly equilibrating antagonists, presumably because their dissociation rates are very slow. The data also suggests that when equilibrium is allowed to be reached, SB-649868 becomes somewhat hOX$_1$R selective, whereas almorexant becomes hOX$_2$R selective. The suvorexant competition curves demonstrated both hOX$_1$R and hOX$_2$R have increasing affinity with time, although the effect on hOX$_2$R was somewhat less pronounced (**Figure 6**). Filorexant shows somewhat different properties, in that equilibrium was slow to be reached at hOX$_2$R. By contrast, time had almost no effect on the affinity of both BBAC and IPSU as measured in the binding experiments. That is, the apparent affinity values measured at 15 min of incubation were at least as high as those measured after 4 h, an indication that they reach steady state at either receptor within a few minutes.

The time-dependent binding translated into differences in the more functional FLIPR® calcium assay in whole cells expressing human, rat, or mouse OX$_1$ and OX$_2$ receptors. Almorexant acted as a pseudo-irreversible or very slowly equilibrating antagonist at human, rat or mouse OX$_2$R, whereas, at OX$_1$R for all three species, almorexant behaved as a fast equilibrating antagonist. This data suggests that although originally described as a dual

antagonist with very similar affinity for both receptors, almorexant is in fact a slowly equilibrating and somewhat selective OX$_2$R antagonist, if sufficient time is given for the ligand to reach equilibrium. Similar findings were made in the calcium experiments with suvorexant, SB-649868 and filorexant, indicating that all display slow equilibration at one and/or the other orexin receptor (see **Tables 1, 2**). By contrast, IPSU (and BBAC) had constant potency values irrespective of the incubation time, again suggesting very fast equilibration at both orexin receptors. On the basis of both the radioligand binding and calcium accumulation data presented here, almorexant is likely to be OX$_2$R selective, a finding that is in agreement with other reports that found almorexant to behave as a dual antagonist only during short incubation times (Malherbe et al., 2009; Mang et al., 2012; Morairty et al., 2012). In addition, we demonstrate in contrast to almorexant, SB-649868, suvorexant, and filorexant have a greater affinity for OX$_1$R with long incubation times.

The differences in binding kinetics between the orexin receptor antagonists demonstrated here are likely to have implications for pharmacodynamics. Suvorexant is a pertinent example: studies of pharmacokinetics revealed a long dose-dependent apparent terminal half-life (between 9 and 12 h, Merck Sharp and Dohme Corporation, 2013a) and next morning residual effects (Sun et al., 2013). It is possible that these residual effects are not only related to half-life, but also longer than expected target/exposure engagement. In addition, the suggestion that suvorexant has a tendency to accumulate after 4 weeks of consecutive treatment is

Table 2 | Ca^{2+} signaling in cells stably transfected with human (CHO), rat (HEK) or mouse (HEK) OX$_2$R in the presence of the endogenous agonist (orexin A) or putative dual orexin receptor antagonists (almorexant, filorexant, suvorexant, SB-649868, and IPSU).

| | OX$_2$R | | | | | | | | | | | |
| | 30 min | | | 1 h | | | 2 h | | | 4 h | | |
	pKi	s.e.m.	n	pKi	s.e.m.	n	pKi	s.e.m.	n	pKi	s.e.m.	n
HUMAN												
Orexin A	8.76	0.05	3	8.79	0.01	548	8.61	0.07	3	8.70	0.02	3
Almorexant	8.33	0.05	6	8.82	0.06	29	8.80	0.15	6	9.09	0.22	6
Filorexant	9.45	0.09	6	9.65	0.06	11	9.73	0.10	6	9.77	0.09	6
Suvorexant	9.00	0.14	6	9.48	0.14	8	9.46	0.19	6	9.53	0.20	6
SB-649868	9.52	0.05	6	9.43	0.09	15	9.77	0.03	6	9.82	0.05	6
IPSU	8.00	0.10	6	7.97	0.07	6	7.82	0.08	6	7.68	0.11	6
RAT												
Orexin A	8.40	0.01	3	8.34	0.07	6	8.48	0.06	3	8.58	0.03	3
Almorexant	8.25	0.08	6	8.65	0.06	6	8.99	0.19	6	9.18	0.10	6
Filorexant	9.13	0.11	6	9.38	0.08	6	9.60	0.11	6	9.75	0.10	6
Suvorexant	8.71	0.19	6	9.06	0.18	6	9.22	0.20	6	9.37	0.22	6
SB-649868	9.34	0.06	6	9.50	0.05	6	9.81	0.07	6	9.85	0.05	6
IPSU	7.63	0.14	6	7.55	0.11	6	7.62	0.12	6	7.55	0.11	6
MOUSE												
Orexin A	8.78	0.07	3	9.05	0.02	53	8.94	0.01	3	9.18	0.02	3
Almorexant	7.72	0.06	5	8.03	0.05	14	8.09	0.05	6	8.38	0.05	6
Filorexant	8.67	0.13	6	8.68	0.06	9	8.84	0.10	6	8.89	0.11	6
Suvorexant	7.99	0.11	6	8.17	0.14	4	8.24	0.11	6	8.35	0.08	6
SB-649868	8.74	0.07	6	8.55	0.08	7	8.93	0.06	6	9.04	0.04	6
IPSU	7.15	0.04	6	7.10	0.09	4	7.26	0.06	6	7.22	0.07	6

not surprising (Farkas, 2013) given 24 h following administration of a single dose, mean plasma levels of suvorexant remain between 0.1 and 0.6 μM (Sun et al., 2013). These results may be explained by a combination of pharmacokinetic effects (slow elimination or metabolism) and pharmacodynamic effects (slow equilibration and off rates), as shown in the present studies.

The Food and Drug Administration (FDA, USA) have concluded that although suvorexant is efficacious, it is not considered safe at doses higher than 20 mg (Farkas, 2013). The key safety concerns raised were rapid onset daytime somnolence, motor impairment, driving impairment, unconscious night time activity such as sleep walking, suicidal ideation, hypnogogic hallucinations and effects resembling mild cataplexy (Farkas, 2013; Radl, 2013; Sun et al., 2013). All of these appeared to be dose and plasma-exposure dependent. In addition, the FDA suggested an effort to find the lowest effective dose may be warranted (Farkas, 2013). Merck has determined that additional clinical studies are not necessary for the 10 mg dose, however, may be required to support a 5 mg dose (Farkas, 2013; Merck Sharp and Dohme Corporation, 2013b).

The individual contribution of orexin receptors to sleep architecture is a matter of debate since, to our knowledge, no selective OX$_1$R or OX$_2$R antagonist has been tested in patients with insomnia. However, rodent models are rather good predictors of the effects of orexin receptor antagonists on sleep. In rodents, OX$_2$R antagonism appears sufficient to induce sleep: almorexant is effective in the OX$_1$R KO whereas it has no effect on the sleep wake cycle in OX$_2$R or in double receptor KO mice (Mang et al., 2012). Further, in rodents with targeted destruction of the orexin neurons of the lateral hypothalamus, treatment with almorexant tends to induce cataplexy (Black et al., 2013). Nevertheless, there are major differences relating to pharmacokinetics and pharmacodynamics between species. One should also keep in mind that whilst narcoleptic/cataplectic dogs have a defect in OX$_2$R, this has never been observed in humans.

In addition to almorexant, SB-649868 and suvorexant have reached phase II clinical trials for the treatment of insomnia. Clinical data suggests that the main effect on total sleep time is largely due to an increase in REM sleep and decreased latency to REM, with modest effects on non-REM or slow wave sleep, if at all (Bettica et al., 2012a,c; Herring et al., 2012a,b; Hoever et al., 2012). In the case of SB-649868, there is strong evidence of sleep onset REM in patients receiving the 60 mg dose (Bettica et al., 2012a). Whilst no clinical evidence exists for filorexant, recent rodent studies demonstrated the filorexant analog, DORA-22, promotes sleep with dose-dependent increases in REM sleep (Fox et al., 2013), suggesting that the mechanism may also be the same for this compound.

Overall, the clinical data appears to confirm the preclinical data collected in mice or rats which demonstrates dual orexin receptor antagonists or dual receptor KOs induce sleep with a very strong REM component, whereas OX$_2$R KO or antagonism has more balanced sleep phenotypes (Willie et al., 2003; Mang et al., 2012; Betschart et al., 2013; Hoyer et al., 2013). Therefore, one may consider OX_1R antagonism to be detrimental and suggest that compounds such as suvorexant and SB-649868, which show very slow kinetics at the OX_1R, are likely to favor REM over non-REM. For SB-649868, clinical studies in healthy volunteers (Bettica et al., 2012b) and insomnia patients (Bettica et al., 2012c) demonstrate that 10, 30, or 60 mg SB-649868 decreases latency to REM and increases REM duration. In a 4 week placebo-controlled study of suvorexant in patients with insomnia, Herring and colleagues observed that increases in total sleep time were mainly due to increased time spent in REM sleep (Herring et al., 2012b). Such compounds may also increase rapid transitions between wake and REM states, especially if the compound is given a relatively long time before bed, as was the case with SB-649868 (90 min, Bettica et al., 2009a, 2012b).

Still, kinetics are of primary importance in sleep and an appropriate balance must be reached for therapeutic efficacy and safety. If target occupancy is too short, the patient will wake up in the middle of the night as happened with early formulations of Z drugs such as zolpidem and zaleplon (Besset et al., 1995; Roth et al., 1995; Greenblatt et al., 1998). Conversely, if target occupancy is too long, there will be "hangover" effects into the next morning, a crucial issue with benzodiazepine hypnotics (Wilson et al., 2010). For compounds that have slow receptor kinetics, pharmacodynamics and pharmacokinetics may not run in parallel, complicating their further development. The current report suggests that all four established "dual" antagonists have very slow kinetics, leading to changes in actual selectivity if equilibrium can be reached *in vivo*; in addition, if equilibrium is reached, slow off rates may result in longer receptor occupancy than may be predicted solely from the pharmacokinetic data.

AUTHOR CONTRIBUTIONS

Gabrielle E. Callander prepared the data for publication and wrote the manuscript. Morenike Olorunda, Dominique Monna, Edi Schuepbach, and Daniel Langenegger have carried out the experiments, contributed to the development of the assays and performed some of the data analysis. Claudia Betschart and Samuel Hintermann have synthesized a number of compounds and led the chemistry efforts and contributed to writing. Emmanuelle Briard contributed to the synthesis of a number of radioligands used in these studies. Dirk Behnke, Simona Cotesta, Grit Laue, and Silvio Ofner have synthesized other compounds and/or have performed a number of analyses in relation to pharmacokinetics. Christine E. Gee, Markus Fendt, and Laura H. Jacobson have performed *in vivo* experiments that led to the concepts developed here and have participated in discussion and writing. Daniel Hoyer has led the team, conceptualized the experimental approach and data interpretation and finalized the writing.

ACKNOWLEDGMENTS

The authors would like to thank T. Cremer and Dr. S. Geisse, (NIBR Basel, Switzerland) and Dr. A. Chen, (GNF, San Diego, CA, USA) for providing cells and cell membranes expressing orexin receptors.

REFERENCES

Besset, A., Tafti, M., Villemin, E., Borderies, P., and Billiard, M. (1995). Effects of zolpidem on the architecture and cyclical structure of sleep in poor sleepers. *Drugs Exp. Clin. Res.* 21, 161–169.

Betschart, C., Hintermann, S., Behnke, D., Cotesta, S., Fendt, M., Gee, C. E., et al. (2013). Identification of a novel series of orexin receptor antagonists with a distinct effect on sleep architecture for the treatment of insomnia. *J. Med. Chem.* 56, 7590–7607. doi: 10.1021/jm4007627

Bettica, P., Nucci, G., Pyke, C., Squassante, L., Zamuner, S., Ratti, E., et al. (2012a). Phase I studies on the safety, tolerability, pharmacokinetics and pharmacodynamics of SB-649868, a novel dual orexin receptor antagonist. *J. Psychopharmacol.* 26, 1058–1070. doi: 10.1177/0269881111408954

Bettica, P., Squassante, L., Groeger, J. A., Gennery, B., Winsky-Sommerer, R., and Dijk, D. J. (2012b). Differential effects of a dual orexin receptor antagonist (SB-649868) and zolpidem on sleep initiation and consolidation, SWS, REM Sleep, and EEG power spectra in a model of situational insomnia. *Neuropsychopharmacology* 37, 1224–1233. doi: 10.1038/npp.2011.310

Bettica, P., Squassante, L., Zamuner, S., Nucci, G., Danker-Hopfe, H., and Ratti, E. (2012c). The orexin antagonist SB-649868 promotes and maintains sleep in men with primary insomnia. *Sleep* 35, 1097–1104. doi: 10.5665/sleep.1996

Bettica, P. U., Lichtenfeld, U., Squassante, L., Shabbir, S., Zuechner, D., Dreykluft, P., et al. (2009a). The orexin antagonist SB-649868 promotes and maintains sleep in healthy volunteers and in patients with primary insomnia. *Sleep* 32, A252–A253.

Bettica, P. U., Squassante, L., Groeger, J. A., Gennery, B., and Dijk, D. (2009b). Hypnotic effects of SB-649868, an orexin antagonist, and zolpidem in a model of situational insomnia. *Sleep* 32, A40.

Beuckmann, C. T., Sinton, C. M., Williams, S. C., Richardson, J. A., Hammer, R. E., Sakurai, T., et al. (2004). Expression of a poly-glutamine-ataxin-3 transgene in orexin neurons induces narcolepsy-cataplexy in the rat. *J. Neurosci.* 24, 4469–4477. doi: 10.1523/jneurosci.5560-03.2004

Beuckmann, C. T., Willie, J. T., Hara, J., Yamanaka, A., Sakurai, T., and Yanagisawa, M. (2002). Orexin neuron-ablated mice fail to increase vigilance and locomotor activity in response to fasting. *Sleep* 25, A353–A354.

Black, S. W., Morairty, S. R., Fisher, S. P., Chen, T. M., Warrier, D. R., and Kilduff, T. S. (2013). Almorexant promotes sleep and exacerbates cataplexy in a murine model of narcolepsy. *Sleep* 36, 325–336. doi: 10.5665/sleep.2442

Brisbare-Roch, C., Dingemanse, J., Koberstein, R., Hoever, P., Aissaoui, H., Flores, S., et al. (2007). Promotion of sleep by targeting the orexin system in rats, dogs and humans. *Nat. Med.* 13, 150–155. doi: 10.1038/nm1544

Buysse, D. J. (2013). Insomnia. *J. Am. Med. Assoc.* 309, 706–716. doi: 10.1001/jama.2013.193

Chemelli, R. M., Willie, J. T., Sinton, C. M., Elmquist, J. K., Scammell, T., Lee, C., et al. (1999). Narcolepsy in orexin knockout mice: molecular genetics of sleep regulation. *Cell* 98, 437–451. doi: 10.1016/s0092-8674(00)81973-x

Cheng, Y., and Prusoff, W. H. (1973). Relationship between the inhibition constant (K1) and the concentration of inhibitor which causes 50 per cent inhibition (I50) of an enzymatic reaction. *Biochem. Pharmacol.* 22, 3099–3108.

Coleman, P. J., Schreier, J. D., Cox, C. D., Breslin, M. J., Whitman, D. B., Bogusky, M. J., et al. (2012). Discovery of (2R,5R)-5-{(5-Fluoropyridin-2-yl)oxy methyl}-2-methylpiperidin-1-yl 5 -methyl-2-(pyrimidin-2-yl)phenyl methanone (MK-6096): a dual orexin receptor antagonist with potent sleep-promoting properties. *ChemMedChem* 7, 415–424. doi: 10.1002/cmdc.201200025

Connor, K., Budd, K., Snavely, D., Liu, K., Hutzel-Mann, J., Benca, R., et al. (2012). Efficacy and safety of suvorexant, an orexin receptor antagonist, in patients with primary insomnia: a 3-month phase 3 trial (trial #1). *J. Sleep Res.* 21, 97.

Cox, C. D., Breslin, M. J., Whitman, D. B., Schreier, J. D., McGaughey, G. B., Bogusky, M. J., et al. (2010). Discovery of the dual orexin receptor antagonist (7R)-4-(5-Chloro-1,3-benzoxazol-2-yl)-7-methyl-1,4-diazepan-1-yl 5-methyl-2-(2H-1,2,3-triazol-2-yl)phenyl methanone (MK-4305) for the treatment of Insomnia. *J. Med. Chem.* 53, 5320–5332. doi: 10.1021/jm100541c

de Lecea, L., Kilduff, T. S., Peyron, C., Gao, X. B., Foye, P. E., Danielson, P. E., et al. (1998). The hypocretins: hypothalamus-specific peptides with neuroexcitatory activity. *Proc. Natl. Acad. Sci. U.S.A.* 95, 322–327. doi: 10.1073/pnas.95.1.322

Farkas, R. (2013). *Suvorexant Safety and Efficacy* [Online]. www.fda.gov: U.S. Food and Drug Administration. Available online at: http://www.fda.gov/downloads/AdvisoryCommittees/CommitteesMeetingMaterials/Drugs/PeripheralandCentralNervousSystemDrugsAdvisoryCommittee/UCM354215.pdf (Accessed on May 08, 2013).

Fox, S. V., Gotter, A. L., Tye, S. J., Garson, S. L., Savitz, A. T., Uslaner, J. M., et al. (2013). Quantitative electroencephalography within sleep/wake states differentiates GABA_A modulators eszopiclone and zolpidem from dual orexin receptor antagonists in rats. *Neuropsychopharmacology* 38, 2401–2408. doi: 10.1038/npp.2013.139

Gotter, A. L., Roecker, A. J., Hargreaves, R., Coleman, P. J., Winrow, C. J., and Renger, J. J. (2012). "Orexin receptors as therapeutic drug targets," in *Orexin/Hypocretin System*, ed A. Shekhar (Amsterdam: Elsevier Science Bv), 163–188.

Greenblatt, D. J., Harmatz, J. S., von Moltke, L. L., Ehrenberg, B. L., Harrel, L., Corbett, K., et al. (1998). Comparative kinetics and dynamics of zaleplon, zolpidem, and placebo. *Clin. Pharmacol. Ther.* 64, 553–561. doi: 10.1016/S0009-9236(98)90139-4

Hara, J., Beuckmann, C. T., Nambu, T., Willie, J. T., Chemelli, R. M., Sinton, C. M., et al. (2001a). Genetic ablation of orexin neurons in mice results in narcolepsy, hypophagia, and obesity. *Neuron* 30, 345–354. doi: 10.1016/s0896-6273(01)00293-8

Hara, J., Nambu, T., Beuckmann, C. T., Goto, K., Yanagisawa, M., and Sakurai, T. (2001b). Genetic ablation of orexin neurons in mice: a mouse model of narcolepsy. *Sleep* 24, A156.

Herring, W. J., Snyder, E., Budd, K., Hutzelmann, J., Snavely, D., Liu, K., et al. (2012a). Orexin receptor antagonism for treatment of insomnia a randomized clinical trial of suvorexant. *Neurology* 79, 2265–2274. doi: 10.1212/WNL.0b013e31827688ee

Herring, W. J., Snyder, E., Paradis, E., Hutzelmann, J., Liu, M. C., Snavely, D., et al. (2012b). Suvorexant, an orexin receptor antagonist, in preventing symptom return in patients with insomnia after 1 year of treatment: a randomised, double-blind, placebo-controlled study. *J. Sleep Res.* 21, 351–351.

Hoever, P., de Haas, S., Dorffner, G., Chiossi, E., van Gerven, J., and Dingemanse, J. (2012). Orexin receptor antagonism: an ascending multiple-dose study with almorexant. *J. Psychopharmacol.* 26, 1071–1080. doi: 10.1177/0269881112448946

Hoyer, D., Dürst, T., Fendt, M., Jacobson, L. H., Betschart, C., Hintermann, S., et al. (2013). Distinct effects of IPSU and suvorexant on mouse sleep architecture. *Front. Neurosci.* 7:235. doi: 10.3389/fnins.2013.00235

Ivgy-May, N., Leibensperger, H., Froman, S., Hutzelmann, J., Snavely, D., Snyder, E., et al. (2012). Efficacy and safety of suvorexant, an orexin receptor antagonist, in patients with primary insomnia: a 3-month phase 3 trial (trial #2). *J. Sleep Res.* 21, 351–352.

Kalogiannis, M., Hsu, E., Willie, J. T., Chemelli, R. M., Kisanuki, Y. Y., Yanagisawa, M., et al. (2011). Cholinergic modulation of narcoleptic attacks in double orexin receptor knockout mice. *PLoS ONE* 6:e18697. doi: 10.1371/journal.pone.0018697

Lin, L., Faraco, J., Li, R., Kadotani, H., Rogers, W., Lin, X. Y., et al. (1999). The sleep disorder canine narcolepsy is caused by a mutation in the hypocretin (orexin) receptor 2 gene. *Cell* 98, 365–376. doi: 10.1016/s0092-8674(00)81965-0

Malherbe, P., Borroni, E., Pinard, E., Wettstein, J. G., and Knoflach, F. (2009). biochemical and electrophysiological characterization of almorexant, a dual orexin 1 receptor (OX(1))/orexin 2 receptor (OX(2)) antagonist: comparison with selective OX(1) and OX(2) antagonists. *Mol. Pharmacol.* 76, 618–631. doi: 10.1124/mol.109.055152

Malherbe, P., Roche, O., Marcuz, A., Kratzeisen, C., Wettstein, J. G., and Bissantz, C. (2010). Mapping the binding pocket of dual antagonist almorexant to human orexin 1 and orexin 2 receptors: comparison with the selective OX1 antagonist SB-674042 and the selective OX2 antagonist N-ethyl-2- (6-methoxy-pyridin-3-yl)-(toluene-2-sulfonyl)-amino -N-pyridi n-3-ylmethyl-acetamide (EMPA). *Mol. Pharmacol.* 78, 81–93. doi: 10.1124/mol.110.064584

Mang, G. M., Durst, T., Burki, H., Imobersteg, S., Abramowski, D., Schuepbach, E., et al. (2012). The dual orexin receptor antagonist almorexant induces sleep and decreases orexin-induced locomotion by blocking orexin 2 receptors. *Sleep* 35, 1625–1635. doi: 10.5665/sleep.2232

Marcus, J. N., Aschkenasi, C. J., Lee, C. E., Chemelli, R. M., Saper, C. B., Yanagisawa, M., et al. (2001). Differential expression of orexin receptors 1 and 2 in the rat brain. *J. Comp. Neurol.* 435, 6–25. doi: 10.1002/cne.1190.

Merck Sharp and Dohme Corporation. (2013a). *Suvorexant Advisory Committee Briefing Document*. Available online at: http://www.fda.gov/downloads/AdvisoryCommittees/CommitteesMeetingMaterials/Drugs/PeripheralandCentralNervousSystemDrugsAdvisoryCommittee/UCM352970.pdf

Merck Sharp and Dohme Corporation. (2013b). *Merck Receives Complete Response Letter for Suvorexant, Merck's Investigational Medicine for Insomnia*. Available online at: http://www.mercknewsroom.com/press-release/research-and-development-news/merck-receives-complete-response-letter-suvorexant-merck.

Morairty, S. R., Revel, F. G., Malherbe, P., Moreau, J. L., Valladao, D., Wettstein, J. G., et al. (2012). Dual hypocretin receptor antagonism is more effective for sleep promotion than antagonism of either receptor alone. *PLoS ONE* 7:e39131. doi: 10.1371/journal.pone.0039131

Nishino, S., Ripley, B., Overeem, S., Lammers, G. J., and Mignot, E. (2000). Hypocretin (orexin) deficiency in human narcolepsy. *Lancet* 355, 39–40. doi: 10.1016/s0140-6736(99)05582-8

Owen, R. T., Castaner, R., Bolos, J., and Estivill, C. (2009). Almorexant dual orexin OX1/OX2 antagonist treatment of sleep disorders. *Drugs Future* 34, 5–10. doi: 10.1358/dof.2009.034.01.1324392

Peyron, C., Tighe, D. K., van den Pol, A. N., de Lecea, L., Heller, H. C., Sutcliffe, J. G., et al. (1998). Neurons containing hypocretin (orexin) project to multiple neuronal systems. *J. Neurosci.* 18, 9996–10015.

Radl, S. (2013). SUVOREXANT dual orexin OX1/OX2 receptor antagonist treatment of sleep disorders. *Drugs Future* 38, 27–36. doi: 10.1358/dof.2013.38.1.1906425

Roecker, A. J., and Coleman, P. J. (2008). Orexin receptor antagonists: medicinal chemistry and therapeutic potential. *Curr. Top. Med. Chem.* 8, 977–987. doi: 10.2174/156802608784936746

Roth, T., Roehrs, T., and Vogel, G. (1995). Zolpidem in the treatment of transient insomnia: a double-blind, randomized comparison with placebo. *Sleep* 18, 246–251.

Sakurai, T. (2007). The neural circuit of orexin (hypocretin): maintaining sleep and wakefulness. *Nat. Rev. Neurosci.* 8, 171–181. doi: 10.1038/nrn2092

Sakurai, T., Amemiya, A., Ishii, M., Matsuzaki, I., Chemelli, R. M., Tanaka, H., et al. (1998). Orexins and orexin receptors: a family of hypothalamic neuropeptides and G protein-coupled receptors that regulate feeding behavior. *Cell* 92, 573–585. doi: 10.1016/s0092-8674(00)80949-6

Scammell, T. E., Estabrooke, I. V., McCarthy, M. T., Chemelli, R. M., Yanagisawa, M., Miller, M. S., et al. (2000). Hypothalamic arousal regions are activated during modafinil-induced wakefulness. *J. Neurosci.* 20, 8620–8628.

Scammell, T. E., and Winrow, C. J. (2011). Orexin receptors: pharmacology and therapeutic opportunities. *Annu. Rev. Pharmacol. Toxicol.* 51, 243–266. doi: 10.1146/annurev-pharmtox-010510-100528

Scatchard, G. (1949). The attractions of proteins for small molecules and ions. *Ann. N.Y. Acad. Sci.* 51, 660–672. doi: 10.1111/j.1749-6632.1949.tb27297.x

Sherin, J. E., Elmquist, J. K., Torrealba, F., and Saper, C. B. (1998). Innervation of histaminergic tuberomammillary neurons by GABAergic and galaninergic neurons in the ventrolateral preoptic nucleus of the rat. *J. Neurosci.* 18, 4705–4721.

Sun, H., Kennedy, W. P., Wilbraham, D., Lewis, N., Calder, N., Li, X. D., et al. (2013). Effects of suvorexant, an orexin receptor antagonist, on sleep parameters as measured by polysomnography in healthy men. *Sleep* 36, 259–267. doi: 10.5665/sleep.2386

Tafti, M. (2007). Reply to 'Promotion of sleep by targeting the orexin system in rats, dogs and humans'. *Nat. Med.* 13, 525–526. doi: 10.1038/nm0507-525

Tafti, M., Maret, S., and Dauvilliers, Y. (2005). Genes for normal sleep and sleep disorders. *Ann. Med.* 37, 580–589. doi: 10.1080/07853890500372047

Tang, J., Chen, J., Ramanjaneya, M., Punn, A., Conner, A. C., and Randeva, H. S. (2008). The signalling profile of recombinant human orexin-2 receptor. *Cell. Signal.* 20, 1651–1661. doi: 10.1016/j.cellsig.2008.05.010

Thannickal, T. C., Moore, R. Y., Nienhuis, R., Ramanathan, L., Gulyani, S., Aldrich, M., et al. (2000). Reduced number of hypocretin neurons in human narcolepsy. *Neuron* 27, 469–474. doi: 10.1016/s0896-6273(00)00058-1

Trivedi, P., Yu, H., MacNeil, D. J., Van der Ploeg, L. H. T., and Guan, X. M. (1998). Distribution of orexin receptor mRNA in the rat brain. *FEBS Lett.* 438, 71–75. doi: 10.1016/s0014-5793(98)01266-6

Uslaner, J. M., Tye, S. J., Eddins, D. M., Wang, X., Fox, S. V., Savitz, A. T., et al. (2013). Orexin receptor antagonists differ from standard sleep drugs by promoting sleep at doses that do not disrupt cognition. *Sci. Transl. Med.* 5, 179ra144. doi: 10.1126/scitranslmed.3005213

Willie, J. T., Chemelli, R. M., Sinston, C. M., Tokita, H., Williams, S. C., Kisanuki, Y. Y., et al. (2003). Distinct narcolepsy syndromes in Orexin receptor-2 and Orexin null mice: molecular genetic dissection of non-REM and REM sleep regulatory processes. *Neuron* 38, 715–730. doi: 10.1016/s0896-6273(03)00330-1

Wilson, S. J., Nutt, D. J., Alford, C., Argyropoulos, S. V., Baldwin, D. S., Bateson, A. N., et al. (2010). British Association for Psychopharmacology consensus statement on evidence-based treatment of insomnia, parasomnias and circadian rhythm disorders. *J. Psychopharmacol.* 24, 1577–1601. doi: 10.1177/0269881110379307

Winrow, C. J., Gotter, A. L., Cox, C. D., Doran, S. M., Tannenbaum, P. L., Breslin, M. J., et al. (2011). Promotion of sleep by suvorexant–a novel dual orexin receptor antagonist. *J. Neurogenet.* 25, 52–61. doi: 10.3109/01677063.2011.566953

Winrow, C. J., Gotter, A. L., Cox, C. D., Tannenbaum, P. L., Garson, S. L., Doran, S. M., et al. (2012). Pharmacological characterization of MK-6096-A dual orexin receptor antagonist for insomnia. *Neuropharmacology* 62, 978–987. doi: 10.1016/j.neuropharm.2011.10.003

Yamanaka, A., Beuckmann, C. T., Willie, J. T., Hara, J., Tsujino, N., Mieda, M., et al. (2003). Hypothalamic orexin neurons regulate arousal according to energy balance in mice. *Neuron* 38, 701–713. doi: 10.1016/s0896-6273(03)00331-3

Zhu, Y., Miwa, Y., Yamanaka, A., Yada, T., Shibahara, M., Abe, Y., et al. (2003). Orexin receptor type-1 couples exclusively to pertussis toxin-insensitive G-proteins, while orexin receptor type-2 couples to both pertussis toxin-sensitive and -insensitive G-proteins. *J. Pharmacol. Sci.* 92, 259–266. doi: 10.1254/jphs.92.259

Conflict of Interest Statement: With the exception of Gabrielle E. Callander, the authors are either past or present Novartis employees, or have been supported by Novartis.

14

Cannabinoid-hypocretin cross-talk in the central nervous system: what we know so far

África Flores, Rafael Maldonado and Fernando Berrendero*

Laboratory of Neuropharmacology, Department of Experimental and Health Sciences, Universitat Pompeu Fabra, Barcelona, Spain

Edited by:
Christopher J. Winrow, Merck, USA

Reviewed by:
Thomas Heinbockel, Howard University College of Medicine, USA
Regina A. Mangieri, The University of Texas at Austin, USA

*Correspondence:
Fernando Berrendero, Laboratory of Neuropharmacology, Department of Experimental and Health Sciences, Universitat Pompeu Fabra, PRBB, C/ Doctor Aiguader 88, 08003 Barcelona, Spain
e-mail: fernando.berrendero@upf.edu

Emerging findings suggest the existence of a cross-talk between hypocretinergic and endocannabinoid systems. Although few studies have examined this relationship, the apparent overlap observed in the neuroanatomical distribution of both systems as well as their putative functions strongly point to the existence of such cross-modulation. In agreement, biochemical and functional studies have revealed the existence of heterodimers between CB1 cannabinoid receptor and hypocretin receptor-1, which modulates the cellular localization and downstream signaling of both receptors. Moreover, the activation of hypocretin receptor-1 stimulates the synthesis of 2-arachidonoyl glycerol culminating in the retrograde inhibition of neighboring cells and suggesting that endocannabinoids could contribute to some hypocretin effects. Pharmacological data indicate that endocannabinoids and hypocretins might have common physiological functions in the regulation of appetite, reward and analgesia. In contrast, these neuromodulatory systems seem to play antagonistic roles in the regulation of sleep/wake cycle and anxiety-like responses. The present review attempts to piece together what is known about this interesting interaction and describes its potential therapeutic implications.

Keywords: hypocretinergic system, endocannabinoid system, heteromerization, reward, energy balance, antinociception, sleep/wake cycle

ENDOCANNABINOIDS AND HYPOCRETINS: TWO ESSENTIAL NEUROMODULATORS

The extracts of the plant *Cannabis sativa* contain about 60 active compounds of which Δ^9-tetrahydrocannabinol (THC) is the main psychoactive component (Hall and Degenhardt, 2009). Although it was initially believed that THC exerted its effects by interacting with the plasma membrane due to its high lipophilic nature (Martin, 1986), the site of action of this substance is an endogenous neuromodulatory system termed endogenous cannabinoid system. The endocannabinoid system is constituted by membrane receptors, their fatty-acid derived endogenous ligands and the enzymatic machinery that synthesizes and degrades these lipidic neurotransmitters.

At least two different cannabinoid receptors have been cloned, termed CB1 and CB2 receptors, which share only 44% amino acid (AA) sequence homology (Matsuda et al., 1990; Munro et al., 1993). The distribution of CB1 and CB2 is markedly different: CB1 is the most abundant G-protein coupled receptor (GPCR) in the central nervous system (CNS) (Herkenham et al., 1990), while CB2 is mainly found in immune cells and peripheral tissues (Munro et al., 1993), although some CB2 expression is detected in the brainstem, cortex and cerebellar neurons and microglia (Núñez et al., 2004; Van Sickle et al., 2005). In addition, cannabinoid compounds are able to activate other "non-CB" receptors, such as GPR55, peroxisome proliferator-activated receptors (PPARs), and vanilloid type TRP channels (Pertwee et al., 2010; Kukkonen, 2011).

Endocannabinoids are arachidonic acid-containing messengers generated by phospholipase action, produced on demand at the site of need and are not usually stored in vesicles like classical neurotransmitters (Di Marzo, 2009). The most important endocannabinoids identified are N-arachidonylethanolamine (anandamide) and 2-arachidonylglycerol (2-AG) (Devane et al., 1992; Sugiura et al., 1995), although other ligands such as noladin ether and virodhamide have also been detected (Hanus et al., 2001; Porter et al., 2002). Endocannabinoids are known to act as retrograde regulators of synaptic transmission. Thus, after being synthesized in postsynaptic neurons in response to a depolarization-induced increase in intracellular Ca^{2+}, and released to act on CB1 expressed in presynaptic and/or nearby neurons, endocannabinoids attenuate presynaptic depolarization and subsequent neurotransmitter release (Kano et al., 2009). After synthesis and release, endocannabinoid signaling is terminated by reuptake into both neurons and glia followed by intracellular hydrolysis of anandamide and 2-AG, carried out by fatty acid amide hydrolase (FAAH) and monoacylglycerol lipase (MAGL), respectively (Muccioli, 2010).

It has been extensively reported that the endocannabinoid system reciprocally modulates other neurotransmitter systems. The interaction with the endogenous opioid system is the most explored of these cross-talks (Robledo et al., 2008; Parolaro et al., 2010), but pharmacological and biochemical data also reveal an interplay at both molecular and functional levels with other neurotransmitters, such as the dopaminergic and adenosinergic systems (Carriba et al., 2007; Ferré et al., 2009; Fernández-Ruiz et al., 2010). Interestingly, emerging evidence points to a cross-modulation between endocannabinoid and hypocretinergic systems, providing a new range of potential therapeutic applications to currently existing drugs targeting these systems.

Hypocretin-1/orexin-A and hypocretin-2/orexin-B are two neuropeptides proteolytically cleaved from the same precursor, prepro-hypocretin/prepro-orexin (de Lecea et al., 1998; Sakurai et al., 1998). Hypocretin-1 is constituted by 33 AA and post-translationally stabilized by two intrachain disulphide bonds, whereas hypocretin-2 consists of 28 AA and remains as a linear peptide (Sakurai et al., 1998). As other neuromodulatory peptides, hypocretins are stored at the axon terminals within secretory vesicles, which release their content in a Ca^{2+}-dependent manner (de Lecea et al., 1998). In contrast to endocannabinoids, hypocretins act mainly as neuroexcitatory modulators. Hypocretins induce neuroexcitation at both pre- and postsynaptic levels: activation of presynaptic Ca^{2+} channels facilitates neurotransmitter release (van den Pol et al., 1998; Li et al., 2002), and regulation of diverse postsynaptic ion channels leads to postsynaptic depolarization (Kukkonen et al., 2002). However, few studies also report hypocretin-induced synaptic inhibition, although the mechanisms underlying this effect remain unclear (Davis et al., 2003; Ma et al., 2007).

So far, two hypocretin receptors with 64% AA sequence homology have been identified: hypocretin or orexin receptor-1 (HcrtR1/OxR1) and hypocretin or orexin receptor-2 (HcrtR2/OxR2) (Sakurai et al., 1998). HcrtR1 displays a 10-fold higher affinity for hypocretin-1 than hypocretin-2, whereas HcrtR2 has equal affinity for both peptides (Smart et al., 2001; Ammoun et al., 2003). Hypocretin-expressing neurons are located exclusively in the hypothalamus, especially in the lateral (LH), perifornical (PFA), and dorsomedial areas (DMH) (de Lecea et al., 1998; Peyron et al., 1998; Sakurai et al., 1998). Despite representing a relatively small population of cells, hypocretinergic neurons send projections widely through the entire neuroaxis of the CNS (Peyron et al., 1998), suggesting that hypocretins modulate the activity of multiple neurotransmitter systems and therefore regulate diverse physiological functions.

COMMON CHARACTERISTICS BETWEEN ENDOCANNABINOID AND HYPOCRETINERGIC SYSTEMS

Anatomical studies have found that CB1 and HcrtRs show an overlapping distribution in several areas of the CNS (Hervieu et al., 2001; Marcus et al., 2001; Mackie, 2005), suggesting a common role in some physiological functions (**Figure 1**). Thus, HcrtR1 and HcrtR2, as well as CB1, are widely expressed within the entire hypothalamus, denoting an important function of these systems in energy homeostasis and central regulation of neuroendocrine and autonomic functions (Wittmann et al., 2007; Tsujino and Sakurai, 2009). Both receptors are also found in diverse areas of the mesocorticolimbic system, such as the ventral tegmental area (VTA), the nucleus accumbens (NAc), the prefrontal cortex (PFC), the septal nuclei and the amygdaloid nuclei, supporting the regulation of natural reward and addiction processes by endocannabinoid and hypocretinergic systems

(Maldonado et al., 2006; Aston-Jones et al., 2010; Plaza-Zabala et al., 2012). The presence of CB1, HcrtR1, and HcrtR2 within diverse brainstem nuclei, including the raphe nuclei, the locus coeruleus, the reticular formation and the periaqueductal gray (PAG), is in agreement with the role of these neuromodulators with the regulation of anxiety-like responses, sleep/wake cycle and nociception (Eriksson et al., 2010; Häring et al., 2012; Wilson-Poe et al., 2012). Nevertheless, the existence of cross-reactivity problems with HcrtR antibodies has hindered the precise location of these receptors (Kukkonen, 2012). Hence, although specific CB1 expression among different neuronal populations has been well characterized (Mackie, 2005), the location of HcrtRs is certainly known only at the level of brain structure since it has been confirmed by *in situ* hybridization studies (Hervieu et al., 2001). As a consequence, direct synaptic connections between CB1 and HcrtRs are not well defined. On the other hand, recent studies have detected certain multifocal expression of CB2 in the brain at levels much lower than those of CB1 receptors (Gong et al., 2006; Onaivi et al., 2006). Among these CB2 expression foci, hippocampus, amygdala and PAG are potentially the most relevant areas to the study of the cannabinoid-hypocretinergic interplay.

CB1 and CB2, as well as HcrtR1 and HcrtR2, belong to the rhodopsin subfamily of GPCR superfamily. The cellular signals triggered upon cannabinoid receptor activation differ from those initiated following the stimulation of hypocretin receptor. However, it seems that diverse signaling pathways are common for cannabinoid and hypocretin receptors (Demuth and Molleman, 2006) (**Figure 2**). Both CB1 and CB2 receptors are associated with the Gi/o family of G-proteins, as most cannabinoid effects are blocked by pertussis toxin (PTX) (Howlett et al., 1986; Slipetz et al., 1995). Subsequent functional inhibition of adenylyl cyclase (AC) activity and decreased cAMP production has been observed in most tissues and cells investigated (Howlett et al., 2002). However, CB1 has been shown to stimulate AC when Gi protein is hardly available, such as under PTX treatment or sequestering by other GPCR receptor activation, indicating that CB1 may be able to couple Gs under these particular experimental conditions (Glass and Felder, 1997; Jarrahian et al., 2004). The modulation of voltage-dependent ion channels by CB1 activation is thought to underlie the cannabinoid-induced inhibition of neurotransmitter release, although it seems that CB1-independent mechanisms of ion channel modulation might also exist (Demuth and Molleman, 2006). CB1 activates inward-rectifying K^+ (Kir) and A-type K^+ channels, triggering the plasmatic membrane repolarization (Deadwyler et al., 1995; Vásquez et al., 2003). This was shown to be mediated by CB1 receptor-mediated reduction in cAMP levels and PKA activation (Deadwyler et al., 1995; Hampson et al., 1995). Additionally, CB1 inhibits N-, P/Q- and L-type voltage-gated Ca^{2+} channels, leading to a decrease in Ca^{2+} influx, mostly by direct Gβγ interaction with the channel (Howlett et al., 2002). CB1 and CB2 activation also leads to the phosphorylation and activation of the MAP kinase cascade (Bouaboula et al., 1995, 1997; Derkinderen et al., 2001), which regulates neuronal gene expression and synaptic plasticity. Diverse transduction pathways leading to activation of different MAP kinases (ERK1/2, JNK, ERK5, and p38) have been proposed, depending on the cell type and the stimulus. MAP kinase activation is mediated

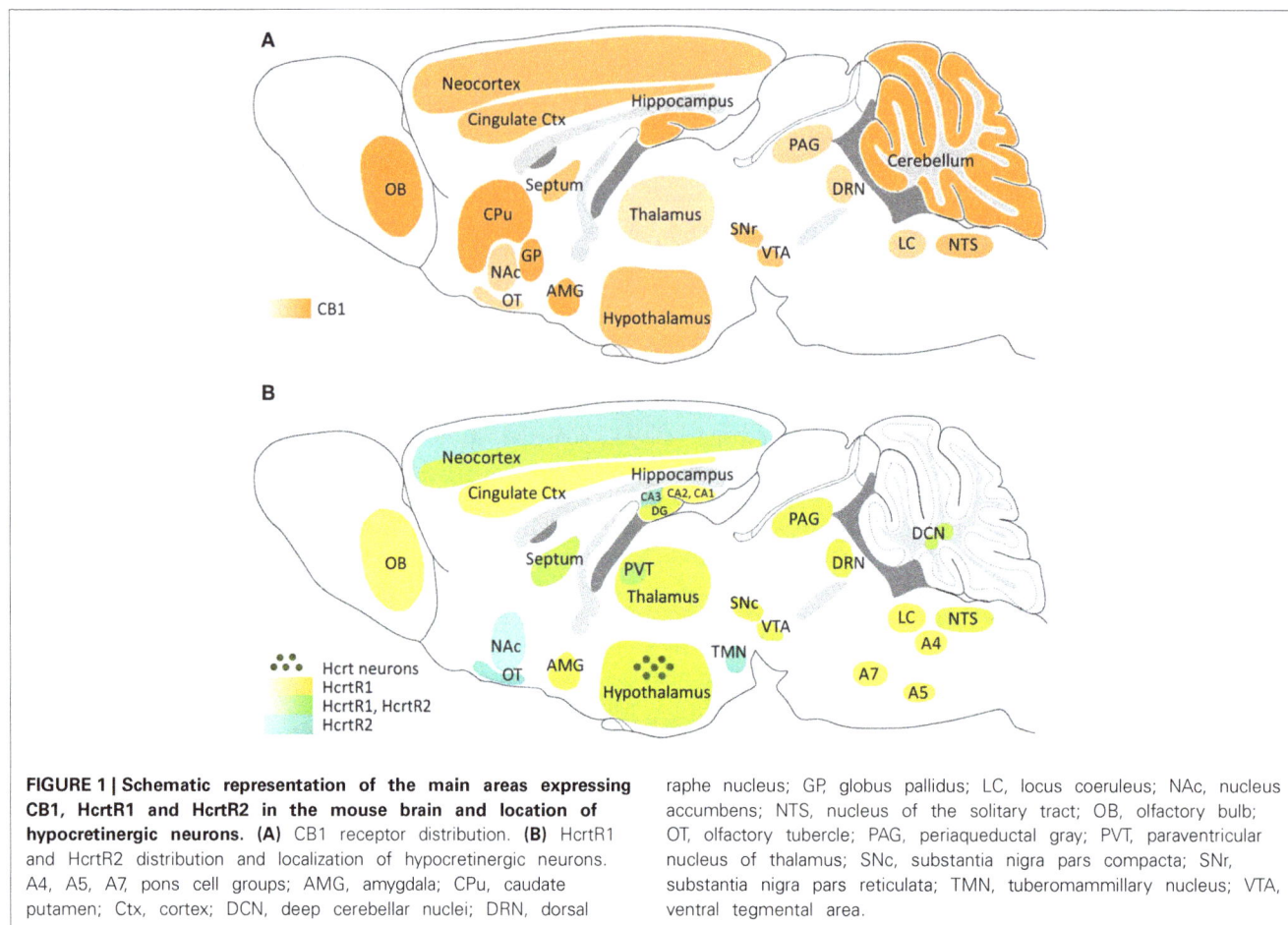

FIGURE 1 | Schematic representation of the main areas expressing CB1, HcrtR1 and HcrtR2 in the mouse brain and location of hypocretinergic neurons. (A) CB1 receptor distribution. **(B)** HcrtR1 and HcrtR2 distribution and localization of hypocretinergic neurons. A4, A5, A7, pons cell groups; AMG, amygdala; CPu, caudate putamen; Ctx, cortex; DCN, deep cerebellar nuclei; DRN, dorsal raphe nucleus; GP, globus pallidus; LC, locus coeruleus; NAc, nucleus accumbens; NTS, nucleus of the solitary tract; OB, olfactory bulb; OT, olfactory tubercle; PAG, periaqueductal gray; PVT, paraventricular nucleus of thalamus; SNc, substantia nigra pars compacta; SNr, substantia nigra pars reticulata; TMN, tuberomammillary nucleus; VTA, ventral tegmental area.

by PI3K pathway in CHO cells (Galve-Roperh et al., 2002), PC-3 cells (Sánchez et al., 2003) and astrocytoma cells (Gómez del Pulgar et al., 2000), through the protein kinase B (PKB/Akt) phosphorylation and Raf-1 activation. Some studies also suggest that decrease in cAMP levels, and consequently reduced inhibitory c-Raf phosphorylation by PKA activity, may participate in the stimulatory effects of CB1 activation on the MAP kinase pathway (Melck et al., 1999; Davis et al., 2003).

On the other hand, both hypocretin receptors are coupled to Gq proteins, which induce the activation of PLC and production of the second messengers DAG and IP3 from PIP2. This triggers the activation of PKC, which phosphorylates and modulates effector ion channels leading to Ca^{2+} entrance (van den Pol et al., 1998; Eriksson et al., 2001), as well as further IP3-mediated entry via store-operated Ca^{2+} channels (Kukkonen and Akerman, 2001; Larsson et al., 2005). In addition, membrane depolarization is facilitated by activation of Na^+/Ca^{2+} exchanger (Burdakov et al., 2003), increase of non-selective cation channel conductances (Liu et al., 2002; Yang and Ferguson, 2002; Murai and Akaike, 2005) and/or blockade of Kir channels (Hwang et al., 2001; Yang and Ferguson, 2003; Ishibashi et al., 2005). It remains to be further elucidated by using selective antagonists the identification of the receptor subtype mediating these effects. Additionally, some studies of lipid signaling pathways activated by HcrtR1-expressing CHO cells have also revealed coupling to PLD

and PLA2 (Turunen et al., 2012). Besides, stimulation of both hypocretin receptors has been suggested to modulate AC activity by coupling other G-proteins, such as Gs-protein as shown by AC activation and cAMP production in neurons (Gorojankina et al., 2007) and astrocytes (Woldan-Tambor et al., 2011), or Gi-protein as observed by hypocretin-1 inhibition of AC via Gi-coupling (Holmqvist et al., 2005; Urbańska et al., 2012). Similar to cannabinoids, hypocretin signaling also activates the MAP kinase pathway. Thus, HcrtR1 challenge leads to ERK1/2 and p38 kinase phosphorylation (Ammoun et al., 2006a). Downstream effectors contributing to ERK1/2 activation after HcrtR1 stimulation include at least Ca^{2+} influx, PLC/PKC, Ras, Src, and PI3K (Ammoun et al., 2006b). Similar results have been recorded in an HcrtR2 expression system (Tang et al., 2008). Thus, cannabinoid and hypocretinergic signaling differ in their modulation of ion channel currents and AC activity, while they converge in the activation of the MAP kinase pathway.

MOLECULAR INTERACTIONS BETWEEN CB1 AND HcrtR1

Direct CB1-HcrtR1 interaction was first proposed in 2003 (Hilairet et al., 2003). Indeed, a 100 fold increase in the potency of hypocretin-1 to activate the ERK signaling was observed when CB1 and HcrtR1 were co-expressed in CHO cells. This effect required a functional CB1 receptor as evidenced by the blockade of hypocretin response by the CB1 antagonist rimonabant,

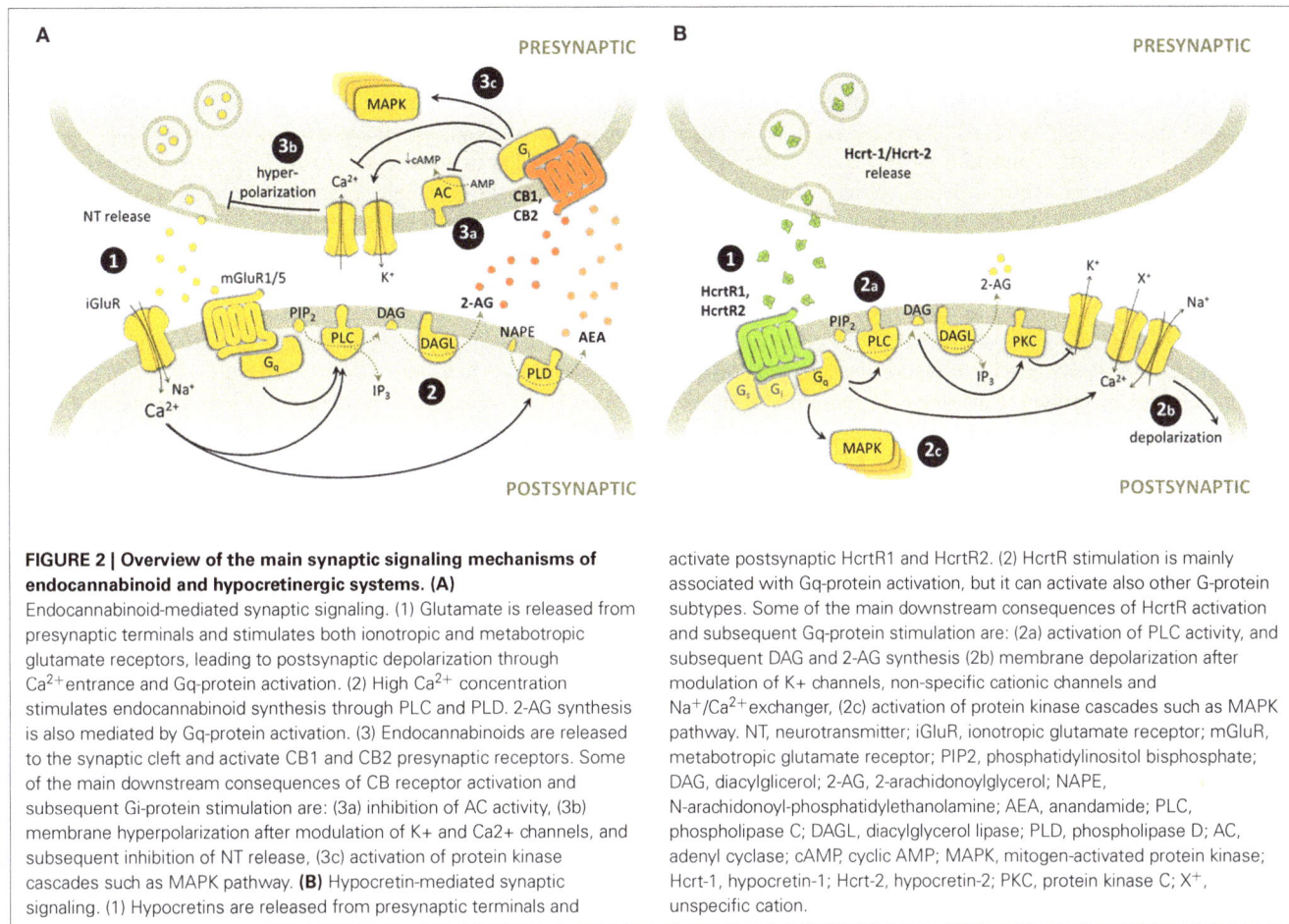

FIGURE 2 | Overview of the main synaptic signaling mechanisms of endocannabinoid and hypocretinergic systems. (A) Endocannabinoid-mediated synaptic signaling. (1) Glutamate is released from presynaptic terminals and stimulates both ionotropic and metabotropic glutamate receptors, leading to postsynaptic depolarization through Ca^{2+} entrance and Gq-protein activation. (2) High Ca^{2+} concentration stimulates endocannabinoid synthesis through PLC and PLD. 2-AG synthesis is also mediated by Gq-protein activation. (3) Endocannabinoids are released to the synaptic cleft and activate CB1 and CB2 presynaptic receptors. Some of the main downstream consequences of CB receptor activation and subsequent Gi-protein stimulation are: (3a) inhibition of AC activity, (3b) membrane hyperpolarization after modulation of K+ and Ca2+ channels, and subsequent inhibition of NT release, (3c) activation of protein kinase cascades such as MAPK pathway. **(B)** Hypocretin-mediated synaptic signaling. (1) Hypocretins are released from presynaptic terminals and activate postsynaptic HcrtR1 and HcrtR2. (2) HcrtR stimulation is mainly associated with Gq-protein activation, but it can activate also other G-protein subtypes. Some of the main downstream consequences of HcrtR activation and subsequent Gq-protein stimulation are: (2a) activation of PLC activity, and subsequent DAG and 2-AG synthesis (2b) membrane depolarization after modulation of K+ channels, non-specific cationic channels and Na^+/Ca^{2+} exchanger, (2c) activation of protein kinase cascades such as MAPK pathway. NT, neurotransmitter; iGluR, ionotropic glutamate receptor; mGluR, metabotropic glutamate receptor; PIP2, phosphatidylinositol bisphosphate; DAG, diacylglicerol; 2-AG, 2-arachidonoylglycerol; NAPE, N-arachidonoyl-phosphatidylethanolamine; AEA, anandamide; PLC, phospholipase C; DAGL, diacylglycerol lipase; PLD, phospholipase D; AC, adenyl cyclase; cAMP, cyclic AMP; MAPK, mitogen-activated protein kinase; Hcrt-1, hypocretin-1; Hcrt-2, hypocretin-2; PKC, protein kinase C; X^+, unspecific cation.

and was blocked by PTX, suggesting a Gi-mediated potentiation. Based on electron microscopy colocalization, the authors inferred the formation of heteromeric complexes by HcrtR1 and CB1 that might explain the enhancement in hypocretin-induced ERK signaling (Hilairet et al., 2003). Importantly, in these colocalization studies specificity problems with anti-HcrtR1 antibodies were avoided by tagging the N-terminus of HcrtR1 with the c-Myc epitope, monitoring its expression using mouse monoclonal anti-Myc antibodies. The possible existence of CB1-HcrtR1 heteromerization has been further assessed by co-expressing these GPCRs in HEK293 cells (Ellis et al., 2006). In this study, rimonabant caused a decrease in the potency of hypocretin-1 to activate the MAP kinases ERK1/2 in cells co-expressing both receptors. Similarly, the HcrtR1 antagonist SB674042 reduced in these cells the potency of the CB1 agonist WIN55,212-2 to phosphorylate ERK1/2. Additionally, co-expression of CB1 and HcrtR1 resulted in coordinated trafficking of these GPCRs. Indeed, following inducible expression in HEK293 cells, HcrtR1 was mainly located in the cell surface, while CB1 constitutive expression resulted in a distribution pattern in intracellular vesicles consistent with spontaneous, agonist-independent internalization. When both receptors were co-expressed, HcrtR1 appeared to be recycled in intracellular vesicles, adopting the location of CB1 inherent to this model. When treated with rimonabant or with SB674042, both

CB1 and HcrtR1 were re-localized at the cell surface. The possible direct protein-protein interaction between CB1 and HcrtR1 deduced from these data was tested by performing single cell fluorescence resonance energy transfer (FRET) imaging studies, which confirmed that CB1 and HcrtR1 were close enough to form veritable heteromers (Ellis et al., 2006). Recently, the same group has demonstrated further evidence of such heteromerization by covalently labeling the extracellular domains of CB1 and HcrtR1 with SNAP-tag® and CLIP-tag™ labeling systems, which consist in two polypeptides that can be fused to a protein of interest and further covalently tagged with a suitable ligand (i.e., a fluorescent dye), allowing a reliable monitorization of these heteromers at the cell surface (Ward et al., 2011a,b). In this study, a higher potency of hypocretin-1 to regulate CB1-HcrtR1 heteromer compared with the HcrtR1-HcrtR1 homomer was reported (Ward et al., 2011b). These data provide unambiguous identification of CB1-HcrtR1 heteromerization, which has a substantial functional impact.

Besides the heteromerization, an additional mechanism has been proposed to explain the increase in the potency of hypocretin-1 to activate the ERK pathway in the presence of CB1 (Jäntti et al., 2013; Kukkonen and Leonard, 2013). Recent studies report that HcrtR1-expressing CHO cells may release 2-AG in response to hypocretin-1 stimulation. In these cells, the activation of PLC is responsible for DAG production, which in turn is used by diacylglycerol lipase (DAGL) as a substrate for 2-AG production (Turunen et al., 2012). Taking into account that both HcrtR1 and CB1 activate ERK upon ligand binding (Bouaboula et al., 1995; Ammoun et al., 2006a), it is possible that 2-AG-mediated stimulation of CB1 could contribute to increase the potency of hypocretin-1 signaling in the CHO cell expression system. In addition, recent evidence supports that endocannabinoids may act in an auto- or paracrine manner, and the influence of endogenously produced endocannabinoids when introducing Gq-coupled receptors to the expression system cannot be discarded (Howlett et al., 2011). Indeed, it has been demonstrated that HcrtR1 stimulation elevates 2-AG in biologically relevant quantities, activating CB1 receptors in nearby cells (Turunen et al., 2012). Importantly, this hypocretin-induced endocannabinoid release might shed light on the mechanisms by which hypocretins mediate synaptic inhibition in certain conditions.

FUNCTIONAL INTERACTION BETWEEN CANNABINOIDS AND HYPOCRETINS: EMERGING STUDIES

Despite anatomical, biochemical and pharmacological evidence supporting the possible existence of a link between cannabinoids and hypocretins, few studies have directly evaluated this crosstalk at the functional level (Table 1). Current research suggests their mutual involvement in the regulation of several physiological responses including appetite, reward, sleep/wake cycle and nociception.

APPETITE AND ENERGY BALANCE

The regulation of energy balance is determined by the control of food intake and energy expenditure. The so-called homeostatic control of energy balance is exerted in response to variations in the nutritional status and energy stores and is autonomic or involuntary, whereas the non-homeostatic control has a cognitive component strongly influenced by the hedonic aspects of eating (Saper et al., 2002; Berthoud, 2007) (see section Regulation of the brain rewarding system). Interestingly, endocannabinoid and hypocretinergic systems appear to be involved in both processes. Recently, the LH has been suggested to constitute a bridge between homeostatic and non-homeostatic brain areas involved in energy balance regulation. Indeed, this region connects the hypothalamic regulators of energy balance [e.g., the arcuate nucleus (Arc) and the paraventricular nucleus (PVN)], to the NAc and the VTA, two key parts of the brain reward system (Berthoud, 2007; Richard et al., 2009).

Endocannabinoids, as well as systemic administration of cannabinoid agonists, stimulate food intake (Williams et al., 1998; Williams and Kirkham, 1999). These effects are mediated by CB1 receptor. Indeed, rimonabant reduces the consumption of standard food in food-deprived animals (Colombo et al., 1998), and CB1-deficient mice consume less food than wild-type littermates and are resistant to diet-induced obesity (Di Marzo et al., 2001; Cota et al., 2003). Accordingly, fasting increases levels of anandamide and 2-AG in the limbic forebrain and, to a lesser extent, of 2-AG in the hypothalamus, whereas feeding declines endocannabinoid levels in these areas (Kirkham et al., 2002). Likewise,

central administration of hypocretin-1 or hypocretin-2 stimulates food consumption, whereas systemic administration of the HcrtR1 antagonist SB334867 reduces feeding (Sakurai et al., 1998; Haynes et al., 2000; Shiraishi et al., 2000). Furthermore, preprohypocretin mRNA is upregulated following fasting (Sakurai et al., 1998) as well as in obese mice during food restriction (Yamanaka et al., 2003). Interestingly, pretreatment with a non-anorectic dose of rimonabant blocks orexigenic actions of hypocretin-1 administered by intracerebroventricular route (icv) in pre-fed rats, suggesting that hypocretin-1 exerts its orexigenic action through CB1 receptor activation (Crespo et al., 2008). However, the increase induced by hypocretin-1 in food intake correlates with an increase in locomotion and wakefulness (Yamanaka et al., 1999; Crespo et al., 2008), leading to the hypothesis that the primary function of this system is promoting arousal in response to food deprivation, which would facilitate the food consumption (Yamanaka et al., 2003; Cason et al., 2010).

One of the main hypothalamic regulators of appetite is the Arc-PVN axis (Girault et al., 2012) (Figure 3). Circulating levels of leptin, produced by adipocytes in proportion to the adipose mass, inhibit neurons in the Arc that co-express the orexigenic neurotransmitters neuropeptide Y (NPY) and agouti-related peptide (AgRP), whereas they activate the anorexic pro-opiomelanocortin (POMC) neurons that co-express cocaine-amphetamine-related transcripts (CART). Grehlin, released during fasting, produces the opposite effect on these neurons. NPY/AgRP and POMC/CART neurons convey their information to second-order neurons in the PVN and LH, such as the corticotrophin-releasing hormone (CRH), the melanin-concentrating hormone (MCH) and hypocretin neurons (Elias et al., 1998). Emerging evidence suggests that NPY and hypocretin neurons have reciprocal excitatory connections. Thus, reduced plasma glucose and leptin and increased grehlin levels induce fasting-related arousal by causing an activation of NPY neurons finally increasing the firing of hypocretin neurons. Additionally, it seems that increased hypocretinergic activity during sleep deprivation may activate NPY neurons resulting in hyperphagia independent from peripheral endocrine and metabolic signaling (Yamanaka et al., 2000).

CB1 receptors colocalize with CART, MCH and hypocretin neurons (Cota et al., 2003). Acute administration of rimonabant induces c-fos in all these neuronal populations including hypocretinergic cells, increases CART and decreases NPY expression, consistent with its anorexic effect. However, the CB1 antagonist has no effect in hypocretin expression suggesting that hypocretins are not likely to be the main mediators of cannabinoid hypothalamic orexigenic effects (Verty et al., 2009). An interesting electrophysiological study in mouse reveals that the cannabinoid agonist WIN55-212,2 depolarizes MCH cells increasing spike frequency while reducing spontaneous firing of hypocretin cells (Huang et al., 2007). CB1-mediated depolarization of MCH cells was a consequence of cannabinoid action on axons arising from LH local inhibitory cells, resulting in reduced synaptic GABA release on MCH neurons. On the contrary, CB1 agonists hyperpolarized hypocretin cells by presynaptic attenuation of glutamate release (Huang et al., 2007). These results are in line with the idea that some of the orexigenic actions of cannabinoids could be explained

Table 1 | Studies investigating the interaction between endocannabinoid and hypocretinergic systems.

Functional interaction	Tools		Techniques	Main result	References
Energy balance	*in vivo* (rat)	Hypocretin-1 CB1 antagonist	Food intake monitoring	Subeffective systemic rimonabant attenuates food intake induced by central hypocretin-1	Crespo et al., 2008
	Rat tissue	CB1 antagonist	LH Immunofluorescence qRT-PCR Western Blot	Rimonabant administration induces Fos expression in hypocretin, MCH, MSH and CART neurons, but does not affect hypocretin mRNA or protein levels	Verty et al., 2009
	ex vivo (mouse)	Obese *ob/ob* mice High-fat diet CB agonist Leptin mTOR inhibitor	Confocal, electron microscopy LH electrophysiology LH immunofluorescence	In obesity, hypocretinergic neurons overexpress DAGL and receive predominantly inhibitory, instead of excitatory, CB1-expressing inputs. These alterations are reversed by leptin administration	Cristino et al., 2013
Reward and Cannabis dependence	*in vivo* (rat)	Cholinergic agonist HcrtR1 antagonist CB1 antagonist	Conditioned place preference	CPP induced by LH-chemical stimulation requires HcrtR1 and CB1 receptor signaling in the VTA	Taslimi et al., 2011
	in vivo (mouse)	HcrtR1 knockout mice CB agonists HcrtR1 and HcrtR2 antagonists	Drug self-administration LH immunofluorescence *In vivo* microdyalisis	Rewarding properties of cannabinoids are modulated by HcrtR1 and activate LH hypocretinergic neurons. HcrtR1 regulates THC-induced dopamine release in Nac	Flores et al., 2013
	in vivo (human)	–	Peripheral blood gene expression and promoter metylation study	THC-smokers show decreased hypocretin expression when compared to cigarette-smokers	Rotter et al., 2012
Antinociception	*ex vivo* and *in vivo* (rat)	Hypocretin-1 HcrtR1 and HcrtR2 antagonists CB1 agonist and antagonist PLC and DAGL inhibitors	PAG electrophysiology PAG Immunofluorescence Hot plate test	Hypocretin-1 inhibits GABA release to PAG neurons through retrograde 2-AG signaling, leading to increased PAG activity. Antinociceptive responses induced by intra-PAG administration of hypocretin-1 are mediated by HcrtR1 and CB1 receptors	Ho et al., 2011
Sleep/wake cycle	*in vivo* (rat)	CB1 agonist and antagonist	EEG and EMG monitoring LH immunofluorescence	Intra-LH administration of 2-AG increases REM sleep and cFos expression in MCH neurons, but does not affect cFos expression in hypocretinergic neurons	Pérez-Morales et al., 2013
	ex vivo (rat)	Hypocretin-2 CB1 agonist and antagonist PLC and DAGL inhibitors	DRN electrophysiology	Hypocretin-2 inhibits glutamate release to DRN serotonergic neurons through retrograde 2-AG signaling	Haj-Dahmane and Shen, 2005
Cellular and molecular interaction	*ex vivo* (mouse)	CB agonist ad antagonist GABAa antagonist iGluR antagonist	LH electrophysiology Immunocytochemistry	Cannabinoids reduce activity of hypocretin neurons by presynaptic attenuation of glutamate release and excite MCH neurons by presynaptic inhibition of GABA release	Huang et al., 2007

(Continued)

Table 1 | Continued

Functional interaction	Tools		Techniques	Main result	References
	in vitro (cell culture)	Hypocretin-1 CB1 antagonist	Confocal, electron microscopy Intracellular signaling assays	CB1-HcrtR1 coexpression potentiates activation of the MAPK pathway induced by hypocretin-1	Hilairet et al., 2003
	in vitro (cell culture)	Hypocretin-1 CB1 agonist and antagonist HcrtR1 antagonist	Redistribution assays Epifluorescence microscopy FRET imaging	CB1-HcrtR1 heteromerization results in coordinated alteration of their cellular localization and downstream signaling	Ellis et al., 2006
	in vitro (cell culture)	CB1 agonist and antagonist HcrtR1 antagonist	Co-immunoprecipitation SNAP and CLIP tagging FRET imaging Intracellular signaling assays	Heteromultimerization of CB1-HcrtR1 is confirmed by co-immunoprecipitation and SNAP/CLIP tagging. Modulation of receptor internalization and MAPK pathway activation is also reproduced	Ward et al., 2011a,b
	in vitro (cell culture)	Hypocretin-1 and -2 CB1 agonist and antagonist DAGL and MAGL inhibitors PLC, PLD and PLA inhibitors HcrtR1 antagonist	Intracellular signaling assays	HcrtR1 stimulation by hypocretin-1 activates PLA2 and DAGL cascades with subsequent release of AA and 2-AG, which acts as paracrine messenger through CB1	Turunen et al., 2012
	in vitro (cell culture)	Hypocretin-1 and -2 CB1 antagonist HcrtR1 antagonist DAGL and MEK inhibitors	Intracellular signaling assays	Release of 2-AG induced by hypocretin-1 stimulates ERK activity in neighboring CB1-expressing cells. HcrtR1-mediated ERK activity is potentiated in cells coexpressing CB1-HcrtR1	Jäntti et al., 2013

Abbreviations: IF, immunofluorescence; EPS, electrophysiology; drug self admin, drug self-administration; EF microscopy, epifluorescence microscopy; co-IP, co-immunoprecipitation.

by their synaptic effects on MCH neurons, which undoubtedly regulate energy balance (Pissios et al., 2006), and are not mediated by hypocretin neurons at least in physiological conditions. However, a recent study shows that the balance between CB1-expressing glutamatergic and GABAergic inputs to hypocretin neurons is altered in obesity (Cristino et al., 2013). In leptin-knockout (ob/ob) obese mice and in diet-induced obese mice, hypocretin neurons appear to receive predominantly inhibitory instead of excitatory CB1-expressing inputs (Cristino et al., 2013). In addition, hypocretin neurons overexpress the main enzyme that synthesizes 2-AG, DAGLα, in these obesity models, in line with previous results reporting elevated hypothalamic levels of endocannabinoids in ob/ob mice and obese Zucker rats (Di Marzo et al., 2001). These alterations could result in a retrograde inhibition of these inhibitory CB1-expressing axon terminals, leading to disinhibition of hypocretinergic neurons and enhancing hypocretin innervation of target brain areas. This remodeling could be a consequence of leptin signaling impairment, since it was reversed by the systemic administration of leptin (Cristino et al., 2013). Therefore, in these pathological conditions, hypocretins could exacerbate obesity as a result of an increased hypocretin release in the hypothalamus, leading to hyperphagia and sleep disorders (Alpár and Harkany, 2013).

Another relevant integrative region in the control of appetite is the nucleus of the solitary tract (NTS) in the hindbrain, which regulates individual meal sizes and the intervals between meals (Valassi et al., 2008). Peripheral satiety signals are relayed to the NTS via vagal afferent neurons, whose cell bodies lie in the nodose ganglia. It has been recently reported that fasting-induced increase in CB1 immunoreactivity has been observed under standard food regime in the nodose ganglia (Cluny et al., 2013). In contrast, OX-1R immunoreactivity is modified by fasting only in rats exposed to high-fat diet, denoting a differential regulation of these neurotransmitter systems in this structure (Cluny et al., 2013). On the other hand, hypocretin-1 depolarizes NTS neurons through regulation of non-selective cationic and K+ conductances in a PKC-dependent manner (Yang et al., 2003; Yang and Ferguson, 2003). It has ben also reported that CB1 receptor activation modulates NTS neuronal activity (Seagard et al., 2005; Endoh, 2006). However, it remains to be investigated whether these neurochemical effects in nodose ganglia and NTS are relevant in the control of feeding behavior, and if there exists an interplay between endocannabinoid and hypocretinergic mechanisms.

Endocannabinoid and hypocretinergic systems seem to play antagonistic roles in the peripheral control of energy balance.

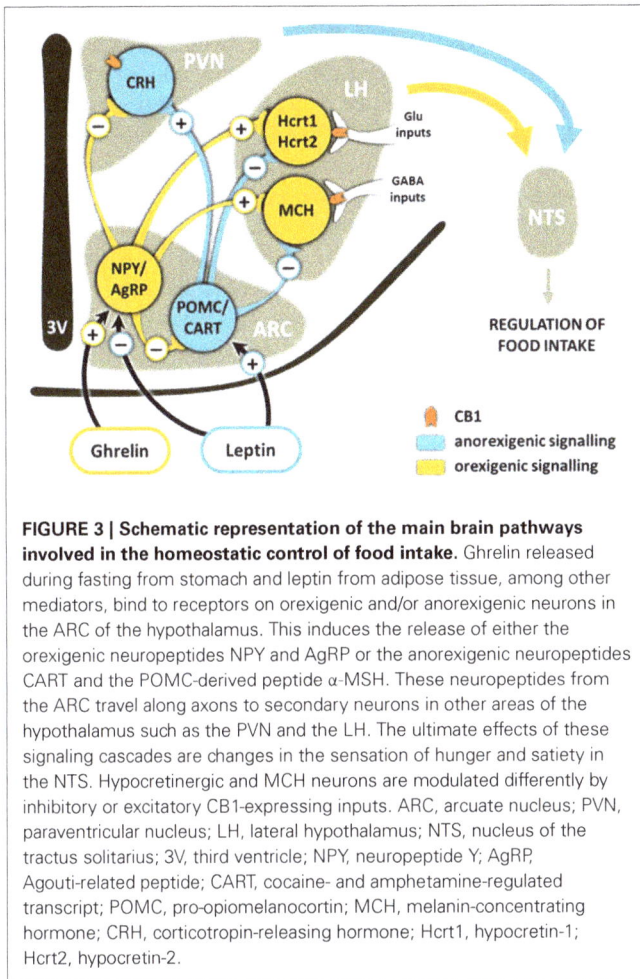

FIGURE 3 | Schematic representation of the main brain pathways involved in the homeostatic control of food intake. Ghrelin released during fasting from stomach and leptin from adipose tissue, among other mediators, bind to receptors on orexigenic and/or anorexigenic neurons in the ARC of the hypothalamus. This induces the release of either the orexigenic neuropeptides NPY and AgRP or the anorexigenic neuropeptides CART and the POMC-derived peptide α-MSH. These neuropeptides from the ARC travel along axons to secondary neurons in other areas of the hypothalamus such as the PVN and the LH. The ultimate effects of these signaling cascades are changes in the sensation of hunger and satiety in the NTS. Hypocretinergic and MCH neurons are modulated differently by inhibitory or excitatory CB1-expressing inputs. ARC, arcuate nucleus; PVN, paraventricular nucleus; LH, lateral hypothalamus; NTS, nucleus of the tractus solitarius; 3V, third ventricle; NPY, neuropeptide Y; AgRP, Agouti-related peptide; CART, cocaine- and amphetamine-regulated transcript; POMC, pro-opiomelanocortin; MCH, melanin-concentrating hormone; CRH, corticotropin-releasing hormone; Hcrt1, hypocretin-1; Hcrt2, hypocretin-2.

The reduction of body weight and fat mass exerted by CB1 antagonists in diet-induced obesity models is partially due to the counteraction of a peripheral stimulation of lipogenesis by endocannabinoids (Di Marzo and Matias, 2005). Moreover, chronic CB1 blockade improves peripheral metabolic parameters of obesity, including a reduction in plasma levels of insulin and leptin. In contrast, mice overproducing the hypocretin peptides exhibit resistance to high-fat diet-induced obesity at least in part by promoting energy expenditure (Tsuneki et al., 2010). These antiobesity metabolic effects have been demonstrated to be mediated by HcrtR2, which has been observed to improve leptin sensitivity (Funato et al., 2009). However, no studies have been yet published assessing whether endocannabinoid and hypocretinergic systems show a cross-modulation in their peripheral control of metabolic rates.

REGULATION OF THE BRAIN REWARD SYSTEM

Endocannabinoid and hypocretinergic systems are also involved in the regulation of the mesocorticolimbic rewarding system, a circuit responsible for the pleasurable feelings associated with natural rewards and the consumption of drugs of abuse. The major components of this reward circuit are the VTA, which contains the dopaminergic cell bodies, and its target areas, including the NAc, amygdala, frontal and limbic cortices (Wise, 2004).

CB1 and HcrtRs receptors are abundant in the brain reward circuitry and participate in the rewarding properties of natural rewards and also in those induced by different drugs of abuse (Maldonado et al., 2006). Acting as a retrograde messenger, endocannabinoids modulate the glutamatergic excitatory and GABAergic inhibitory synaptic inputs into the dopaminergic neurons of the VTA and the glutamate transmission in the NAc. Thus, the activation of CB1 receptors present on axon terminals of GABAergic neurons in the VTA inhibits GABA transmission, removing this inhibitory input on dopaminergic neurons (Riegel and Lupica, 2004). Glutamate synaptic transmission in the VTA and NAc, mainly from neurons of the PFC, is similarly modulated by the activation of CB1 receptors (Melis et al., 2004). The final effect of endocannabinoids on the modulation of dopaminergic activity, which depends on the functional balance between these GABAergic and glutamatergic inputs, is predominantly excitatory (Maldonado et al., 2006). On the other hand, hypocretins regulate reward seeking also by modulating VTA dopaminergic transmission. In agreement, intra-VTA infusion of hypocretin-1 and -2 increased dopamine release in NAc and PFC as measured by microdialysis or voltammetry (Vittoz et al., 2008; España et al., 2011). Hypocretins elicit their influence on VTA dopamine cell firing not only via direct depolarization of dopamine neurons (Korotkova et al., 2003), but also interacting with other neurotransmitters within the VTA, such as glutamate (Borgland et al., 2006). Thus, intra-VTA infusion of hypocretin-1 increased both glutamate and dopamine release, which was attenuated by the AMPA/NMDA antagonist kynurenic acid, suggesting that hypocretin has a profound influence on dopamine neurons by affecting glutamatergic activity (Wang et al., 2009). Hypocretin-1 enhanced glutamatergic synaptic strength on dopamine neurons in VTA slices (Borgland et al., 2006). In accordance, the control of this limbic structure by the PFC projections was improved by hypocretin-1 in rats (Mahler et al., 2013).

This considerable modulation of the reward circuit by endocannabinoid and hypocretinergic systems reveal their important role in the non-homeostatic control of food intake. CB1 receptor antagonists have been reported to reduce the conditioned place preference (CPP) for food (Chaperon et al., 1998), and the motivation for food in a progressive ratio schedule of food self-administration in rats (Gallate and McGregor, 1999). According to this, null mutant CB1 mice show a reduced motivation to work for food compared to wild-type littermates (Sanchis-Segura et al., 2004). CB1 receptor blockade also decreases the reinforcing properties of chocolate and sweets (Maccioni et al., 2008). In addition, intra-NAc injections of anandamide enhance the reward associated with sweets (Mahler et al., 2007). Similarly, several data support a role for hypocretins in food-seeking and taking. Thus, chronic administration of the HcrtR1 antagonist SB334867 altered standard food self-administration in food-restricted mice (Sharf et al., 2010), although this effect was not observed in rats after acute administration of the HcrtR1 antagonist (Borgland et al., 2009). Indeed, it seems that hypocretinergic control of food-related reward is more relevant when it involves particularly palatable foods (Mahler et al., 2012). In agreement, SB334867 reduces both motivational and primary reinforcing effects in rats trained to self-administer high-fat food, both under food-restriction or satiation (Nair et al., 2008; Choi et al., 2010). So far, no studies have investigated if endocannabinoid and hypocretinergic systems have common mechanisms in the modulation of natural reward. However, it seems that both neurotransmitter systems regulate food intake especially when particularly palatable/or salient food is involved or higher effort is required to obtain this natural reinforcer.

Similarly, the addictive properties of several drugs of abuse are modulated by hypocretinergic and endocannabinoid systems. Hypocretin transmission regulates the primary reinforcing effects of opioids (Narita et al., 2006; Smith and Aston-Jones, 2012), nicotine (Hollander et al., 2008; LeSage et al., 2010) and alcohol (Lawrence et al., 2006; Moorman and Aston-Jones, 2009). However, the involvement of the hypocretin system in the rewarding properties of psychostimulants seems to be relevant only under conditions that require a high effort to obtain the drug (Boutrel et al., 2005; España et al., 2011). This distinct regulation could be due to differences among the mechanism of action by which these drugs of abuse alter the mesolimbic function (Plaza-Zabala et al., 2012). Opioids, nicotine and alcohol increase extracellular levels of dopamine in the NAc by enhancing dopaminergic firing rates in the VTA, whereas psychostimulants directly inhibit dopamine uptake in the NAc (Di Chiara et al., 2004). Thus, rewarding effects of drugs of abuse that depend on increased VTA dopaminergic activity may require hypocretinergic transmission, as the VTA appears to be an essential site of action for hypocretins to modulate these effects. In contrast, the mechanism of action of psychostimulants avoids this critical site of action of hypocretins. Intriguingly, a similar phenomenon occurs with the modulatory role of the endocannabinoid system on the primary rewarding effects of drugs of abuse. Thus, opioid (Navarro et al., 2001, 2004), cannabinoid (Maldonado et al., 2006), nicotine (Castañé et al., 2002; Cohen et al., 2002) and alcohol (Hungund et al., 2003; Wang et al., 2003) reinforcement depend on endocannabinoid signaling in the VTA, but primary rewarding effects of psychostimulants remain unaffected in the absence of CB1 receptors (Martin et al., 2000; Soria et al., 2005). However, the endocannabinoid system is important for maintaining psychostimulants seeking behavior when higher effort is required to obtain the drug, probably by the modulation of other mechanisms independent from release of dopamine in the NAc (Soria et al., 2005). It has been recently reported that CPP induced by chemical stimulation of the LH with the cholinergic agonist carbachol is regulated by HcrtR1 activation in the VTA. Thus, unilateral intra-VTA administration of the HcrtR1 antagonist SB334867 dose-dependently inhibited this behavioral response (Taslimi et al., 2011). Interestingly, intra-VTA administration of rimonabant also decreased CPP induced by LH-stimulation in a dose-dependent manner. Co-administration of effective doses of both HcrtR1 and CB1 antagonists into the VTA reduced CPP in a non-additive manner, suggesting that these receptors regulate this effect by a common mechanism (Taslimi et al., 2011). Nevertheless, future experiments showing the specific location of HcrtR1 and CB1 receptors within the VTA neurons will be necessary to better understand the interaction between the endocannabinoid and hypocretin systems in the regulation of the reward circuit.

A relevant but almost unexplored aspect of hypocretin-cannabinoid interplay is the role of the hypocretinergic system in the addictive properties of cannabinoids, whose recreational use has progressively increased in developed countries in the last decade (Murray et al., 2007). Therefore, the identification of new therapeutic targets to improve treatment outcomes for cannabis dependence is imperative considering that no effective pharmacotherapeutic approaches for this disorder are currently available. Although operant responding for self-infused THC has not been consistently reported in rodents, intravenous self-administration of the synthetic cannabinoid WIN55,212-2 has been observed in rats and mice (Fattore et al., 2001; Mendizábal et al., 2006). The reinforcing properties of cannabinoids have been related to their capability to enhance dopamine extracellular levels in the NAc shell (Fadda et al., 2006; Lecca et al., 2006), although other neurochemical systems have also been involved in cannabinoid reward, such as opioid, noradrenaline, serotonine, acetylcholine and adenosine systems (Maldonado et al., 2011).

Recently, the hypocretinergic system has also been reported to contribute to cannabinoid-induced reward. Indeed, genetic deletion or pharmacological blockade of HcrtR1 reduced the reinforcing effects of WIN55,212-2, as revealed by impaired intravenous self-administration of this synthetic cannabinoid in mice (Flores et al., 2013). In contrast, the HcrtR2 antagonist TCSOX229 had no effect in these behavioral responses. The enhancement in dopamine extracellular levels in the nucleus accumbens induced by THC was also blocked in mice lacking the HcrtR1, suggesting that cannabinoids require hypocretinergic transmission to induce dopamine release in the NAc. Moreover, contingent WIN55,212-2 self-administration, but not passive exposure to the cannabinoid, increased the percentage of hypocretin neurons expressing FosB/ΔFosB in the LH, revealing that this activation was mainly due to operant seeking for the reinforcing effects of this drug and not to its pharmacological responses (Flores et al., 2013). Cannabinoid-induced activation of hypocretin neurons reported in this study differs from previous electrophysiological data supporting that cannabinoids inhibit hypocretin neurons by CB1-mediated attenuation of glutamate release in these cells (Huang et al., 2007), but possible clarification of this divergence has recently emerged. As previously mentioned, a switch in CB1-mediated control of GABAergic and glutamatergic inputs is observed in obese mice (Cristino et al., 2013). It is thus reasonable that if this synaptic remodeling takes place in determined pathological conditions, such as obesity, the development of drug addiction might entail similar consequences by different mechanisms. However, this possibility still remains to be elucidated. Other recent evidence supports the relationship between hypocretins and cannabis dependence. It has been reported that hypocretin-1 expression in peripheral blood cells is modified in cannabis-dependent smokers when compared to nicotine-dependent smokers and non-smokers (Rotter et al., 2012). However, these data provide poor functional information, as peripheral hypocretin mRNA levels do not necessarily reflect the situation in the CNS. Moreover, it is likely that these differences are more related to peripheral actions of THC and not to the central effects involved in the development of dependence.

NOCICEPTION

Analgesia is one of the main therapeutic targets of cannabinoids. CB1 receptors are highly expressed in pain transmission and modulation regions such as PAG, rostroventral medulla (RVM), spinal cord and primary afferent fibers (Hohmann and Suplita, 2006). Consistent with this anatomic location, several animal studies demonstrated that both endogenous and exogenous cannabinoids produce antinociceptive effects in different animal models mainly through the activation of CB1 receptors (Martin et al., 1993; Herzberg et al., 1997; Dogrul et al., 2002). Moreover, CB2 receptors have been reported to contribute to antinociception in some chronic pain models (Racz et al., 2008; La Porta et al., 2013). Cannabinoid-mediated antinociception takes places at peripheral, spinal and supraspinal levels. One of the best characterized mechanisms of pain modulation is the descending inhibitory pathway. This descending modulatory mechanism originates in the PAG, which activates neurons in the RVM, the main relay station between the PAG and spinal cord. RVM neurons send inhibitory projections to the dorsal horn of the spinal cord via dorsolateral funiculus (DLF) and modulate pain perception at the spinal level (Ren and Dubner, 2008). The demonstration that cannabinoid antinociceptive effects are diminished following surgical DLF lesion provides evidence that descending pain modulatory pathways play a crucial role in these responses (Lichtman and Martin, 1991). Thus, microinjection of the cannabinoid agonists HU210 and WIN55,212-2 into the PAG elicits antinociception mediated by CB1 receptor activation (Lichtman et al., 1996; Finn et al., 2003). This effect is the result of disinhibition of GABAergic output neurons in the PAG that leads to activation of descending inhibitory pain pathways (Vaughan et al., 2000). Similarly, local injection of CB1 agonists into RVM had antinociceptive effects due to presynaptic inhibition of GABAergic tone (Vaughan et al., 2000). Moreover, anandamide and 2-AG levels were increased in RVM in some models of chronic pain, presumably as an adaptive mechanism to counteract pain transmission (Petrosino et al., 2007).

Antinociceptive effects of hypocretins have been shown in several pain models (Chiou et al., 2010). Thus, hypocretin-1 administration by central or systemic route reduces the nociceptive responses in mice in response to thermal, mechanical and chemical stimuli (Mobarakeh et al., 2005). Hypocretin-2 has also been reported to induce antinociceptive effects in some pain models, but with lower potency than hypocretin-1 (Mobarakeh et al., 2005). Hypocretin-induced antinociception seems to be mainly mediated by HcrtR1, as revealed by using selective antagonists (Bingham et al., 2001). Hypocretin-containing fibers and HcrtRs are densely distributed in several regions of the CNS involved in the regulation of pain, including the PAG and spinal dorsal horn (Peyron et al., 1998; Marcus et al., 2001). Like cannabinoids, hypocretins appear to modulate pain perception at both spinal and supraspinal levels, but the mechanism of action remains unclear. The midbrain PAG is one of the possible supraspinal sites of hypocretin antinociception. Interestingly, PAG c-fos expression was elevated following central hypocretin administration (Date et al., 1999). In agreement, microinjection of hypocretin-1 into the PAG reduced hot-plate nociceptive responses in mice (Lee and Chiou, 2009) and

formalin-induced nociceptive behaviors in rats (Yamamoto et al., 2002). A recent study in PAG slices revealed that hypocretin-1 induces inhibition of GABAergic transmission, producing an overall excitatory effect on evoked postsynaptic potentials and hence increasing PAG neuronal activity (Ho et al., 2011). This effect was blocked by the HcrtR1 antagonist SB334867, but not by the HcrtR2 antagonist TCSOX229. Moreover, the CB1 antagonist AM251 reversed the effect of hypocretin-1. Administration of U73122 and tetrahydrolipstatin, inhibitors of PLC and DAGL respectively, blocked the inhibition of GABAergic tone induced by hypocretin-1, while the inhibitor of the enzymatic degradation of 2-AG, URB602, enhanced this hypocretin effect. Therefore, hypocretin-1 may produce antinociception in part by activating postsynaptic HcrtR1 receptors and stimulating synthesis of 2-AG through a PLC–DAGL enzymatic cascade, culminating in retrograde inhibition of GABA release in the PAG. The *in vivo* existence of such analgesic mechanism was confirmed by systemic administration of SB334867 and AM251 after intra-PAG microinjection of hypocretin-1, which almost fully reversed the antinociceptive responses in the hot-plate test in rats (Ho et al., 2011). Importantly, this 2-AG-mediated antinociception induced by hypocretin signaling may contribute to stress-induced analgesia, since hypocretins have been reported to modulate this response to stress (Watanabe et al., 2005; Xie et al., 2008) and endocannabinoids within the PAG are also believed to be involved in this effect (Hohmann and Suplita, 2006). Therefore, under stressful conditions, activation of HcrtR1 may lead to PAG stimulation and produce analgesia through 2-AG via the CB1–PLC–DAGL cascade.

Both endocannabinoid and hypocretinergic systems exert also antinociceptive effects at the spinal (Drew et al., 2000; Grudt et al., 2002) and peripheral levels (Millns et al., 2001; Yan et al., 2008), but no data are available regarding a possible contribution of endocannabinoids in spinal or peripheral hypocretin-induced analgesia. Moreover, the possible modulation of cannabinoid-induced antinociception by hypocretins has not been studied yet.

SLEEP/WAKE CYCLE

Several data indicates that the hypocretinergic system is involved in the regulation of sleep-wake cycle. Thus, hypocretin neurons fire at maximal rate in wakefulness and remain silent in rapid eye movement (REM) sleep (Lee et al., 2005). Likewise, pharmacological stimulation of the hypocretinergic system increases wakefulness and reduces REM sleep (Akanmu and Honda, 2005). Accordingly, the dysfunction of this system is linked to narcolepsy, as revealed in dogs with mutated HcrtR2 gene and mice lacking hypocretins or HcrtR2 (Lin et al., 1999; Willie et al., 2003). On the other hand, endocannabinoids are also involved in sleep regulation and have been shown to be strong sleep-inducers (Cravatt et al., 1995). Besides, systemic administration of rimonabant increases wakefulness and decreases REM sleep in rats (Santucci et al., 1996), whereas acute (Murillo-Rodríguez et al., 2001), subchronic (Herrera-Solís et al., 2010) and intrahippocampal (Rueda-Orozco et al., 2010) administration of anandamide has the opposite effect.

Few studies have investigated the possible mechanisms shared by the hypocretinergic and endocannabinoid systems in the regulation of sleep and wakefulness. The finding that cannabinoid signaling leads to hyperpolarization of hypocretin neurons and depolarization of MCH neurons in *in vitro* preparations (Huang et al., 2007) encouraged the idea that endocannabinoids could interact with these hypothalamic neurons to regulate sleep. Indeed, intra-hypothalamic administration of 2-AG increases REM sleep in rats through CB1 receptor and MCH signaling, since 2-AG slightly decreased c-fos expression in hypocretin neurons and activated MCH neurons (Pérez-Morales et al., 2013). Endocannabinoid and hypocretinergic systems could be involved in the modulation of sleep/wake cycle by acting in dorsal raphe nucleus (DRN) serotonergic neurons, closely linked to REM sleep and arousal. Thus, these neurons discharge at a high frequency during waking, at a lower rate during non-REM sleep and become silent during REM sleep (McGinty and Harper, 1976; Portas et al., 1996). Activation of HcrtRs increases activity of DRN serotonergic neurons (Brown et al., 2001; Liu et al., 2002). However, an electrophysiological study performed in rat DRN slices has reported that hypocretin-2 also inhibits glutamatergic transmission to serotonergic neurons of the DRN via retrograde endocannabinoid messengers (Haj-Dahmane and Shen, 2005). Although the functional implications of this retrograde synaptic modulation are not clear, the authors propose that it could prevent excessive excitation of DRN serotonergic neurons to provide a homeostatic control, contributing to the stable firing activity of these arousal-related neurons. Therefore, the loss of the hypocretin signal could lead to the disorganized activity and fragmented wakefulness observed in narcolepsy (Haj-Dahmane and Shen, 2005). However, further studies should be carried out to clarify the relevance of the possible interactions between cannabinoid and hypocretinergic systems in sleep modulation.

CONCLUDING REMARKS

The existence of a cross-talk between the hypocretinergic and endocannabinoid systems is strongly supported by their partially overlapping anatomical distribution and common role in several physiological and pathological processes. However, little is known about the mechanisms underlying this interaction. The formation of heteromers between HcrtR1 and CB1 receptors has been demonstrated *in vitro*, which alters the cellular localization and downstream signaling of both receptors. However, the biological significance of these heteromers remains unknown, and further studies are needed to verify whether the two receptors are expressed on the same target neurons and if they form heteromers *in vivo*. In this regard, better tools should be developed to determine the specific location of HcrtRs due to the cross-reactivity problems of the currently available antibodies (Kukkonen, 2012). On the other hand, hypocretin signaling has been reported to stimulate the synthesis of 2-AG leading to retrograde inhibition, which suggests that endocannabinoids might contribute to several hypocretin effects. Recent evidence denotes that this endocannabinoid-mediated retrograde inhibition is present in diverse brain regions *in vivo*, being of special relevance in the regulation of the analgesic effects induced by hypocretins. Interesting data also point to a collaboration of endocannabinoid and hypocretinergic systems in the central

control of food intake and obesity. The hypocretinergic transmission is overstimulated in this pathological condition, and HcrtR antagonists might be useful in the control of appetite and other disorders associated with obesity, such as anxiety and sleep deregulations. However, the apparent antiobesity role of HcrtR2 in the peripheral control of energy balance should be taken into account and would possibly require the use of selective HcrtR1 antagonists for this specific purpose. Blockade of HcrtR1 signaling has demonstrated also its therapeutic potential against cannabinoid dependence by interfering with the rewarding effects of this drug. Nevertheless, the variety of hypocretin and endocannabinoid signaling implies that their manipulation to regulate a specific physiological process would probably produce several side effects. To avoid this problem, efforts should be focused on the development of selective agonists/antagonists for the different receptors and/or with site specific activity. Some authors defend that diverse GPCR heteromers are diseasespecific and/or exhibit unique tissue specificity (Gomes et al., 2013). If this would be the case of CB1-HcrtR1 heteromers, they would serve as ideal drug targets with potentially lesser side effects that the single receptors. Although research about the cannabinoid-hypocretinergic interplay has only taken the first steps, future investigation in this field will lead to a better understanding of the therapeutic potential of this interesting interaction.

ACKNOWLEDGMENTS

This work was supported by the Instituto de Salud Carlos III grants, #PI07/0559, #PI10/00316 and #RD06/001/001 (RTA-RETICS), by the Spanish Ministry of Science and Technology, Consolider-C #SAF2007-64062 and #SAF2011-29864, the Catalan Government (SGR2009-00731), and by the Catalan Institution for Research and Advanced Studies (ICREA Academia program). África Flores is recipient of a predoctoral fellowship from the Spanish Ministry of Education.

REFERENCES

Akanmu, M. A., and Honda, K. (2005). Selective stimulation of orexin receptor type 2 promotes wakefulness in freely behaving rats. *Brain Res.* 1048, 138–145. doi: 10.1016/j.brainres.2005.04.064

Alpár, A., and Harkany, T. (2013). Orexin neurons use endocannabinoids to break obesity-induced inhibition. *Proc. Natl. Acad. Sci. U.S.A.* 110, 9625–9626. doi: 10.1073/pnas.1307389110

Ammoun, S., Holmqvist, T., Shariatmadari, R., Oonk, H. B., Detheux, M., Parmentier, M. et al. (2003). Distinct recognition of OX1 and OX2 receptors by orexin peptides. *J. Pharmacol. Exp. Ther.* 305, 507–514. doi: 10.1124/jpet.102.048025

Ammoun, S., Johansson, L., Ekholm, M. E., Holmqvist, T., Danis, A. S., Korhonen, L., et al. (2006b). OX1 orexin receptors activate extracellular signal-regulated kinase in Chinese hamster ovary cells via multiple mechanisms: the role of Ca2+ influx in OX1 receptor signaling. *Mol. Endocrinol.* 20, 80–99. doi: 10.1210/me.2004-0389

Ammoun, S., Lindholm, D., Wootz, H., Akerman, K. E., and Kukkonen, J. P. (2006a). G-protein-coupled OX1 orexin/hcrtr-1 hypocretin receptors induce caspase-dependent and -independent cell death through p38 mitogen-/stress-activated protein kinase. *J. Biol. Chem.* 281, 834 842. doi: 10.1074/jbc.M508603200

Aston-Jones, G., Smith, R. J., Sartor, G. C., Moorman, D. E., Massi, L., Tahsili-Fahadan, P. et al. (2010). Lateral hypothalamic orexin/hypocretin neurons: a role in reward-seeking and addiction. *Brain Res.* 1314, 74–90. doi: 10.1016/j.brainres.2009.09.106

Berthoud, H. R. (2007). Interactions between the "cognitive" and "metabolic" brain in the control of food intake. *Physiol Behav.* 91, 486–498. doi: 10.1016/j.physbeh.2006.12.016

Bingham, S., Davey, P. T., Babbs, A. J., Irving, E. A., Sammons, M. J., Wyles, M., et al. (2001). Orexin-A, an hypothalamic peptide with analgesic properties. *Pain* 92, 81–90. doi: 10.1016/S0304-3959(00)00470-X

Borgland, S. L., Chang, S. J., Bowers, M. S., Thompson, J. L., Vittoz, N., Floresco, S. B., et al. (2009). Orexin A/hypocretin-1 selectively promotes motivation for positive reinforcers. *J. Neurosci.* 29, 11215–11225. doi: 10.1523/JNEUROSCI.6096-08.2009

Borgland, S. L., Taha, S. A., Sarti, F., Fields, H. L., and Bonci, A. (2006). Orexin A in the VTA is critical for the induction of synaptic plasticity and behavioral sensitization to cocaine. *Neuron* 49, 589–601. doi: 10.1016/j.neuron.2006.01.016

Bouaboula, M., Perrachon, S., Milligan, L., Canat, X., Rinaldi-Carmona, M., Portier, M., et al. (1997). A selective inverse agonist for central cannabinoid receptor inhibits mitogen-activated protein kinase activation stimulated by insulin or insulin-like growth factor 1. Evidence for a new model of receptor/ligand interactions. *J Biol. Chem.* 272, 22330–22339. doi: 10.1074/jbc.272.35.22330

Bouaboula, M., Poinot-Chazel, C., Bourrié, B., Canat, X., Calandra, B., Rinaldi-Carmona, M., et al. (1995). Activation of mitogen-activated protein kinases by stimulation of the central cannabinoid receptor CB1. *Biochem. J.* 312, 637–641.

Boutrel, B., Kenny, P. J., Specio, S. E., Martin-Fardon, R., Markou, A., Koob, G. F., et al. (2005). Role for hypocretin in mediating stress-induced reinstatement of cocaine-seeking behavior. *Proc. Natl. Acad. Sci. U.S.A.* 102, 19168–19173. doi: 10.1073/pnas.0507480102

Brown, R. E., Sergeeva, O., Eriksson, K. S., and Haas, H. L. (2001). Orexin A excites serotonergic neurons in the dorsal raphe nucleus of the rat. *Neuropharmacology* 40, 457–459. doi: 10.1016/S0028-3908(00)00178-7

Burdakov, D., Liss, B., and Ashcroft, F. M. (2003). Orexin excites GABAergic neurons of the arcuate nucleus by activating the sodium—calcium exchanger. *J. Neurosci.* 23, 4951–4957.

Carriba, P., Ortiz, O., Patkar, K., Justinova, Z., Stroik, J., Themann, A. et al. (2007). Striatal adenosine A2A and cannabinoid CB1 receptors form functional heteromeric complexes that mediate the motor effects of cannabinoids. *Neuropsychopharmacology* 32, 2249–2259. doi: 10.1038/sj.npp.1301375

Cason, A. M., Smith, R. J., Tahsili-Fahadan, P., Moorman, D. E., Sartor, G. C., and Aston-Jones, G. (2010). Role of orexin/hypocretin in reward-seeking and addiction: implications for obesity. *Physiol Behav.* 100, 419–428. doi: 10.1016/j.physbeh.2010.03.009

Castañé, A., Valjent, E., Ledent, C., Parmentier, M., Maldonado, R., and Valverde, O. (2002). Lack of CB1 cannabinoid receptors modifies nicotine behavioural responses, but not nicotine abstinence. *Neuropharmacology* 43, 857–867. doi: 10.1016/S0028-3908(02)00118-1

Chaperon, F., Soubrié, P., Puech, A. J., and Thiébot, M. H. (1998). Involvement of central cannabinoid (CB1) receptors in the establishment of place conditioning in rats. *Psychopharmacology (Berl.)* 135, 324–332. doi: 10.1007/s002130050518

Chiou, L. C., Lee, H. J., Ho, Y. C., Chen, S. P., Liao, Y. Y., Ma, C. H., et al. (2010). Orexins/hypocretins: pain regulation and cellular actions. *Curr. Pharm. Des.* 16, 3089–3100. doi: 10.2174/138161210793292483

Choi, D. L., Davis, J. F., Fitzgerald, M. E., and Benoit, S. C. (2010). The role of orexin-A in food motivation, reward-based feeding behavior and food-induced neuronal activation in rats. *Neuroscience* 167, 11–20. doi: 10.1016/j.neuroscience.2010.02.002

Cluny, N. L., Baraboi, E. D., Mackie, K., Burdyga, G., Richard, D., Dockray, G. J., et al. (2013). High fat diet and body weight have different effects on cannabinoid CB1 receptor expression in rat nodose ganglia. *Auton. Neurosci.* 179, 122–130. doi: 10.1016/j.autneu.2013.09.015

Cohen, C., Perrault, G., Voltz, C., Steinberg, R., and Soubrié, P. (2002). SR141716, a central cannabinoid (CB(1)) receptor antagonist, blocks the motivational and dopamine-releasing effects of nicotine in rats. *Behav Pharmacol.* 13, 451–463. doi: 10.1097/00008877-200209000-00018

Colombo, G., Agabio, R., Diaz, G., Lobina, C., Reali, R., and Gessa, G. L. (1998). Appetite suppression and weight loss after the cannabinoid antagonist SR 141716. *Life Sci.* 63, PL113–117. doi: 10.1016/S0024-3205(98)00322-1

Cota, D., Marsicano, G., Lutz, B., Vicennati, V., Stalla, G. K., Pasquali, R., et al. (2003). Endogenous cannabinoid system as a modulator of food intake. *Int. J. Obes. Relat. Metab. Disord.* 27, 289–301. doi: 10.1038/sj.ijo.0802250

Cravatt, B. F., Prospero-Garcia, O., Siuzdak, G., Gilula, N. B., Henriksen, S. J., Boger, D. L., et al. (1995). Chemical characterization of a family of brain lipids that induce sleep. *Science* 268, 1506–1509. doi: 10.1126/science.7770779

Crespo, I., Gómez de Heras, R., Rodríguez de Fonseca, F., and Navarro, M. (2008). Pretreatment with subeffective doses of Rimonabant attenuates orexigenic actions of orexin A-hypocretin 1. *Neuropharmacology* 54, 219–225. doi: 10.1016/j.neuropharm.2007.05.027

Cristino, L., Busetto, G., Imperatore, R., Ferrandino, I., Palomba, L., Silvestri, C., et al. (2013). Obesity-driven synaptic remodeling affects endocannabinoid control of orexinergic neurons. *Proc. Natl. Acad. Sci. U.S.A.* 110, E2229–E2238. doi: 10.1073/pnas.1219485110

Date, Y., Ueta, Y., Yamashita, H., Yamaguchi, H., Matsukura, S., Kangawa, K., et al. (1999). Orexins, orexigenic hypothalamic peptides, interact with autonomic, neuroendocrine and neuroregulatory systems. *Proc. Natl. Acad. Sci. U.S.A.* 96, 748–753. doi: 10.1073/pnas.96.2.748

Davis, S. F., Williams, K. W., Xu, W., Glatzer, N. R., and Smith, B. N. (2003). Selective enhancement of synaptic inhibition by hypocretin (orexin) in rat vagal motor neurons: implications for autonomic regulation. *J. Neurosci.* 23, 3844–3854.

Deadwyler, S. A., Hampson, R. E., Mu, J., Whyte, A., and Childers, S. (1995). Cannabinoids modulate voltage sensitive potassium A-current in hippocampal neurons via a cAMP-dependent process. *J. Pharmacol. Exp. Ther.* 273, 734–743.

de Lecea, L., Kilduff, T. S., Peyron, C., Gao, X., Foye, P. E., Danielson, P. E. et al. (1998). The hypocretins: hypothalamus-specific peptides with neuroexcitatory activity. *Proc. Natl. Acad. Sci. U.S.A.* 95, 322–327. doi: 10.1073/pnas.95.1.322

Demuth, D. G., and Molleman, A. (2006). Cannabinoid signalling. *Life Sci.* 78, 549–563. doi: 10.1016/j.lfs.2005.05.055

Derkinderen, P., Ledent, C., Parmentier, M., and Girault, J. A. (2001). Cannabinoids activate p38 mitogen-activated protein kinases through CB1 receptors in hippocampus. *J. Neurochem.* 77, 957–960. doi: 10.1046/j.1471-4159.2001.00333.x

Devane, W. A., Hanus, L., Breuer, A., Pertwee, R. G., Stevenson, L. A., Griffin, G., et al. (1992). Isolation and structure of a brain constituent that binds to the cannabinoid receptor. *Science* 258, 1946–1949. doi: 10.1126/science.1470919

Di Chiara, G., Bassareo, V., Fenu, S., De Luca, M. A., Spina, L., Cadoni, C., et al. (2004). Dopamine and drug addiction: the nucleus accumbens shell connection. *Neuropharmacology* 47(Suppl. 1), 227–241. doi: 10.1016/j.neuropharm.2004.06.032

Di Marzo, V. (2009). The endocannabinoid system: its general strategy of action, tools for its pharmacological manipulation and potential therapeutic exploitation. *Pharmacol Res.* 60, 77–84. doi: 10.1016/j.phrs.2009.02.010

Di Marzo, V., Goparaju, S. K., Wang, L., Liu, J., Bátkai, S., Járai, Z., et al. (2001). Leptin-regulated endocannabinoids are involved in maintaining food intake. *Nature* 410, 822–825. doi: 10.1038/35071088

Di Marzo, V., and Matias, I. (2005). Endocannabinoid control of food intake and energy balance. *Nat. Neurosci.* 8, 585–589. doi: 10.1038/nn1457

Dogrul, A., Gardell, L. R., Ma, S., Ossipov, M. H., Porreca, F., and Lai, J. (2002). "Knock-down" of spinal CB1 receptors produces abnormal pain and elevates spinal dynorphin content in mice. *Pain* 100, 203–209. doi: 10.1016/S0304-3959(02)00302-0

Drew, L. J., Harris, J., Millns, P. J., Kendall, D. A., and Chapman, V. (2000). Activation of spinal cannabinoid 1 receptors inhibits C-fibre driven hyperexcitable neuronal responses and increases [35S]GTPgammaS binding in the dorsal horn of the spinal cord of noninflamed and inflamed rats. *Eur. J. Neurosci.* 12, 2079–2086. doi: 10.1046/j.1460-9568.2000.00101.x

Elias, C. F., Saper, C. B., Maratos-Flier, E., Tritos, N. A., Lee, C., Kelly, J., et al. (1998). Chemically defined projections linking the mediobasal hypothalamus and the lateral hypothalamic area. *J. Comp. Neurol.* 402, 442–459. doi: 10.1002/(SICI)1096-9861(19981228)402:4<442::AID-CNE2>3.3.CO;2-I

Ellis, J., Pediani, J. D., Canals, M., Milasta, S., and Milligan, G. (2006). Orexin-1 receptor-cannabinoid CB1 receptor heterodimerization results in both ligand-dependent and -independent coordinated alterations of receptor localization and function. *J. Biol. Chem.* 281, 38812–38824. doi: 10.1074/jbc.M602494200

Endoh, T. (2006). Pharmacological characterization of inhibitory effects of post-synaptic opioid and cannabinoid receptors on calcium currents in neonatal rat nucleus tractus solitarius. *Br. J. Pharmacol.* 147, 391–401. doi: 10.1038/sj.bjp.0706623

Eriksson, K. S., Sergeeva, O., Brown, R. E., and Haas, H. L. (2001). Orexin/hypocretin excites the histaminergic neurons of the tuberomammillary nucleus. *J. Neurosci.* 21, 9273–9279.

Eriksson, K. S., Sergeeva, O. A., Haas, H. L., and Selbach, O. (2010). Orexins/hypocretins and aminergic systems. *Acta Physiol. (Oxf.)* 198, 263–275. doi: 10.1111/j.1748-1716.2009.02015.x

España, R. A., Melchior, J. R., Roberts, D. C., and Jones, S. R. (2011). Hypocretin 1/orexin A in the ventral tegmental area enhances dopamine responses to cocaine and promotes cocaine self-administration. *Psychopharmacology (Berl.)* 214, 415–426. doi: 10.1007/s00213-010-2048-8

Fadda, P., Scherma, M., Spano, M. S., Salis, P., Melis, V., Fattore, L., et al. (2006). Cannabinoid self-administration increases dopamine release in the nucleus accumbens. *Neuroreport* 17, 1629–1632. doi: 10.1097/01.wnr.00002 36853.40221.8e

Fattore, L., Cossu, G., Martellotta, C. M., and Fratta, W. (2001). Intravenous self-administration of the cannabinoid CB1 receptor agonist WIN 55,212-2 in rats. *Psychopharmacology (Berl.)* 156, 410–416. doi: 10.1007/s002130100734

Fernández-Ruiz, J., Hernández, M., and Ramos, J. A. (2010). Cannabinoid-dopamine interaction in the pathophysiology and treatment of CNS disorders. *CNS Neurosci. Ther.* 16, e72–e91. doi: 10.1111/j.1755-5949.2010.00144.x

Ferré, S., Lluís, C., Justinova, Z., Quiroz, C., Orru, M., Navarro, G. et al. (2009). Adenosine-cannabinoid receptor interactions. Implications for striatal function. *Br. J. Pharmacol.* 160, 443–453. doi: 10.1111/j.1476-5381.2010.00723.x

Finn, D. P., Jhaveri, M. D., Beckett, S. R., Roe, C. H., Kendall, D. A., Marsden, C. A., et al. (2003). Effects of direct periaqueductal gray administration of a cannabinoid receptor agonist on nociceptive and aversive responses in rats. *Neuropharmacology* 45, 594–604. doi: 10.1016/S0028-3908(03) 00235-1

Flores, Á., Maldonado, R., and Berrendero, F. (2013). The hypocretin/orexin receptor-1 as a novel target to modulate cannabinoid reward. *Biol. Psychiatry.* doi: 10.1016/j.biopsych.2013.06.012. [Epub ahead of print].

Funato, H., Tsai, A. L., Willie, J. T., Kisanuki, Y., Williams, S. C., Sakurai, T., et al. (2009). Enhanced orexin receptor-2 signaling prevents diet-induced obesity and improves leptin sensitivity. *Cell Metab.* 9, 64–76. doi: 10.1016/j.cmet.2008.10.010

Gallate, J. E., and McGregor, I. S. (1999). The motivation for beer in rats: effects of ritanserin, naloxone and SR 141716. *Psychopharmacology (Berl.)* 142, 302–308. doi: 10.1007/s002130050893

Galve-Roperh, I., Rueda, D., Gómez del Pulgar, T., Velasco, G., and Guzmán, M. (2002). Mechanism of extracellular signal-regulated kinase activation by the CB(1) cannabinoid receptor. *Mol. Pharmacol.* 62, 1385–1392. doi: 10.1124/mol.62.6.1385

Girault, E. M., Yi, C. X., Fliers, E., and Kalsbeek, A. (2012). Orexins, feeding, and energy balance. *Prog. Brain Res.* 198, 47–64. doi: 10.1016/B978-0-444-59489-1.00005-7

Glass, M., and Felder, C. C. (1997). Concurrent stimulation of cannabinoid CB1 and dopamine D2 receptors augments cAMP accumulation in striatal neurons: evidence for a Gs linkage to the CB1 receptor. *J. Neurosci.* 17, 5327–5333.

Gomes, I., Fujita, W., Chandrakala, M. V., and Devi, L. A. (2013). Disease-specific heteromerization of G-protein-coupled receptors that target drugs of abuse. *Prog. Mol. Biol. Transl. Sci.* 117, 207–265. doi: 10.1016/B978-0-12-386931-9.00009-X

Gómez del Pulgar, T., Velasco, G., and Guzmán, M. (2000). The CB1 cannabinoid receptor is coupled to the activation of protein kinase B/Akt. *Biochem. J.* 347, 369–373. doi: 10.1042/0264-6021:3470369

Gong, J. P., Onaivi, E. S., Ishiguro, H., Liu, Q. R., Tagliaferro, P. A., Brusco, A., et al. (2006). Cannabinoid CB2 receptors: immunohistochemical localization in rat brain. *Brain Res.* 1071, 10–23. doi: 10.1016/j.brainres.2005.11.035

Gorojankina, T., Grébert, D., Salesse, R., Tanfin, Z., and Caillol, M. (2007). Study of orexins signal transduction pathways in rat olfactory mucosa and in olfactory sensory neurons-derived cell line Odora: multiple orexin signalling pathways. *Regul. Pept.* 141, 73–85. doi: 10.1016/j.regpep.2006.12.012

Grudt, T. J., van den Pol, A. N., and Perl, ER. (2002). Hypocretin-2 (orexin-B) modulation of superficial dorsal horn activity in rat. *J. Physiol.* 538, 517–525. doi: 10.1113/jphysiol.2001.013120

Haj-Dahmane, S., and Shen, R. Y. (2005). The wake-promoting peptide orexin-B inhibits glutamatergic transmission to dorsal raphe nucleus serotonin neurons through retrograde endocannabinoid signaling. *J. Neurosci.* 25, 896–905. doi: 10.1523/JNEUROSCI.3258-04.2005

Hall, W., and Degenhardt, L. (2009). Adverse health effects of non-medical cannabis use. *Lancet* 374, 1383–1391. doi: 10.1016/S0140-6736(09) 61037-0

Hampson, R. E., Evans, G. J., Mu, J., Zhuang, S. Y., King, V. C., Childers, S. R, et al. (1995). Role of cyclic AMP dependent protein kinase in cannabinoid receptor modulation of potassium "A-current" in cultured rat hippocampal neurons. *Life Sci.* 56, 2081–2088. doi: 10.1016/0024-3205(95)00192-9

Hanus, L., Abu-Lafi, S., Fride, E., Breuer, A., Vogel, Z., Shalev, D. E., et al. (2001). 2-arachidonyl glyceryl ether, an endogenous agonist of the cannabinoid CB1 receptor. *Proc. Natl. Acad. Sci. U.S.A.* 98, 3662–3665. doi: 10.1073/pnas.0610 29898

Häring, M., Guggenhuber, S., and Lutz, B. (2012). Neuronal populations mediating the effects of endocannabinoids on stress and emotionality. *Neuroscience* 204, 145–158. doi: 10.1016/j.neuroscience.2011.12.035

Haynes, A. C., Jackson, B., Chapman, H., Tadayyon, M., Johns, A., Porter, R. A. et al. (2000). A selective orexin-1 receptor antagonist reduces food consumption in male and female rats. *Regul. Pept.* 96, 45–51. doi: 10.1016/S0167-0115(00)00199-3

Herkenham, M., Lynn, A. B., Little, M. D., Johnson, M. R., Melvin, L. S., de Costa, B. R., et al. (1990). Cannabinoid receptor localization in brain. *Proc. Natl. Acad. Sci. U.S.A.* 87, 1932–1936. doi: 10.1073/pnas.87.5.1932

Herrera-Solís, A., Vásquez, K. G., and Prospéro-García, O. (2010). Acute and subchronic administration of anandamide or oleamide increases REM sleep in rats. *Pharmacol. Biochem. Behav.* 95, 106–112. doi: 10.1016/j.pbb.2009.12.014

Hervieu, G. J., Cluderay, J. E., Harrison, D. C., Roberts, J. C., and Leslie, R. A. (2001). Gene expression and protein distribution of the orexin-1 receptor in the rat brain and spinal cord. *Neuroscience* 103, 777–797. doi: 10.1016/S0306-4522(01)00033-1

Herzberg, U., Eliav, E., Bennett, G. J., and Kopin, I. J. (1997). The analgesic effects of R(+)-WIN 55,212-2 mesylate, a high affinity cannabinoid agonist, in a rat model of neuropathic pain. *Neurosci. Lett.* 221, 157–160. doi: 10.1016/S0304-3940(96)13308-5

Hilairet, S., Bouaboula, M., Carrière, D., Le Fur, G., and Casellas, P. (2003). Hypersensitization of the Orexin 1 receptor by the CB1 receptor: evidence for cross-talk blocked by the specific CB1 antagonist, SR141716. *J. Biol Chem.* 278, 23731–23737. doi: 10.1074/jbc.M212369200

Ho, Y. C., Lee, H. J., Tung, L. W., Liao, Y. Y., Fu, S. Y., Teng, S. F., et al. (2011). Activation of orexin 1 receptors in the periaqueductal gray of male rats leads to antinociception via retrograde endocannabinoid (2-arachidonoylglycerol)-induced disinhibition. *J. Neurosci.* 31, 14600–14610. doi: 10.1523/JNEUROSCI.2671-11.2011

Hohmann, A. G., and Suplita, R. L. 2nd. (2006). Endocannabinoid mechanisms of pain modulation. *AAPS J.* 8, E693–E708. doi: 10.1208/aapsj080479

Hollander, J. A., Lu, Q., Cameron, M. D., Kamenecka, T. M., and Kenny, P. J. (2008). Insular hypocretin transmission regulates nicotine reward. *Proc. Natl. Acad. Sci. U.S.A.* 105, 19480–19485. doi: 10.1073/pnas.0808023105

Holmqvist, T., Johansson, L., Ostman, M., Ammoun, S., Akerman, K. E., and Kukkonen, J. P. (2005). OX1 orexin receptors couple to adenylyl cyclase regulation via multiple mechanisms. *J. Biol. Chem.* 280, 6570–6579. doi: 10.1074/jbc.M407397200

Howlett, A. C., Barth, F., Bonner, T. I., Cabral, G., Casellas, P., Devane, W. A., et al. (2002). International Union of Pharmacology. XXVII. Classification of cannabinoid receptors. *Pharmacol. Rev.* 54, 161–202. doi: 10.1124/pr.54.2.161

Howlett, A. C., Qualy, J. M., and Khachatrian, L. L. (1986). Involvement of Gi in the inhibition of adenylate cyclase by cannabimimetic drugs. *Mol. Pharmacol.* 29, 307–313.

Howlett, A. C., Reggio, P. H., Childers, S. R., Hampson, R. E., Ulloa, N. M., and Deutsch, D. G. (2011). Endocannabinoid tone versus constitutive activity of cannabinoid receptors. *Br. J. Pharmacol.* 163, 1329–1343. doi: 10.1111/j.1476-5381.2011.01364.x

Huang, H., Acuna-Goycolea, C., Li, Y., Cheng, H. M., Obrietan, K., and van den Pol, A. N. (2007). Cannabinoids excite hypothalamic melanin-concentrating hormone but inhibit hypocretin/orexin neurons: implications for cannabinoid actions on food intake and cognitive arousal. *J. Neurosci.* 27, 4870–4881. doi: 10.1523/JNEUROSCI.0732-07.2007

Hungund, B. L., Szakall, I., Adam, A., Basavarajappa, B. S., and Vadasz, C. (2003). Cannabinoid CB1 receptor knockout mice exhibit markedly reduced voluntary alcohol consumption and lack alcohol-induced dopamine release in the nucleus accumbens. *J. Neurochem.* 84, 698–704. doi: 10.1046/j.1471-4159.2003.01576.x

Hwang, L. L., Chen, C. T., and Dun, N. J. (2001). Mechanisms of orexin-induced depolarizations in rat dorsal motor nucleus of vagus neurones *in vitro*. *J. Physiol.* 537, 511–520. doi: 10.1111/j.1469-7793.2001.00511.x

Ishibashi, M., Takano, S., Yanagida, H., Takatsuna, M., Nakajima, K., Oomura, Y., et al. (2005). Effects of orexins/hypocretins on neuronal activity in the paraventricular nucleus of the thalamus in rats *in vitro*. *Peptides* 26, 471–481. doi: 10.1016/j.peptides.2004.10.014

Jäntti, M. H., Putula, J., Turunen, P. M., Näsman, J., Reijonen, S., Lindqvist, C., et al. (2013). Autocrine endocannabinoid signaling through CB1 receptors potentiates OX1 orexin receptor signaling. *Mol. Pharmacol.* 83, 621–632. doi: 10.1124/mol.112.080523

Jarrahian, A., Watts, V. J., and Barker, E. L. (2004). D2 dopamine receptors modulate Galpha-subunit coupling of the CB1 cannabinoid receptor. *J. Pharmacol. Exp. Ther.* 308, 880–886. doi: 10.1124/jpet.103.057620

Kano, M., Ohno-Shosaku, T., Hashimotodani, Y., Uchigashima, M., and Watanabe, M. (2009). Endocannabinoid-mediated control of synaptic transmission. *Physiol. Rev.* 89, 309–380. doi: 10.1152/physrev.00019.2008

Kirkham, T. C., Williams, C. M., Fezza, F., and Di Marzo, V. (2002). Endocannabinoid levels in rat limbic forebrain and hypothalamus in relation to fasting, feeding and satiation: stimulation of eating by 2-arachidonoyl glycerol. *Br. J. Pharmacol.* 36, 550–557. doi: 10.1038/sj.bjp.0704767

Korotkova, T. M., Sergeeva, O. A., Eriksson, K. S., Haas, H. L., and Brown, R. E. (2003). Excitation of ventral tegmental area dopaminergic and nondopaminergic neurons by orexins/hypocretins. *J. Neurosci.* 23, 7–11.

Kukkonen, J. P. (2011). A ménage à trois made in heaven: G-protein-coupled receptors, lipids and TRP channels. *Cell Calcium.* 50, 9–26. doi: 10.1016/j.ceca.2011.04.005

Kukkonen, J. P. (2012). Physiology of the orexinergic/hypocretinergic system: a revisit in 2012. *Am. J. Physiol. Cell Physiol.* 304, C2–C32. doi: 10.1152/ajpcell.00227.2012

Kukkonen, J. P., and Akerman, K. E. (2001). Orexin receptors couple to Ca2+ channels different from store-operated Ca2+ channels. *Neuroreport* 12, 2017–2020. doi: 10.1097/00001756-200107030-00046

Kukkonen, J. P., Holmqvist, T., Ammoun, S., and Akerman, K. E. (2002). Functions of the orexinergic/hypocretinergic system. *Am. J. Physiol. Cell Physiol.* 283, C1567–C1591. doi: 10.1152/ajpcell.00055.2002

Kukkonen, J. P., and Leonard, C. S. (2013). Orexin/hypocretin receptor signalling cascades. *Br. J. Pharmacol.* doi: 10.1111/bph.12324. [Epub ahead of print].

La Porta, C., Bura, S. A., Aracil-Fernández, A., Manzanares, J., and Maldonado, R. (2013). Role of CB1 and CB2 cannabinoid receptors in the development of joint pain induced by monosodium iodoacetate. *Pain.* 154, 160–174. doi: 10.1016/j.pain.2012.10.009

Larsson, K. P., Peltonen, H. M., Bart, G., Louhivuori, L. M., Penttonen, A., Antikainen, M., et al. (2005). Orexin-A-induced Ca2+ entry: evidence for involvement of trpc channels and protein kinase C regulation. *J. Biol. Chem.* 280, 1771–1781. doi: 10.1074/jbc.M406073200

Lawrence, A. J., Cowen, M. S., Yang, H. J., Chen, F., and Oldfield, B. (2006). The orexin system regulates alcohol-seeking in rats. *Br. J. Pharmacol.* 148, 752–759. doi: 10.1038/sj.bjp.0706789

Lecca, D., Cacciapaglia, F., Valentini, V., and Di Chiara, G. (2006). Monitoring extracellular dopamine in the rat nucleus accumbens shell and core during acquisition and maintenance of intravenous WIN 55,212-2 self-administration. *Psychopharmacology (Berl.)* 188, 63–74. doi: 10.1007/s00213-006-0475-3

Lee, H. J., and Chiou, L. C. (2009). Orexins reduce nociceptive response via endocannabinoid signaling in the midbrain ventrolateral periaqueductal gray. Chicago, IL., USA. *Neuroscience* Prog. No. 458.14.

Lee, M. G., Hassani, O. K., and Jones, B. E. (2005). Discharge of identified orexin/hypocretin neurons across the sleep-waking cycle. *J. Neurosci.* 25, 6716–6720. doi: 10.1523/JNEUROSCI.1887-05.2005

LeSage, M. G., Perry, J. L., Kotz, C. M., Shelley, D., and Corrigall, W. A. (2010). Nicotine self-administration in the rat: effects of hypocretin antagonists and changes in hypocretin mRNA. *Psychopharmacology (Berl.)* 209, 203–212. doi: 10.1007/s00213-010-1792-0

Li, Y., Gao, X. B., Sakurai, T., and van den Pol, A. N. (2002). Hypocretin/Orexin excites hypocretin neurons via a local glutamate neuron-A potential mechanism for orchestrating the hypothalamic arousal system. *Neuron* 36, 1169–1181. doi: 10.1016/S0896-6273(02)01132-7

Lichtman, A. H., Cook, S. A., and Martin, B. R. (1996). Investigation of brain sites mediating cannabinoid-induced antinociception in rats: evidence supporting periaqueductal gray involvement. *J. Pharmacol. Exp. Ther.* 276, 585–593.

Lichtman, A. H., and Martin, B. R. (1991). Spinal and supraspinal components of cannabinoid-induced antinociception. *J. Pharmacol. Exp. Ther.* 258, 517–523.

Lin, L., Faraco, J., Li, R., Kadotani, H., Rogers, W., Lin, X., et al. (1999). The sleep disorder canine narcolepsy is caused by a mutation in the hypocretin (orexin) receptor 2 gene. *Cell* 98, 365–376. doi: 10.1016/S0092-8674(00)81965-0

Liu, R. J., van den Pol, A. N., and Aghajanian, G. K. (2002). Hypocretins (orexins) regulate serotonin neurons in the dorsal raphe nucleus by excitatory direct and inhibitory indirect actions. *J. Neurosci.* 22, 9453–9464.

Ma, X., Zubcevic, L., Brüning, J. C., Ashcroft, F. M., and Burdakov, D. (2007). Electrical inhibition of identified anorexigenic POMC neurons by orexin/hypocretin. *J. Neurosci.* 27, 1529–1533. doi: 10.1523/JNEUROSCI.3583-06.2007

Maccioni, P., Pes, D., Carai, M. A., Gessa, G. L., and Colombo, G. (2008). Suppression by the cannabinoid CB1 receptor antagonist, rimonabant, of the reinforcing and motivational properties of a chocolate-flavoured beverage in rats. *Behav. Pharmacol.* 19, 197–209. doi: 10.1097/FBP.0b013e3282fe8888

Mackie, K. (2005). Distribution of cannabinoid receptors in the central and peripheral nervous system. *Handb. Exp. Pharmacol.* 168, 299–325. doi: 10.1007/3-540-26573-2_10

Mahler, S. V., Smith, K. S., and Berridge, K. C. (2007). Endocannabinoid hedonic hotspot for sensory pleasure: anandamide in nucleus accumbens shell enhances "liking" of a sweet reward. *Neuropsychopharmacology* 32, 2267–2278. doi: 10.1038/sj.npp.1301376

Mahler, S. V., Smith, R. J., and Aston-Jones, G. (2013). Interactions between VTA orexin and glutamate in cue-induced reinstatement of cocaine seeking in rats. *Psychopharmacology (Berl.)* 226, 687–698. doi: 10.1007/s00213-012-2681-5

Mahler, S. V., Smith, R. J., Moorman, D. E., Sartor, G. C., and Aston-Jones, G. (2012). Multiple roles for orexin/hypocretin in addiction. *Prog. Brain Res.* 198, 79–121. doi: 10.1016/B978-0-444-59489-1.00007-0

Maldonado, R., Berrendero, F., Ozaita, A., and Robledo, P. (2011). Neurochemical basis of cannabis addiction. *Neuroscience* 181, 1–17. doi: 10.1016/j.neuroscience.2011.02.035

Maldonado, R., Valverde, O., and Berrendero, F. (2006). Involvement of the endocannabinoid system in drug addiction. *Trends Neurosci.* 29, 225–232. doi: 10.1016/j.tins.2006.01.008

Marcus, J. N., Aschkenasi, C. J., Lee, C. E., Chemelli, R. M., Saper, C. B., Yanagisawa, M. et al. (2001). Differential expression of orexin receptors 1 and 2 in the rat brain. *J. Comp. Neurol.* 435, 6–25. doi: 10.1002/cne.1190

Martin, B. R. (1986). Cellular effects of cannabinoids. *Pharmacol. Rev.* 38, 45–74.

Martin, M., Ledent, C., Parmentier, M., Maldonado, R., and Valverde, O. (2000). Cocaine, but not morphine, induces conditioned place preference and sensitization to locomotor responses in CB1 knockout mice. *Eur. J. Neurosci.* 11, 4038–4046. doi: 10.1046/j.1460-9568.2000.00287.x

Martin, W. J., Lai, N. K., Patrick, S. L., Tsou, K., and Walker, J. M. (1993). Antinociceptive actions of cannabinoids following intraventricular administration in rats. *Brain Res.* 629, 300–304. doi: 10.1016/0006-8993(93)91334-O

Matsuda, L. A., Lolait, S. J., Brownstein, M. J., Young, A. C., and Bonner, T. I. (1990). Structure of a cannabinoid receptor and functional expression of the cloned cDNA. *Nature* 346, 561–564. doi: 10.1038/346561a0

McGinty, D. J., and Harper, R. M. (1976). Dorsal raphe neurons: depression of firing during sleep in cats. *Brain Res.* 101, 569–575. doi: 10.1016/0006-8993(76)90480-7

Melck, D., Rueda, D., Galve-Roperh, I., De Petrocellis, L., Guzmán, M., and Di Marzo, V. (1999). Involvement of the cAMP/protein kinase A pathway and of mitogen-activated protein kinase in the anti-proliferative effects of anandamide in human breast cancer cells. *FEBS Lett.* 463, 235–240. doi: 10.1016/S0014-5793(99)01639-7

Melis, M., Pistis, M., Perra, S., Muntoni, A. L., Pillolla, G., and Gessa, G. L. (2004). Endocannabinoids mediate presynaptic inhibition of glutamatergic transmission in rat ventral tegmental area dopamine neurons through activation of CB1 receptors. *J. Neurosci.* 24, 53–62. doi: 10.1523/JNEUROSCI.4503-03.2004

Mendizábal, V., Zimmer, A., and Maldonado, R. (2006). Involvement of kappa/dynorphin system in WIN 55,212-2 self-administration in mice. *Neuropsychopharmacology* 31, 1957–1966. doi: 10.1038/sj.npp.1300957

Millns, P. J., Chapman, V., and Kendall, D. A. (2001). Cannabinoid inhibition of the capsaicin-induced calcium response in rat dorsal root ganglion neurones. *Br. J. Pharmacol.* 132, 969–971. doi: 10.1038/sj.bjp.0703919

Mobarakeh, J. I., Takahashi, K., Sakurada, S., Nishino, S., Watanabe, H., Kato, M., et al. (2005). Enhanced antinociception by intracerebroventricularly and intrathecally-administered orexin A and B (hypocretin-1 and -2) in mice. *Peptides* 26, 767–777. doi: 10.1016/j.peptides.2005.01.001

Moorman, D. E., and Aston-Jones, G. (2009). Orexin-1 receptor antagonism decreases ethanol consumption and preference selectively in high-ethanol—preferring Sprague—Dawley rats. *Alcohol.* 43, 379–386. doi: 10.1016/j.alcohol.2009.07.002

Muccioli, G. G. (2010). Endocannabinoid biosynthesis and inactivation, from simple to complex. *Drug Discov. Today* 15, 474–483. doi: 10.1016/j.drudis.2010.03.007

Munro, S., Thomas, K. L., and Abu-Shaar, M. (1993). Molecular characterization of a peripheral receptor for cannabinoids. *Nature* 365, 61–65. doi: 10.1038/365061a0

Murai, Y., and Akaike, T. (2005). Orexins cause depolarization via nonselective cationic and K+ channels in isolated locus coeruleus neurons. *Neurosci. Res.* 51, 55–65. doi: 10.1016/j.neures.2004.09.005

Murillo-Rodríguez, E., Cabeza, R., Méndez-Díaz, M., Navarro, L., and Prospéro-García, O. (2001). Anandamide-induced sleep is blocked by SR141716A, a CB1 receptor antagonist and by U73122, a phospholipase C inhibitor. *Neuroreport* 12, 2131–2136. doi: 10.1097/00001756-200107200-00018

Murray, R. M., Morrison, P. D., Henquet, C., and Di Forti, M. (2007). Cannabis, the mind and society: the hash realities. *Nat. Rev. Neurosci.* 8, 885–895. doi: 10.1038/nrn2253

Nair, S. G., Golden, S. A., and Shaham, Y. (2008). Differential effects of the hypocretin 1 receptor antagonist SB 334867 on high-fat food self-administration and reinstatement of food seeking in rats. *Br. J. Pharmacol.* 154, 406–416. doi: 10.1038/bjp.2008.3

Narita, M., Nagumo, Y., Hashimoto, S., Narita, M., Khotib, J., Miyatake, M., et al. (2006). Direct involvement of orexinergic systems in the activation of the mesolimbic dopamine pathway and related behaviors induced by morphine. *J. Neurosci.* 26, 398–405. doi: 10.1523/JNEUROSCI.2761-05.2006

Navarro, M., Carrera, M. R., Del Arco, I., Trigo, J. M., Koob, G. F., and Rodríguez de Fonseca, F. (2004). Cannabinoid receptor antagonist reduces heroin self-administration only in dependent rats. *Eur. J. Pharmacol.* 501, 235–237. doi: 10.1016/j.ejphar.2004.08.022

Navarro, M., Carrera, M. R., Fratta, W., Valverde, O., Cossu, G., Fattore, L., et al. (2001). Functional interaction between opioid and cannabinoid receptors in drug self-administration. *J. Neurosci.* 21, 5344–5350.

Núñez, E., Benito, C., Pazos, M. R., Barbachano, A., Fajardo, O., González, S., et al. (2004). Cannabinoid CB2 receptors are expressed by perivascular microglial cells in the human brain: an immunohistochemical study. *Synapse* 53, 208–213. doi: 10.1002/syn.20050

Onaivi, E. S., Ishiguro, H., Gong, J. P., Patel, S., Perchuk, A., Meozzi, P. A., et al. (2006). Discovery of the presence and functional expression of cannabinoid CB2 receptors in brain. *Ann. N.Y. Acad. Sci.* 1074, 514–536. doi: 10.1196/annals.1369.052

Parolaro, D., Rubino, T., Viganò, D., Massi, P., Guidali, C., and Realini, N. (2010). Cellular mechanisms underlying the interaction between cannabinoid and opioid system. *Curr. Drug Targets* 11, 393–405. doi: 10.2174/138945010790980367

Pérez-Morales, M., De La Herrán-Arita, A. K., Méndez-Díaz, M., Ruiz-Contreras, A. E., Drucker-Colín, R., and Prospéro-García, O. (2013). 2-AG into the lateral hypothalamus increases REM sleep and cFos expression in melanin concentrating hormone neurons in rats. *Pharmacol. Biochem. Behav.* 108, 1–7. doi: 10.1016/j.pbb.2013.04.006

Pertwee, R. G., Howlett, A. C., Abood, M. E., Alexander, S. P., Di Marzo, V., Elphick, M. R., et al. (2010). International Union of Basic and Clinical Pharmacology. LXXIX. Cannabinoid receptors and their ligands: beyond CB1 and CB2. *Pharmacol. Rev.* 62, 588–631. doi: 10.1124/pr.110.003004

Petrosino, S., Palazzo, E., de Novellis, V., Bisogno, T., Rossi, F., Maione, S., et al. (2007). Changes in spinal and supraspinal endocannabinoid levels in neuropathic rats. *Neuropharmacology* 52, 415–422. doi: 10.1016/j.neuropharm.2006.08.011

Peyron, C., Tighe, D. K., van den Pol, A. N., de Lecea, L., Heller, H. C., Sutcliffe, J. G. et al. (1998). Neurons containing hypocretin (orexin) project to multiple neuronal systems. *J. Neurosci.* 18, 9996–10015.

Pissios, P., Bradley, R. L., and Maratos-Flier, E. (2006). Expanding the scales: the multiple roles of MCH in regulating energy balance and other biological functions. *Endocr. Rev.* 27, 606–620. doi: 10.1210/er.2006-0021

Plaza-Zabala, A., Maldonado, R., and Berrendero, F. (2012). The hypocretin/orexin system: implications for drug reward and relapse. *Mol. Neurobiol.* 45, 424–439. doi: 10.1007/s12035-012-8255-z

Portas, C. M., Thakkar, M., Rainnie, D., and McCarley, R. W. (1996). Microdialysis perfusion of 8-hydroxy-2-(di-n-propylamino)tetralin (8-OH-DPAT) in the dorsal raphe nucleus decreases serotonin release and increases rapid eye movement sleep in the freely moving cat. *J. Neurosci.* 16, 2820–2828.

Porter, A. C., Sauer, J. M., Knierman, M. D., Becker, G. W., Berna, M. J., Bao, J., et al. (2002). Characterization of a novel endocannabinoid, virodhamine, with antagonist activity at the CB1 receptor. *J. Pharmacol. Exp. Ther.* 301, 1020–1024. doi: 10.1124/jpet.301.3.1020

Racz, I., Nadal, X., Alferink, J., Baños, J. E., Rehnelt, J., Martín, M., et al. (2008). Crucial role of CB(2) cannabinoid receptor in the regulation of central immune responses during neuropathic pain. *J. Neurosci.* 28, 12125–12135. doi: 10.1523/JNEUROSCI.3400-08.2008.

Ren, K., and Dubner, R. (2008). Neuron-glia crosstalk gets serious: role in pain hypersensitivity. *Curr. Opin. Anaesthesiol.* 21, 570–579. doi: 10.1097/ACO.0b013e32830edbdf

Richard, D., Guesdon, B., and Timofeeva, E. (2009). The brain endocannabinoid system in the regulation of energy balance. *Best Pract. Res. Clin. Endocrinol. Metab.* 23, 17–32. doi: 10.1016/j.beem.2008.10.007

Riegel, A. C., and Lupica, C. R. (2004). Independent presynaptic and postsynaptic mechanisms regulate endocannabinoid signaling at multiple synapses in the ventral tegmental area. *J. Neurosci.* 24, 11070–11078. doi: 10.1523/JNEUROSCI.3695-04.2004

Robledo, P., Berrendero, F., Ozaita, A., and Maldonado, R. (2008). Advances in the field of cannabinoid-opioid cross-talk. *Addict. Biol.* 13, 213–224. doi: 10.1111/j.1369-1600.2008.00107.x

Rotter, A., Bayerlein, K., Hansbauer, M., Weiland, J., Sperling, W., Kornhuber, J., et al. (2012). Orexin A expression and promoter methylation in patients with cannabis dependence in comparison to nicotine-dependent cigarette smokers and nonsmokers. *Neuropsychobiology* 66, 126–133. doi: 10.1159/000339457

Rueda-Orozco, P. E., Soria-Gómez, E., Montes-Rodríguez, C. J., Pérez-Morales, M., and Prospéro-García, O. (2010). Intrahippocampal administration of anandamide increases REM sleep. *Neurosci. Lett.* 473, 158–162. doi: 10.1016/j.neulet.2010.02.044

Sakurai, T., Amemiya, A., Ishii, M., Matsuzaki, I., Chemelli, R. M., Tanaka, H. et al. (1998). Orexins and orexin receptors: a family of hypothalamic neuropeptides and G protein-coupled receptors that regulate feeding behavior. *Cell* 92, 573–585. doi: 10.1016/S0092-8674(00)80949-6

Sánchez, M. G., Ruiz-Llorente, L., Sánchez, A. M., and Díaz-Laviada, I. (2003). Activation of phosphoinositide 3-kinase/PKB pathway by CB(1) and CB(2) cannabinoid receptors expressed in prostate PC-3 cells. Involvement in Raf-1 stimulation and NGF induction. *Cell Signal.* 15, 851–859. doi: 10.1016/S0898-6568(03)00036-6

Sanchis-Segura, C., Cline, B. H., Marsicano, G., Lutz, B., and Spanagel, R. (2004). Reduced sensitivity to reward in CB1 knockout mice. *Psychopharmacology (Berl.)* 176, 223–232. doi: 10.1007/s00213-004-1877-8

Santucci, V., Storme, J. J., Soubrié, P., and Le Fur, G. (1996). Arousal-enhancing properties of the CB1 cannabinoid receptor antagonist SR 141716A in rats as assessed by electroencephalographic spectral and sleep-waking cycle analysis. *Life Sci.* 58, PL103– PL110. doi: 10.1016/0024-3205(95)02319-4

Saper, C. B., Chou, T. C., and Elmquist, J. K. (2002). The need to feed: homeostatic and hedonic control of eating. *Neuron* 36, 199–211 doi: 10.1016/S0896-6273(02)00969-8

Seagard, J. L., Hopp, F. A., Hillard, C. J., and Dean, C. (2005). Effects of endocannabinoids on discharge of baroreceptive NTS neurons. *Neurosci. Lett.* 381, 334–339. doi: 10.1016/j.neulet.2005.02.044

Sharf, R., Sarhan, M., Brayton, C. E., Guarnieri, D. J., Taylor, J. R., and DiLeone, R. J. (2010). Orexin signaling via the orexin 1 receptor mediates operant responding for food reinforcement. *Biol. Psychiatry* 67, 753–760. doi: 10.1016/j.biopsych.2009.12.035

Shiraishi, T., Oomura, Y., Sasaki, K., and Wayner, M. J. (2000). Effects of leptin and orexin-A on food intake and feeding related hypothalamic neurons. *Physiol. Behav.* 71, 251–261. doi: 10.1016/S0031-9384(00)00341-3

Slipetz, D. M., O'Neill, G. P., Favreau, L., Dufresne, C., Gallant, M., Gareau, Y., et al. (1995). Activation of the human peripheral cannabinoid receptor results in inhibition of adenylyl cyclase. *Mol. Pharmacol.* 48, 352–361.

Smart, D., Sabido-David, C., Brough, S. J., Jewitt, F., Johns, A., Porter, R. A., et al. (2001). SB-334867-A: the first selective orexin-1 receptor antagonist. *Br. J. Pharmacol.* 132, 1179–1182. doi: 10.1038/sj.bjp.0703953

Smith, R. J., and Aston-Jones, G. (2012). Orexin/hypocretin 1 receptor antagonist reduces heroin self-administration and cue-induced heroin seeking. *Eur. J. Neurosci.* 35, 798–804. doi: 10.1111/j.1460-9568.2012.08013.x

Soria, G., Mendizábal, V., Touriño, C., Robledo, P., Ledent, C., Parmentier, M., et al. (2005). Lack of CB1 cannabinoid receptor impairs cocaine self-administration. *Neuropsychopharmacology* 30, 1670–1680. doi.org/10.1038/sj.npp.1300707

Sugiura, T., Kondo, S., Sukagawa, A., Nakane, S., Shinoda, A., Itoh, K., et al. (1995). 2-Arachidonoylglycerol: a possible endogenous cannabinoid receptor ligand in brain. *Biochem. Biophys. Res. Commun.* 215, 89–97. doi: 10.1006/bbrc.1995.2437

Tang, J., Chen, J., Ramanjaneya, M., Punn, A., Conner, A. C., and Randeva, H. S. (2008). The signalling profile of recombinant human orexin-2 receptor. *Cell Signal.* 20, 1651–1661. doi: 10.1016/j.cellsig.2008.05.010

Taslimi, Z., Haghparast, A., Hassanpour-Ezatti, M., and Safari, M. S. (2011). Chemical stimulation of the lateral hypothalamus induces conditioned place preference in rats: involvement of OX1 and CB1 receptors in the ventral tegmental area. *Behav. Brain Res.* 217, 41–46. doi: 10.1016/j.bbr.2010.10.007

Tsujino, N., and Sakurai, T. (2009). Orexin/hypocretin: a neuropeptide at the interface of sleep, energy homeostasis, and reward system. *Pharmacol. Rev.* 61, 162–176. doi: 10.1124/pr.109.001321

Tsuneki, H., Wada, T., and Sasaoka, T. (2010). Role of orexin in the regulation of glucose homeostasis. *Acta Physiol. (Oxf.)* 198, 335–348. doi: 10.1111/j.1748-1716.2009.02008.x

Turunen, P. M., Jäntti, M. H., and Kukkonen, J. P. (2012). OX1 orexin/hypocretin receptor signaling through arachidonic acid and endocannabinoid release. *Mol. Pharmacol.* 82, 156–167. doi: 10.1124/mol.112.078063

Urbańska, A., Sokołowska, P., Woldan-Tambor, A., Biegańska, K., Brix, B., Jöhren, O., et al. (2012). Orexins/hypocretins acting at Gi protein-coupled OX 2 receptors inhibit cyclic AMP synthesis in the primary neuronal cultures. *J. Mol. Neurosci.* 46, 10–17. doi: 10.1007/s12031-011-9526-2

Valassi, E., Scacchi, M., and Cavagnini, F. (2008). Neuroendocrine control of food intake. *Nutr. Metab. Cardiovasc. Dis.* 18, 158–168. doi: 10.1016/j.numecd.2007.06.004

van den Pol, A. N., Gao, X. B., Obrietan, K., Kilduff, T. S., and Belousov, A. B. (1998). Presynaptic and postsynaptic actions and modulation of neuroendocrine neurons by a new hypothalamic peptide, hypocretin/orexin. *J. Neurosci.* 18, 7962–7671.

Van Sickle, M. D., Duncan, M., Kingsley, P. J., Mouihate, A., Urbani, P., Mackie, K., et al. (2005). Identification and functional characterization of brainstem cannabinoid CB2 receptors. *Science* 310, 329–332. doi: 10.1126/science.1115740

Vásquez, C., Navarro-Polanco, R. A., Huerta, M., Trujillo, X., Andrade, F., Trujillo-Hernández, B., et al. (2003). Effects of cannabinoids on endogenous K+ and Ca2+ currents in HEK293 cells. *Can. J. Physiol. Pharmacol.* 81, 436–442. doi: 10.1139/y03-055

Vaughan, C. W., Connor, M., Bagley, E. E., and Christie, M. J. (2000). Actions of cannabinoids on membrane properties and synaptic transmission in rat periaqueductal gray neurons *in vitro*. *Mol. Pharmacol.* 57, 288–295.

Verty, A. N., Allen, A. M., and Oldfield, B. J. (2009). The effects of rimonabant on brown adipose tissue in rat: implications for energy expenditure. *Obesity (Silver Spring)*. 17, 254–261. doi: 10.1038/oby.2008.509

Vittoz, N. M., Schmeichel, B., and Berridge, C. W. (2008). Hypocretin/orexin preferentially activates caudomedial ventral tegmental area dopamine neurons. *Eur. J. Neurosci.* 28, 1629–1640. doi: 10.1111/j.1460-9568.2008.06453.x

Wang, B., You, Z. B., and Wise, R. A. (2009). Reinstatement of cocaine seeking by hypocretin (orexin) in the ventral tegmental area: independence from the local corticotropin-releasing factor network. *Biol. Psychiatry.* 65, 857–862. doi: 10.1016/j.biopsych.2009.01.018

Wang, L., Liu, J., Harvey-White, J., Zimmer, A., and Kunos, G. (2003). Endocannabinoid signaling via cannabinoid receptor 1 is involved in ethanol preference and its age-dependent decline in mice. *Proc. Natl. Acad. Sci. U.S.A.* 100, 1393–1398. doi: 10.1073/pnas.0336351100

Ward, R. J., Pediani, J. D., and Milligan, G. (2011a). Heteromultimerization of cannabinoid CB(1) receptor and orexin OX(1) receptor generates a unique complex in which both protomers are regulated by orexin A. *J. Biol. Chem.* 286, 37414–37428. doi: 10.1074/jbc.M111.287649

Ward, R. J., Pediani, J. D., and Milligan, G. (2011b). Ligand-induced internalization of the orexin OX(1) and cannabinoid CB(1) receptors assessed via N-terminal SNAP and CLIP-tagging. *Br. J. Pharmacol.* 162, 1439–1452. doi: 10.1111/j.1476-5381.2010.01156.x

Watanabe, S., Kuwaki, T., Yanagisawa, M., Fukuda, Y., and Shimoyama. M. (2005). Persistent pain and stress activate pain-inhibitory orexin pathways. *Neuroreport* 16, 5–8. doi: 10.1097/00001756-200501190-00002

Williams, C. M., and Kirkham, T. C. (1999). Anandamide induces overeating: mediation by central cannabinoid (CB1) receptors. *Psychopharmacology (Berl.)* 143, 315–317. doi: 10.1007/s002130050953

Williams, C. M., Rogers, P. J., and Kirkham, T. C. (1998). Hyperphagia in pre-fed rats following oral delta9-THC. *Physiol. Behav.* 65, 343–346. doi: 10.1016/S0031-9384(98)00170-X

Willie, J. T., Chemelli, R. M., Sinton, C. M., Tokita, S., Williams, S. C., Kisanuki, Y. Y., et al. (2003). Distinct narcolepsy syndromes in Orexin receptor-2 and Orexin null mice: molecular genetic dissection of Non-REM and REM sleep regulatory processes. *Neuron* 38, 715–730. doi: 10.1016/S0896-6273(03)00330-1

Wilson-Poe, A. R., Morgan, M. M., Aicher, S. A., and Hegarty, D. M. (2012). Distribution of CB1 cannabinoid receptors and their relationship with mu-opioid receptors in the rat periaqueductal gray. *Neuroscience* 213, 191–200. doi: 10.1016/j.neuroscience.2012.03.038

Wise, R. A. (2004). Dopamine, learning and motivation. *Nat. Rev. Neurosci.* 5, 483–94. doi: 10.1038/nrn1406

Wittmann, G., Deli, L., Kalló, I., Hrabovszky, E., Watanabe, M., Liposits, Z., et al. (2007). Distribution of type 1 cannabinoid receptor (CB1)-immunoreactive axons in the mouse hypothalamus. *J. Comp. Neurol.* 503, 270–279. doi: 10.1002/cne.21383

Woldan-Tambor, A., Biegańska, K., Wiktorowska-Owczarek, A., and Zawilska, J. B. (2011). Activation of orexin/hypocretin type 1 receptors stimulates cAMP synthesis in primary cultures of rat astrocytes. *Pharmacol Rep.* 63, 717–723.

Xie, X., Wisor, J. P., Hara, J., Crowder, T. L., LeWinter, R., Khroyan, T. V., et al. (2008). Hypocretin/orexin and nociceptin/orphanin FQ coordinately regulate analgesia in a mouse model of stress-induced analgesia. *J. Clin. Invest.* 118, 2471–2481. doi: 10.1172/JCI35115

Yamamoto, T., Nozaki-Taguchi, N., and Chiba, T. (2002). Analgesic effect of intrathecally administered orexin-A in the rat formalin test and in the rat hot plate test. *Br. J. Pharmacol.* 137, 170–176. doi: 10.1038/sj.bjp.0704851

Yamanaka, A., Beuckmann, C. T., Willie, J. T., Hara, J., Tsujino, N., Mieda, M., et al. (2003). Hypothalamic orexin neurons regulate arousal according to energy balance in mice. *Neuron* 38, 701–713. doi: 10.1016/S0896-6273(03)00331-3

Yamanaka, A., Kunii, K., Nambu, T., Tsujino, N., Sakai, A., Matsuzaki, I., et al. (2000). Orexin-induced food intake involves neuropeptide Y pathway. *Brain Res.* 859, 404–409. doi: 10.1016/S0006-8993(00)02043-6

Yamanaka, A., Sakurai, T., Katsumoto, T., Yanagisawa, M., and Goto, K. (1999). Chronic intracerebroventricular administration of orexin-A to rats increases food intake in daytime, but has no effect on body weight. *Brain Res.* 849, 248–252. doi: 10.1016/S0006-8993(99)01905-8

Yan, J. A., Ge, L., Huang, W., Song, B., Chen, X. W., and Yu, Z. P. (2008). Orexin affects dorsal root ganglion neurons: a mechanism for regulating the spinal nociceptive processing. *Physiol. Res.* 57, 797–800.

Yang, B., and Ferguson, A. V. (2002). Orexin-A depolarizes dissociated rat area postrema neurons through activation of a nonselective cationic conductance. *J. Neurosci.* 22, 6303–6308.

Yang, B., and Ferguson, A. V. (2003). Orexin-A depolarizes nucleus tractus solitarius neurons through effects on nonselective cationic and K+ conductances. *J. Neurophysiol.* 89, 2167–2175. doi: 10.1152/jn.01088.2002

Yang, B., Samson, W. K., and Ferguson, A. V. (2003). Excitatory effects of orexin-A on nucleus tractus solitarius neurons are mediated by phospholipase C and protein kinase C. *J. Neurosci.* 23, 6215–6222.

Conflict of Interest Statement: The authors declare that the research was conducted in the absence of any commercial or financial relationships that could be construed as a potential conflict of interest.

15

LSN2424100: a novel, potent orexin-2 receptor antagonist with selectivity over orexin-1 receptors and activity in an animal model predictive of antidepressant-like efficacy

Thomas E. Fitch*, **Mark J. Benvenga**, **Cynthia D. Jesudason**, **Charity Zink**, **Amy B. Vandergriff**, **Michelle M. Menezes**, **Douglas A. Schober** and **Linda M. Rorick-Kehn**

Lilly Research Laboratories, Department of Neuroscience, Eli Lilly and Company, Indianapolis, IN, USA

Edited by:
Michel A. Steiner, Actelion Pharmaceuticals Ltd., Switzerland

Reviewed by:
J. M. Monti, Clinics Hospital, Uruguay
Selena Bartlett, Translational Research Institute, Australia
Christine E. Gee, University Medical Center Eppendorf-Hamburg, Germany

*Correspondence:
Thomas E. Fitch, Lilly Corporate Center DC0510, Eli Lilly and Company, Indianapolis, IN 46285, USA
e-mail: fitch_thomas@lilly.com

We describe a novel, potent and selective orexin-2 (OX2)/hypocretin-2 receptor antagonist with *in vivo* activity in an animal model predictive of antidepressant-like efficacy. *N*-biphenyl-2-yl-4-fluoro-*N*-(1H-imidazol-2-ylmethyl) benzenesulfonamide HCl (LSN2424100) binds with high affinity to recombinant human OX2 receptors ($Ki = 4.5$ nM), and selectivity over OX1 receptors ($Ki = 393$ nM). LSN2424100 inhibited OXA-stimulated intracellular calcium release in HEK293 cells expressing human and rat OX2 receptors ($Kb = 0.44$ and 0.83 nM, respectively) preferentially over cells expressing human and rat OX1 ($Kb = 90$ and 175 nM, respectively). LSN2424100 exhibits good exposure in Sprague–Dawley rats after IP, but not PO, administration of a 30 mg/kg dose ($AUC_{0-6h} = 1300$ and 269 ng*h/mL, respectively). After IP administration in rats and mice, LSN2424100 produces dose-dependent antidepressant-like activity in the delayed-reinforcement of low-rate (DRL) assay, a model predictive of antidepressant-like efficacy. Efficacy in the DRL model was lost in mice lacking OX2, but not OX1 receptors, confirming OX2-specific activity. Importantly, antidepressant-like efficacy of the tricyclic antidepressant, imipramine, was maintained in both OX1 and OX2 receptor knock-out mice. In conclusion, the novel OX2 receptor antagonist, LSN2424100, is a valuable tool compound that can be used to explore the role of OX2 receptor-mediated signaling in mood disorders.

Keywords: hypocretin, orexin, neuropeptide, OX2 antagonist, antidepressant, DRL, rat, mouse

INTRODUCTION

The orexin (or hypocretin) family of neuropeptides, termed orexin-A (OXA) and orexin-B (OXB), and the receptors to which they bind, were first identified in the late 1990's (De Lecea et al., 1998; Sakurai et al., 1998). The orexin peptides bind to two G-protein coupled receptors, orexin-1 (OX1) and orexin-2 (OX2), with OXA showing roughly equal affinity for OX1 and OX2 receptors and OXB binding preferentially to OX2 receptors (Spinazzi et al., 2006). Although orexin-containing neurons are predominantly localized in the lateral and posterior hypothalamus, they send widespread projections throughout the neuro-axis (Spinazzi et al., 2006). Orexin has been demonstrated to play a role in mediating feeding (Sakurai et al., 1998), regulation of sleep/wake states (Chemelli et al., 1999), addiction and reward-seeking behavior (Richards et al., 2008; Aston-Jones et al., 2009), monoaminergic transmission (Borgland et al., 2008; Ortega et al., 2012), and stress modulation (Boutrel et al., 2005). That many of these functions are often dysregulated in depression has led researchers to propose that orexins may be involved in the pathophysiology of depression (reviewed in Nollet and Leman, 2013).

The exact role of orexins in modulating mood and depressive disorders has proven more difficult to delineate. Early clinical studies evaluating the potential role of orexin in depressive disorders indicated that depressed patients had a blunted diurnal variation in CSF orexin-A levels accompanied by higher orexin-A levels at night, and that these differences were improved with antidepressant treatment, suggesting a link between disrupted orexin signaling and HPA axis disruption associated with depression (Salomon et al., 2003). However, later studies reported contradictory findings, specifically that CSF orexin-A levels were decreased in depressed patients who had attempted suicide (Brundin et al., 2007). To better understand the role of orexin signaling in depression, some researchers turned to putative genetic animal models of depression, although these studies also produced seemingly contradictory findings. For example, it has been demonstrated that Wistar–Kyoto rats, long-regarded as a genetic model of depression based on enhanced sensitivity to stress and reduced sensitivity to selective serotonin reuptake inhibitors (SSRIs; Lopez-Rubalcava and Lucki, 2000), exhibit reduced numbers of orexin neurons, as well as smaller soma size, lower prepro-orexin mRNA expression, and lower OXA levels in various brain areas (Taheri et al., 2001; Allard et al., 2004). The Flinders Sensitive Line (FSL) is another line of selectively bred animals with a prodepressive phenotype characterized by reduced body weight, reduced sexual behavior, disrupted sleep/wake patterns (particularly REM sleep) and exaggerated immobility responses in the Porsolt Forced swim test (Overstreet and Wegener, 2013). In contrast to results in Wistar–Kyoto rats, the FSL rats were found to have a higher number of OX-immunopositive hypothalamic neurons associated with higher immobility in the forced swim test (Mikrouli et al., 2011). Recently, Nollet et al. (2011) reported that unpredictable chronic mild stress was associated with increased aggression and activation of orexin neurons in the dorsomedial hypothalamus, along with concomitant reductions in the number of OX2, but not OX1, receptors in ventral hippocampus, thalamus and hypothalamus. Interestingly, these effects were reversed by chronic treatment with the SSRI antidepressant, fluoxetine (Nollet et al., 2011). The dual orexin receptor antagonist, almorexant, has also been shown to produce antidepressant-like effects in the chronic unpredictable mild stress model (Nollet et al., 2012). While accumulating evidence suggests that orexin neurotransmission may play a role in modulating mood states, little is known about the molecular mechanisms involved.

A more thorough understanding of the involvement of the orexin system in mediating depression, a complex disorder with multiple behavioral sequelae, would benefit from the availability of precise pharmacological probes from multiple chemical scaffolds. These, in turn, could lead to the development of novel pharmacotherapies targeting the orexin system that could prove beneficial in treating depressive disorders. The OX1 antagonist SB334867 (Smart et al., 2001), and the dual orexin antagonist, almorexant (Brisbare-Roch et al., 2007), have been broadly utilized in preclinical experiments. Although OX2-selective antagonists have been reported in the literature, including TCS-OX2-29 (Hirose et al., 2003), JNJ-10397049 (McAtee et al., 2004), and EMPA (Malherbe et al., 2009), very little has been published on these molecules, especially with regard to antidepressant-like efficacy.

Here, we describe a novel OX2 receptor antagonist N-((1H-imidazol-2-yl)methyl)-N-([1,1'-biphenyl]-2-yl)-4-fluorobenzenesulfonamide hydrochloride (LSN2424100, **Figure 1**), and characterize it in terms of its *in vitro* binding affinity, functional selectivity, and pharmacokinetic properties, and further examine its effects on c-fos expression in the rat prefrontal cortex, a brain region implicated in the pathophysiology of depression (Drevets et al., 2008), in response to restraint stress. We then contrast the effects of this compound in an established animal model predictive of antidepressant-like efficacy, the differential reinforcement of low-rate (DRL) schedule of reinforcement, in both rat (DRL-72; O'Donnell et al., 2005), and mouse (DRL-36; Zhang et al., 2009), as well as mice lacking OX1 and OX2 receptors. The DRL model has been pharmacologically validated for detecting antidepressant-like efficacy using clinical antidepressants across multiple pharmacological classes, including tricyclic antidepressants, SSRIs, norepinephrine reuptake inhibitors, and monoamine oxidase inhibitors as indicated by reduced impulsivity, improved response inhibition, and improved response timing (O'Donnell et al., 2005; Zhang et al., 2009).

MATERIALS AND METHODS
DRUGS AND REAGENTS
N-((1H-imidazol-2-yl)methyl)-N-([1,1'-biphenyl]-2-yl)-4-fluorobenzenesulfonamide hydrochloride (LSN2424100), SB334867, and both (S)-almorexant (ACT-078573; Weller et al., 2005)

and its inactive enantiomer (R)-almorexant were synthesized at Lilly Research Laboratories (Indianapolis, IN; see **Figure 1**). LSN2424100 and SB334867 were suspended in a solution of 1% carboxymethylcellulose, 0.25% polysorbate 80, and 0.05% Dow antifoam and injected IP in a volume of 10 ml/kg body weight for mice and 1 ml/kg in rat (LSN2424100 was injected in a 2 ml/kg volume for c-fos studies). (S)-almorexant and (R)-almorexant were suspended in a solution of 1% carboxymethylcellulose, 0.25% polysorbate 80, and 0.05% Dow antifoam and dosed PO in a volume of 2 ml/kg in rat (dosed IP at 10 ml/kg for mice). Imipramine and alprazolam were purchased from Sigma-Aldrich (St. Louis, MO). Imipramine was dissolved in sterile water. Alprazolam was dissolved in 10% 2-hydroxypropyl-β-cyclodextrin. Drugs were mixed fresh on the day of the experiment and doses were calculated based on the free base weight.

SUBJECTS
Adult Male Sprague–Dawley rats weighing 200–225 g (Harlan, Indianapolis, IN for c-fos experiments) were housed 4 per cage with *ad libitum* access to food (Teklad 4% Rat Diet; Harlan Teklad, Madison, WI) and water (except during experimental sessions) and maintained on a 12 h light:dark cycle (lights on at 0600 h). Rats were acclimated to housing conditions for 4 days, followed by sham dosing once daily for 3 days, prior to the experiment. For DRL experiments, male Sprague–Dawley rats weighing between 300 and 350 g at the beginning of the behavioral experiments (Holtzman, Madison, WI) were housed in pairs. For mouse DRL studies, male C57Bl/6 mice (Taconic Farms, Hudson, NY) or mice lacking either OX1 or OX2 receptors, around 8 weeks of age, were obtained from private breeding colonies at Taconic Farms

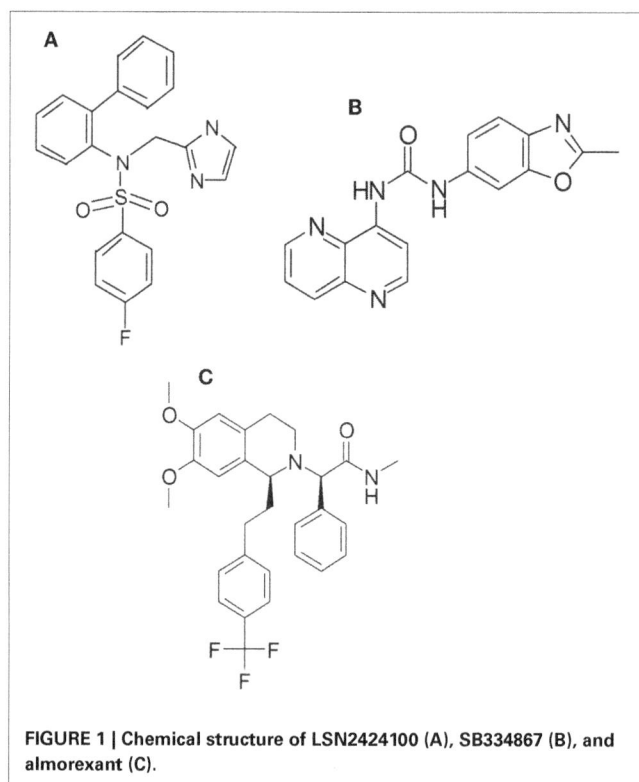

FIGURE 1 | Chemical structure of LSN2424100 (A), SB334867 (B), and almorexant (C).

(Hudson, NY). OX1 and OX2 receptor knockout mice were generated using *in vitro* fertilization of embryos in C57Bl/6 female mice with sperm harvested from male mice obtained from the University of Texas Southwestern Medical Center (Dallas, TX), and backcrossed for at least 10 generations. Mice and rats were housed in separate colony rooms, which were maintained at 22°C and 60% relative humidity. For rat DRL experiments, water was available for a 20-min period following the daily behavioral session. Based on recommendations from the animal care and use committee, the mouse DRL assay was developed using food deprivation rather than water deprivation. Mice had free access to water except during experimental sessions, were maintained at 85% of free-feeding weight, and received 1 h of free-feeding after each experimental session. All experiments were conducted during the light cycle and in compliance with the Guide for the Care and Use of Laboratory Animals under protocols approved by a local animal care and use committee.

RADIOLIGAND BINDING

Recombinant human OX1 or OX2 receptors were stably expressed in HEK293 cells and grown in DMEM/F-12 (3:1) supplemented with 5% FBS, 20 mM HEPES, 100 ug/ml Penn/Strep, and 500 ug/ml geneticin. Briefly, the membranes were isolated by homogenizing cell pellet in 30 ml (w/v) 50 mM Tris buffer (pH 7.4) containing Roche Complete EDTA free protease tablets. Membranes were incubated with $\sim$0.25 nM [^{125}I]-Orexin A (PerkinElmer, Inc., Waltham, MA) for 90 min at 22°C in polystyrene 96-deep well plates. All binding studies were conducted at a final volume of 200 µl. The assay buffer contained 25 mM HEPES, 2.5 mM $CaCl_2$, 1.0 mM $MgCl_2$, 0.5% BSA, and 0.125% BSA (pH 7.4). To generate binding affinity (Ki), 11 different compound concentrations were incubated with $\sim$15 µg of OX1 membrane or $\sim$50 µg of OX2 membrane in the presence of [^{125}I]-Orexin A. Compounds were solubilized to make a 10 mM stock in DMSO then diluted to 40 µM by placing 4 µl into 996 µl binding assay buffer. Then 300 µl of this solution was placed in column B on a Nunc polypropylene 96-well plate (Thermo Fisher Scientific, Inc., Rochester, NY). Serial dilutions were then made using a Biomek 2000 (Beckman Coulter, Inc., Fullerton, CA) from a starting concentration of 40 µM. Non-specific binding was determined in these experiments using 10 µM SB-334867 and LSN2158312 for OX1 and OX2, respectively. All binding was terminated by rapid filtration using a TOMTEC 96-well cell harvester (Hamden, CT) through GF/A filters that had been presoaked with 0.3% polyethyleneimine. The filters were washed with 5.0 ml ice-cold 50 mM Tris buffer (pH 7.4) and air-dried overnight. The dried filters were treated with MeltiLex A (PerkinElmer, Inc., Waltham, MA) melt-on scintillator sheets, and the radioactivity retained on the filters counted using a Wallac 1205 Betaplate (PerkinElmer, Inc., Waltham, MA) scintillation counter. Protein concentrations were measured using Coomassie Protein Plus Assay Reagent (Pierce, Rockford, IL) and serum albumin standards. Ki-values from displacement of [^{125}I]-orexin-A binding were calculated based on 11-point dilution curves using ActivityBase templates (ID Business Solutions, Ltd., Guildford, Surrey, UK). Reported values are shown as a mean ± the standard error of the mean (s.e.m.).

INTRACELLULAR CALCIUM MOBILIZATION

Recombinant human OX1 and OX2 receptors were stably expressed in HEK293 cells, or rat recombinant OX1 and OX2 receptors stably expressed in AV12 cells, and assessed for intracellular calcium mobilization using Fluo-3 dye (Molecular Probes, Eugene, OR). Fluo-3 dye was made at 2.2 mM in equal parts of Pluronic f-127 (Molecular Probes, Eugene, OR) and 100% DMSO. It was further diluted to 8 mM in 2.5 mM probenecid loading buffer which was made as described below. The human cell line was grown in DMEM/F-12 (3:1) supplemented with 10% FBS (heat-inactivated), 20 mM HEPES, 1% Penn/Strep, and 4 µg/ml Blasticidin (35,000 cells/well). The rat cell line was grown in DMEM supplemented with 10% FBS (heat-inactivated), 20 mM HEPES, 1% Penn/Strep, 4 µg/ml Blasticidin, and 1 mM sodium pyruvate (60,000 cells/well). Cells were plated in Biocoat black poly-d-lysine coated clear bottom 96-well plates (Becton Dickinson, Bedford, MA), allowed to attach for 30 min at room temperature, and then grown overnight at 37°C and 5% CO_2 in a humidified incubator. Probenecid loading buffer was made at 250 mM in equal parts of 1 N NaOH and HBSS. It was further diluted to 2.5 mM in HBSS containing calcium and magnesium +20 mM HEPES. The agonist used in this study was Orexin-A (Bachem/Peninsula Laboratories, San Carlos, CA) dissolved in de-ionized water at a stock concentration of 80 µM. An EC_{70} concentration of orexin A in 0.1% BSA (Sigma Aldrich, St. Louis, MO) in HBSS with calcium and magnesium, was used to challenge the antagonists. Compounds were serial diluted 1:3 from a 10 mM stock in DMSO on a Biomek (Beckman Coulter, Inc., Fullerton, CA) and further diluted in HBSS containing calcium and magnesium +0.04% Bacitracin (USB Corp., Cleveland, OH). The assay was performed with the following steps: (1) growth medium was removed and cells were washed with 30 µl HBSS (with calcium and magnesium) and then removed. Next, 30 µl of dye was added to the wells, and cell plates were incubated in the dark at room temperature for 60 min; dye was removed, cells were washed with 30 µl probenecid loading buffer and removed, and then 50 µl of probenecid loading buffer was added to the wells. Finally, plates were read on a fluorescence imaging plate reader (FLIPR; Molecular Devices, LLC, Sunnyvale, CA) instrument with a 50 µl addition of antagonist; cells were placed in the dark at room temperature for an additional 15 min; then read on FLIPR instrument with a 100 µl addition of an EC_{70} concentration of orexin A (for a total volume of 200 µl). Final concentrations of the test compounds were 20 µM in 1.25% DMSO and 10 µM in 0.625% DMSO for the two different FLIPR reads, respectively. Kb-values were calculated based on 10-point dilution curves using ActivityBase templates (ID Business Solutions, Ltd., Guildford, Surrey, UK). Reported values are shown as a mean ± the standard error of the mean (s.e.m.).

RAT EXPOSURE AND UNBOUND FRACTION

Two male cannulated rats were administered a single 30 mg/kg intraperitoneal (IP) or 30 mg/kg oral (PO) dose of LSN2424100 to determine the pharmacokinetic parameters. Plasma samples were collected at 0.5, 1, 1.5, 2, 4, and 6 h post-dose and analyzed by liquid chromatography coupled to tandem mass spectral detection

(LC-MS/MS) to determine the concentrations of LSN2424100. Two cohorts of rats were used in each study, with samples taken from one cohort at 0.5, 1, and 2 h post-dose, and samples taken from the second cohort at 1.5, 4, and 6 h post-dose. The first cohort of animals was sacrificed at 2 h post-dose, and the second at 6 h post-dose to allow for collection of brain samples. The plasma and brain binding of LSN2424100 were determined by equilibrium dialysis at 1 μM which were used to calculate unbound concentrations in brain and plasma at 2 h post-dose (Zamek-Gliszczynski et al., 2011).

RESTRAINT-STRESS-INDUCED c-FOS ACTIVATION

Beginning at 0830 h on the day of the study, groups of rats ($n = 8$ per group) received IP injections of vehicle, 30 mg/kg LSN2424100, or 3 mg/kg alprazolam in a counter-balanced manner and were returned to the home cage. Thirty min later, rats were restrained in a rigid plastic flat-bottom restraint tube (Braintree Scientific, Inc.; Braintree, MA, USA) for 20 min. After the 20 min stress period, rats were moved to a new cage and housed individually. Rats were sacrificed 2 h after stress onset. Separate groups of control animals ($n = 6 - 8$ each) received either vehicle or 30 mg/kg LSN2424100 and were returned to their home cage until sacrifice. Immediately after sacrifice, brains were removed, the medial prefrontal cortex (mPFC), a brain area implicated in the pathophysiology of depression, was dissected from both hemispheres and frozen in 1.5 ml centrifuge tubes in dry ice, and stored at −80°C for later analysis.

c-Fos ELISA ANALYSIS

Frozen mPFC tissues were removed from the −80°C freezer and placed on ice. Tissue was homogenized with a dounce homogenizer. The nuclear extract was prepared from the homogenized samples as per manufacturer's instructions using a CHEMICON®Nuclear Extraction Kit (Millipore; Billerica, MA, USA). Protein concentrations were determined in the nuclear extracts using the Pierce BCA Protein Assay kit (Pierce Biotechnology, Inc., Rockford, IL, USA). Nuclear fractions were then assayed for Fos protein levels using the Pierce c-Fos Transcription Factor Kit (Pierce Biotechnology, Inc., Rockford, IL, USA), according to the manufacturer's instructions. A Wallac 1420 VICTOR luminometer (PerkinElmer; Waltham, MA, USA) was used to measure chemiluminesence in the ELISA plates. Data were analyzed and plotted using GraphPad Prism (GraphPad Software, Inc.; La Jolla, CA, USA).

RAT APPARATUS AND TRAINING

Sixteen operant-conditioning chambers (30.5 × 24.1 × 29.2 cm; MED Associates, St. Albans, VT) were utilized in conducting the DRL experiments. Each chamber was enclosed in a melamine sound-attenuating cubicle. A white noise generator provided masking noise. The interior of each chamber consisted of three levers mounted on one wall with a house light mounted on the opposite wall. The house light was turned on at initiation of each test session and was turned off at the termination of each session. A water access port was situated next to the lever in the middle of the wall, wherein a reinforced response caused a clicker apparatus to sound paired with a dipper (0.02-ml cup) to be lifted from a water trough to an opening in the floor of the access port for 4 s.

Rats were water deprived for ~22.5 h before each session. Rats were initially trained under an alternative fixed ratio 1 water reinforcement schedule with a fixed 1-min time schedule for automatic reinforcement. Thus, each response was reinforced, with water also provided every minute in the absence of a response. Rats that did not acquire lever-pressing behavior following three daily 1-h sessions under this schedule were trained using the method of successive approximation. Following acquisition of lever-pressing behavior, rats were trained daily on DRL 18-s sessions for ~2 weeks, following which they were advanced to DRL 72-s sessions. Responding on these sessions became stable after ~8 weeks. Experimental test sessions lasted for 1 h and were conducted 5 days/week during light hours.

MOUSE APPARATUS AND TRAINING

Twelve operant-conditioning chambers (30.5 × 24.1 × 29.2 cm; MED Associates, St. Albans, VT) were used for the DRL experiments. The levers in these chambers were mounted on one wall with an adjacent food magazine next to the lever in the middle of the wall. A reinforced response caused a clicker apparatus to activate and the pellet feeder to deposit one 45-mg sucrose pellet (BioServ, Frenchtown, NJ) into the food magazine. The house light, which was mounted on the ceiling, was turned on when the session began, remained on throughout the entire session, and was turned off at the end of the session. Each experimental chamber was enclosed in a melamine sound-attenuating cubicle and equipped with a white noise generator to provide masking noise.

Each mouse was initially trained under a variable time 60-s operant schedule for 5 days, followed by fixed ratio-1 ratio schedule for 5 days. After the mice had acquired lever-pressing behavior, they were trained during daily DRL 6-s sessions for ~1 week, then mice progressed through weekly ascending DRL requirements (12, 18, 24, 30 s) before moving to DRL 36-s sessions. The responding on these sessions became stable after ~6 weeks. Experimental sessions lasted for 45 min and were conducted 5 days/week during light hours.

DELAYED REINFORCEMENT OF LOW-RATE (DRL) DATA ANALYSES

Drugs were administered to the animals once or twice weekly with at least 1 week between subsequent drugs to minimize possible carryover effects. Drug treatments were administered on Tuesdays and Fridays. No treatments were administered on other test days. Wednesdays were control days. "Control" behavior was calculated as the pooled mean lever presses or reinforcers received during Wednesday sessions across all Wednesdays for the duration of each study. Performance was normalized to percent of control by dividing total responses (or reinforcers) for each drug or vehicle treatment by the mean number of responses (reinforcers) in the respective pooled control condition, multiplied by 100.

The data analyses were conducted on the raw response and reinforcement data. All behavioral data are expressed as the mean ± s.e.m. normalized to the control condition. The effects of LSN2424100 (3–40 mg/kg), SB334867 (3–40 mg/kg), almorexant (10–100 mg/kg) along with its inactive enantiomer (100 mg/kg), and imipramine (1–15 mg/kg) were analyzed using separate One-Way repeated measures ANOVAs on responses and reinforcements, followed by Dunnett's *post-hoc* tests (alpha = 0.05).

Table 1 | *In vitro* binding and functional activity at human recombinant OX1 and OX2 receptors.

Compound	Receptor binding affinity, Ki(nM)[a]		Functional antagonist activity, Kb (nM)[b]			
	OX1	OX2	hOX1	hOX2	rOX1	rOX2
LSN2424100	393 ± 47 (3)	4.49 ± 1.39 (3)	90.3 ± 17.7 (2)	0.44 ± 0.11 (3)	175 ± 41 (2)	0.83 ± 0.19 (2)
SB334867	173 ± 11 (3)	>10,000 (3)	8.68 ± 1.76 (3)	>10,000 (3)	7.1 ± 0.71 (3)	>10,000 (3)
Almorexant (S)	21 ± 3.2 (2)	6.9 ± 0.18 (2)	2.32 ± 0.18 (3)	1.73 ± 0.35 (3)	3.2 ± 0.7 (4)	4.4 ± 1.6 (4)
Almorexant (R)	>10,000 (2)	>10,000 (2)	>10,000 (2)	>10,000 (2)	NT	NT

[a]*Radioligand binding was performed using HEK293 membranes expressing either human OX1 or OX2 receptors in the presence of $[^{125}I]$-orexin A with a 90 min incubation time. Data represent the mean ± s.e.m. performed on separate occasions with the number of independent experiments in parenthesis. (R) is the inactive enantiomer of almorexant.*

[b]*Inhibition of calcium mobilization from HEK293 cells stably expressing human or rat OX1 or OX2 receptors, respectively. Functional antagonist activity was determined by measuring the effects of an EC_{70} concentration of orexin-A. Data represent the mean ± s.e.m. performed on separate occasions with the number of independent experiments in parenthesis. NT = not tested.*

RESULTS

RADIOLIGAND BINDING AND INTRACELLULAR CALCIUM MOBILIZATION

Using both an orexin filtration binding assay and a functional intracellular calcium mobilization assay performed in antagonist mode, LSN2424100 demonstrated selectivity for human OX2 receptors stably expressed in HEK293 cells over OX1 receptors (**Table 1**). LSN2424100 was approximately 87-fold more potent at OX2 with a Ki of 4.49 nM (OX1 Ki = 393 nM) in the receptor binding assay. In the functional assay, LSN2424100 was over 200-fold more potent for human OX2 with a $Kb = 0.44$ nM whereas the Kb for human OX1 was 90.3 nM. Similar results were obtained in the rat OX receptor cell lines, with rat OX2 and OX1 $Kb = 0.83$ and 175 nM, respectively, indicating 210-fold selectivity. Conversely, SB334867 was more selective for the human OX1 receptor (**Table 1**). SB334867 was completely inactive at the OX2 receptor in both the *in vitro* assays. The measured binding affinity of SB334867 for the OX1 receptor was 173 nM. SB334867 showed potent inhibition of intracellular calcium mobilization, with OX1 Kb in human and rat = 8.68 and 7.1 nM, respectively. In addition to testing selective orexin agents, we also evaluated the non-selective orexin antagonist, almorexant. The more active S-enantiomer of almorexant demonstrated balanced activity for both human OX1 and OX2 receptors (**Table 1**). The binding affinities of (S)-almorexant for OX1 and OX2 receptors were 21 and 6.9 nM, respectively. Similarly, in the functional assay, (S)-almorexant showed roughly equal potency at inhibiting intracellular calcium mobilization in cells expressing hOX1 and hOX2 receptors, with Kb-values of 2.32 and 1.73 nM, respectively. The (R)-enantiomer of almorexant was inactive in both assays.

RAT EXPOSURE AND UNBOUND FRACTION

Pharmacokinetic data for LSN2424100 in rats are summarized in **Table 2**. LSN2424100 exhibits good exposure in Sprague–Dawley rats after IP, but not PO, administration of a 30 mg/kg dose (AUC_{0-6h} = 1300 and 269 ng*h/mL, respectively). Mean maximum plasma concentrations observed following a single 30 mg/kg IP and PO dose were 1170 and 196 ng/ml, respectively at 0.5 h post injection. Mean brain concentrations observed following a single 30 mg/kg IP and PO dose were 77.2 and 33.5 ng/g,

Table 2 | Pharmacokinetic datafor LY2424100[a].

Parameter[b]	30 mg/kg IP	30 mg/kg PO
AUC_{0-6h} (ng*h/ml)	1300	269
C_{max} (ng/ml)	1170	196
t_{max} (hr)	0.5	0.5
Brain concentration[c] (ng/g)	77.2	33.5
Plasma concentration[c] (ng/ml)	149	45.8
Brain:plasma ratio[c]	0.52	0.72
F_u (brain/plasma)	0.0089/0.0341	
C_u^c (brain/plasma, nM)	5.93/2.99	0.67/3.52

[a]*n = 2 cannulated rats/dose.*

[b]*Abbreviations: AUC_{0-6h}, area under the concentration vs. time curve from time 0–6 h; C_{max}, maximum observed drug concentration; t_{max}, time to maximum observed drug concentration; F_u, fraction unbound in brain/plasma; C_u (unbound or free concentration) = $C_{total} \times F_u$.*

[c]*Two hours post treatment.*

respectively, at 2 h post injection. Unbound fraction in plasma and brain were determined to be 0.0341 and 0.0089, respectively.

c-Fos EXPRESSION

Administration of LSN2424100 to subjects in home cages produced no effects on c-fos protein levels in the rat prefrontal cortex, compared to vehicle treated subjects ($p > 0.05$; **Figure 2**). However, restraint stress invoked a significant increase in c-fos expression in vehicle treated rats [$F_{(4, 28)} = 23.19$; $p < 0.001$], and this effect was attenuated by pre-treatment with either LSN2424100 or alprazolam ($p < 0.05$; **Figure 2**).

DRL

In rats, imipramine produced a significant antidepressant-like response, characterized by a decrease in total lever presses emitted (51% of control responding) at 10 mg/kg [$F_{(3, 68)} = 10.16$, $p < 0.0001$] with a concomitant increase in reinforcers received [210% of control responding; $F_{(3, 68)} = 14.47$, $p < 0.001$; **Figure 3A**]. Doses of 1 and 3 mg/kg had no significant effect on behavior. Raw (non-normalized) data for all DRL experiments are provided in Supplementary Table S1. In mice, imipramine also produced an antidepressant-like signature, with an increase in reinforcers received (330% of control, **Figure 3B**) at 15 mg/kg [$F_{(4, 60)} = 7.32, p < 0.001$], and a concomitant decrease in lever presses emitted [70% of control; $F_{(4, 60)} = 4.2, p < 0.005$]. The antidepressant-like effect of imipramine was maintained in mice lacking OX1 receptors, as demonstrated by a dose-dependent increase in reinforcers received up to 15 mg/kg [206% of control; $F_{(3, 44)} = 3.33, p = 0.028$; **Figure 3C**], and a decrease in lever presses emitted (63% of control) but this difference did not quite reach statistical significance [$F_{(3, 44)} = 2.64, p = 0.06$; Dunnett's *post-hoc* test, $p = 0.02$; **Figure 3C**]. Lower doses of imipramine did not affect lever pressing in mice lacking OX1 receptors. Similarly, imipramine produced antidepressant-like effects in mice lacking OX2 receptors, with a significant effect in both lever presses emitted [$F_{(3, 44)} = 6.63, p < 0.001$] and reinforcers received [$F_{(3, 44)} = 7.58, p < 0.001$; 70 and 140% of control, respectively, at 15 mg/kg; **Figure 3D**].

In rats, SB334867 did not produce a significant change in either reinforcers received or total lever presses made, at doses up to 30 mg/kg (**Figure 4A**). Importantly, the positive control used in this test, imipramine, significantly increased reinforcers received [160% of control, $F_{(4, 24)} = 9.22, p < 0.001$] and decreased lever presses [64% of control, $F_{(4, 24)} = 16.21, p < 0.001$]. In mice, SB334867 did not significantly affect lever presses emitted or reinforcers received up to 40 mg/kg ($p > 0.05$; **Figure 4B**). In mice lacking OX1 receptors, SB334867 produced a significant decrease in lever presses emitted at 20 and 40 mg/kg (75 and 35% of control, respectively; $F_{(5, 58)} = 10.5, p < 0.001$), while only producing a significant increase in reinforcers received at 20 mg/kg [166% of control; $F_{(5, 58)} = 3.95, p < 0.005$; **Figure 4C**]. Although an increase reinforcers received was observed at 40 mg/kg (123%), this was not significant. In mice lacking OX2 receptors, SB334867 only produced a disruption of lever pressing at 40 mg/kg [$F_{(5, 58)} = 17.79, p < 0.001$; **Figure 4D**]. At this dose, lever presses emitted were less than 20% of control, while reinforcers received were 75% of control, indicative of the animals' inability to behave within the scheduled operant parameters.

(S)-Almorexant treatment in rats produced a significant increase in reinforcers received [$F_{(3, 30)} = 4.09, p < 0.02$; **Figure 5A**], while the reduction in lever presses emitted did not reach statistical significance ($p > 0.05$). The inactive enantiomer (R)-almorexant produced no effect on behavior at 100 mg/kg ($ps > 0.05$). In mice, (S)-almorexant produced a significant increase in reinforcers received [>400% of control; $F_{(4, 28)} = 5.95, p = 0.001$], while also producing a significant dose-related decrease in lever presses emitted [47% of control; $F_{(4, 28)} = 6.46, p < 0.001$; **Figure 5B**]. Again, (R)-almorexant produced no significant effects on behavior at 100 mg/kg. In mice lacking OX1 receptors, all doses of (S)-almorexant reduced the number of lever presses emitted [10–60 mg/kg; $F_{(4, 51)} = 10.16, p < 0.001$] while a significant increase in reinforcers received was observed at 10 and 40 mg/kg [$F_{(4, 51)} = 4.39, p < 0.004$; **Figure 5C**], although these effects do not appear to be dose-dependent. In these animals, (R)-almorexant also produced effects similar to (S)-almorexant, with significant increases in reinforcers received and a concomitant significant decrease in

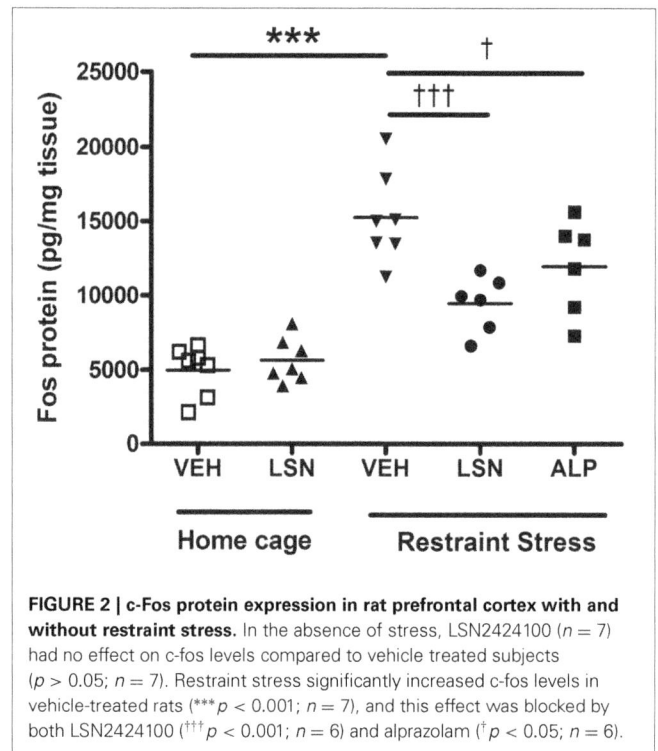

FIGURE 2 | c-Fos protein expression in rat prefrontal cortex with and without restraint stress. In the absence of stress, LSN2424100 ($n = 7$) had no effect on c-fos levels compared to vehicle treated subjects ($p > 0.05$; $n = 7$). Restraint stress significantly increased c-fos levels in vehicle-treated rats (***$p < 0.001$; $n = 7$), and this effect was blocked by both LSN2424100 (†††$p < 0.001$; $n = 6$) and alprazolam (†$p < 0.05$; $n = 6$).

lever pressing [$t_{(54)} = 2.04, p < 0.05$ and $t_{(54)} = 2.04, p < 0.05$, respectively]. In mice lacking OX2 receptors, the effect of (S)-almorexant was completely abolished ($ps > 0.05$; **Figure 5D**). In these mice, (R)-almorexant (100 mg/kg) produced a significant decrease in lever presses emitted [65% of control; $t_{(54)} = 2.04, p < 0.05$], but did not significantly affect the number of reinforcers received.

When administered to rats, LSN2424100 produced a significant increase in reinforcers received [**Figure 6A**; 170% of control; $F_{(4, 24)} = 3.13, p = 0.033$] at 30 mg/kg, along with a significant decrease in lever presses made [60 and 70 of control; $F_{(4, 24)} = 4.64, p = 0.006$] at 10 and 30 mg/kg, respectively. In mice, LSN2424100 produced an increase in reinforcers received (up to 225% of control, **Figure 6B**), but this effect did not reach statistical significance. LSN2424100 treatment did produce a significant decrease in lever presses emitted at 10 mg/kg [50% of control; $F_{(3, 35)} = 3.28, p = 0.032$]. A higher dose of 20 mg/kg produced a decrease in lever presses emitted, but this result did not reach statistical significance (**Figure 6B**). In mice lacking OX1 receptors, the antidepressant-like efficacy of LSN2424100 was maintained, as demonstrated by a statistically significant increase in reinforcers received at 20 mg/kg [200% of control; $F_{(3, 36)} = 2.98, p = 0.044$], and a significant decrease in lever presses emitted at this dose [50% of control; **Figure 6C**; $F_{(3, 36)} = 4.73, p = 0.007$]. In mice lacking OX2 receptors, however, there was no significant change either in reinforcers received or lever presses emitted with LSN2424100 doses administered up to 40 mg/kg (**Figure 6D**), indicating complete loss of antidepressant-like efficacy in OX2 knockout mice.

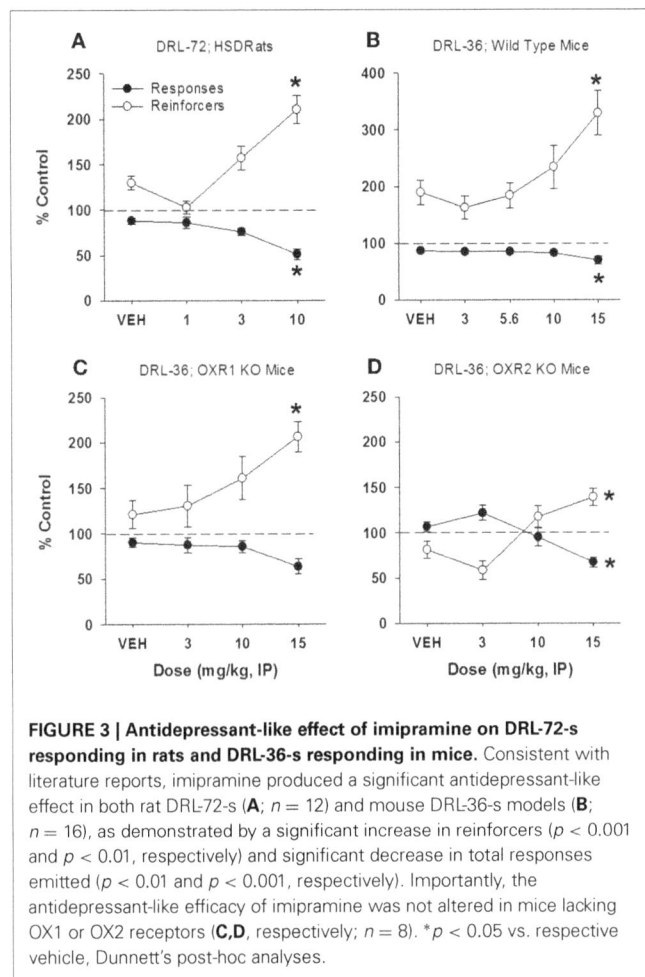

FIGURE 3 | Antidepressant-like effect of imipramine on DRL-72-s responding in rats and DRL-36-s responding in mice. Consistent with literature reports, imipramine produced a significant antidepressant-like effect in both rat DRL-72-s (**A**; $n = 12$) and mouse DRL-36-s models (**B**; $n = 16$), as demonstrated by a significant increase in reinforcers ($p < 0.001$ and $p < 0.01$, respectively) and significant decrease in total responses emitted ($p < 0.01$ and $p < 0.001$, respectively). Importantly, the antidepressant-like efficacy of imipramine was not altered in mice lacking OX1 or OX2 receptors (**C,D**, respectively; $n = 8$). *$p < 0.05$ vs. respective vehicle, Dunnett's post-hoc analyses.

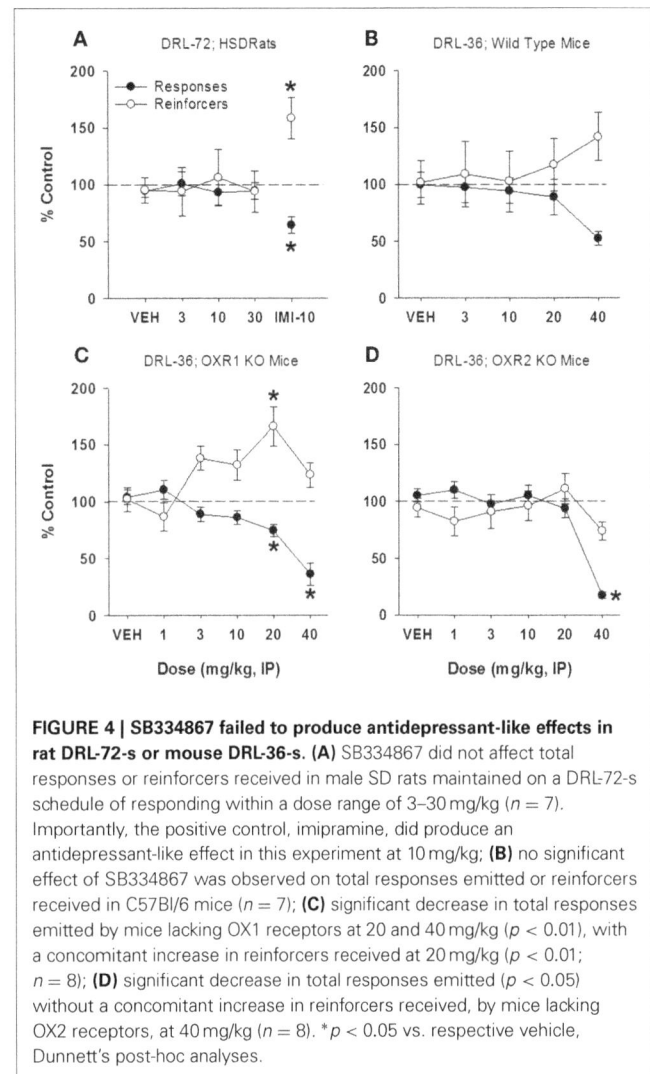

FIGURE 4 | SB334867 failed to produce antidepressant-like effects in rat DRL-72-s or mouse DRL-36-s. (**A**) SB334867 did not affect total responses or reinforcers received in male SD rats maintained on a DRL-72-s schedule of responding within a dose range of 3–30 mg/kg ($n = 7$). Importantly, the positive control, imipramine, did produce an antidepressant-like effect in this experiment at 10 mg/kg; (**B**) no significant effect of SB334867 was observed on total responses emitted or reinforcers received in C57Bl/6 mice ($n = 7$); (**C**) significant decrease in total responses emitted by mice lacking OX1 receptors at 20 and 40 mg/kg ($p < 0.01$), with a concomitant increase in reinforcers received at 20 mg/kg ($p < 0.01$; $n = 8$); (**D**) significant decrease in total responses emitted ($p < 0.05$) without a concomitant increase in reinforcers received, by mice lacking OX2 receptors, at 40 mg/kg ($n = 8$). *$p < 0.05$ vs. respective vehicle, Dunnett's post-hoc analyses.

DISCUSSION

Herein, we describe the pharmacological characterization of a structurally-novel OX2 receptor antagonist, LSN2424100, with high affinity and selectivity for OX2 over OX1 receptors. *In vitro* selectivity data for OX2 over OX1 receptors obtained using radioligand binding and intracellular calcium mobilization assays showed 87- and 205-fold selectivity, respectively (210-fold selectivity in the rat functional assay). Results showed that the two comparator compounds, SB334867 and (S)-almorexant, possessed *in vitro* profiles in the expected ranges, wherein SB334867 showed high affinity and selectivity for OX1 receptors, while the dual orexin antagonist, almorexant, showed roughly equal affinity for OX1 and OX2 receptors. Pharmacokinetic data indicated that LSN2424100 exhibits good exposure in male Sprague–Dawley rats after IP, but not PO, administration of a 30 mg/kg dose ($AUC_{0-6h} = 1300$ and 269 ng*h/mL, respectively), suggesting its use as a tool compound to evaluate the role of OX2 receptor signaling mechanisms in preclinical models.

Here, we report that orexin-2 receptor antagonists, including LSN2424100 and almorexant, exhibit antidepressant-like efficacy in the rat DRL-72 sec model, at 20–30 and 100 mg/kg, respectively, as indicated by significant reductions in total lever presses emitted along with concomitant increases in reinforcers received. Our data are consistent with previous reports that increased OX signaling produced anhedonia-like symptoms in rats (measured by intracranial self-stimulation) (Boutrel et al., 2005), whereas almorexant produced antidepressant-like effects in a model of chronic unpredictable mild stress (Nollet et al., 2012). Interestingly, Nollet et al. (2011) demonstrated that chronic unpredictable mild stress increased activation of dorsomedial hypothalamus/perifornical area (DMH-PFA), where orexin cell bodies are localized. Moreover, they reported that chronic treatment with the SSRI, fluoxetine, reversed the DMH-PFA activation, suggesting a role for orexin signaling in the pathophysiology of depression and antidepressant treatment response (Nollet et al., 2011). The OX1 antagonist SB334867 did not produce antidepressant-like effects in the assays studied here. Together, the pharmacological data suggest that OX2 receptor signaling may be involved in modulating mood states. The results presented here contradict other studies suggesting that increases in orexin-dependent signaling may produce antidepressant-like effects (Ito et al., 2008; Lutter et al., 2008; Scott et al., 2011). The

FIGURE 5 | Antidepressant-like effect of almorexant on DRL-72-s responding in rats and DRL-36-s responding in mice. (A) dose-dependent increase in the number of reinforcers obtained by male SD rats in DRL-72-s, with significant effects at 100 mg/kg ($p < 0.05$), as well as a lack of effect of the inactive enantiomer at 100 mg/kg ($n = 11$); (B) dose-dependent and significant increase in the number of reinforcers obtained ($p < 0.05$) by C57Bl/6 mice in DRL-36-s at 100 mg/kg and a significant decrease ($p < 0.05$) in total responses emitted at 100 mg/kg, as well as lack of effect of the inactive enantiomer at 100 mg/kg ($n = 8$); (C) significant decrease in responses emitted at all doses tested ($p < 0.05$) with a concomitant increase in reinforcers received at doses of 10 and 40 mg/kg ($p < 0.05$) in mice lacking OX1 receptors ($n = 8$). However, 100 mg/kg of the inactive enantiomer also produced significantly fewer responses ($p < 0.05$) with a concomitant increase in reinforcers received ($p < 0.05$) in mice lacking OX1 receptors; (D) almorexant failed to produce antidepressant-like effects in mice lacking OX2 receptors, up to 100 mg/kg ($n = 8$). The inactive enantiomer (100 mg/kg) significantly reduced total responses emitted in mice lacking OX2 receptors ($p < 0.05$), without significantly affecting reinforcers earned ($n = 8$). *$p < 0.05$ vs. respective vehicle, Dunnett's post-hoc analyses.

FIGURE 6 | Antidepressant-like effects of LSN2424100 on DRL-72-s responding in rats and DRL-36-s responding in mice. (A) dose-dependent increase in the number of reinforcers obtained by male SD rats in DRL-72-s ($n = 7$), with a significant effect at 30 mg/kg ($p < 0.05$) and a significant decrease in total responses emitted at 10 and 30 mg/kg ($p < 0.05$); (B) a significant decrease in total responses emitted by C57Bl/6 mice in DRL-36-s at 10 mg/kg ($p < 0.05$; $n = 8$); (C) antidepressant-like efficacy of LSN2424100 is maintained in mice lacking OX1 receptors, with a significant increase in reinforcers obtained and a significant decrease in responses at 20 mg/kg ($p < 0.05$; $n = 8$); (D) antidepressant-like effect of LSN2424100 is lost in mice lacking OX2 receptors, as illustrated by lack of significant effects in either responses emitted or reinforcers received at all doses ($n = 8$). *$p < 0.05$ vs. respective vehicle, Dunnett's post-hoc analyses.

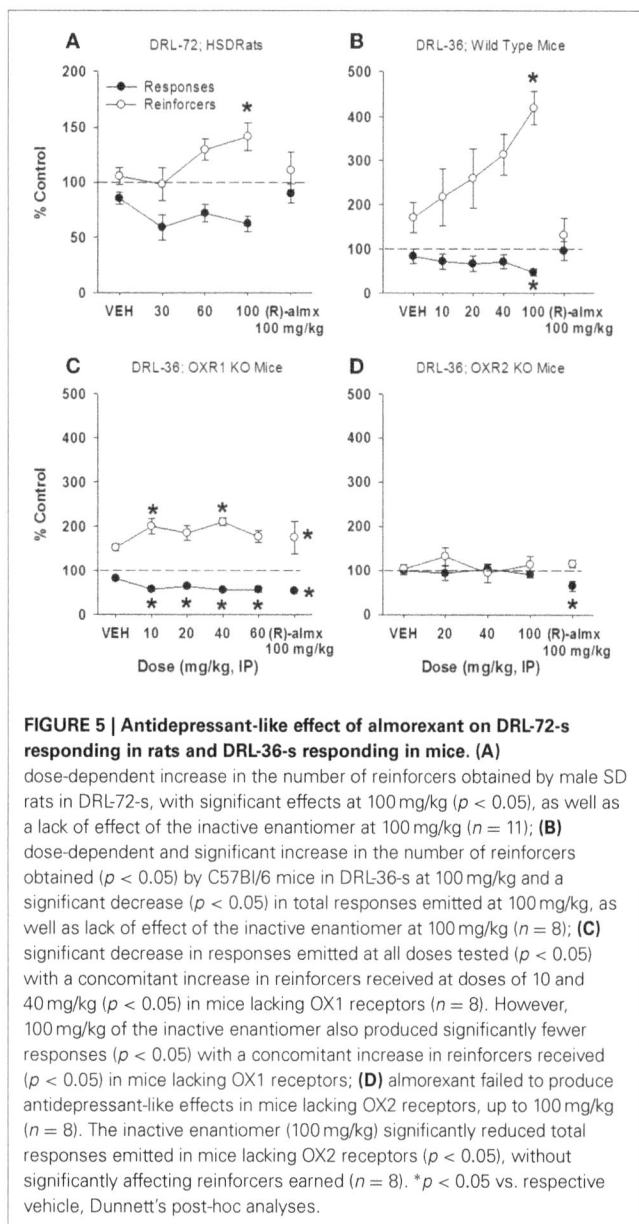

reason for this difference is unclear, but may be related to methodological differences between labs. Efficacy in the forced swim test, although useful in many respects, does not always translate to clinical antidepressant efficacy (De Pablo et al., 1989). The DRL model used here has strong construct and predictive validity, and is less likely to produce false positive results (O'Donnell et al., 2005; Zhang et al., 2009). Although less susceptible to false positive results due to motor effects, drugs that dramatically affect food intake, as has been reported for orexin antagonists (Mieda et al., 2006; Boutrel et al., 2010), can affect behavior in the DRL model. However, LSN2424100 was found to have no direct effects on food or water intake (Fitch et al., unpublished results; and see Anderson et al., under review). Alternatively, differences between our study and previous reports may be related to the use of mice lacking the orexin peptide (Lutter et al., 2008) vs. mice lacking individual OX1 or OX2 receptors (current study).

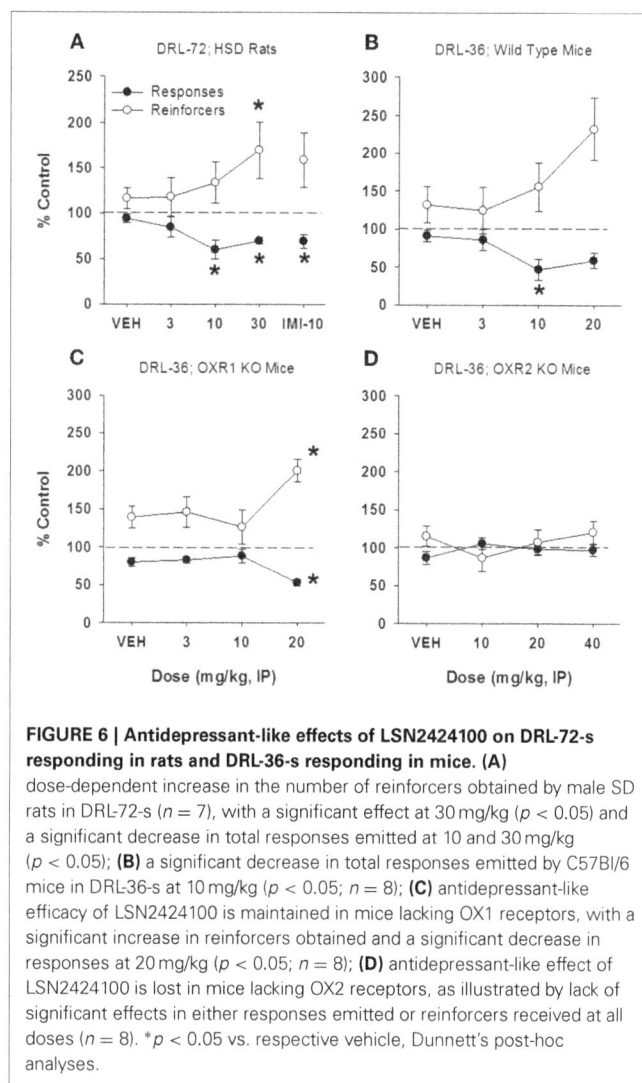

In addition to demonstrating antidepressant-like efficacy of OX2 antagonists in the rat DRL-72 s model, we extend the findings to demonstrate efficacy in a mouse DRL-36 s schedule of reinforcement. Importantly, we demonstrate similar antidepressant-like efficacy of imipramine in the mouse that closely resembles effects observed in the rat DRL model. In the mouse DRL model, LSN2424100 and almorexant produced antidepressant-like effects, similar to the effects observed in rats (Figures 5, 6). Moreover, the antidepressant-like effects of LSN2424100 and almorexant were completely abolished in mice lacking OX2 receptors, confirming the critical role of OX2 receptor signaling in mediating mood and antidepressant-like efficacy of the orexin antagonists tested here. Importantly, the effects of imipramine were found to be similar in mice lacking either OX1 or OX2 receptors, although efficacy appeared to be blunted in mice lacking OX2 receptors (Figure 3D). It is possible that the antidepressant-like phenotype observed in mice lacking OX2 receptors (see non-normalized data in Supplementary Table S1) may be responsible for the apparent blunted efficacy in the normalized data. Nonetheless, the efficacy of imipramine was not lost in mice lacking OX2 receptors, indicating that the antidepressant-like effects of imipramine are not mediated through orexin signaling mechanisms. By extension, our data further suggest that the antidepressant-like efficacy of OX2 and dual orexin receptor antagonists are mechanistically distinct from monoamine-based antidepressants. Considering the sleep disturbances often experienced by depressed individuals, the known side effect of SSRIs to exacerbate or even produce sleep disruption in depressed patients, and the robust sleep-enhancing properties of orexin antagonists (Mayers and Baldwin, 2005; Riemann, 2007; Thase et al., 2010), it seems plausible that selectively inhibiting OX2 receptor signaling may provide additional clinical benefits by simultaneously improving mood and sleep.

The OX1 antagonist, SB334867, appeared void of antidepressant-like activity in rats and mice, although antidepressant-like effects were observed in mice lacking OX1 receptors. Our results differ from previous reports that SB334867 produced antidepressant-like efficacy in the mouse forced swim test and tail suspension test (Scott et al., 2011). It has also been reported that mice lacking OX1 receptors had an antidepressant-like phenotype, an effect which we failed to replicate (Fitch et al., unpublished observations). The reason for the apparent antidepressant-like efficacy of SB334867 in mice lacking OX1 receptors is not known, but could involve either compensatory upregulation of OX2 receptors in mice with constitutive deletion of OX1 receptors, or perhaps some off-target, non-orexin pharmacology of SB334867 that may be either amplified or unmasked in the absence of OX1 receptors. Indeed, off-target pharmacology of SB334867 has already been reported by others, including activity at targets that may produce antidepressant-like effects, such as monoamine transporters, norepinephrine transporter, and 5-HT2C receptors (Gotter et al., 2012). Thus, data from our lab supports previous suggestions that SB334867 should not be considered OX1-selective. At the highest dose of 40 mg/kg, SB334867 produced behavioral disruption in mice lacking OX2 receptors, as indicated by strong reductions in total responding and concomitant reductions in reinforcers received. The mechanism by which SB334867 disrupted behavior in these mice is not known, but may be related to compensatory upregulation of OX1 receptors in these mice, an increase in functional sensitivity of OX1 receptors in the absence of OX2 receptors, or some unidentified off-target pharmacology of SB334867. Further studies will be required to understand these effects in the knockout mice.

Stress is a major trigger of depression and relapse to recurrent depressive episodes (Mazure, 1998). In rats, restraint stress stimulates ventral tegmental area (VTA) dopamine cell activity and c-fos expression in the mPFC, an area with dense reciprocal connections to the VTA that is known to be disrupted in depression (Drevets et al., 2008; Valenti et al., 2011). We demonstrate here that restraint stress-induced c-fos activation in the PFC was significantly attenuated by pre-treatment with LSN2424100. Our data are consistent with previous studies demonstrating that restraint-stress induced mPFC activation, as measured by c-fos expression in both rats and mice (Radley et al., 2006; O'Mahony et al., 2010; Valenti et al., 2011), and extend those results to demonstrate that orexin signaling may be involved in mediating

stress responses within corticolimbic circuits. Although we and others have reported c-fos activation in the PFC in response to restraint stress, others have reported that restraint stress did not produce robust c-fos activation of hypothalamic orexin cells (Furlong et al., 2009), suggesting that the orexin system may modulate stress responses in the PFC through indirect pathways rather than by direct connections from hypothalamic cells where orexin is synthesized. While the importance of the PFC in regulating mood is well-established, the potential role of orexin in modulating these circuits is unclear. Further studies will be required to explore the exact mechanism by which orexin signaling may modulate prefrontal cortical activation following restraint stress, which may involve modulation of dopaminergic and noradrenergic neurotransmission (Borgland et al., 2008; Del Cid-Pellitero and Garzon, 2011).

Elucidating the role of the orexin system in modulating the complex physiological and behavioral traits associated with psychiatric disorders, including depression, has been a complex undertaking, confounded by a dearth of selective pharmacological tools. With its suggested involvement in the regulation of vigilance states, feeding and energy homeostasis, drug-seeking behavior, and emotional processing (Mieda et al., 2006; Richards et al., 2008; Aston-Jones et al., 2009; Boutrel et al., 2010; Sinton, 2011; Nollet and Leman, 2013), the orexin system appears to play a critical role in maintaining equilibrium in the mammalian nervous system (Sinton, 2011). In pathological states related to mood, arousal, or consummatory behaviors, the orexin system may present opportunities for pharmacological intervention with potentially beneficial outcomes. Recent research has begun to shed light on the diverse signaling properties of orexins. For example, it is known that OX1 and OX2 receptors can couple, either directly or indirectly, to several G-protein effectors, including G_q, $G_{i/o}$, and G_s, with the potential to confer diverse signaling properties of either OXA or OXB through various intracellular pathways including phospholipase C, adenylyl cyclase, phospholipase A2, and phospholipase D (reviewed recently by Leonard and Kukkonen, 2014). However, little is known about which molecular pathways mediate the diverse physiological effects of orexins reported in the literature. Research focused on elucidating these mechanisms will benefit from an array of tools providing precise control of component function, including OX2-selective antagonists, which have not been widely tested to date with regard to potential antidepressant-like efficacy. Pharmacological tools, in particular, afford the investigator with an accessible, fast-acting and straightforward methodology for manipulation of receptor functioning to gain insight into the dynamics of receptor-ligand interactions, downstream physiological processes, signaling mechanisms, and behavioral output in preclinical models.

We demonstrate here that LSN2424100 is a novel orexin receptor antagonist with high affinity and selectivity for OX2 receptors and favorable pharmacokinetics following IP doses up to 30 mg/kg, and propose its use as a structurally-unique, synthetically-accessible tool for probing the role of OX2-dependent signaling in rodent models. Moreover, we demonstrate that LSN2424100 blocks stress-induced c-fos activation in the mPFC and produces antidepressant-like efficacy in an established animal model of depression in both rats and mice. Moreover, the antidepressant-like efficacy of LSN2424100 was completely abolished in mice lacking OX2, but not OX1, receptors, indicating a critical role of OX2-receptor-mediated signaling. In conclusion, LSN2424100 represents a functional tool compound for the investigation of OX2-receptor-mediated function, particularly in mood disorders.

SUPPLEMENTARY MATERIAL

The Supplementary Material for this article can be found online at: http://www.frontiersin.org/journal/10.3389/fnins.2014.00005/abstract

ACKNOWLEDGMENTS

The authors would like to thank Stephen F. Chaney and Lisa A. Foltz for their excellent technical assistance.

REFERENCES

Allard, J. S., Tizabi, Y., Shaffery, J. P., Trouth, C. O., and Manaye, K. (2004). Stereological analysis of the hypothalamic hypocretin/orexin neurons in an animal model of depression. *Neuropeptides* 38, 311–315. doi: 10.1016/j.npep.2004.06.004

Aston-Jones, G., Smith, R. J., Moorman, D. E., and Richardson, K. A. (2009). Role of lateral hypothalamic orexin neurons in reward processing and addiction. *Neuropharmacology* 56(Suppl. 1), 112–121. doi: 10.1016/j.neuropharm.2008.06.060

Borgland, S. L., Storm, E., and Bonci, A. (2008). Orexin B/hypocretin 2 increases glutamatergic transmission to ventral tegmental area neurons. *Eur. J. Neurosci.* 28, 1545–1556. doi: 10.1111/j.1460-9568.2008.06397.x

Boutrel, B., Cannella, N., and De Lecea, L. (2010). The role of hypocretin in driving arousal and goal-oriented behaviors. *Brain Res.* 1314, 103–111. doi: 10.1016/j.brainres.2009.11.054

Boutrel, B., Kenny, P. J., Specio, S. E., Martin-Fardon, R., Markou, A., Koob, G. F., et al. (2005). Role for hypocretin in mediating stress-induced reinstatement of cocaine-seeking behavior. *Proc. Natl. Acad. Sci. U.S.A.* 102, 19168–19173. doi: 10.1073/pnas.0507480102

Brisbare-Roch, C., Dingemanse, J., Koberstein, R., Hoever, P., Aissaoui, H., Flores, S., et al. (2007). Promotion of sleep by targeting the orexin system in rats, dogs and humans. *Nat. Med.* 13, 150–155. doi: 10.1038/nm1544

Brundin, L., Bjorkqvist, M., Petersen, A., and Traskman-Bendz, L. (2007). Reduced orexin levels in the cerebrospinal fluid of suicidal patients with major depressive disorder. *Eur. Neuropsychopharmacol.* 17, 573–579. doi: 10.1016/j.euroneuro.2007.01.005

Chemelli, R. M., Willie, J. T., Sinton, C. M., Elmquist, J. K., Scammell, T., Lee, C., et al. (1999). Narcolepsy in orexin knockout mice: molecular genetics of sleep regulation. *Cell* 98, 437–451. doi: 10.1016/S0092-8674(00)81973-X

Del Cid-Pellitero, E., and Garzon, M. (2011). Hypocretin1/OrexinA-containing axons innervate locus coeruleus neurons that project to the Rat medial prefrontal cortex. Implication in the sleep-wakefulness cycle and cortical activation. *Synapse* 65, 843–857. doi: 10.1002/syn.20912

De Lecea, L., Kilduff, T. S., Peyron, C., Gao, X., Foye, P. E., Danielson, P. E., et al. (1998). The hypocretins: hypothalamus-specific peptides with neuroexcitatory activity. *Proc. Natl. Acad. Sci. U.S.A.* 95, 322–327. doi: 10.1073/pnas.95.1.322

De Pablo, J. M., Parra, A., Segovia, S., and Guillamon, A. (1989). Learned immobility explains the behavior of rats in the forced swimming test. *Physiol. Behav.* 46, 229–237. doi: 10.1016/0031-9384(89)90261-8

Drevets, W. C., Price, J. L., and Furey, M. L. (2008). Brain structural and functional abnormalities in mood disorders: implications for neurocircuitry models of depression. *Brain Struct. Funct.* 213, 93–118. doi: 10.1007/s00429-008-0189-x

Furlong, T. M., Vianna, D. M., Liu, L., and Carrive, P. (2009). Hypocretin/orexin contributes to the expression of some but not all forms of stress and arousal. *Eur. J. Neurosci.* 30, 1603–1614. doi: 10.1111/j.1460-9568.2009.06952.x

Gotter, A. L., Webber, A. L., Coleman, P. J., Renger, J. J., and Winrow, C. J. (2012). International union of basic and clinical pharmacology. LXXXVI. orexin receptor function, nomenclature and pharmacology. *Pharmacol. Rev.* 64, 389–420. doi: 10.1124/pr.111.005546

Hirose, M., Egashira, S., Goto, Y., Hashihayata, T., Ohtake, N., Iwaasa, H., et al. (2003). N-acyl 6,7-dimethoxy-1,2,3,4-tetrahydroisoquinoline: the first orexin-2 receptor selective non-peptidic antagonist. *Bioorg. Med. Chem. Lett.* 13, 4497–4499. doi: 10.1016/j.bmcl.2003.08.038

Ito, N., Yabe, T., Gamo, Y., Nagai, T., Oikawa, T., Yamada, H., et al. (2008). I.c.v. administration of orexin-A induces an antidepressive-like effect through hippocampal cell proliferation. *Neuroscience* 157, 720–732. doi: 10.1016/j.neuroscience.2008.09.042

Leonard, C. S., and Kukkonen, J. P. (2014). Orexin/hypocretin receptor signalling: a functional perspective. *Br. J. Pharmacol.* 171, 294–313. doi: 10.1111/bph.12296

Lopez-Rubalcava, C., and Lucki, I. (2000). Strain differences in the behavioral effects of antidepressant drugs in the rat forced swimming test. *Neuropsychopharmacology* 22, 191–199. doi: 10.1016/S0893-133X(99)00100-1

Lutter, M., Krishnan, V., Russo, S. J., Jung, S., Mcclung, C. A., and Nestler, E. J. (2008). Orexin signaling mediates the antidepressant-like effect of calorie restriction. *J. Neurosci.* 28, 3071–3075. doi: 10.1523/JNEUROSCI.5584-07.2008

Malherbe, P., Borroni, E., Gobbi, L., Knust, H., Nettekoven, M., Pinard, E., et al. (2009). Biochemical and behavioural characterization of EMPA, a novel high-affinity, selective antagonist for the OX(2) receptor. *Br. J. Pharmacol.* 156, 1326–1341. doi: 10.1111/j.1476-5381.2009.00127.x

Mayers, A. G., and Baldwin, D. S. (2005). Antidepressants and their effect on sleep. *Hum. Psychopharmacol.* 20, 533–559. doi: 10.1002/hup.726

Mazure, C. M. (1998). Life stressors as risk factors in depression. *Clin. Psychol. Sci. Pract.* 5, 291–313. doi: 10.1111/j.1468-2850.1998.tb00151.x

McAtee, L. C., Sutton, S. W., Rudolph, D. A., Li, X., Aluisio, L. E., Phong, V. K., et al. (2004). Novel substituted 4-phenyl-[1,3]dioxanes: potent and selective orexin receptor 2 (OX(2)R) antagonists. *Bioorg. Med. Chem. Lett.* 14, 4225–4229. doi: 10.1016/j.bmcl.2004.06.032

Mieda, M., Williams, S. C., Richardson, J. A., Tanaka, K., and Yanagisawa, M. (2006). The dorsomedial hypothalamic nucleus as a putative food-entrainable circadian pacemaker. *Proc. Natl. Acad. Sci. U.S.A.* 103, 12150–12155. doi: 10.1073/pnas.0604189103

Mikrouli, E., Wortwein, G., Soylu, R., Mathe, A. A., and Petersen, S. (2011). Increased numbers of orexin/hypocretin neurons in a genetic rat depression model. *Neuropeptides* 45, 401–406. doi: 10.1016/j.npep.2011.07.010

Nollet, M., Gaillard, P., Minier, F., Tanti, A., Belzung, C., and Leman, S. (2011). Activation of orexin neurons in dorsomedial/perifornical hypothalamus and antidepressant reversal in a rodent model of depression. *Neuropharmacology* 61, 336–346. doi: 10.1016/j.neuropharm.2011.04.022

Nollet, M., Gaillard, P., Tanti, A., Girault, V., Belzung, C., and Leman, S. (2012). Neurogenesis-independent antidepressant-like effects on behavior and stress axis response of a dual orexin receptor antagonist in a rodent model of depression. *Neuropsychopharmacology* 37, 2210–2221. doi: 10.1038/npp.2012.70

Nollet, M., and Leman, S. (2013). Role of orexin in the pathophysiology of depression: potential for pharmacological intervention. *CNS Drugs* 27, 411–422. doi: 10.1007/s40263-013-0064-z

O'Donnell, J. M., Marek, G. J., and Seiden, L. S. (2005). Antidepressant effects assessed using behavior maintained under a differential-reinforcement-of-low-rate (DRL) operant schedule. *Neurosci. Biobehav. Rev.* 29, 785–798. doi: 10.1016/j.neubiorev.2005.03.018

O'Mahony, C. M., Sweeney, F. F., Daly, E., Dinan, T. G., and Cryan, J. F. (2010). Restraint stress-induced brain activation patterns in two strains of mice differing in their anxiety behaviour. *Behav. Brain Res.* 213, 148–154. doi: 10.1016/j.bbr.2010.04.038

Ortega, J. E., Katner, J., Davis, R., Wade, M., Nisenbaum, L., Nomikos, G. G., et al. (2012). Modulation of neurotransmitter release in orexin/hypocretin-2 receptor knockout mice: a microdialysis study. *J. Neurosci. Res.* 90, 588–596. doi: 10.1002/jnr.22781

Overstreet, D. H., and Wegener, G. (2013). The flinders sensitive line rat model of depression–25 years and still producing. *Pharmacol. Rev.* 65, 143–155. doi: 10.1124/pr.111.005397

Radley, J. J., Arias, C. M., and Sawchenko, P. E. (2006). Regional differentiation of the medial prefrontal cortex in regulating adaptive responses to acute emotional stress. *J. Neurosci.* 26, 12967–12976. doi: 10.1523/JNEUROSCI.4297-06.2006

LSN2424100: a novel, potent orexin-2 receptor antagonist with selectivity over orexin-1 receptors and activity...

143

Richards, J. K., Simms, J. A., Steensland, P., Taha, S. A., Borgland, S. L., Bonci, A., et al. (2008). Inhibition of orexin-1/hypocretin-1 receptors inhibits yohimbine-induced reinstatement of ethanol and sucrose seeking in Long-Evans rats. *Psychopharmacology (Berl.)* 199, 109–117. doi: 10.1007/s00213-008-1136-5

Riemann, D. (2007). Insomnia and comorbid psychiatric disorders. *Sleep Med.* 8(Suppl. 4), S15–S20. doi: 10.1016/S1389-9457(08)70004-2

Sakurai, T., Amemiya, A., Ishii, M., Matsuzaki, I., Chemelli, R. M., Tanaka, H., et al. (1998). Orexins and orexin receptors: a family of hypothalamic neuropeptides and G protein-coupled receptors that regulate feeding behavior. *Cell* 92, 573–585. doi: 10.1016/S0092-8674(00)80949-6

Salomon, R. M., Ripley, B., Kennedy, J. S., Johnson, B., Schmidt, D., Zeitzer, J. M., et al. (2003). Diurnal variation of cerebrospinal fluid hypocretin-1 (Orexin-A) levels in control and depressed subjects. *Biol. Psychiatry* 54, 96–104. doi: 10.1016/S0006-3223(02)01740-7

Scott, M. M., Marcus, J. N., Pettersen, A., Birnbaum, S. G., Mochizuki, T., Scammell, T. E., et al. (2011). Hcrtr1 and 2 signaling differentially regulates depression-like behaviors. *Behav. Brain Res.* 222, 289–294. doi: 10.1016/j.bbr.2011.02.044

Sinton, C. M. (2011). Orexin/hypocretin plays a role in the response to physiological disequilibrium. *Sleep Med. Rev.* 15, 197–207. doi: 10.1016/j.smrv.2010.12.003

Smart, D., Sabido-David, C., Brough, S. J., Jewitt, F., Johns, A., Porter, R. A., et al. (2001). SB-334867-A: the first selective orexin-1 receptor antagonist. *Br. J. Pharmacol.* 132, 1179–1182. doi: 10.1038/sj.bjp.0703953

Spinazzi, R., Andreis, P. G., Rossi, G. P., and Nussdorfer, G. G. (2006). Orexins in the regulation of the hypothalamic-pituitary-adrenal axis. *Pharmacol. Rev.* 58, 46–57. doi: 10.1124/pr.58.1.4

Taheri, S., Gardiner, J., Hafizi, S., Murphy, K., Dakin, C., Seal, L., et al. (2001). Orexin A immunoreactivity and preproorexin mRNA in the brain of Zucker and WKY rats. *Neuroreport* 12, 459–464. doi: 10.1097/00001756-200103050-00008

Thase, M. E., Murck, H., and Post, A. (2010). Clinical relevance of disturbances of sleep and vigilance in major depressive disorder: a review. *Prim. Care Companion J. Clin. Psychiatry* 12. e1–e10. doi: 10.4088/PCC.08m00676gry

Valenti, O., Lodge, D. J., and Grace, A. A. (2011). Aversive stimuli alter ventral tegmental area dopamine neuron activity via a common action in the ventral hippocampus. *J. Neurosci.* 31, 4280–4289. doi: 10.1523/JNEUROSCI.5310-10.2011

Weller, T., Koberstein, R., Aissaoui, H., Clozel, M., and Fischli, W. (2005). "Substituted 1,2,3,4-tetrahydroisoquinoline derivatives," in *International Patent # WO2005118548. Issued to Actelion Pharmaceuticals, Ltd.* (Allschwil, CH).

Zamek-Gliszczynski, M. J., Ruterbories, K. J., Ajamie, R. T., Wickremsinhe, E. R., Pothuri, L., Rao, M. V., et al. (2011). Validation of 96-well equilibrium dialysis with non-radiolabeled drug for definitive measurement of protein binding and application to clinical development of highly-bound drugs. *J. Pharm. Sci.* 100, 2498–2507. doi: 10.1002/jps.22452

Zhang, H. T., Whisler, L. R., Huang, Y., Xiang, Y., and O'Donnell, J. M. (2009). Postsyanptic α-2 adrenergic receptors are critical for the anti-depressant like effects of desipramine on behavior. *Neuropsychopharmacology* 34, 1067–1077. doi: 10.1038/npp.2008.184

Conflict of Interest Statement: All authors are employees of, and stockholders in, Eli Lilly and Company. Financial support for the research conducted in this manuscript was provided by Eli Lilly and Company.

16

OX$_1$ and OX$_2$ orexin/hypocretin receptor pharmacogenetics

Miles D. Thompson[1]*, Henri Xhaard[2], Takeshi Sakurai[3], Innocenzo Rainero[4] and Jyrki P. Kukkonen[5]

[1] *University of Toronto Epilepsy Research Program, Department of Pharmacology, University of Toronto, Toronto, ON, Canada*
[2] *Faculty of Pharmacy, Centre for Drug Research, University of Helsinki, Helsinki, Finland*
[3] *Department of Molecular Neuroscience and Integrative Physiology, Faculty of Medicine, Kanazawa University, Kanazawa, Japan*
[4] *Department of Neuroscience, University of Turin, Torino, Italy*
[5] *Biochemistry and Cell Biology, Department of Veterinary Biosciences, University of Helsinki, Helsinki, Finland*

Edited by:
Christopher J. Winrow, Merck, USA

Reviewed by:
Michiru Hirasawa, Memorial University, Canada
Robyn Mary Brown, Florey Neuroscience Institutes, Australia

*Correspondence:
Miles D. Thompson, University of Toronto Epilepsy Research Program, Department of Pharmacology, University of Toronto, 1 King's College Circle, Medical Sciences Building, Toronto, ON M5S 1A8, Canada
e-mail: miles.thompson@ utoronto.ca

Orexin/hypocretin peptide mutations are rare in humans. Even though human narcolepsy is associated with orexin deficiency, this is only extremely rarely due to mutations in the gene coding prepro-orexin, the precursor for both orexin peptides. In contrast, coding and non-coding variants of the OX$_1$ and OX$_2$ orexin receptors have been identified in many human populations; sometimes, these have been associated with disease phenotype, although most confer a relatively low risk. In most cases, these studies have been based on a candidate gene hypothesis that predicts the involvement of orexins in the relevant pathophysiological processes. In the current review, the known human OX$_1$/*HCRTR1* and OX$_2$/*HCRTR2* genetic variants/polymorphisms as well as studies concerning their involvement in disorders such as narcolepsy, excessive daytime sleepiness, cluster headache, polydipsia-hyponatremia in schizophrenia, and affective disorders are discussed. In most cases, the functional cellular or pharmacological correlates of orexin variants have not been investigated—with the exception of the possible impact of an amino acid 10 Pro/Ser variant of OX$_2$ on orexin potency—leaving conclusions on the nature of the receptor variant effects speculative. Nevertheless, we present perspectives that could shape the basis for further studies. The pharmacology and other properties of the orexin receptor variants are discussed in the context of GPCR signaling. Since orexinergic therapeutics are emerging, the impact of receptor variants on the affinity or potency of ligands deserves consideration. This perspective (pharmacogenetics) is also discussed in the review.

Keywords: orexin, hypocretin, G protein-coupled receptor, polymorphism, pharmacogenetics

INTRODUCTION

The orexin/hypocretin system was identified by two groups. de Lecea with colleagues described two putative peptide transmitters, encoded by a propeptide, the gene for which is located at human chromosome 17q21.2 (de Lecea et al., 1998). The hypocretin peptides were named for their expression in the synaptic vesicles in the hypothalamus and for the homology of hypocretin-2/orexin-B with some incretin peptides. The hypocretin-2/orexin-B peptide was shown to be markedly neuroexcitatory in neuronal cultures (de Lecea et al., 1998). Contemporaneously, Sakurai and co-workers deorphanized the putative G protein-coupled receptor (GPCR), HFGAN72, and identified the two peptide transmitters that activated the receptor, the common precursor peptide and its gene and, finally, a second receptor based on a sequence homology search (Sakurai et al., 1998). Peptide–receptor pharmacology was established and mRNA expression and peptide distribution in the central nervous system (CNS) was mapped.

Orexin-A/hypocretin-1 and orexin-B/hypocretin-2 are 33- and 28-residue hypothalamic peptides, respectively, derived from a 130 (or 131, depending on species)-amino acid precursor, prepro-orexin (PPO). The peptides were found to be linked to the regulation of feeding behavior based on evidence that they stimulated food intake upon intracerebroventricular administration, and increased peptide mRNA expression in the hypothalamus upon fasting. Sakurai et al. termed the peptides orexins for their orexinergic function, and the receptors OX$_1$ and OX$_2$ receptors (Sakurai et al., 1998).

Subsequently, genetic and disease-based studies supplied major findings concerning the physiological role of orexins in the regulation of wakefulness and sleep pattern. Mignot and co-workers isolated two OX$_2$ receptor gene frame-shift mutations responsible for hereditary canine narcolepsy (Lin et al., 1999). The frame shifts generate a premature in-frame stop codon, and the truncated receptors remain cytosolic and do not traffic at all to the plasma membrane (Hungs et al., 2001). Simultaneously, Yanagisawa and co-workers showed that knockout of the precursor peptide, PPO, causes narcoleptic phenotype in mice (Chemelli et al., 1999). In 2000, a report found orexin-A to be at very low or undetectable levels in the cerebrospinal fluid (CSF) of human narcoleptics with cataplexy (Nishino et al., 2000). In contrast, mutations in PPO gene have been identified in only a few patients (Peyron et al., 2000; Gencik et al., 2001).

Further studies have established that the neurobiology of the orexin system is complex, having possible roles in stress responses, reward/addiction, analgesia, in addition to sleep and wakefulness and appetite/metabolism (Kukkonen, 2013). In the CNS, the complexity is primarily created by the wide range of orexin neuron projections. On the cellular level, orexin receptor activation produces highly diverse cellular signals. This is likely a result of orexin receptor coupling to several families of heterotrimeric G proteins and other proteins that ultimately regulate entities such as ion channels, phospholipases and protein kinases, which impact on neuronal excitation, synaptic plasticity, and cell death, to mention a few (Kukkonen, 2013; Kukkonen and Leonard, 2014; Leonard and Kukkonen, 2014). The selection of signal cascade in each case is likely determined by the expression profile of signaling components, signal complexes and other concurrent signals. The possibly distinct role of the two orexin peptides and two orexin receptors is not resolved.

Gene variants for the orexin peptides and, especially, their G protein-coupled receptors, OX1 and OX2, have been identified (**Figures 1, 2**), and investigated in many CNS disorders, including sleep and wakefulness (Lin et al., 1999), polydipsia in schizophrenia (Meerabux et al., 2005; Fukunaka et al., 2007), panic disorder (Annerbrink et al., 2011), mood disorders (Rainero et al., 2011a), migraine (Schürks et al., 2007b; Rainero et al., 2011b), and cluster headache (Rainero et al., 2004). The associations under investigation will ultimately benefit from the clarification, possible from genome-wide association studies (GWAS).

In the current report, we review the known gene variants of orexin receptors. The major focus is on the investigations of association of the variants with disease phenotypes. Before presenting those data, we present the theoretical basis of the impact of DNA and amino acid sequence variations on the protein (here orexin receptor) expression, structure, function and regulation. In general, however, definitive evidence for the functional significance of orexin receptor variants is lacking.

HOW CAN GENETIC VARIATION AFFECT PEPTIDE TRANSMITTERS AND THEIR RECEPTORS?

Gene sequence variation for a peptide transmitter may cause alterations in signaling at several stages. The first level could be the gene structural level, i.e., sequence effect on the chromatin structure with impact on the transcriptional activity. mRNA stability and processing is affected by its secondary structure. Translation may proceed at different pace depending on the codon usage. For correct translation, packing and proteolytic processing, the signal sequence is of great importance. Finally, the sequence may affect the structure and the breakdown process of the transmitter. For receptors, although mRNA issues are similar, there are specific alterations in the potentially very vulnerable processes of protein processing (folding, glycosylation), trafficking (including wrong subcellular localization), dimerization, ligand binding, signaling, and desensitization and down-regulation. A significant bottle-neck of the production lies in the folding and processing; some other issues, such as codon usage, may be of minor importance.

Since there is limited knowledge of the processing of orexin peptides and receptors, and few studies that evaluate orexin receptor variants in an expression system, it is difficult to predict a role for most of these processes for the orexin peptides or receptors. One notable exception is the Leu16Arg mutant of the signal peptide of human PPO, which impairs its processing (Peyron et al., 2000). The best characterized orexin receptor mutants are the three OX2 mutants found in narcoleptic canines: the two most extreme ones cause truncation and subsequent gross protein folding failure, while the Glu54Lys variant is associated with proper membrane localization but shows a notable loss of ligand binding and dramatically diminished calcium signaling (Hungs et al., 2001). While these mutations (recessively) produce a strong narcoleptic phenotype in affected animals, the human receptor variants seem to confer significantly milder phenotypes (see below).

IMPACT OF THE GENETIC VARIATION ON THE OREXIN RECEPTOR LIGAND BINDING

The most dramatic GPCR mutations—if we disregard the grossly disruptive mutations such as truncations—may result in (a) altered sensitivity to native ligands or drugs (e.g., variants of follicle-stimulating hormone receptor causing ovarian dysgenesis; Thompson et al., 2008b) or (b) disruption to the receptor's interaction with the signal transduction machinery (e.g., G protein-binding site mutations found in the β_1-adrenoceptor; Thompson et al., 2008c). GPCRs share a common three dimensional structure composed of seven transmembrane helices (TMs). Like other family A GPCRs, orexin receptors are assumed to bind their peptide and non-peptide ligands mainly in a partially hydrophilic, partially hydrophobic cleft with possible contribution from more extracellular portion of the receptor. While orexin receptor crystal structures have not been published, mutagenesis studies have been performed and receptor models constructed (Malherbe et al., 2010; Putula et al., 2011; Tran et al., 2011; Heifetz et al., 2012; Putula and Kukkonen, 2012). Out of the 11 variable sites found and described in this review, only three—$OX_1{}^{167}$ [transmembrane helix (TM) 4, closer to intracellular side of receptor], $OX_2{}^{193}$ (TM) 4, near the putative binding cavity and $OX_2{}^{308}$ (TM6, closer to intracellular side) (**Figures 1, 2**)—are within the predicted transmembrane helix domain forming this cavity. Among these sites, only $OX_2{}^{193}$ is located in the putative binding cleft, where it might have a direct effect on receptor pharmacology. The other two sites are less likely to act through direct molecular contacts since they are located toward the intracellular ends of TM regions. Unfortunately, the impact of these polymorphisms has not been determined in heterologous expression studies, and neither have these sites been targeted in the point-mutation studies (Malherbe et al., 2010; Tran et al., 2011; Heifetz et al., 2012).

Most GPCR polymorphisms are found in the loops and in the N- and C-terminal. This is consistent with general observation that loops connecting helices are much more variable—and in some case hypervariable—in comparison to the transmembrane core of GPCRs (Madsen et al., 2002; Jaakola et al., 2005), and does not as such necessarily imply a functional significance. However, amino acids located outside the (predicted)

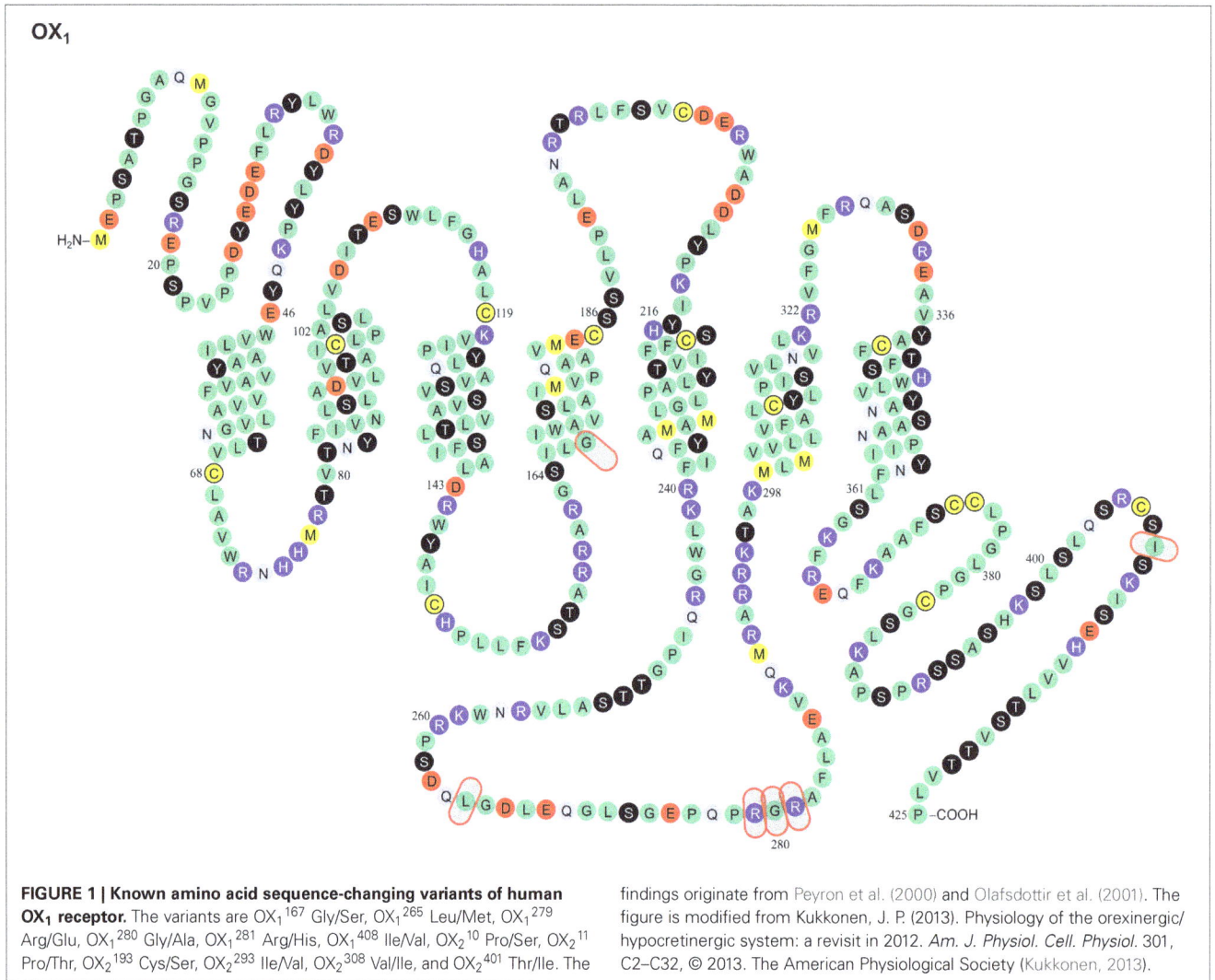

FIGURE 1 | Known amino acid sequence-changing variants of human OX$_1$ receptor. The variants are OX$_1$[167] Gly/Ser, OX$_1$[265] Leu/Met, OX$_1$[279] Arg/Glu, OX$_1$[280] Gly/Ala, OX$_1$[281] Arg/His, OX$_1$[408] Ile/Val, OX$_2$[10] Pro/Ser, OX$_2$[11] Pro/Thr, OX$_2$[193] Cys/Ser, OX$_2$[293] Ile/Val, OX$_2$[308] Val/Ile, and OX$_2$[401] Thr/Ile. The findings originate from Peyron et al. (2000) and Olafsdottir et al. (2001). The figure is modified from Kukkonen, J. P. (2013). Physiology of the orexinergic/hypocretinergic system: a revisit in 2012. *Am. J. Physiol. Cell. Physiol.* 301, C2–C32, © 2013. The American Physiological Society (Kukkonen, 2013).

binding cavity may also have consequences on the binding affinities measured in pharmacological assays, as exemplified by the canine OX$_2$ Glu54Lys mutation (see above) (Hungs et al., 2001). Polymorphism at the N-terminal of OX$_2$ (Pro10Ser and Pro11Thr; **Figures 1, 2**) may, similarly, act directly on ligand binding or indirectly via receptor structure. However, also other effects are possible, as discussed below.

Orexin-B was 2.7-fold less potent as an activator of the OX$_2$[10] Ser receptor by comparison with the wild-type OX$_2$[10] Pro receptor in calcium measurements in recombinant COS-7 cells (Thompson et al., 2004). However, this may also relate to the signaling or receptor expression/maturation; as a result, no firm conclusions can be drawn as yet, although the finding is interesting.

IMPACT OF THE GENETIC VARIATION ON OREXIN RECEPTOR SIGNALING

Orexin receptors are able to couple to multiple G proteins. Experimental evidence suggests that OX$_2$ receptors in human adrenal cortex activate G$_i$, G$_s$, and G$_q$ proteins (Karteris et al., 2001; Randeva et al., 2001). Mixed orexin receptor populations

in rat adrenal cortex or hypothalamus couple to G$_i$, G$_o$, G$_s$, and G$_q$ (Karteris et al., 2005). In recombinant systems, OX$_1$ receptors easily couple to all these three G protein families (Holmqvist et al., 2005; Magga et al., 2006). In summary, both orexin receptors are likely capable of coupling to G$_{i/o}$, G$_s$, and G$_q$ family G proteins; however, this may be subject to tissue- and context-specific regulation (Kukkonen, 2013). For G protein coupling, the most central receptor domains are usually the 2nd and 3rd intracellular loops, while also the 1st intracellular loop and the receptor's C-terminus are sometimes implicated based on mutagenesis studies (Wess, 1998); orexin receptors themselves have not been examined for this. Like other GPCRs (Ritter and Hall, 2009), orexin receptors may also couple to other proteins, like β-arrestin and dynein light chain Tctex-type 1 (Milasta et al., 2005; Dalrymple et al., 2011; Duguay et al., 2011). Coupling to both these proteins is suggested to take place on the receptor's C-terminus. Variations in these regions may directly impact orexin receptor interaction with effectors while also indirectly modifying effector coupling as a result of alterations in the receptor configuration that determines the specificity of these interactions. Among the identified variable sites, OX$_1$[265], OX$_1$[279], OX$_1$[280], OX$_1$[281], OX$_1$[408], OX$_2$[293],

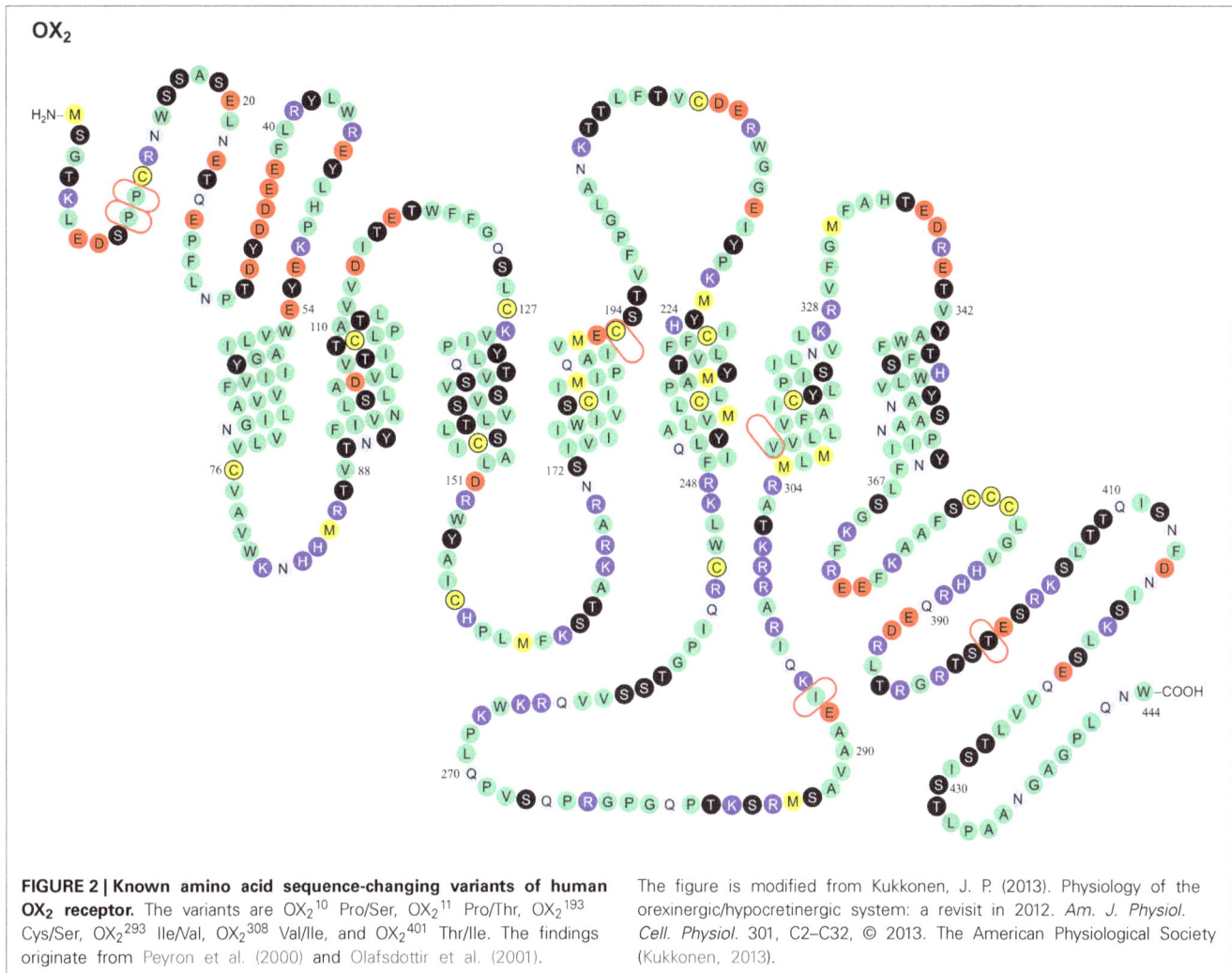

FIGURE 2 | Known amino acid sequence-changing variants of human OX₂ receptor. The variants are OX$_2$^{10} Pro/Ser, OX$_2$^{11} Pro/Thr, OX$_2$^{193} Cys/Ser, OX$_2$^{293} Ile/Val, OX$_2$^{308} Val/Ile, and OX$_2$^{401} Thr/Ile. The findings originate from Peyron et al. (2000) and Olafsdottir et al. (2001). The figure is modified from Kukkonen, J. P. (2013). Physiology of the orexinergic/hypocretinergic system: a revisit in 2012. *Am. J. Physiol. Cell. Physiol.* 301, C2–C32, © 2013. The American Physiological Society (Kukkonen, 2013).

and OX$_2$^{401} (**Figures 1, 2**) may thus be implicated in G protein and/or other protein coupling of orexin receptors.

Further complexity in the trafficking, ligand interaction and signaling of GPCR is introduced by the fact that many GPCRs have been shown to dimerize (Bulenger et al., 2005; Milligan, 2009). In fact, some models predict that all functional GPCRs form dimers. Orexin receptors are known to homo- and hetero-dimerize/oligomerize in recombinant expression systems (Ellis et al., 2006; Ward et al., 2011; Xu et al., 2011; Jäntti et al., 2014). It should be noted, however, that there is no evidence for such interactions in native cells thus far.

GPCRs may utilize both extracellular and intracellular parts as well as the hydrophobic outer surfaces of the transmembrane helices for interaction during dimerization (see, e.g., Liang et al., 2003; Wu et al., 2010; Huang et al., 2013). One region involved in receptor–receptor interaction, at least according to X-ray crystal structure-based modeling of the CXCR4 (Wu et al., 2010) and the β$_1$-adrenoceptor (Huang et al., 2013), is near the palmitoylated C-terminal region. An analogous structure is present in the human orexin receptors. It may form a coiled coil motif in the putative helix 8 (parallel to membrane) that would allow OX$_1$ and OX$_2$ dimerization. The impact of OX$_1$^{408} and OX$_2$^{401} (**Figures 1, 2**) on receptor dimerization is unknown; in

any case, they are well downstream from the potential palmitoylation sites. The importance of dimerization/oligomerization for most GPCRs, however, is unclear (Bulenger et al., 2005; Milligan, 2009). Notable exceptions to this among GPCR family A receptors are the opioid receptors, whose pharmacology and trafficking is significantly affected by dimerization. OX$_1$–CB$_1$ dimerization was suggested to strongly potentiate orexin receptor signaling, but a likely explanation for the signal potentiation is, instead, offered by the ability of OX$_1$ receptor signaling to produce 2-arachidonoyl glycerol, a CB$_1$ receptor ligand, and a subsequent co-signaling of the receptors (Haj-Dahmane and Shen, 2005; Turunen et al., 2012; Jäntti et al., 2013). However, this does not preclude dimerization.

Phosphorylation (or other similar protein interaction) differences may be seen between the variants. Hydroxyl group-containing amino acids Ser, Thr and Tyr may be direct substrates for phosphorylation, but other amino acids can also affect the kinase consensus sequences. These sites have not been targeted in the point mutagenesis studies. Scansite (http://scansite.mit. edu/) (Obenauer et al., 2003) motif search suggest that some of the polymorphisms at OX$_1$^{167}, OX$_1$^{265}, OX$_1$^{279}, OX$_1$^{280}, OX$_1$^{408}, and OX$_2$^{401} (**Figures 1, 2**) may impact kinase or other protein binding. Because these predictions are solely based on the amino acid sequence, however, they should be treated with caution. It is also unclear whether all these sites, especially OX_1^{167}, are accessible for interaction.

IMPACT OF GENETIC VARIATION ON THE OREXIN PEPTIDE AND RECEPTOR PROCESSING, FOLDING AND HALF-LIFE

It is very difficult to predict the sites affecting receptor folding; in principle, every residue can influence receptor folding on the local or a more general level. A major change in the amino acid size, conformation, polarity and, especially, charge is likely to have a more pronounced effect of this type. Such an impact could be most pronounced for OX_1^{279} Arg/Glu. Glycosylation, found on the extracellular GPCR surfaces, could be affected by the availability of Asn and Ser/Thr residues (and other sites in the putative consensus sequence). This could be relevant for the OX_2^{10} Pro/Ser, OX_2^{11} Pro/Thr, and OX_2^{193} Cys/Ser variants (**Figures 1, 2**).

Posttranslational modifications are also necessary for the peptides for proper ligand function. For orexins, these include cyclization of N-terminal Glu and correct formation of the two disulphide bridges in orexin-A, and amidation of the free C-terminus of both peptides (Sakurai et al., 1998). With the very limited knowledge of the processing of orexin peptides and receptors as well as the very few studies which evaluate the orexin receptor variants in heterologous expression systems, it is difficult to predict a role for most of these processes in human disease. The one notable exception is the Leu16Arg mutant of the signal peptide of PPO, which impairs the processing of the PPO (Peyron et al., 2000), stressing the importance of the signal sequence for correct translation, packing and proteolytic processing.

For both receptors and peptides, the amino acid sequence may impact the trafficking and half-life. Receptor internalization from the plasma membrane is involved both in signaling and degradation, and requires interaction with other proteins (see above). Therefore, mutations may, for instance, decrease or increase the half-life of the receptor protein or redirect signal cascades.

OREXIN PHARMACOGENETICS

Coding and non-coding variants of the OX_1 and OX_2 orexin receptors have been identified in many human populations and phenotypes. Due to the emerging market for drugs targeting OX_1 and OX_2 receptors, knowledge of genetic variation in the human genes coding for these receptors, *HCRTR1* and *HCRTR2*, respectively, is of pharmacogenetic interest. Although canine *HCRTR2* mutations are associated with narcolepsy (Lin et al., 1999; Hungs et al., 2001), mutations in human orexin receptor genes have been associated only with rather moderately elevated disease risks—and, in some cases, the associations have not been met with consensus. **Table 1** presents a selection of the studies of OX_1 and OX_2 orexin receptor variants examined in human disease states.

With respect to drug development, the orexin receptor variants may be particularly relevant. Dual orexin antagonists, such as almorexant and suvorexant (**Figure 3**), as well as OX_2-selective antagonists, have been developed for use as sleep aids. Orexin receptor antagonists seem to act to turn off wakefulness instead of inducing sleep, *per se* (Winrow et al., 2011). While the development of almorexant by Actelion Pharmaceuticals has been

curtailed, Merck and Co. has continued the development of suvorexant (MK-4305) (Cox et al., 2010; Mieda and Sakurai, 2013; Winrow and Renger, 2014). Suvorexant completed three Phase III trials in 2013 (Winrow and Renger, 2014). The U.S. Food and Drug Administration's (FDA) peripheral and CNS advisory committee found the drug generally safe and effective for treating sleep maintenance and latency. Although it has a promising side-effect profile, the FDA review suggested that suvorexant is associated with increased somnolence the day after use, and that higher doses may be associated with an increased rate of suicidal ideation (Mieda and Sakurai, 2013). Pharmacogenetic considerations may assist in establishing the correct dosing for patients. Conversely, orexin receptor-activating therapy may become available for narcolepsy. Some recent findings support this therapeutic concept (Liu et al., 2011; Kantor et al., 2013). Narcolepsy may, however, not be the only disorder where such therapy may be beneficial, as indicated by some results briefly presented below and in Kukkonen (2012) and Kukkonen (2013).

Given the frequency of OX_1 and OX_2 receptor amino acid sequence variants, there is a clear rationale for examining the pharmacology of the agents at the variants *in vitro*. These results may, in turn, justify studying drug response in patients carrying receptor variants. For many human GPCRs, amino acid variants are well known to confer distinct pharmacological properties (Thompson et al., 2005, 2008a); however, the pharmacological data is generally unavailable for the human orexin receptor variants (Kukkonen, 2013).

OREXIN RECEPTOR VARIANTS IDENTIFIED IN SLEEP/WAKEFULNESS DISORDERS

Genetic variants of the orexin system have been identified only rarely in narcolepsy. For example, the Leu16Arg mutation in the signal peptide of PPO (Peyron et al., 2000; Gencik et al., 2001) disrupts a region of neutral, hydrophobic polyleucine amino acids in the PPO, which, in turn, limits the biologically active products, orexin-A and -B (Peyron et al., 2000). In contrast, the DNA or amino acid sequence variants of human HCRTR1/OX_1 and HCRTR2/OX_2 receptors (**Figures 1, 2**) do not seem to be involved in narcolepsy (Peyron et al., 2000; Olafsdottir et al., 2001)

OX_2^{11} Thr variant was identified in two DQB1*0602-negative excessive daytime sleepiness (EDS) patients and an OX_2^{10} Ser variant in a Tourette's syndrome patient comorbid with attention deficit hyperactivity disorder (ADHD) (Thompson et al., 2004). OX_2^{10} Ser or OX_2^{11} Thr variants were not identified in the 110 control individuals assessed, suggesting a possible association with sleep disorders. The fact that Tourette's syndrome patients diagnosed comorbid with ADHD frequently experience sleep disorders (Allen et al., 1992; Freeman et al., 2000; Cohrs et al., 2001), suggest that the OX_2^{10} Ser might be involved in the aetiology of some sleep abnormalities. Furthermore, while the OX_2^{10} Ser and OX_2^{11} Thr variants were reported to be more common in HLA DQB1*0602-negative narcoleptics compared with controls, these variants were reported to be benign with respect to narcolepsy (Peyron et al., 2000). The presence of these variants in EDS and Tourette's syndrome patients, however, suggests that they should be evaluated *in vitro* for functional differences that may contribute to sleep dysregulation. In this context, it is interesting to

Table 1 | Summary of OX$_1$ and OX$_2$ orexin receptor variants: investigations in disease.

OX$_1$ aa	Corresponding aa in OX$_2$	Location	SNP (or other access code)	Numbering/ peyron	Numbering/ olafsdottir	Findings	References
167 Gly/Ser	Ile	TM4	rs144603792		652 G/A	Not linked with narcolepsy	Olafsdottir et al., 2001
265 Leu/Met	[a]	IC3		793 C/A		Not linked with narcolepsy	Peyron et al., 2000
279 Arg/Gln	[a]	IC3	rs7516785		989 G/A	Not linked with narcolepsy	Olafsdottir et al., 2001
280 Gly/Ala	[a]	IC3	NP_001516 (C), AF041243 (G)				
281 Arg/His	[a]	IC3	rs41439244	842 G/A	995 G/A	Not linked with narcolepsy	Peyron et al., 2000; Olafsdottir et al., 2001
408 Ile/Val	[a]	C-terminus	rs2271933	1222 G/A	1375 G/A	Not linked with narcolepsy	Peyron et al., 2000; Olafsdottir et al., 2001
						A allele associated with 1.4-fold risk of migraine	Rainero et al., 2011b
						1.6-fold increased risk of major mood disorders	Rainero et al., 2011a
						Association with polydipsia–hyponatremia in schizophrenia possible	Meerabux et al., 2005; Fukunaka et al., 2007
						No allele associations in panic disorder	Annerbrink et al., 2011

OX$_2$ aa	Corresponding aa in OX$_1$	Location	SNP	Numbering/ peyron	Numbering/ olafsdottir	Findings	References
10 Pro/Ser	Pro	N-terminus	rs41271310	28 C/T	352 C/T	Not linked with narcolepsy	Peyron et al., 2000; Olafsdottir et al., 2001; Thompson et al., 2004
11 Pro/Thr	[a]	N-terminus	rs41271312	31 C/A	355 C/A	Not linked with narcolepsy	Peyron et al., 2000; Olafsdottir et al., 2001; Thompson et al., 2004
						Tourette syndrome/ADHD/sleep disorder 1.6 and 2.7-fold shifts in EC$_{50}$ for orexin-A and -B	
193 Cys/Ser	[a]	TM4		577 T/A		Not linked with narcolepsy	Peyron et al., 2000
293 Ile/Val	[a]	IC3			1201 G/A	Not linked with narcolepsy	Olafsdottir et al., 2001
308 Ile/Val	Val	TM6	rs265334	922 G/A	1246 G/A	Not linked with narcolepsy	Peyron et al., 2000; Olafsdottir et al., 2001
						Ile variant associated with panic disorder in female patients	Annerbrink et al., 2011
						Migraine not associated. Association with CH found in some but not in all studies	Baumber et al., 2006; Schürks et al., 2006; Rainero et al., 2008
						Does not affect migraine drug response	Schürks et al., 2007a
401 Thr/Ile	[a]	C-terminus		1202 C/T		Not linked with narcolepsy	Peyron et al., 2000

aa, amino acid; IC, intracellular loop; SNP, single nucleotide polymorphism; TM, transmembrane helix.

[a] The corresponding amino acids can be defined with certainty only for TM regions.

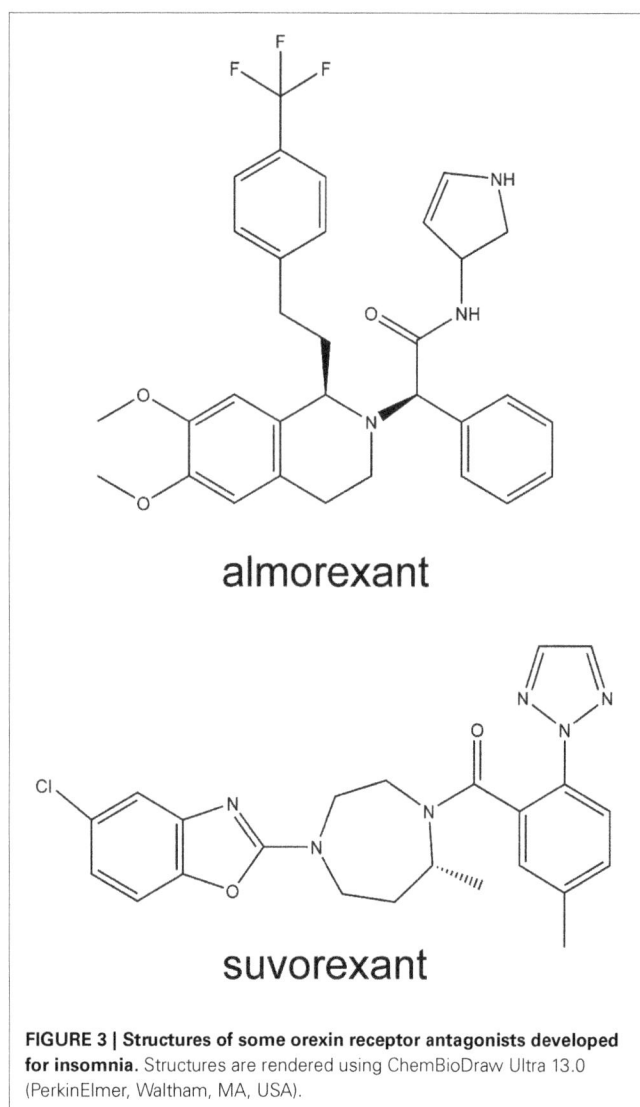

FIGURE 3 | Structures of some orexin receptor antagonists developed for insomnia. Structures are rendered using ChemBioDraw Ultra 13.0 (PerkinElmer, Waltham, MA, USA).

note that orexin-A/orexin-B pharmacology was suggested to be altered in OX_2^{10} Ser as compared to the wild-type OX_2^{10} Pro variant (see Impact of the genetic variation on the orexin receptor ligand binding).

Thus, orexin receptor sequence variation may contribute to sleep disorders (OX_2^{11} Thr, possibly OX_2^{10} Ser). This is by no means surprising; it may rather be unexpected that so few findings of this type have been described. However, dramatic orexin receptor mutations might have such a detrimental effect on the regulation of wakefulness that they have been eliminated from the population, while milder phenotypes persist.

THE ROLE OF THE OREXIN SYSTEM IN HEADACHES

The orexin system has been examined in various forms of headache including migraine and cluster headache. While cluster headache is a rare, extremely debilitating headache that occurs in groups (or clusters) during seasonal changes (Goadsby, 2002), migraines are comparatively common headaches that are comparatively more treatable with non-steroid anti-inflammatory drugs or specific serotonergic drugs. Migraines often run in families where as cluster headaches are more sporadic

(Benoliel and Eliav, 2013). While genome-wide studies have resulted in better understanding of migraine (Thompson et al., 2012), many complex traits, including cluster headache, have been less amenable to study—possibly due to their heterogeneity (Rainero et al., 2011b).

Cluster headache consists of attacks of sudden, severe, unilateral periorbital pain, accompanied by restlessness and cranial autonomic symptoms, and is characterized by a strikingly unique circadian and circannual rhythmicity (Goadsby, 2002). There is increasing evidence that cluster headache may have a significant genetic component. Genetic epidemiological studies have suggested that first-degree relatives of cluster headache probands are more likely to have cluster headache than the general population (Russell et al., 1996; Leone et al., 2001; El Amrani et al., 2002). Cluster headache has been found to be an autosomal dominant trait in some affected families, but despite numerous attempts, no clear molecular genetic basis has been identified for cluster headache (Russell, 2004). Segregation analysis suggests that cluster headache is a complex disease: several genetic factors may result in cluster headache when the correct environmental conditions are present (Pinessi et al., 2005).

Since there is no major gene effect for the orexin *loci* linked to migraine, the orexins have tended to be studied more frequently in cluster headache, where a model of complex genetic traits suggests multifactorial involvement that may include orexin *loci*. Numerous common polymorphisms of *HCRTR1* and *HCRTR2* have been studied in cluster headache (below), though the frequency and physiological significance of these variants is still being investigated (Rainero et al., 2004; Schürks et al., 2007a; Rainero et al., 2011b).

A number of studies provide evidence that orexins are involved in pain modulation within brain structures in the midbrain, indicating a possible link between orexins and the nociceptive phenomena observed in primary headache disorders (Bingham et al., 2001; Kajiyama et al., 2005; Mobarakeh et al., 2005). Orexin-producing neurons of CNS are also specifically located to the postero- and dorsolateral hypothalamus, regions implicated in cluster headache (May et al., 1998, 1999). The role of orexins in noradrenergic activation, shown by innervation and stimulation of the locus coeruleus in rats, monkeys and cats (Hagan et al., 1999; Horvath et al., 1999; Diano et al., 2003), may implicate changes in blood flow in cluster headache, although this evidence is not conclusive (Cohen and Goadsby, 2004). This suggests complexity of the cluster headache etiology.

OX₁ RECEPTORS IN MIGRAINE

In addition to synonymous SNPs (rs10914456, rs4949449), a non-synonymous *HCRTR1* polymorphism of G1222A in exon 7 (rs2271933) encoding an OX_1 Ile408Val substitution, has been implicated in migraine. Genotype and allele frequencies of the rs2271933 non-synonymous polymorphism have been associated with a 1.4-fold risk of migraine (Rainero et al., 2011b). The functional significance of this common OX_1 receptor variant is not fully understood, however. While OX_1^{408} in the receptor's C-terminus resides is likely to be located within the region for interaction with other proteins (below), it has not been experimentally resolved whether the mutation changes the receptor's expression level, coupling to effectors, or homo- or heterodimerization. Neither $OX_1{}^{408}$ variant correlates with human narcolepsy (Peyron et al., 2000; Olafsdottir et al., 2001).

OX₂ RECEPTORS IN CLUSTER HEADACHE

While the literature on the OX_2/*HCRTR2* polymorphisms (rs1049880, rs3122156T, rs9357855G, rs2653342A, rs2653349G) is large, it remains inconclusive (Rainero et al., 2004, 2008). In particular, homozygosity for the common G allele of rs2653349 (1246 G/A), encoding $OX_2{}^{308}$ Val, has been associated with an increased disease risk for cluster headache—as compared to the $OX_2{}^{308}$ Ile variant—in some, but not all studies. The association was confirmed in a large study from Germany—showing that homozygous carriers of the G allele had a 2-fold increase in cluster headache risk (Schürks et al., 2006)—but not in a GWAS study of cluster headache patients of Danish, Swedish, and British origin (Baumber et al., 2006).

Additionally five intronic polymorphisms, covering more than 75% of the entire 108.35 kb sequence of the *HCRTR2* gene, were used to evaluate the association between cluster headache and the OX_2/*HCRTR2* (Rainero et al., 2008). A significant difference between cluster headache cases and controls was found for 3 out of the 5 examined polymorphisms. Carriage of the GTAAGG haplotype—defined as a combination of the intronic positions Rs2653349, Rs3122156, Rs9357855, Rs2653342 and Rs3800539, and the exonic Rs2653349 (above)—was shown to be associated with cluster headache, resulting in a 3.7-fold increased risk. Sequence analysis of genomic DNA for the entire coding region of the OX_2/*HCRTR2* gene in 11 cluster headache patients, identified no additional coding sequence difference besides rs2653349. The functional relevance of these intronic variants and how they impact cluster headache, remains to be determined (Rainero et al., 2008). In another study, neither one of the rs2653349 alleles ($OX_2{}^{308}$ Val or Ile) was associated with response to drugs, such as triptans, in cluster headache (Schürks et al., 2007a).

In conclusion, orexin receptor variants $OX_1{}^{408}$ Val and $OX_2{}^{308}$ Val have been associated with a somewhat elevated risk for migraine and cluster headache, respectively. While the intracellular $OX_1{}^{408}$ may affect the receptor interaction with other intracellular or plasma membrane proteins, and the TM6 $OX_2{}^{308}$ ligand binding, it is not known whether variants at these amino acids result in distinct functional properties, or if the difference might be found in differential processing etc., as suggested by co-segregation of $OX_2{}^{308}$ Val with the intronic *HCRTR2* polymorphisms. Future studies should address the significance of co-inheritance of variants of both receptors.

OREXIN RECEPTOR VARIANTS IN PSYCHIATRIC DISORDERS
ANXIETY DISORDERS

The role of the orexins in anxiety disorders is currently unclear because orexins have been suggested to be both anxiogenic and anxiolytic—or possibly even neutral—in investigations in rodent models (Kukkonen, 2013). Nevertheless, orexinergic interventions into panic disorder are currently under investigation (Perna et al., 2011). Panic disorder is an anxiety disorder characterized by unexpected attacks of fear with enhanced arousal and somatic symptoms (Meuret et al., 2011). The heritability of panic disorder has been estimated to be 50% (Hettema

et al., 2001); however, the inheritance is most likely multifactorial. The rational for examining the involvement of orexins in panic disorder also reflects indications of orexin-mediated regulation of respiration (Kuwaki, 2008; Williams and Burdakov, 2008)—dysregulation of respiration is a hallmark of panic attacks. Orexin neurons innervate brain nuclei, such as the reticular formation of the medulla, that control respiration (Peyron et al., 1998). PPO knockout mice exhibit a decreased response to CO_2 that is partly restored by supplementation with orexin (Deng et al., 2007). OX_1 receptor antagonist, SB-334867, mimics the PPO knockout phenotype when administered to wild-type mice. Intracerebroventricular administration of orexin promotes respiration in rodents (Zhang et al., 2005; Johnson et al., 2012); in rats, this has been shown to be blocked by SB-334867 (Johnson et al., 2012).

$OX_2{}^{308}$ Ile variant has been associated with panic disorder in female patients (Annerbrink et al., 2011). In contrast, neither male nor female populations showed a risk associated with either variant (Val or Ile) of $OX_1{}^{408}$ (Annerbrink et al., 2011). Functional analysis of variant orexin receptors may provide insight into these allele associations.

MOOD DISORDERS

Studies in rodents have suggested that orexins may also be involved in the pathogenesis of mood disorders. Wistar-Kyoto rats, an animal model of depression, have a reduced number of hypothalamic cells expressing orexin immunoreactivity (Allard et al., 2007). Furthermore, neonatal administration of the tricyclic antidepressant clomipramine may result in decreased orexin concentrations in brain regions such as the hypothalamus (Feng et al., 2008).

Consistent with this, intracerebroventricular administration of orexin-A has a long-term antidepressessive effect in some rodent depression paradigms; an effect that may involve hippocampal neurogenesis (Ito et al., 2008). Activation of orexinergic neurons leads to the excitation of major monoaminergic nuclei of the brain stem, including raphe nuclei (serotonin), locus coeruleus (norepinephrine), and the ventral tegmental area (dopamine) (Peyron et al., 1998; Leonard and Kukkonen, 2014). Furthermore, orexin knockout mice show a significant reduction in the dopamine turnover rate and a compensatory increase of serotoninergic activity possibly suggesting a relationship between monoamines and orexins (Mori et al., 2010).

The role of orexins in drug addiction and reward (Aston-Jones et al., 2010; Boutrel et al., 2010; Thompson and Borgland, 2011) may be linked to the proposed involvement of orexins in mood regulation, and the tendency of depressed patients to self-medication. The few studies conducted in humans suggest decreases in CSF orexin-A concentrations or its rhythmicity in depression (Salomon et al., 2003; Brundin et al., 2007).

The possible contribution of orexin receptor variants to axis I disorders, however, has not been widely studied. For example, the functional $OX_2{}^{11}$ Ser variant identified in Tourette's syndrome has not been examined in other patient cohorts. By comparison, studies of the $OX_1{}^{408}$ Val variant have reported it to be associated with a 1.6-fold increased risk of major mood disorders as compared to the $OX_1{}^{408}$ Ile (Rainero et al., 2011a). Patients homozygous for the Val-coding allele (1222A; rs2271933)—in comparison with those homozygous for the Ile-coding allele (1222G)—have an even higher, 2.5-fold increased risk for mood disorders, as also confirmed by haplotype analysis (Rainero et al., 2011a). Functional analysis of variant orexin receptors may confirm the relevance of these findings.

SCHIZOPHRENIA

OX_1^{408} Ile/Val polymorphism has been studied in schizophrenia patients. Specifically, variation was associated with polydipsia–hyponatremia in schizophrenic patients when compared with non-polydipsic patients (Meerabux et al., 2005; Fukunaka et al., 2007); however, the associations were found for the opposite variants in the two studies.

Orexin regulation of water intake has been suggested by the anatomy of orexinergic projections to, for instance, subfornical organ and area postrema (Kukkonen et al., 2002). Intracerebroventricular infusion of orexin-A, more potently, but also of orexin-B, acutely increases water intake and drinking in rats (Kunii et al., 1999; Rodgers et al., 2000; Takano et al., 2004; Zheng et al., 2005; Kis et al., 2012), while in the continuous treatment (7 or 14 days), the effect wanes (Lin et al., 2002). PPO mRNA expression in the hypothalamus is upregulated upon water deprivation (Kunii et al., 1999). Orexin-A also excites subfornical organ neurons (Ono et al., 2008). Orexin-A alone does not affect baseline vasopressin release, but inhibits histamine-induced release in OX_1 receptor-dependent manner (Russell et al., 2001; Kis et al., 2012). In golden hamster, infusion of orexin-B, but not orexin-A, in the amygdala stimulates water intake (Avolio et al., 2012).

Thus, one physiological role of orexins may be in the regulation of water intake. Whether this has a role in schizophrenia-associated polydipsia, remains to be shown. However, the dopamine D_2-type receptor agonist, quinpirole, increases water intake, which is further enhanced by blocking OX_1 receptors with SB-334867 (Milella et al., 2010), which would rather suggest an opposite role for orexin signaling under these conditions.

CONCLUSIONS AND PERSPECTIVES

Human orexin receptor sequence variation has been investigated in the context of disease-based targeted approaches, first with narcolepsy and then with other diseases. Variants have been identified, some with an apparent relevance for the disease(s) under investigation, some not. Interestingly, the same variants that are putatively associated with headaches, namely OX_1^{408} and OX_2^{308} have been implicated in panic disorder, mood disorders and in polydipsia in schizophrenia. The "overrepresentation" of these variants in many disorders, however, may be an artifact from the candidate gene rational used to select these *loci*. However, in none of the cases has a very high risk been identified. Nevertheless, we suggest that the full functional phenotype of each receptor variant should be established; currently of greatest interest are the OX_1^{408}, OX_2^{10}, OX_2^{11}, and OX_2^{308} variants. In the absence of these data, the reasons behind the observations are difficult to speculate on.

So far, none of the orexin receptor variants has conferred a very high disease risk or apparently a very grave phenotype. Is this because the two orexin receptor subtypes are simply too

redundant; are the data sets confounded by a lack of valid disease phenotype classifications and an inadequate consideration of contributing environmental factors; or are the phenotypes carried by the known human orexin receptor gene variants simply rather mild? Currently, we cannot resolve this dilemma. We might assume, however, that any genotype grossly hampering orexin receptor function would be eliminated from the population due to its strong impact on the wakefulness, and thus the genotypes present only confer mild phenotypes. In essentially all cases we have to recognize the fact that cellular phenotypes of the orexin receptor variants have not been investigated, and conclusions based on this are thus vague. Evidence for a significant association of certain haplotypes of orexin genes with disease will inevitably be re-evaluated from a genome-wide perspective (GWAS) and with respect to the risk factors posed by other genetic and environmental variables. Although orexin receptor mutations may, alone, not confer highly increased risk (or protection) for a disease, these findings may propel studies concerning the physiological roles of orexins, and therefor also identify novel therapeutic approaches.

More complete study of orexins pharmacogenetics may facilitate novel areas of orexin research. This approach may help to refine drug design by targeting variant receptors. The continued study of orexin pharmacogenetics and receptor function at the cellular level is necessary before the role of orexinergic ligands in the treatment of disorders such as migraine, cluster headache, EDS and even idiopathic narcolepsy can be predicted fully. The emergence of dual orexin receptor antagonists, as well the possible OX_2-selective ones (Dugovic et al., 2009; Etori et al., 2014), reinforces evidence for the partly overlapping and partly distinct roles of orexin receptors in the regulation of sleep/wakefulness states. Characterization of variant receptor pharmacology may be of further use in establishing pharmacogenetic profiles for the drugs. Specific groups of sleep disorder patients may benefit from these compounds. For example, the sleep disturbances characteristic of Parkinson's and Alzheimer's diseases may be amenable to orexinergic drugs. Parkinson's disease patients frequently complain of sleep disturbances and loss of muscle tone during rapid-eye-movement (REM) sleep. A more complete evaluation of the pharmacology of orexin receptor variants may facilitate the development of orexin receptor agonists.

AUTHOR CONTRIBUTIONS

Every author contributed to the writing. Jyrki P. Kukkonen made the figures.

ACKNOWLEDGMENTS

This work was supported by grants from the Scottish Rite Foundation of Canada and the Ontario Brain Institute (OBI) *Eplink* Drug Discovery Project, The Canadian Institutes of Health Research (CIHR) and Epilepsy Canada (Miles D. Thompson), and the Liv and Hälsa Foundation (Jyrki P. Kukkonen).

REFERENCES

Allard, J. S., Tizabi, Y., Shaffery, J. P., and Manaye, K. (2007). Effects of rapid eye movement sleep deprivation on hypocretin neurons in the hypothalamus of a rat model of depression. *Neuropeptides* 41, 329–337. doi: 10.1016/j.npep.2007.04.006

Allen, R. P., Singer, H. S., Brown, J. E., and Salam, M. M. (1992). Sleep disorders in Tourette syndrome: a primary or unrelated problem? *Pediatr. Neurol.* 8, 275–280.

Annerbrink, K., Westberg, L., Olsson, M., Andersch, S., Sjodin, I., Holm, G., et al. (2011). Panic disorder is associated with the Val308Iso polymorphism in the hypocretin receptor gene. *Psychiatr. Genet.* 21, 85–89. doi: 10.1097/YPG.0b013e328341a3db

Aston-Jones, G., Smith, R. J., Sartor, G. C., Moorman, D. E., Massi, L., Tahsili-Fahadan, P., et al. (2010). Lateral hypothalamic orexin/hypocretin neurons: a role in reward-seeking and addiction. *Brain Res.* 1314, 74–90. doi: 10.1016/j.brainres.2009.09.106

Avolio, E., Alo, R., Mele, M., Carelli, A., Canonaco, A., Bucarelli, L., et al. (2012). Amygdalar excitatory/inhibitory circuits interacting with orexinergic neurons influence differentially feeding behaviors in hamsters. *Behav. Brain Res.* 234, 91–99. doi: 10.1016/j.bbr.2012.06.013

Baumber, L., Sjostrand, C., Leone, M., Harty, H., Bussone, G., Hillert, J., et al. (2006). A genome-wide scan and HCRTR2 candidate gene analysis in a European cluster headache cohort. *Neurology* 66, 1888–1893. doi: 10.1212/01.wnl.0000219765.95038.d7

Benoliel, R., and Eliav, E. (2013). Primary headache disorders. *Dent. Clin. North Am.* 57, 513–539. doi: 10.1016/j.cden.2013.04.005

Bingham, S., Davey, P. T., Babbs, A. J., Irving, E. A., Sammons, M. J., Wyles, M., et al. (2001). Orexin-A, an hypothalamic peptide with analgesic properties. *Pain* 92, 81–90. doi: 10.1016/S0304-3959(00)00470-X

Boutrel, B., Cannella, N., and de Lecea, L. (2010). The role of hypocretin in driving arousal and goal-oriented behaviors. *Brain Res.* 1314, 103–111. doi: 10.1016/j.brainres.2009.11.054

Brundin, L., Bjorkqvist, M., Petersen, A., and Traskman-Bendz, L. (2007). Reduced orexin levels in the cerebrospinal fluid of suicidal patients with major depressive disorder. *Eur. Neuropsychopharmacol.* 17, 573–579. doi: 10.1016/j.euroneuro.2007.01.005

Bulenger, S., Marullo, S., and Bouvier, M. (2005). Emerging role of homo- and heterodimerization in G-protein-coupled receptor biosynthesis and maturation. *Trends. Pharmacol. Sci.* 26, 131–137. doi: 10.1016/j.tips.2005.01.004

Chemelli, R. M., Willie, J. T., Sinton, C. M., Elmquist, J. K., Scammell, T., Lee, C., et al. (1999). Narcolepsy in orexin knockout mice: molecular genetics of sleep regulation. *Cell* 98, 437–451. doi: 10.1016/S0092-8674(00)81973-X

Cohen, A. S., and Goadsby, P. J. (2004). Functional neuroimaging of primary headache disorders. *Curr. Neurol. Neurosci. Rep.* 4, 105–110. doi: 10.1007/s11910-004-0023-7

Cohrs, S., Rasch, T., Altmeyer, S., Kinkelbur, J., Kostanecka, T., Rothenberger, A., et al. (2001). Decreased sleep quality and increased sleep related movements in patients with Tourette's syndrome. *J. Neurol. Neurosurg. Psychiatry* 70, 192–197. doi: 10.1136/jnnp.70.2.192

Cox, C. D., Breslin, M. J., Whitman, D. B., Schreier, J. D., McGaughey, G. B., Bogusky, M. J., et al. (2010). Discovery of the dual orexin receptor antagonist [(7R)-4-(5-chloro-1,3-benzoxazol-2-yl)-7-methyl-1,4-diazepan-1-yl][5-methyl-2-(2H -1,2,3-triazol-2-yl)phenyl]methanone (MK-4305) for the treatment of insomnia. *J. Med. Chem.* 53, 5320–5332. doi: 10.1021/jm100541c

Dalrymple, M. B., Jaeger, W. C., Eidne, K. A., and Pfleger, K. D. (2011). Temporal profiling of orexin receptor-arrestin-ubiquitin complexes reveals differences between receptor subtypes. *J. Biol. Chem.* 286, 16726–16733. doi: 10.1074/jbc.M111.223537

de Lecea, L., Kilduff, T. S., Peyron, C., Gao, X., Foye, P. E., Danielson, P. E., et al. (1998). The hypocretins: hypothalamus-specific peptides with neuroexcitatory activity. *Proc. Natl. Acad. Sci. U.S.A.* 95, 322–327.

Deng, B. S., Nakamura, A., Zhang, W., Yanagisawa, M., Fukuda, Y., and Kuwaki, T. (2007). Contribution of orexin in hypercapnic chemoreflex: evidence from genetic and pharmacological disruption and supplementation studies in mice. *J. Appl. Physiol.* 103, 1772–1779. doi: 10.1152/japplphysiol.00075.2007

Diano, S., Horvath, B., Urbanski, H. F., Sotonyi, P., and Horvath, T. L. (2003). Fasting activates the nonhuman primate hypocretin (orexin) system and its postsynaptic targets. *Endocrinology* 144, 3774–3778. doi: 10.1210/en.2003-0274

Dugovic, C., Shelton, J. E., Aluisio, L. E., Fraser, I. C., Jiang, X., Sutton, S. W., et al. (2009). Blockade of orexin-1 receptors attenuates orexin-2 receptor antagonism-induced sleep promotion in the rat. *J. Pharmacol. Exp. Ther.* 330, 142–151. doi: 10.1124/jpet.109.152009

Duguay, D., Belanger-Nelson, E., Mongrain, V., Beben, A., Khatchadourian, A., and Cermakian, N. (2011). Dynein light chain Tctex-type 1 modulates orexin signaling through its interaction with orexin 1 receptor. *PLoS ONE* 6:e26430. doi: 10.1371/journal.pone.0026430

El Amrani, M., Ducros, A., Boulan, P., Aidi, S., Crassard, I., Visy, J. M., et al. (2002). Familial cluster headache: a series of 186 index patients. *Headache* 42, 974–977. doi: 10.1046/j.1526-4610.2002.02226.x

Ellis, J., Pediani, J. D., Canals, M., Milasta, S., and Milligan, G. (2006). Orexin-1 receptor-cannabinoid CB1 receptor heterodimerization results in both ligand-dependent and -independent coordinated alterations of receptor localization and function. *J. Biol. Chem.* 281, 38812–38824. doi: 10.1074/jbc.M602494200

Etori, K., Saito, Y. C., Tsujino, N., and Sakurai, T. (2014). Effects of a newly developed potent orexin-2 receptor-selective antagonist, compound 1 m, on sleep/wakefulness states in mice. *Front. Neurosci.* 8:8. doi: 10.3389/fnins.2014.00008

Feng, P., Vurbic, D., Wu, Z., Hu, Y., and Strohl, K. P. (2008). Changes in brain orexin levels in a rat model of depression induced by neonatal administration of clomipramine. *J. Psychopharmacol.* 22, 784–791. doi: 10.1177/0269881106082899

Freeman, R. D., Fast, D. K., Burd, L., Kerbeshian, J., Robertson, M. M., and Sandor, P. (2000). An international perspective on Tourette syndrome: selected findings from 3,500 individuals in 22 countries. *Dev. Med. Child Neurol.* 42, 436–447. doi: 10.1017/S0012162200000839

Fukunaka, Y., Shinkai, T., Hwang, R., Hori, H., Utsunomiya, K., Sakata, S., et al. (2007). The orexin 1 receptor (HCRTR1) gene as a susceptibility gene contributing to polydipsia-hyponatremia in schizophrenia. *Neuromol. Med.* 9, 292–297. doi: 10.1007/s12017-007-8001-2

Gencik, M., Dahmen, N., Wieczorek, S., Kasten, M., Bierbrauer, J., Anghelescu, I., et al. (2001). A prepro-orexin gene polymorphism is associated with narcolepsy. *Neurology* 56, 115–117. doi: 10.1212/WNL.56.1.115

Goadsby, P. J. (2002). Pathophysiology of cluster headache: a trigeminal autonomic cephalgia. *Lancet Neurol.* 1, 251–257. doi: 10.1016/S1474-4422(02)00104-7

Hagan, J. J., Leslie, R. A., Patel, S., Evans, M. L., Wattam, T. A., Holmes, S., et al. (1999). Orexin A activates locus coeruleus cell firing and increases arousal in the rat. *Proc. Natl. Acad. Sci. U.S.A.* 96, 10911–10916. doi: 10.1073/pnas.96.19.10911

Haj-Dahmane, S., and Shen, R. Y. (2005). The wake-promoting peptide orexin-B inhibits glutamatergic transmission to dorsal raphe nucleus serotonin neurons through retrograde endocannabinoid signaling. *J. Neurosci.* 25, 896–905. doi: 10.1523/JNEUROSCI.3258-04.2005

Heifetz, A., Morris, G. B., Biggin, P. C., Barker, O., Fryatt, T., Bentley, J., et al. (2012). Study of human Orexin-1 and -2 G-protein-coupled receptors with novel and published antagonists by modeling, molecular dynamics simulations, and site-directed mutagenesis. *Biochemistry* 51, 3178–3197. doi: 10.1021/bi300136h

Hettema, J. M., Neale, M. C., and Kendler, K. S. (2001). A review and meta-analysis of the genetic epidemiology of anxiety disorders. *Am. J. Psychiatry* 158, 1568–1578. doi: 10.1176/appi.ajp.158.10.1568

Holmqvist, T., Johansson, L., Östman, M., Ammoun, S., Åkerman, K. E., and Kukkonen, J. P. (2005). OX_1 orexin receptors couple to adenylyl cyclase regulation via multiple mechanisms. *J. Biol. Chem.* 280, 6570–6579. doi: 10.1074/jbc.M407397200

Horvath, T. L., Peyron, C., Diano, S., Ivanov, A., Aston-Jones, G., Kilduff, T. S., et al. (1999). Hypocretin (orexin) activation and synaptic innervation of the locus coeruleus noradrenergic system. *J. Comp. Neurol.* 415, 145–159.

Huang, J., Chen, S., Zhang, J. J., and Huang, X. Y. (2013). Crystal structure of oligomeric beta1-adrenergic G protein-coupled receptors in ligand-free basal state. *Nat. Struct. Mol. Biol.* 20, 419–425. doi: 10.1038/nsmb.2504

Hungs, M., Fan, J., Lin, L., Lin, X., Maki, R. A., and Mignot, E. (2001). Identification and functional analysis of mutations in the hypocretin (orexin) genes of narcoleptic canines. *Genome Res.* 11, 531–539. doi: 10.1101/gr.161001

Ito, N., Yabe, T., Gamo, Y., Nagai, T., Oikawa, T., Yamada, H., et al. (2008). I.c.v. administration of orexin-A induces an antidepressive-like effect through hippocampal cell proliferation. *Neuroscience* 157, 720–732. doi: 10.1016/j.neuroscience.2008.09.042

Jaakola, V. P., Prilusky, J., Sussman, J. L., and Goldman, A. (2005). G protein-coupled receptors show unusual patterns of intrinsic unfolding. *Protein Eng. Des. Sel.* 18, 103–110. doi: 10.1093/protein/gzi004

Jäntti, M. H., Mandrika, I., and Kukkonen, J. P. (2014). Human orexin/hypocretin receptors form constitutive homo- and heteromeric complexes with each other and with human CB1 cannabinoid receptors. *Biochem. Biophys. Res. Commun.* 445, 486–490. doi: 10.1016/j.bbrc.2014.02.026

Jäntti, M. H., Putula, J., Turunen, P. M., Näsman, J., Reijonen, S., and Kukkonen, J. P. (2013). Autocrine endocannabinoid signaling potentiates orexin receptor signaling upon CB1 cannabinoid-OX_1 orexin receptor coexpression. *Mol. Pharmacol.* 83, 621–632. doi: 10.1124/mol.112.080523

Johnson, P. L., Samuels, B. C., Fitz, S. D., Lightman, S. L., Lowry, C. A., and Shekhar, A. (2012). Activation of the orexin 1 receptor is a critical component of CO2-mediated anxiety and hypertension but not bradycardia. *Neuropsychopharmacology* 37, 1911–1922. doi: 10.1038/npp.2012.38

Kajiyama, S., Kawamoto, M., Shiraishi, S., Gaus, S., Matsunaga, A., Suyama, H., et al. (2005). Spinal orexin-1 receptors mediate anti-hyperalgesic effects of intrathecally-administered orexins in diabetic neuropathic pain model rats. *Brain Res.* 1044, 76–86. doi: 10.1016/j.brainres.2005.03.007

Kantor, S., Mochizuki, T., Lops, S. N., Ko, B., Clain, E., Clark, E., et al. (2013). Orexin gene therapy restores the timing and maintenance of wakefulness in narcoleptic mice. *Sleep* 36, 1129–1138. doi: 10.5665/sleep.2870

Karteris, E., Machado, R. J., Chen, J., Zervou, S., Hillhouse, E. W., and Randeva, H. S. (2005). Food deprivation differentially modulates orexin receptor expression and signalling in the rat hypothalamus and adrenal cortex. *Am. J. Physiol. Endocrinol. Metab.* 288, E1089–E1100. doi: 10.1152/ajpendo.00351.2004

Karteris, E., Randeva, H. S., Grammatopoulos, D. K., Jaffe, R. B., and Hillhouse, E. W. (2001). Expression and coupling characteristics of the crh and orexin type 2 receptors in human fetal adrenals. *J. Clin. Endocrinol. Metab.* 86, 4512–4519

Kis, G. K., Molnar, A. H., Daruka, L., Gardi, J., Rakosi, K., Laszlo, F., et al. (2012). The osmotically and histamine-induced enhancement of the plasma vasopressin level is diminished by intracerebroventricularly administered orexin in rats. *Pflugers Arch.* 463, 531–536. doi: 10.1007/s00424-012-1080-4

Kukkonen, J. P. (2012). Recent progress in orexin/hypocretin physiology and pharmacology. *Biomol. Concepts* 3, 447–463. doi: 10.1515/bmc-2012-0013

Kukkonen, J. P. (2013). Physiology of the orexinergic/hypocretinergic system: a revisit in 2012. *Am. J. Physiol. Cell Physiol.* 304, C2–C32. doi: 10.1152/ajpcell.00227.2012

Kukkonen, J. P., Holmqvist, T., Ammoun, S., and Åkerman, K. E. (2002). Functions of the orexinergic/hypocretinergic system. *Am. J. Physiol. Cell. Physiol.* 283, C1567–C1591. doi: 10.1152/ajpcell.00055.2002

Kukkonen, J. P., and Leonard, C. S. (2014). Orexin/hypocretin receptor signalling cascades. *Br. J. Pharmacol.* 171, 294–313. doi: 10.1111/bph.12324

Kunii, K., Yamanaka, A., Nambu, T., Matsuzaki, I., Goto, K., and Sakurai, T. (1999). Orexins/hypocretins regulate drinking behaviour. *Brain Res.* 842, 256–261. doi: 10.1016/S0006-8993(99)01884-3

Kuwaki, T. (2008). Orexinergic modulation of breathing across vigilance states. *Respir. Physiol. Neurobiol.* 164, 204–212. doi: 10.1016/j.resp.2008.03.011

Leonard, C. S., and Kukkonen, J. P. (2014). Orexin/hypocretin receptor signalling: a functional perspective. *Br. J. Pharmacol.* 171, 294–313. doi: 10.1111/bph.12296

Leone, M., Russell, M. B., Rigamonti, A., Attanasio, A., Grazzi, L., D'Amico, D., et al. (2001). Increased familial risk of cluster headache. *Neurology* 56, 1233–1236. doi: 10.1212/WNL.56.9.1233

Liang, Y., Fotiadis, D., Filipek, S., Saperstein, D. A., Palczewski, K., and Engel, A. (2003). Organization of the G protein-coupled receptors rhodopsin and opsin in native membranes. *J. Biol. Chem.* 278, 21655–21662. doi: 10.1074/jbc.M302536200

Lin, L., Faraco, J., Li, R., Kadotani, H., Rogers, W., Lin, X., et al. (1999). The sleep disorder canine narcolepsy is caused by a mutation in the hypocretin (orexin) receptor 2 gene. *Cell* 98, 365–376. doi: 10.1016/S0092-8674(00)81965-0

Lin, Y., Matsumura, K., Tsuchihashi, T., Abe, I., and Iida, M. (2002). Chronic central infusion of orexin-A increases arterial pressure in rats. *Brain Res. Bull.* 57, 619–622. doi: 10.1016/S0361-9230(01)00756-0

Liu, M., Blanco-Centurion, C., Konadhode, R., Begum, S., Pelluru, D., Gerashchenko, D., et al. (2011). Orexin gene transfer into zona incerta neurons suppresses muscle paralysis in narcoleptic mice. *J. Neurosci.* 31, 6028–6040. doi: 10.1523/JNEUROSCI.6069-10.2011

Madsen, O., Willemsen, D., Ursing, B. M., Arnason, U., and de Jong, W. W. (2002). Molecular evolution of the mammalian alpha 2B adrenergic receptor. *Mol. Biol. Evol.* 19, 2150–2160. doi: 10.1093/oxfordjournals.molbev.a004040

Magga, J., Bart, G., Oker-Blom, C., Kukkonen, J. P., Åkerman, K. E., and Näsman, J. (2006). Agonist potency differentiates G protein activation and Ca2+ signalling by the orexin receptor type 1. *Biochem. Pharmacol.* 71, 827–836. doi: 10.1016/j.bcp.2005.12.021

Malherbe, P., Roche, O., Marcuz, A., Kratzeisen, C., Wettstein, J. G., and Bissantz, C. (2010). Mapping the binding pocket of dual antagonist almorexant to human orexin 1 and orexin 2 receptors: comparison with the selective OX_1 (SB-674042) and OX_2 (EMPA) antagonists. *Mol. Pharmacol.* 78, 81–93. doi: 10.1124/mol.110.064584

May, A., Ashburner, J., Buchel, C., McGonigle, D. J., Friston, K. J., Frackowiak, R. S., et al. (1999). Correlation between structural and functional changes in brain in an idiopathic headache syndrome. *Nat. Med.* 5, 836–838. doi: 10.1038/10561

May, A., Bahra, A., Buchel, C., Frackowiak, R. S., and Goadsby, P. J. (1998). Hypothalamic activation in cluster headache attacks. *Lancet* 352, 275–278. doi: 10.1016/S0140-6736(98)02470-2

Meerabux, J., Iwayama, Y., Sakurai, T., Ohba, H., Toyota, T., Yamada, K., et al. (2005). Association of an orexin 1 receptor 408Val variant with polydipsia-hyponatremia in schizophrenic subjects. *Biol. Psychiatry* 58, 401–407. doi: 10.1016/j.biopsych.2005.04.015

Meuret, A. E., Rosenfield, D., Wilhelm, F. H., Zhou, E., Conrad, A., Ritz, T., and Roth, W. T. (2011). Do unexpected panic attacks occur spontaneously? *Biol. Psychiatry* 70, 985–991. doi: 10.1016/j.biopsych.2011.05.027

Mieda, M., and Sakurai, T. (2013). Orexin (hypocretin) receptor agonists and antagonists for treatment of sleep disorders. Rationale for development and current status. *CNS Drugs* 27, 83–90. doi: 10.1007/s40263-012-0036-8

Milasta, S., Evans, N. A., Ormiston, L., Wilson, S., Lefkowitz, R. J., and Milligan, G. (2005). The sustainability of interactions between the orexin-1 receptor and beta-arrestin-2 is defined by a single C-terminal cluster of hydroxy amino acids and modulates the kinetics of ERK MAPK regulation. *Biochem. J.* 387, 573–584. doi: 10.1042/BJ20041745

Milella, M. S., Passarelli, F., De Carolis, L., Schepisi, C., Nativio, P., Scaccianoce, S., et al. (2010). Opposite roles of dopamine and orexin in quinpirole-induced excessive drinking: a rat model of psychotic polydipsia. *Psychopharmacology* 211, 355–366. doi: 10.1007/s00213-010-1909-5

Milligan, G. (2009). G protein-coupled receptor hetero-dimerization: contribution to pharmacology and function. *Br. J. Pharmacol.* 158, 5–14. doi: 10.1111/j.1476-5381.2009.00169.x

Mobarakeh, J. I., Takahashi, K., Sakurada, S., Nishino, S., Watanabe, H., Kato, M., et al. (2005). Enhanced antinociception by intracerebroventricularly administered orexin A in histamine H1 or H2 receptor gene knockout mice. *Pain* 118, 254–262. doi: 10.1016/j.pain.2005.08.024

Mori, T., Ito, S., Kuwaki, T., Yanagisawa, M., Sakurai, T., and Sawaguchi, T. (2010). Monoaminergic neuronal changes in orexin deficient mice. *Neuropharmacology* 58, 826–832. doi: 10.1016/j.neuropharm.2009.08.009

Nishino, S., Ripley, B., Overeem, S., Lammers, G. J., and Mignot, E. (2000). Hypocretin (orexin) deficiency in human narcolepsy. *Lancet* 355, 39–40. doi: 10.1016/S0140-6736(99)05582-8

Obenauer, J. C., Cantley, L. C., and Yaffe, M. B. (2003). Scansite 2.0: Proteome-wide prediction of cell signaling interactions using short sequence motifs. *Nucleic Acids Res.* 31, 3635–3641. doi: 10.1093/nar/gkg584

Olafsdottir, B. R., Rye, D. B., Scammell, T. E., Matheson, J. K., Stefansson, K., and Gulcher, J. R. (2001). Polymorphisms in hypocretin/orexin pathway genes and narcolepsy. *Neurology* 57, 1896–1899. doi: 10.1212/WNL.57.10.1896

Ono, K., Kai, A., Honda, E., and Inenaga, K. (2008). Hypocretin-1/orexin-A activates subfornical organ neurons of rats. *Neuroreport* 19, 69–73. doi: 10.1097/WNR.0b013e3282f32d64

Perna, G., Guerriero, G., and Caldirola, D. (2011). Emerging drugs for panic disorder. *Expert Opin. Emerg. Drugs* 16, 631–645. doi: 10.1517/14728214.2011.628313

Peyron, C., Faraco, J., Rogers, W., Ripley, B., Overeem, S., Charnay, Y., et al. (2000). A mutation in a case of early onset narcolepsy and a generalized absence of hypocretin peptides in human narcoleptic brains. *Nat. Med.* 6, 991–997. doi: 10.1038/79690

Peyron, C., Tighe, D. K., van den Pol, A. N., de Lecea, L., Heller, H. C., Sutcliffe, J. G., et al. (1998). Neurons containing hypocretin (orexin) project to multiple neuronal systems. *J. Neurosci.* 18, 9996–10015.

Pinessi, L., Rainero, I., Rivoiro, C., Rubino, E., and Gallone, S. (2005). Genetics of cluster headache: an update. *J. Headache Pain* 6, 234–236. doi: 10.1007/s10194-005-0194-x

Putula, J., and Kukkonen, J. P. (2012). Mapping of the binding sites for the OX(1) orexin receptor antagonist, SB-334867, using orexin/hypocretin receptor chimaeras. *Neurosci. Lett.* 506, 111–115. doi: 10.1016/j.neulet.2011.10.061

Putula, J., Turunen, P. M., Johansson, L., Näsman, J., Ra, R., Korhonen, L., et al. (2011). Orexin/hypocretin receptor chimaeras reveal structural features important for orexin peptide distinction. *FEBS Lett.* 585, 1368–1374. doi: 10.1016/j.febslet.2011.04.020

Rainero, I., Gallone, S., Rubino, E., Ponzo, P., Valfre, W., Binello, E., et al. (2008). Haplotype analysis confirms the association between the HCRTR2 gene and cluster headache. *Headache* 48, 1108–1114. doi: 10.1111/j.1526-4610.2008.01080.x

Rainero, I., Gallone, S., Valfre, W., Ferrero, M., Angilella, G., Rivoiro, C., et al. (2004). A polymorphism of the hypocretin receptor 2 gene is associated with cluster headache. *Neurology* 63, 1286–1288. doi: 10.1212/01.WNL.0000142424.65251.DB

Rainero, I., Ostacoli, L., Rubino, E., Gallone, S., Picci, L. R., Fenoglio, P., et al. (2011a). Association between major mood disorders and the hypocretin receptor 1 gene. *J. Affect. Disord.* 130, 487–491. doi: 10.1016/j.jad.2010.10.033

Rainero, I., Rubino, E., Gallone, S., Fenoglio, P., Picci, L. R., Giobbe, L., et al. (2011b). Evidence for an association between migraine and the hypocretin receptor 1 gene. *J. Headache Pain* 12, 193–199. doi: 10.1007/s10194-011-0314-8

Randeva, H. S., Karteris, E., Grammatopoulos, D., and Hillhouse, E. W. (2001). Expression of orexin-A and functional orexin type 2 receptors in the human adult adrenals: implications for adrenal function and energy homeostasis. *J. Clin. Endocrinol. Metab.* 86, 4808–4813. doi: 10.1210/jc.86.10.4808

Ritter, S. L., and Hall, R. A. (2009). Fine-tuning of GPCR activity by receptor-interacting proteins. *Nat. Rev. Mol. Cell Biol.* 10, 819–830. doi: 10.1038/nrm2803

Rodgers, R. J., Halford, J. C., Nunes de Souza, R. L., Canto de Souza, A. L., Piper, D. C., Arch, J. R., et al. (2000). Dose-response effects of orexin-A on food intake and the behavioural satiety sequence in rats. *Regul. Pept.* 96, 71–84. doi: 10.1016/S0167-0115(00)00203-2

Russell, M. B. (2004). Epidemiology and genetics of cluster headache. *Lancet Neurol.* 3, 279–283. doi: 10.1016/S1474-4422(04)00735-5

Russell, M. B., Andersson, P. G., and Iselius, L. (1996). Cluster headache is an inherited disorder in some families. *Headache* 36, 608–612.

Russell, S. H., Small, C. J., Dakin, C. L., Abbott, C. R., Morgan, D. G., Ghatei, M. A., et al. (2001). The central effects of orexin-A in the hypothalamic-pituitary-adrenal axis *in vivo* and *in vitro* in male rats. *J. Neuroendocrinol.* 13, 561–566. doi: 10.1046/j.1365-2826.2001.00672.x

Sakurai, T., Amemiya, A., Ishii, M., Matsuzaki, I., Chemelli, R. M., Tanaka, H., et al. (1998). Orexins and orexin receptors: a family of hypothalamic neuropeptides and G protein-coupled receptors that regulate feeding behavior. *Cell* 92, 573–585. doi: 10.1016/S0092-8674(00)80949-6

Salomon, R. M., Ripley, B., Kennedy, J. S., Johnson, B., Schmidt, D., Zeitzer, J. M., et al. (2003). Diurnal variation of cerebrospinal fluid hypocretin-1 (Orexin-A) levels in control and depressed subjects. *Biol. Psychiatry* 54, 96–104. doi: 10.1016/S0006-3223(02)01740-7

Schürks, M., Kurth, T., Geissler, I., Tessmann, G., Diener, H. C., and Rosskopf, D. (2006). Cluster headache is associated with the G1246A polymorphism in the hypocretin receptor 2 gene. *Neurology* 66, 1917–1919. doi: 10.1212/01.wnl.0000215852.35329.34

Schürks, M., Kurth, T., Geissler, I., Tessmann, G., Diener, H. C., and Rosskopf, D. (2007a). The G1246A polymorphism in the hypocretin receptor 2 gene is not associated with treatment response in cluster headache. *Cephalalgia* 27, 363–367. doi: 10.1111/j.1468-2982.2007.01287.x

Schürks, M., Limmroth, V., Geissler, I., Tessmann, G., Savidou, I., Engelbergs, J., et al. (2007b). Association between migraine and the G1246A polymorphism in the hypocretin receptor 2 gene. *Headache* 47, 1195–1199. doi: 10.1111/j.1526-4610.2007.00863.x

Takano, S., Kanai, S., Hosoya, H., Ohta, M., Uematsu, H., and Miyasaka, K. (2004). Orexin-A does not stimulate food intake in old rats. *Am. J. Physiol. Gastrointest. Liver Physiol.* 287, G1182–1187. doi: 10.1152/ajpgi.00218.2004

Thompson, J. L., and Borgland, S. L. (2011). A role for hypocretin/orexin in motivation. *Behav. Brain Res.* 217, 446–453. doi: 10.1016/j.bbr.2010.09.028

Thompson, M. D., Burnham, W. M., and Cole, D. E. (2005). The G protein-coupled receptors: pharmacogenetics and disease. *Crit. Rev. Clin. Lab. Sci.* 42, 311–392. doi: 10.1080/10408360591001895

Thompson, M. D., Cole, D. E., and Jose, P. A. (2008a). Pharmacogenomics of G protein-coupled receptor signaling: insights from health and disease. *Methods Mol. Biol.* 448, 77–107. doi: 10.1007/978-1-59745-205-2_6

Thompson, M. D., Comings, D. E., Abu-Ghazalah, R., Jereseh, Y., Lin, L., Wade, J., et al. (2004). Variants of the orexin2/hcrt2 receptor gene identified in patients with excessive daytime sleepiness and patients with Tourette's syndrome comorbidity. *Am. J. Med. Genet. B Neuropsychiatr. Genet.* 129, 69–75. doi: 10.1002/ajmg.b.30047

Thompson, M. D., Noble-Topham, S., Percy, M. E., Andrade, D. M., and Ebers, G. C. (2012). Chromosome 1p36 in migraine with aura: association study of the 5HT(1D) locus. *Neuroreport* 23, 45–48. doi: 10.1097/WNR.0b013e32834e5af3

Thompson, M. D., Percy, M. E., McIntyre Burnham, W., and Cole, D. E. (2008b). G protein-coupled receptors disrupted in human genetic disease. *Methods Mol. Biol.* 448, 109–137. doi: 10.1007/978-1-59745-205-2_7

Thompson, M. D., Siminovitch, K. A., and Cole, D. E. (2008c). G protein-coupled receptor pharmacogenetics. *Methods Mol. Biol.* 448, 139–185. doi: 10.1007/978-1-59745-205-2_8

Tran, D. T., Bonaventure, P., Hack, M., Mirzadegan, T., Dvorak, C., Letavic, M., et al. (2011). Chimeric, mutant orexin receptors show key interactions between orexin receptors, peptides and antagonists. *Eur. J. Pharmacol.* 667, 120–128. doi: 10.1016/j.ejphar.2011.05.074

Turunen, P. M., Jäntti, M. H., and Kukkonen, J. P. (2012). OX1 orexin/hypocretin receptor signaling via arachidonic acid and endocannabinoid release. *Mol. Pharmacol.* 82, 156–167. doi: 10.1124/mol.112.078063

Ward, R. J., Pediani, J. D., and Milligan, G. (2011). Hetero-multimerization of the cannabinoid CB1 receptor and the orexin OX1 receptor generates a unique complex in which both protomers are regulated by orexin A. *J. Biol. Chem.* 286, 37414–37428. doi: 10.1074/jbc.M111.287649

Wess, J. (1998). Molecular basis of receptor/G-protein-coupling selectivity. *Pharmacol. Ther.* 80, 231–264. doi: 10.1016/S0163-7258(98)00030-8

Williams, R. H., and Burdakov, D. (2008). Hypothalamic orexins/hypocretins as regulators of breathing. *Expert Rev. Mol. Med.* 10, e28. doi: 10.1017/S1462399408000823

Winrow, C. J., Gotter, A. L., Cox, C. D., Doran, S. M., Tannenbaum, P. L., Breslin, M. J., et al. (2011). Promotion of sleep by suvorexant-a novel dual orexin receptor antagonist. *J. Neurogenet.* 25, 52–61. doi: 10.3109/01677063.2011.566953

Winrow, C. J., and Renger, J. J. (2014). Discovery and development of orexin receptor antagonists as therapeutics for insomnia. *Br. J. Pharmacol.* 171, 283–293. doi: 10.1111/bph.12261

Wu, B., Chien, E. Y., Mol, C. D., Fenalti, G., Liu, W., Katritch, V., et al. (2010). Structures of the CXCR4 chemokine GPCR with small-molecule and cyclic peptide antagonists. *Science* 330, 1066–1071. doi: 10.1126/science.1194396

Xu, T. R., Ward, R. J., Pediani, J. D., and Milligan, G. (2011). The orexin OX1 receptor exists predominantly as a homodimer in the basal state: potential regulation of receptor organization by both agonist and antagonist ligands. *Biochem. J.* 439, 171–183. doi: 10.1042/BJ20110230

Zhang, W., Fukuda, Y., and Kuwaki, T. (2005). Respiratory and cardiovascular actions of orexin-A in mice. *Neurosci. Lett.* 385, 131–136. doi: 10.1016/j.neulet.2005.05.032

Zheng, H., Patterson, L. M., and Berthoud, H. R. (2005). Orexin-A projections to the caudal medulla and orexin-induced c-Fos expression, food intake, and autonomic function. *J. Comp. Neurol.* 485, 127–142. doi: 10.1002/cne.20515

Conflict of Interest Statement: The authors declare that the research was conducted in the absence of any commercial or financial relationships that could be construed as a potential conflict of interest.

17

Orexin A and orexin receptor 1 axonal traffic in dorsal roots at the CNS/PNS interface

Damien Colas[1,2]*, Annalisa Manca[2], Jean-Dominique Delcroix[2] and Philippe Mourrain[3,4]*

[1] Department of Biology, Stanford University, Stanford, CA, USA
[2] Laboratory of Neurodegeneration and Axon Dynamics, European Brain Research Institute, Rome, Italy
[3] Department of Psychiatry and Behavioral Sciences, Center for Sleep Sciences, Beckman Center, Stanford University, Stanford, CA, USA
[4] INSERM 1024, Ecole Normale Supérieure, Paris, France

Edited by:
Christopher J. Winrow, Merck, USA

Reviewed by:
Gabriella Gobbi, McGill University,
Canada
Daya S. Gupta, Camden County
College, USA
Kyle Baumbauer, University of
Pittsburgh Medical School, USA
Chloe Alexandre, Beth Israel
Deaconess Medical Center, USA

*Correspondence:
Damien Colas, Department of
Biology, Stanford University, 371
Serra Mall, Stanford, CA 94305, USA
e-mail: colas@stanford.edu;
Philippe Mourrain, Center for Sleep
Sciences, Beckman Center, Stanford
University, 279 Campus Drive,
Room B201, Stanford, CA 94305,
USA
e-mail: mourrain@stanford.edu

Hypothalamic orexin/hypocretin neurons send long axonal projections through the dorsal spinal cord in lamina I–II of the dorsal horn (DH) at the interface with the peripheral nervous system (PNS). We show that in the DH OXA fibers colocalize with substance P (SP) positive afferents of dorsal root ganglia (DRG) neurons known to mediate sensory processing. Further, OR1 is expressed in p75[NTR] and SP positive DRG neurons, suggesting a potential signaling pathway between orexin and DRG neurons. Interestingly, DRG sensory neurons have a distinctive bifurcating axon where one branch innervates the periphery and the other one the spinal cord (pseudo-unipolar neurons), allowing for potential functional coupling of distinct targets. We observe that OR1 is transported selectively from DRG toward the spinal cord, while OXA is accumulated retrogradely toward the DRG. We hence report a rare situation of asymmetrical neuropeptide receptor distribution between axons projected by a single neuron. These molecular and cellular data are consistent with the role of OXA/OR1 in sensory processing, including DRG neuronal modulation, and support the potential existence of an OX/HCRT circuit between CNS and PNS.

Keywords: orexin, hypocretin, receptor 1, dorsal root ganglia, axonal transport, nociception, substance P

INTRODUCTION

Orexin A and B (OXA and B also known as hypocretin 1 and 2, HCRT1 and 2) are neuropeptides produced within the lateral/perifornical hypothalamus, derived from a single prepropeptide (de Lecea et al., 1998; Sakurai et al., 1998). While their cell bodies form a compact cluster within the hypothalamus, OX/HCRT neurons project widely throughout the central nervous system (CNS) from the olfactory bulbs to the spinal cord in both mammals and fishes (Cutler et al., 1999; van den Pol, 1999; Appelbaum et al., 2009; de Lecea, 2010). These widespread projections are matched by the expression of the two orexin receptors (OR1 and 2) (Hervieu et al., 2001; Marcus et al., 2001). OR1 displays higher affinity for OXA than OXB, whereas OR2 has equal affinity for both ligands. Orexins play a crucial role in orchestrating mechanisms related to the level of arousal such as feeding, reward-seeking, metabolism, and energy expenditure (for review see Tsujino and Sakurai, 2013). This neuropeptidergic system is particularly well known for stabilizing the sleep-wake states and is responsible for narcolepsy when disrupted (Peyron et al., 2000; Sakurai, 2013; Sorensen et al., 2013). As such, OX innervations of other sleep-regulating brain nuclei are extensively studied. While it is well known that OX axons project throughout the dorsal spinal cord (Cutler et al., 1999; van den Pol, 1999; Appelbaum et al., 2009; de Lecea, 2010), the interaction of the central OX system with the peripheral nervous system (PNS) including the dorsal root ganglia (DRG) (Hervieu et al., 2001) has

been less explored. Interestingly, several studies have shown that OXA and OR1 can modulate sensory and nociception processing (for review Chiou et al., 2010).

DRG neurons are pseudo-unipolar neurons that have the unique property of projecting axon branches toward the spinal cord and toward peripheral targets (**Figure 1A**) (Kandel et al., 2000). In the periphery, DRG neurons innervate the skin and muscle (Kandel et al., 2000). In the spinal cord, afferents of proprioceptive DRG neurons terminate in the ventral horn, afferents of cutaneous mechanoreceptive DRG neurons terminate in the deep dorsal horn (DH) and afferents of nociceptive and thermoreceptive DRG neurons terminate in the superficial (lamina I/II) DH (Kandel et al., 2000). The difference between projection areas of DRG neurons in the central and the PNS prompted us to question whether neurotransmission material present in both axon branches was identical (Delcroix et al., 2004). Here, we show that in the DH of the spinal cord lamina I and II, DRG afferents closely appose with the OXA descending innervation arising from the hypothalamus. We also observed that OR1 is expressed in DRG neuron cell bodies and detected in the dorsal root (DR) connecting the DRG to the spinal cord but not in the sciatic nerve (SN). This data suggests that the anterograde axonal transport of OR1 can be directed toward one axon branch and not the other. Consistent with this finding, OXA is also detected in the DRG neuron cell bodies suggesting a retrograde transport from the spinal cord to the DRG. This body of

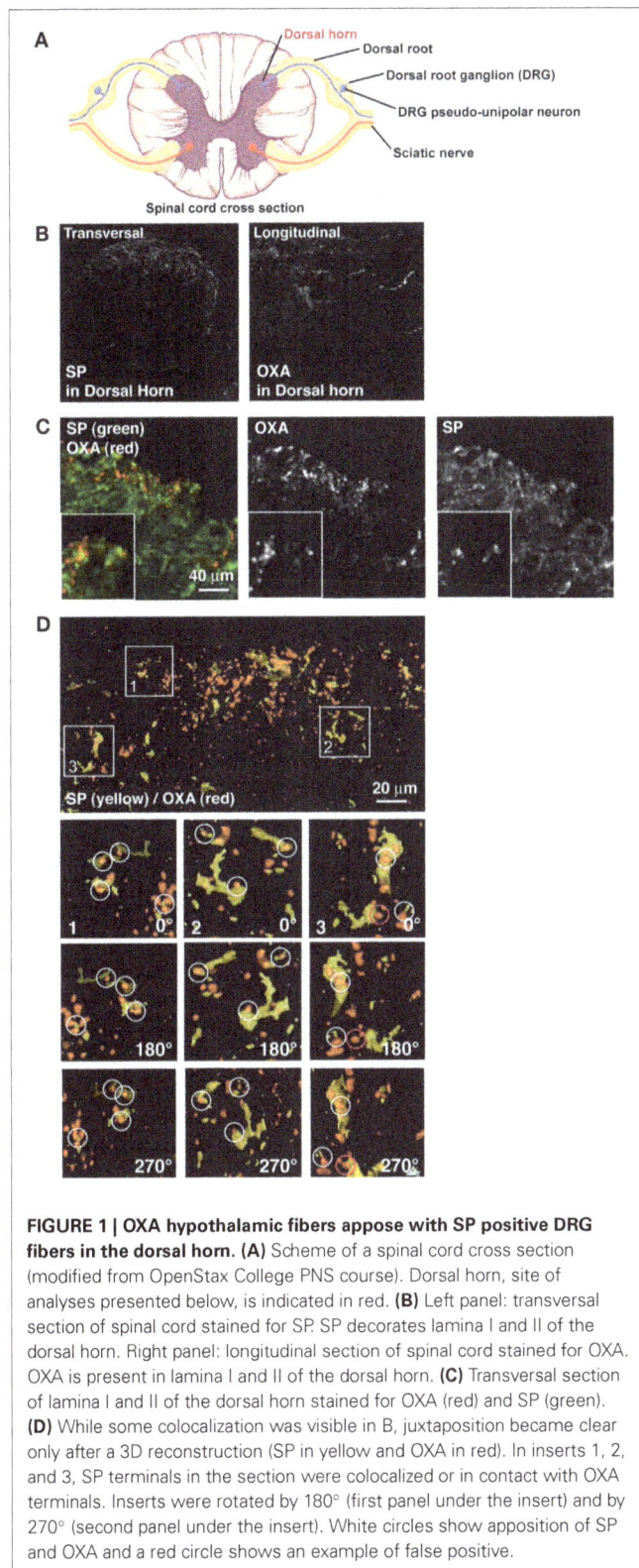

FIGURE 1 | OXA hypothalamic fibers appose with SP positive DRG fibers in the dorsal horn. (A) Scheme of a spinal cord cross section (modified from OpenStax College PNS course). Dorsal horn, site of analyses presented below, is indicated in red. **(B)** Left panel: transversal section of spinal cord stained for SP. SP decorates lamina I and II of the dorsal horn. Right panel: longitudinal section of spinal cord stained for OXA. OXA is present in lamina I and II of the dorsal horn. **(C)** Transversal section of lamina I and II of the dorsal horn stained for OXA (red) and SP (green). **(D)** While some colocalization was visible in B, juxtaposition became clear only after a 3D reconstruction (SP in yellow and OXA in red). In inserts 1, 2, and 3, SP terminals in the section were colocalized or in contact with OXA terminals. Inserts were rotated by 180° (first panel under the insert) and by 270° (second panel under the insert). White circles show apposition of SP and OXA and a red circle shows an example of false positive.

work supports at the cellular level the existence of an interaction between the central hypothalamic orexin neurons and the PNS. Understanding the influence of orexins on the PNS physiology is not only important for its function in arousal threshold changes

but also potentially relevant to OXA anti-nociceptive function (Dauvilliers et al., 2011; Doghramji, 2012; Roehrs et al., 2012).

RESULTS

OREXIN A AXONAL FIBERS AND SP POSITIVE FIBERS FROM DRG ARE JUXTAPOSED IN SPINAL CORD LAMINA I AND II

CNS OX/HCRT neurons are well known for their long axonal projections to the dorsal spinal cord (Cutler et al., 1999; van den Pol, 1999; Appelbaum et al., 2009). Similarly, PNS axons coming from the DRG and releasing Substance P (SP) connect the CNS in lamina I and II of the spinal cord DH (Nichols et al., 1999), suggesting a possible interaction with the OX/HCRT circuit in these layers. Thus, we first inquired if afferents of SP neurons in the spinal cord were in physical contact with OXA-positive fibers arising from the hypothalamus. Axons expressing OXA propagate into lamina I and II by spreading longitudinally (**Figure 1B**) (Cutler et al., 1999; van den Pol, 1999) whereas the SP positive fibers branch and spread robustly in a coronal fashion in these layers (**Figure 1B**). OXA and SP double immunofluorescent histochemistry staining suggested colocalization of these fibers (**Figure 1C**), but due to these innervation orthogonal characteristics it was difficult to analyze the extent of the apposition between SP and OXA either in coronal sections or in longitudinal sections. 3D reconstructions of coronal sections (see **Figure 1D**) clearly showed that OXA and SP terminals are juxtaposed in lamina I and II (**Figure 1D**). We found that $22 \pm 4\%$ (from 4 rats, 2 sections taken from the DH) of OXA terminals colocalized with SP terminals, whereas $75 \pm 6\%$ (from 4 rats, 2 sections taken from the DH) of SP terminals colocalized with OXA terminals.

OREXIN RECEPTOR 1 IS EXPRESSED IN DORSAL ROOT GANGLIA p75^{NTR}/SP NEURONS

Since the OXA positive terminals were potentially in contact with SP positive fibers, we tested if OR1 was present in DRG neurons (see schematic **Figure 2A**) expressing SP or p75 neurotrophin receptor (p75^{NTR}), another marker for sensory neurons (Delcroix et al., 1998, 2003) (**Figure 2B**). Staining for p75^{NTR} and OR1 was neuronal since the nuclei of satellite cells stained with DAPI did not show OR1 staining (**Figure 2B**). The percentage of p75^{NTR}-positive cells was $43 \pm 4\%$ (from 4 rats, 2 sections taken from the middle of the DRG). The percentage of OR1-positive cells was $57 \pm 5\%$ (from 4 rats, 2 sections taken from the middle of the DRG). The neuroanatomical analysis showed that p75^{NTR}-positive neurons were predominantly small and medium sized neurons (cell bodies ranging from 250 to 750 μm^2, **Figure 2E**). The size of OR1-positive neurons was also small and medium (**Figures 2E,F**). This size and morphology distribution was consistent with our previous characterization of the DRG p75^{NTR} and trkA-expressing sensory neurons (Delcroix et al., 1998, 2003).

Importantly, double staining of DRGs shows that most, if not all, of the p75^{NTR}-positive neurons express OR1 (**Figure 2B**), even if it was also clear that neurons other than p75^{NTR}-positive neurons were OR1 positive. DRG sections were also immunostained for OR1 and SP (**Figure 2C**) and we observed that all SP positive cells also expressed OR1 (**Figure 2C**). The large co-expression of OR1 with p75^{NTR} and SP markers hence further supports a potential interaction between the OXA terminals and

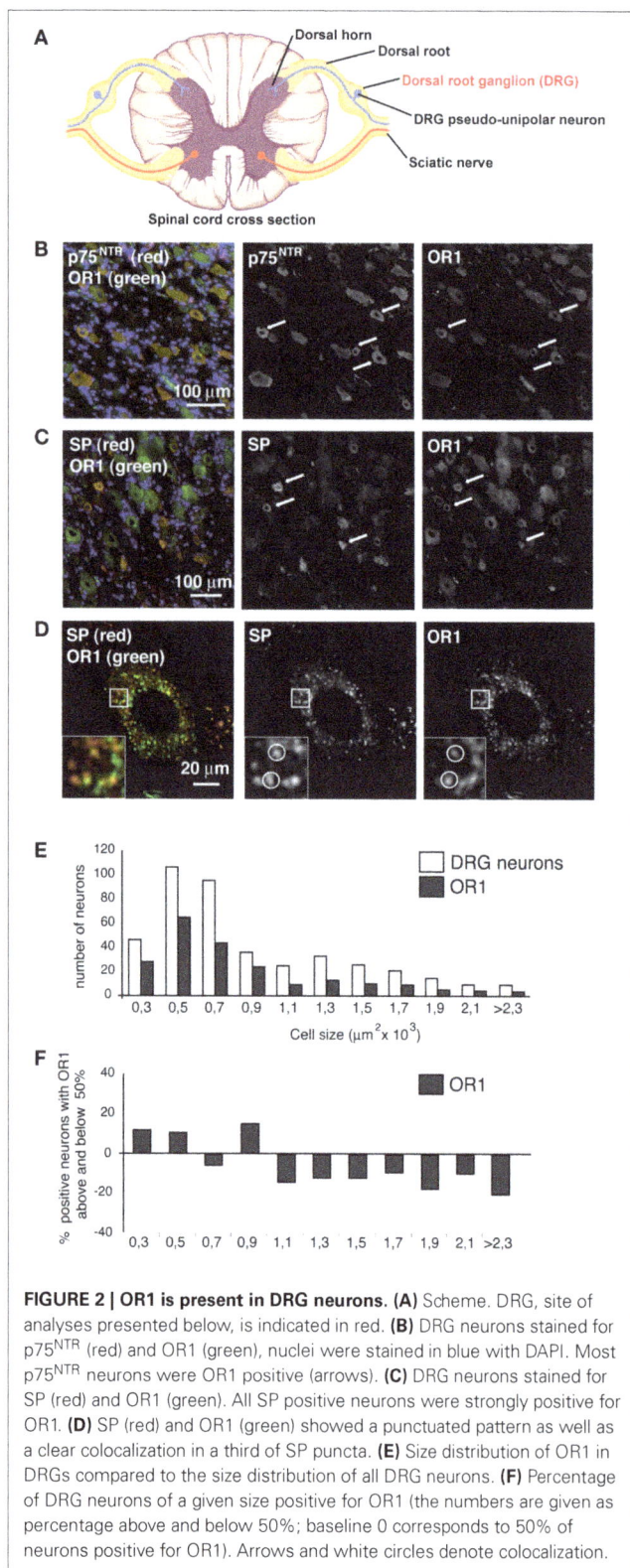

FIGURE 2 | OR1 is present in DRG neurons. (A) Scheme. DRG, site of analyses presented below, is indicated in red. **(B)** DRG neurons stained for $p75^{NTR}$ (red) and OR1 (green), nuclei were stained in blue with DAPI. Most $p75^{NTR}$ neurons were OR1 positive (arrows). **(C)** DRG neurons stained for SP (red) and OR1 (green). All SP positive neurons were strongly positive for OR1. **(D)** SP (red) and OR1 (green) showed a punctuated pattern as well as a clear colocalization in a third of SP puncta. **(E)** Size distribution of OR1 in DRGs compared to the size distribution of all DRG neurons. **(F)** Percentage of DRG neurons of a given size positive for OR1 (the numbers are given as percentage above and below 50%; baseline 0 corresponds to 50% of neurons positive for OR1). Arrows and white circles denote colocalization.

SP. Because of the secreted nature of the SP neuropeptide, the cytoplasmic colocalization of OR1 with SP prompted us to investigate whether OR1 expressed in DRG neurons was present in the trafficking pathway that sends material toward nerve terminals.

OR1 IS ANTEROGRADELY ACCUMULATED FROM DRG TO THE SPINAL CORD WHILE OXA IS RETROGRADELY ACCUMULATED FROM THE SPINAL CORD TO THE DRG

Since the OXA positive terminals colocalize with SP positive fibers in the spinal cord and OR1 is expressed in DRG neurons, we then tested whether OR1 was anterogradely accumulated/transported from the DRG to the spinal cord (see principle in **Figure 3A**). We used the nerve crush method and axonal transport analysis described in our previous works on nerve growth factor effects on sensory neurons (Delcroix et al., 1998, 2003). We performed laminectomies (bone removal allowing access to DRG and DR) on rats and crushed the dorsal roots (DRs) arising from lumbar 4 and 5 (L_4 and L_5) DRGs (**Figure 3A**). Nerve crush leads to accumulation of normally transported material on both sides of the crush (**Figure 3A**). The DRs were collected at 3 time points, 0, 3, and 6 h (3 animals were used for each time point), and the proximal section of the crushed DR was run on an SDS-Page gel (**Figure 3B**, right panel). OR1 accumulated over time (**Figure 3B**, right panel). As a control, DRG was also tested and as expected, OR1 was expressed in the ganglia. In striking contrast, OR1 was not accumulated in the SN toward the periphery even after 12 h (**Figure 3B**, right panel). We do not know whether it involves a passive or active transport, however this data clearly suggests that OR1 is selectively accumulated toward the spinal cord and not the periphery. This data further strengthens the possibility of an orexin/hypocretin neurotransmission between the CNS and PNS/DRG. More importantly, from a more general neurobiological perspective, this observation is also a rare case of asymmetrical neuropeptide receptor distribution between axons projected by a single neuronal cell type.

We next tested whether OXA secreted by hypothalamus-originating fiber terminals could be taken up by afferents arising from the DRG. We looked for retrogradely transported OXA by withdrawing material accumulated at the crush site of DRs arising from L_4 and L_5 DRGs (retrograde accumulation was harvested after 6 h) (**Figure 3B**, left panel). OXA accumulated at the crush site ($n = 3$ animals) as opposed to intact DRs (0 h transport) (**Figure 3B**, left panel). Furthermore, we found that retrograde transport of OXA was specific, as it was present in DRG neuron cell bodies always colocalizing with its receptor (**Figure 3C**). Altogether these results suggest the existence of neurotransmission between the central OX/HCRT neurons and the peripheral SP neurons. The existence of a functional circuit between OX/HCRT and DRG neurons is yet to be fully demonstrated.

DISCUSSION

The discovery of molecular motors, and in particular kinesin, has led to the realization that cell trafficking was a highly controlled phenomenon (Vale et al., 1985). Despite our present extended knowledge of cellular trafficking, our comprehension of transport events in neurons is incomplete. Moreover, the possibility of transport directed toward specific axon branches poses a

the DRG neurons. Higher magnification analysis of SP and OR1 double staining showed a robust punctate pattern in neuron cell bodies (**Figure 2D**). 32 $\pm$ 6% ($n = 10$ neurons in 4 different animals) of OR1 positive puncta in those cells colocalized with

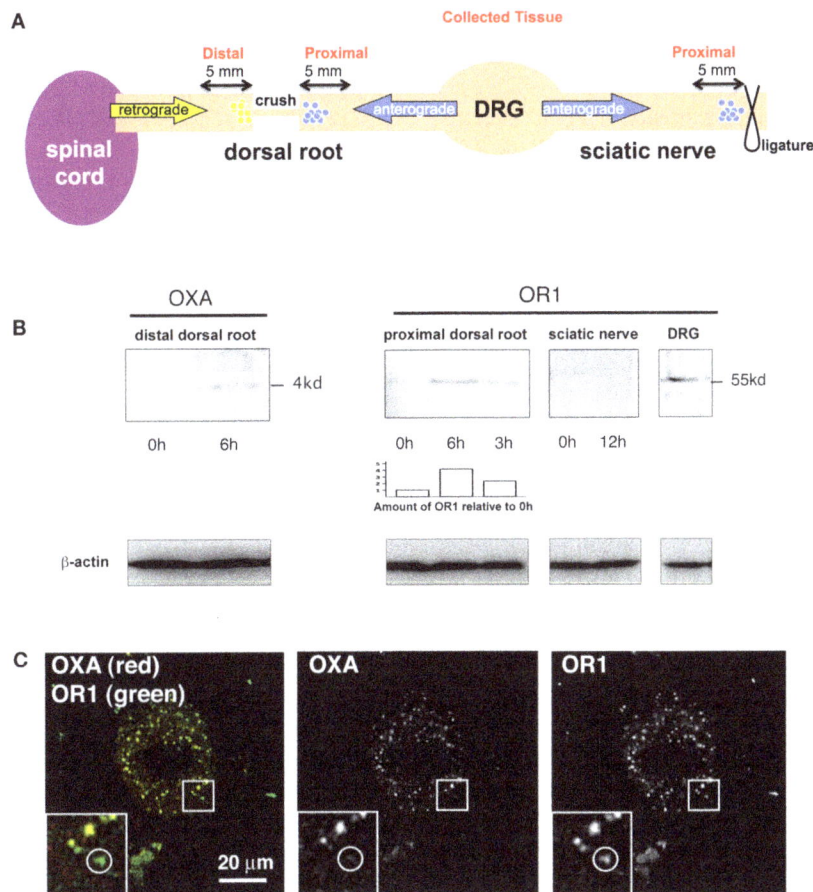

FIGURE 3 | OR1 and OXA are transported in dorsal root axons.
(A) Scheme illustrating the crush and ligature experiments and indicating the sites where tissue samples were collected to measure OXA and OR1 accumulation. (B) Transport analysis (based on our previous work Delcroix et al., 2003). Left panel, OXA is accumulated after 6 h in the dorsal root suggesting a retrograde transport. Right panel, 6 and 3 h OR1 accumulation proximal at a crush site in the dorsal roots. The 0 h lane has been loaded with an intact root from the same animal. Blot analysis and accumulation of OR1 was determined using ImageJ and normalized to the 0 h value (see bar chart). Note the progressive accumulation over time of OR1 suggesting an anterograde transport. 12 h accumulation in the SN did not show OR1 accumulation. DRG tissue was used as positive control. Lower panels, β-actin was used as an internal loading control. (C) OXA (red) was present in the DRG and always colocalized with OR1 (green) whereas OR1 could be found without OXA (see white circle).

clear challenge to our understanding of axonal transport toward specific targets. In this work we show that indeed a specific protein, OR1, can be transported—via a mechanism yet to be deciphered—in one axon branch (DR) but not in the other (SN). Much evidence points to the existence of changes in transport flux in axon branches. Goldberg and Schacher showed that cultured *Aplysia californica* cerebral neurons grow from both ends of both branches (Goldberg and Schacher, 1987). When a branch was next to a target cell, bidirectional fast axonal transport of organelles was more robust in that branch. A similar observation was made in hippocampal neurons by Ruthel and Hollenbeck (2003). Indirect evidence also pointed to differential axonal transport *in vivo*. Schreyer and Skene showed that injuries of the SN or the DR did have different effects in DRG neurons, implying the existence of a different retrograde signal that might be linked to a different composition in the proteins anterogradely transported in both axon branches (Schreyer and Skene, 1993). Differential transport in axon branches might also be linked to morphological

changes occurring in network rearrangements during embryonic and adult life (for review see Luo and O'Leary, 2005). It is unclear what mechanism mediates differential transport in axon branches and it is beyond the scope of this study. Nevertheless, in this work we link differential OR1 accumulation to an OXA/SP network that only exists in the spinal cord and not in the periphery.

OXA was retrogradely accumulated from the spinal cord to the DRG and was always detected in the DRG in the presence of its receptor. The potential retrograde transport of a receptor-bound neuropeptide may be an important process, which conveys information from the synapse to the DRG cell bodies. OXA could also play a role in the regulation of cell mechanisms as shown for neuropeptide Y that regulates axonal transport of organelles in neurites of cultured DRGs (Hiruma et al., 2002). In addition, OR1 is a G protein-coupled receptor (GPCR). Its binding to OXA and potential subsequent internalization in SP-positive synapses might have a similar role to the one played by the internalization of other DRG GPCRs. For instance, the opioid receptor-like receptor controls the availability of calcium channels through internalization and consequently modulates long-term pain related signaling (Altier et al., 2006).

We do not demonstrate here the existence of a functional circuit between central OX/HCRT neurons and peripheral DRG neurons, however we bring evidence suggesting a potential interaction between these neurons. While we do not show synaptic connections, the paracrine release of OX/HCRT neuropeptides in close proximity to DRG neuron fibers expressing OR1 could suffice for neurotransmission. This hypothesis is substantiated by the axon-specific accumulation of OR1 in DRG pseudo-unipolar neurons and the presence of its ligand OXA in the cell bodies. We believe that the presence of OXA neuropeptide in the DRG neurons is due to its uptake and not to its cell-autonomous expression in these neurons. Besides the lateral hypothalamus, OX/HCRT mRNA has indeed never been detected in the nervous system elsewhere in all species studied so far, including fishes (zebrafish Faraco et al., 2006; Appelbaum et al., 2009, goldfish Nakamachi et al., 2006), birds (chicken Ohkubo et al., 2002, quail Phillips-Singh et al., 2003), and mammals (de Lecea et al., 1998; Sakurai et al., 1998 and Luis de Lecea pers. commun.). Of course, we cannot rule out a sub-threshold expression of OX/HCRT transcript in the DRG, but it seems less likely compared to its uptake in the dorsal spinal cord.

Finally, a potential network between the CNS and PNS may account for the involvement of the OX/HCRT in the modulation of sensorial processing. An increasing body of knowledge shows that the orexin system is involved in pain regulation and orexin peptides exert antinociceptive actions (Bingham et al., 2001; Holland et al., 2005, 2006; Kajiyama et al., 2005; Mobarakeh et al., 2005; Yan et al., 2008; Ho et al., 2011; Feng et al., 2012) and for review Chiou et al. (2010). In particular, OXA decreases nociception mostly via OR1 both at spinal and supra-spinal levels in various models of pain. For instance, in an acute model of pain (hot plate test), intrathecal injections of OXA proved to be anti-nociceptive (Yamamoto et al., 2002). In addition, in a model of chronic neuropathic pain (chronic constrictive injury of SN), Jeong and Holden showed that stimulation of posterior hypothalamus induces anti-nociception and that the anti-nociceptive effect is mediated in part by the OR-1 receptor in the spinal cord DH. Their findings, in combination with our findings suggest a possible role of axonal transport of OR-1 and OXA in pain models of chronic constrictive nerve injuries (Jeong and Holden, 2009). Cellular effects of orexins on pain mechanisms have scarcely been studied so far, but it has been shown that orexins modulate the electrophysiological properties of key pain modulatory centers, such as the spinal cord DH and the ventro-lateral peri-aqueductal gray vlPAG (Grudt et al., 2002; Ho et al., 2011). Further, the anti-nociceptive effects of OXA were endocannabinoid dependent in the vlPAG (Ho et al., 2011) and endonncannabinoid independent in the DH (Bingham et al., 2001). Moreover, orexin mediates the analgesia in the model of stress-induced analgesia (Xie et al., 2008; Gerashchenko et al., 2011). Surprisingly, in some instances anti-nociceptive effects of peripheral OXA injections have also been shown (Bingham et al., 2001; Holland et al., 2005, 2006). Importantly, patients suffering from narcolepsy with

cataplexy, a condition associated with a disrupted OX/HCRT system, experience a higher frequency of pain (Dauvilliers et al., 2011). Anatomical and cellular studies may account for those peripheral effects as OR1 and OXA have indeed been found in DRG (Bingham et al., 2001) and OXA directly modulates the DRG neuronal activity (Yan et al., 2008).

Our data also allow us to speculate on the mechanism underlying the possible analgesic effects of peripheral OXA injections. Indeed, OXA might affect SP-positive DRG neurons by binding to OR1, thus changing the DRG-mediated nociceptive action and/or chronically adapting the pain sensation threshold. Such findings may have practical importance in the wake of current hypnotic drug development aiming at blocking orexin receptors using peripheral routes (Scammell and Winrow, 2011).

MATERIALS AND METHODS
ANIMALS
Adult (6-month-old) male Wistar rats (300–350 g) were purchased from Harlan (Italy), and all experiments were performed according to the national and international laws for laboratory animal welfare and experimentation (EEC council directive 86/609, 12 December 1987) under a license issued by the Local Animal Ethics Committee. Rats were kept under a 12-h dark–light cycle, at $23 \pm 1°C$, with food and water *ad libitum*.

SURGERY
Rats were anesthetized with chloral hydrate at 500 mg/kg and subjected to a laminectomy. Axonal transport was measured in DRs 3 or 6 h after the application of crushes on the right side of the animal (Raivich et al., 1991; Delcroix et al., 1997) (*Nota bene*: because of the thin nature of the DR tissue, crush was favored over ligature). Crushes were made with watchmaker's forceps, with compression for a period of 30 s and repeated twice as in our previous work (Delcroix et al., 1997, 2003). After the laminectomy, the wound was closed with Michel clips and the animal was monitored for recovery. Axonal transport was measured in the SN by placement of 2 tight ligatures using surgical silk for 12 h at mid thigh as described elsewhere (Raivich et al., 1991; Delcroix et al., 1997). At the end of the procedure 5 mm of DRs was harvested on both sides of the crush, proximal and distal to the DRG. Five millimeter of SN was harvested on the side of the ligature proximal to DRG (see schematic **Figure 3A**).

HOMOGENIZATION AND WESTERN BLOTTING
A similar volume of tissue samples from the DRs, SN, and lumbar 4 and lumbar 5 (L_4 and L_5) DRGs was homogenized as described previously (Filliatreau et al., 1988; Delcroix et al., 2003) using a polytron (Kinematica, Luzern, Switzerland) in 200 μl of protein extraction buffer [0.1 mM PBS (pH 7.4), 1.0 mM of NaF, 1.0 mM NaVO$_4$, 2.0 mM EDTA, 0.5% Triton X-100, 1.0 mM phenyl methylsulphonyl fluoride (PMSF), and 10 μg/ml aprotinin]. Total protein content was determined using Bio-Rad protein assay (Bradford method). SDS-Page gels were then loaded with the same amount of material proportionally to 5 mm of collected sample [10 μg (~20 μl) of total proteins from DR, SN, and DRG tissues]. The separated proteins were transferred to PVDF (Millipore, Billerica, Massachusetts, USA) using a Biorad Mini

Trans-blot (30 V overnight, at 4°C). The blots were incubated with a 1:200 dilution of OR1 (Santa Cruz antibodies #SC-8073, Santa Cruz, California, USA) goat polyclonal antibody or with a 1:200 dilution of OXA (Phoenix peptide #H-003-30, Belmont, California) rabbit polyclonal antibody (Santa Cruz antibodies, Santa Cruz, California, USA). Blots were then incubated with the secondary antibody (anti-rabbit HRP conjugate or anti-goat HRP conjugate from Jackson Immunoresearch Europe, UK) at 1:2000 for 60 min at room temperature. Detection was achieved using a Bio-rad Versadoc image analyzer (Bio-rad, Hercules, California, USA). Band signal quantification was achieved using ImageJ (NIH, Bethesda). Monoclonal mouse anti-actin antibody (Sigma Aldrich) was then used as a loading control for western blot analysis of proteins from rat DRG, SN, and DR.

IMMUNOCYTOCHEMISTRY

Wistar rats (6 months old) were prepared for immunohistochemical analysis using standard techniques. Anesthesia was induced with chloral hydrate (700 mg/kg); animals were perfused through the ascending aorta with saline followed by 300 ml of 4% paraformaldehyde in 0.1 M phosphate buffer, pH 7.4. L_4 and L_5 DRGs and the lumbar spinal cord were removed, postfixes overnight at 4°C in the same fixative and then cryoprotected in 30% sucrose overnight. DRGs and spinal cord were frozen and sectioned with a thickness of 10 μm. Sections were stained using indirect immunofluorescence histochemistry with a rabbit polyclonal antibody directed against OXA (Phoenix peptide #H-003-30, Belmont, California) diluted at 1:250, a rabbit polyclonal antibody against p75^{NTR} (#1405-41-0 Promega, Madison, Wisconsin, USA) diluted at 1:250, a mouse monoclonal antibody against SP (abcam #14184-50, Cambridge, UK) diluted at 1:250, a goat polyclonal antibody directed against OR1 at 1:250 (Santa Cruz antibodies #SC-8073, Santa Cruz, California, USA). For detection of primary polyclonal antibodies, a donkey anti-rabbit or a donkey anti-goat Cy3 or Cy2 conjugated secondary antiserum (1:250; Jackson Immunoresearch, Cambridge, UK) was used; for detection of monoclonal antibodies, a donkey anti-mouse Cy3 or Cy2 conjugate was used (Jackson Immunoresearch). Double labeling of SP together with OR1 was achieved using standard indirect immunofluorescence as described elsewhere (Merighi and Carmignoto, 2002). After final washes in phosphate buffered saline (PBS), sections were coverslipped in a PBS/glycerol solution (1:3) containing 2.5% 1,4 diazobicyclo (2,2,2) octane (antifading agent; Sigma). Immunoreactivity was visualized on a Nikon 90i epifluorescence microscope linked to a C1 confocal system.

3D reconstructions as shown in **Figure 1** were produced using the software Osirix, a freeware used for tomography (http://homepage.mac.com/rossetantoine/osirix/Index2.html). Twenty optical sections were taken every 0.4 μm and were then reconstructed in 3D.

CELL QUANTIFICATION

Cell size and cell density was calculated with ImageJ (NIH, Bethesda). Cell size and staining intensity were quantified when a clear nuclei was visible in the image. To decide if a cell was p75^{NTR} or OR1 positive, the following criteria was applied: an average background was obtained by quantifying the average intensity of 5 fields that did not show any staining in the image. Then, if the intensity measured for a given neuron was 3 fold above background, the cell was considered positive for p75^{NTR} or OR1. For OXA and for p75^{NTR} we quantified from 4 rats 2 sections taken from the middle of the DRG. Numerical data are expressed as mean ± standard deviation.

ACKNOWLEDGMENTS

We would like to thank Profs. Paul Fernyhough and William C. Mobley's laboratory for their advice during the experimental phase of this work. We would also like to acknowledge Drs. Maria d'Onofrio, Hélène Marie, and Alberto Bacci for fruitful discussions. We thank Dr. Louis Leung and Kerry Breuer for their helpful comments on the manuscript. Jean-Dominique Delcroix's work was financed by the Ministero della Sanità (Italy), and the Fondazione Rita Levi-Montalcini. Philippe Mourrain's work on hypocretin/orexin is supported by the National Institutes of Health (NS062798).

REFERENCES

Altier, C., Khosravani, H., Evans, R. M., Hameed, S., Peloquin, J. B., Vartian, B. A., et al. (2006). ORL1 receptor-mediated internalization of N-type calcium channels. *Nat. Neurosci.* 9, 31–40. doi: 10.1038/nn1605

Appelbaum, L., Wang, G. X., Maro, G. S., Mori, R., Tovin, A., Marin, W., et al. (2009). Sleep-wake regulation and hypocretin-melatonin interaction in zebrafish. *Proc. Natl. Acad. Sci. U.S.A.* 106, 21942–21947. doi: 10.1073/pnas.906637106

Bingham, S., Davey, P. T., Babbs, A. J., Irving, E. A., Sammons, M. J., Wyles, M., et al. (2001). Orexin-A, an hypothalamic peptide with analgesic properties. *Pain* 92, 81–90. doi: 10.1016/S0304-3959(00)00470-X

Chiou, L. C., Lee, H. J., Ho, Y. C., Chen, S. P., Liao, Y. Y., Ma, C. H., et al. (2010). Orexins/hypocretins: pain regulation and cellular actions. *Curr. Pharm. Des.* 16, 3089–3100. doi: 10.2174/138161210793292483

Cutler, D. J., Morris, R., Sheridhar, V., Wattam, T. A., Holmes, S., Patel, S., et al. (1999). Differential distribution of orexin-A and orexin-B immunoreactivity in the rat brain and spinal cord. *Peptides* 20, 1455–1470. doi: 10.1016/S0196-9781(99)00157-6

Dauvilliers, Y., Bayard, S., Shneerson, J. M., Plazzi, G., Myers, A. J., and Garcia-Borreguero, D. (2011). High pain frequency in narcolepsy with cataplexy. *Sleep Med.* 12, 572–577. doi: 10.1016/j.sleep.2011.01.010

Delcroix, J. D., Michael, G. J., Priestley, J. V., Tomlinson, D. R., and Fernyhough, P. (1998). Effect of nerve growth factor treatment on p75NTR gene expression in lumbar dorsal root ganglia of streptozotocin-induced diabetic rats. *Diabetes* 47, 1779–1785. doi: 10.2337/diabetes.47.11.1779

Delcroix, J. D., Tomlinson, D. R., and Fernyhough, P. (1997). Diabetes and axotomy-induced deficits in retrograde axonal transport of nerve growth factor correlate with decreased levels of p75LNTR protein in lumbar dorsal root ganglia. *Brain Res. Mol. Brain Res.* 51, 82–90. doi: 10.1016/S0169-328X(97)00215-5

Delcroix, J. D., Valletta, J., Wu, C., Howe, C. L., Lai, C. F., Cooper, J. D., et al. (2004). Trafficking the NGF signal: implications for normal and degenerating neurons. *Prog. Brain Res.* 146, 3–23. doi: 10.1016/S0079-6123(03)46001-9

Delcroix, J. D., Valletta, J. S., Wu, C., Hunt, S. J., Kowal, A. S., and Mobley, W. C. (2003). NGF signaling in sensory neurons: evidence that early endosomes carry NGF retrograde signals. *Neuron* 39, 69–84. doi: 10.1016/S0896-6273(03)00397-0

de Lecea, L. (2010). A decade of hypocretins: past, present and future of the neurobiology of arousal. *Acta Physiol. (Oxf.)* 198, 203–208. doi: 10.1111/j.1748-1716.2009.02004.x

de Lecea, L., Kilduff, T. S., Peyron, C., Gao, X., Foye, P. E., Danielson, P. E., et al. (1998). The hypocretins: hypothalamus-specific peptides with neuroexcitatory activity. *Proc. Natl. Acad. Sci. U.S.A.* 95, 322–327. doi: 10.1073/pnas.95.1.322

Doghramji, K. (2012). Sleep extension in sleepy individuals reduces pain sensitivity: new evidence regarding the complex, reciprocal relationship between sleep and pain. *Sleep* 35, 1587–1588. doi: 10.5665/sleep.2220

Faraco, J. H., Appelbaum, L., Marin, W., Gaus, S. E., Mourrain, P., and Mignot, E. (2006). Regulation of hypocretin (orexin) expression in embryonic zebrafish. *J. Biol. Chem.* 281, 29753–29761. doi: 10.1074/jbc.M605811200

Feng, X. M., Mi, W. L., Xia, F., Mao-Ying, Q. L., Jiang, J. W., Xiao, S., et al. (2012). Involvement of spinal orexin A in the electroacupuncture analgesia in a rat model of post-laparotomy pain. *BMC Complement. Altern. Med.* 12:225. doi: 10.1186/1472-6882-12-225

Filliatreau, G., Denoulet, P., de Nechaud, B., and Di Giamberardino, L. (1988). Stable and metastable cytoskeletal polymers carried by slow axonal transport. *J. Neurosci.* 8, 2227–2233.

Gerashchenko, D., Horvath, T. L., and Xie, X. S. (2011). Direct inhibition of hypocretin/orexin neurons in the lateral hypothalamus by nociceptin/orphanin FQ blocks stress-induced analgesia in rats. *Neuropharmacology* 60, 543–549. doi: 10.1016/j.neuropharm.2010.12.026

Goldberg, D. J., and Schacher, S. (1987). Differential growth of the branches of a regenerating bifurcate axon is associated with differential axonal transport of organelles. *Dev. Biol.* 124, 35–40. doi: 10.1016/0012-1606(87)90456-8

Grudt, T. J., van den Pol, A. N., and Perl, E. R. (2002). Hypocretin-2 (orexin-B) modulation of superficial dorsal horn activity in rat. *J. Physiol.* 538, 517–525. doi: 10.1113/jphysiol.2001.013120

Hervieu, G. J., Cluderay, J. E., Harrison, D. C., Roberts, J. C., and Leslie, R. A. (2001). Gene expression and protein distribution of the orexin-1 receptor in the rat brain and spinal cord. *Neuroscience* 103, 777–797. doi: 10.1016/S0306-4522(01)00033-1

Hiruma, H., Saito, A., Kusakabe, T., Takenaka, T., and Kawakami, T. (2002). Neuropeptide Y inhibits axonal transport of particles in neurites of cultured adult mouse dorsal root ganglion cells. *J. Physiol.* 543, 85–97. doi: 10.1113/jphysiol.2002.020578

Ho, Y. C., Lee, H. J., Tung, L. W., Liao, Y. Y., Fu, S. Y., Teng, S. F., et al. (2011). Activation of orexin 1 receptors in the periaqueductal gray of male rats leads to antinociception via retrograde endocannabinoid (2-arachidonoylglycerol)-induced disinhibition. *J. Neurosci.* 31, 14600–14610. doi: 10.1523/JNEUROSCI.2671-11.2011

Holland, P. R., Akerman, S., and Goadsby, P. J. (2005). Orexin 1 receptor activation attenuates neurogenic dural vasodilation in an animal model of trigeminovascular nociception. *J. Pharmacol. Exp. Ther.* 315, 1380–1385. doi: 10.1124/jpet.105.090951

Holland, P. R., Akerman, S., and Goadsby, P. J. (2006). Modulation of nociceptive dural input to the trigeminal nucleus caudalis via activation of the orexin 1 receptor in the rat. *Eur. J. Neurosci.* 24, 2825–2833. doi: 10.1111/j.1460-9568.2006.05168.x

Jeong, Y., and Holden, J. E. (2009). The role of spinal orexin-1 receptors in posterior hypothalamic modulation of neuropathic pain. *Neuroscience* 159, 1414–1421. doi: 10.1016/j.neuroscience.2009.02.006

Kajiyama, S., Kawamoto, M., Shiraishi, S., Gaus, S., Matsunaga, A., Suyama, H., et al. (2005). Spinal orexin-1 receptors mediate anti-hyperalgesic effects of intrathecally-administered orexins in diabetic neuropathic pain model rats. *Brain Res.* 1044, 76–86. doi: 10.1016/j.brainres.2005.03.007

Kandel, E., Schwartz, J., and Jessell, T. (2000). *Principles of Neural Science.* New York, NY: McGraw-Hill.

Luo, L., and O'Leary, D. D. (2005). Axon retraction and degeneration in development and disease. *Annu. Rev. Neurosci.* 28, 127–156. doi: 10.1146/annurev.neuro.28.061604.135632

Marcus, J. N., Aschkenasi, C. J., Lee, C. E., Chemelli, R. M., Saper, C. B., Yanagisawa, M., et al. (2001). Differential expression of orexin receptors 1 and 2 in the rat brain. *J. Comp. Neurol.* 435, 6–25. doi: 10.1002/cne.1190

Merighi, A., and Carmignoto, G. (2002). *Cellular and Molecular Methods in Neuroscience Research.* New York, NY: Springer. doi: 10.1007/b98863

Mobarakeh, J. I., Takahashi, K., Sakurada, S., Nishino, S., Watanabe, H., Kato, M., et al. (2005). Enhanced antinociception by intracerebroventricularly and intrathecally-administered orexin A and B (hypocretin-1 and -2) in mice. *Peptides* 26, 767–777. doi: 10.1016/j.peptides.2005.01.001

Nakamachi, T., Matsuda, K., Maruyama, K., Miura, T., Uchiyama, M., Funahashi, H., et al. (2006). Regulation by orexin of feeding behaviour and locomotor activity in the goldfish. *J. Neuroendocrinol.* 18, 290–297. doi: 10.1111/j.1365-2826.2006.01415.x

Nichols, M. L., Allen, B. J., Rogers, S. D., Ghilardi, J. R., Honore, P., Luger, N. M., et al. (1999). Transmission of chronic nociception by spinal neurons expressing the substance P receptor. *Science* 286, 1558–1561. doi: 10.1126/science.286.5444.1558

Ohkubo, T., Boswell, T., and Lumineau, S. (2002). Molecular cloning of chicken prepro-orexin cDNA and preferential expression in the chicken hypothalamus. *Biochim. Biophys. Acta* 1577, 476–480. doi: 10.1016/S0167-4781(02)00483-9

Peyron, C., Faraco, J., Rogers, W., Ripley, B., Overeem, S., Charnay, Y., et al. (2000). A mutation in a case of early onset narcolepsy and a generalized absence of hypocretin peptides in human narcoleptic brains. *Nat. Med.* 6, 991–997. doi: 10.1038/79690

Phillips-Singh, D., Li, Q., Takeuchi, S., Ohkubo, T., Sharp, P. J., and Boswell, T. (2003). Fasting differentially regulates expression of agouti-related peptide, pro-opiomelanocortin, prepro-orexin, and vasoactive intestinal polypeptide mRNAs in the hypothalamus of Japanese quail. *Cell Tissue Res.* 313, 217–225. doi: 10.1007/s00441-003-0755-8

Raivich, G., Hellweg, R., and Kreutzberg, G. W. (1991). NGF receptor-mediated reduction in axonal NGF uptake and retrograde transport following sciatic nerve injury and during regeneration. *Neuron* 7, 151–164. doi: 10.1016/0896-6273(91)90083-C

Roehrs, T. A., Harris, E., Randall, S., and Roth, T. (2012). Pain sensitivity and recovery from mild chronic sleep loss. *Sleep* 35, 1667–1672. doi: 10.5665/sleep.2240

Ruthel, G., and Hollenbeck, P. J. (2003). Response of mitochondrial traffic to axon determination and differential branch growth. *J. Neurosci.* 23, 8618–8624.

Sakurai, T. (2013). Orexin deficiency and narcolepsy. *Curr. Opin. Neurobiol.* 23, 760–766. doi: 10.1016/j.conb.2013.04.007

Sakurai, T., Amemiya, A., Ishii, M., Matsuzaki, I., Chemelli, R. M., Tanaka, H., et al. (1998). Orexins and orexin receptors: a family of hypothalamic neuropeptides and G protein-coupled receptors that regulate feeding behavior. *Cell* 92, 573–585. doi: 10.1016/S0092-8674(00)80949-6

Scammell, T. E., and Winrow, C. J. (2011). Orexin receptors: pharmacology and therapeutic opportunities. *Annu. Rev. Pharmacol. Toxicol.* 51, 243–266. doi: 10.1146/annurev-pharmtox-010510-100528

Schreyer, D. J., and Skene, J. H. (1993). Injury-associated induction of GAP-43 expression displays axon branch specificity in rat dorsal root ganglion neurons. *J. Neurobiol.* 24, 959–970. doi: 10.1002/neu.480240709

Sorensen, G. L., Knudsen, S., and Jennum, P. (2013). Sleep transitions in hypocretin-deficient narcolepsy. *Sleep* 36, 1173–1177. doi: 10.5665/sleep.2880

Tsujino, N., and Sakurai, T. (2013). Role of orexin in modulating arousal, feeding, and motivation. *Front. Behav. Neurosci.* 7:28. doi: 10.3389/fnbeh.2013.00028

Vale, R. D., Reese, T. S., and Sheetz, M. P. (1985). Identification of a novel force-generating protein, kinesin, involved in microtubule-based motility. *Cell* 42, 39–50. doi: 10.1016/S0092-8674(85)80099-4

van den Pol, A. N. (1999). Hypothalamic hypocretin (orexin): robust innervation of the spinal cord. *J. Neurosci.* 19, 3171–3182.

Xie, X., Wisor, J. P., Hara, J., Crowder, T. L., LeWinter, R., Khroyan, T. V., et al. (2008). Hypocretin/orexin and nociceptin/orphanin FQ coordinately regulate analgesia in a mouse model of stress-induced analgesia. *J. Clin. Invest.* 118, 2471–2481. doi: 10.1172/JCI35115

Yamamoto, T., Nozaki-Taguchi, N., and Chiba, T. (2002). Analgesic effect of intrathecally administered orexin-A in the rat formalin test and in the rat hot plate test. *Br. J. Pharmacol.* 137, 170–176. doi: 10.1038/sj.bjp.0704851

Yan, J. A., Ge, L., Huang, W., Song, B., Chen, X. W., and Yu, Z. P. (2008). Orexin affects dorsal root ganglion neurons: a mechanism for regulating the spinal nociceptive processing. *Physiol. Res.* 57, 797–800.

Conflict of Interest Statement: The authors declare that the research was conducted in the absence of any commercial or financial relationships that could be construed as a potential conflict of interest.

18

Effects of a newly developed potent orexin-2 receptor-selective antagonist, compound 1 m, on sleep/wakefulness states in mice

Keishi Etori, Yuki C. Saito, Natsuko Tsujino and Takeshi Sakurai*

Department of Molecular Neuroscience and Integrative Physiology, Faculty of Medicine, Institute of Medical, Pharmaceutical and Health Sciences, Kanazawa University, Kanazawa, Japan

Edited by:
Michel A. Steiner, Actelion Pharmaceuticals Ltd., Switzerland

Reviewed by:
Stephen Morairty, SRI International, USA
Catherine Brisbare-Roch, Actelion Pharmaceuticals Ltd., Switzerland

*Correspondence:
Takeshi Sakurai, Department of Molecular Neuroscience and Integrative Physiology, Institute of Medical, Pharmaceutical and Health Sciences, 13-1 Takara-machi, Kanazawa, Ishikawa 920-8640, Japan
e-mail: tsakurai@med.kanazawa-u.ac.jp

Orexins (also known as hypocretins) play critical roles in the regulation of sleep/wakefulness states by activating two G-protein coupled receptors (GPCRs), orexin 1 (OX_1R) and orexin 2 receptors (OX_2R). In order to understand the differential contribution of both receptors in regulating sleep/wakefulness states we compared the pharmacological effects of a newly developed OX_2R antagonist (2-SORA), Compound 1 m (C1 m), with those of a dual orexin receptor antagonist (DORA), suvorexant, in C57BL/6J mice. After oral administration in the dark period, both C1m and suvorexant decreased wakefulness time with similar efficacy in a dose-dependent manner. While C1m primarily increased total non-rapid eye movement (NREM) sleep time without affecting episode durations and with minimal effects on REM sleep, suvorexant increased both total NREM and REM sleep time and episode durations with predominant effects on REM sleep. Fos-immunostaining showed that both compounds affected the activities of arousal-related neurons with different patterns. The number of Fos-IR noradrenergic neurons in the locus coeruleus was lower in the suvorexant group as compared with the control and C1m-treated groups. In contrast, the numbers of Fos-IR neurons in histaminergic neurons in the tuberomamillary nucleus and serotonergic neurons in the dorsal raphe were reduced to a similar extent in the suvorexant and C1m groups as compared with the vehicle-treated group. Together, these results suggest that an orexin-mediated suppression of REM sleep via potential activation of OX_1Rs in the locus coeruleus may possibly contribute to the differential effects on sleep/wakefulness exerted by a DORA as compared to a 2-SORA.

Keywords: orexin receptor antagonists, sleep, wakefulness, REM sleep, orexin

INTRODUCTION

A series of studies have suggested that loss of hypothalamic neurons producing orexin (orexin neurons) causes narcolepsy in humans and other mammalian species, showing that orexin plays an extremely important role in the regulation of sleep/wakefulness states, especially in the maintenance of wakefulness (Sakurai and Mieda, 2011). Because orexin is an arousal-promoting factor, it is reasonable to hypothesize that orexin receptor antagonists will be effective as drugs for the treatment of insomnia. Indeed, several orexin receptor antagonists with different pharmacological characteristics are under development as next generation sleep-inducing drugs.

A dual orexin receptor antagonist (DORA), almorexant (ACT-078573), blocks both OX_1R and OX_2R with similar potency (IC_{50} 16 and 15 nM, respectively). Almorexant was reported to shorten the time spent awake and maintain sleep in rats, dogs, and humans (Brisbare-Roch et al., 2007; Hoever et al., 2010). Almorexant significantly improved the primary parameter of sleep efficiency in humans (time spent sleeping while confined to bed during an 8 h period at night) in a dose-dependent manner. Almorexant decreased the latency to sleep onset and

the number of wakefulness bouts after sleep onset. Importantly, almorexant not only changed these physiological sleep parameters, but also significantly improved subjective sleep quality. Effective or even higher doses of almorexant did not cause any significant negative effects on next-day performance (assessed by fine motor testing and mean reaction time). In addition, it was reported that rats administered a high dose of almorexant (300 mg/kg, p.o.) were fully capable of spatial and avoidance learning (Dietrich and Jenck, 2010). Notably, almorexant was well tolerated with no sign of cataplexy, suggesting that acute, short-lived, intermittent temporary blockade of orexin receptors will not result in a narcolepsy-like phenotype (Neubauer, 2010).

Phase III clinical trials of suvorexant (MK-4305), a DORA developed by Merck & Co., for the modulation of sleep have been completed (Cox et al., 2010). Suvorexant is a potent DORA with excellent potency in cell-based calcium mobilization assays (OX_1R $IC_{50} = 50$ nM, OX_2R $IC_{50} = 56$ nM) (Winrow and Renger, 2013). Recent studies showed that patients taking the drug fell asleep faster and slept longer than those on placebo, with no major adverse effects (Hopkins, 2012; Mieda and Sakurai,

2013). Suvorexant is expected to be available for clinical use in 2014.

Recently, administration of a selective OX_2R antagonist (2-SORA), JNJ-10397049, in rats was also shown to decrease the latency to persistent sleep and to increase NREM sleep time more potently than did almorexant (Dugovic et al., 2009), while a selective OX_1R antagonist, SB-408124, had no effect on sleep parameters. Rather, SB-408124 attenuated the sleep-promoting effects of the OX_2R antagonist when simultaneously administered, possibly by increasing dopamine release in the prefrontal cortex. However, the effectiveness of DORA and 2-SORA is a controversial issue, because another report suggested that almorexant is more effective for sleep promotion than is antagonism of either receptor alone (Morairty et al., 2012). Further research using selective antagonists with different pharmacological characteristics is required to reach a conclusion on the effectiveness, advantages and disadvantages of these compounds.

In this study, we compared the effects of a newly-developed potent OX_2R-selective antagonist (2-SORA), Compound 1m (C1m), with those of suvorexant. C1m showed potent OX_2R antagonistic activity (IC_{50} 27 nM) and good selectivity against OX_1R (IC_{50} 3000 nM, determined by cell-based calcium mobilization assay using receptor-expressing cells). C1m is an amphiphilic molecule simultaneously possessing high water solubility and lipophilicity, to which its good oral availability is attributable (Fujimoto et al., 2011). Furthermore, this compound showed excellent metabolic stability in human and rat liver microsomes (Fujimoto et al., 2011).

We found C1m had comparable efficacy to that of suvorexant in increasing NREM sleep time, but showed little effect on REM sleep amount, while suvorexant significantly increased REM sleep. Suvorexant induced longer NREM and REM sleep episode durations as compared with C1m. Suvorexant and C1m affected the number of Fos-positive monoaminergic neurons in the brain stem with differential patterns. These results suggest differential roles of OX_1R and OX_2R in sleep/wakefulness regulation.

MATERIALS AND METHODS
ANIMALS
All mice used in this study had a C57B6/J genetic background and were 12–15 weeks of age and weighed 25–30 g. They were fed *ad libitum* and housed under conditions where temperature (22°C) and humidity were controlled with a 12-h light/dark cycle (lights on at 8:45 a.m., off at 8:45 p.m.). All experimental procedures were approved by the Animal Experimental and Use Committee of Kanazawa University (AP-132649) and were in accordance with NIH guidelines. All efforts were made to minimize animal suffering and discomfort and to reduce the number of animals used.

SUBSTANCES AND ADMINISTRATION
C1m, a novel potent 2-SORA, was provided by Takeda Pharmaceutical, Co., Ltd. (Japan) (Fujimoto et al., 2011). A DORA, [(7R)-4-(5-chloro-1,3-benzoxazol-2-yl)-7-methyl-1,4-diazepan-1-yl][5-methyl-2-(2H-1,2,3-triazol-2-yl)phenyl]methanone (suvorexant) was synthesized according to a previously reported procedure (Cox et al., 2010) (lot # 130301, NARD

Institute, Amagasaki, Japan). Drugs were suspended in 1% methylcellulose (Sigma) and administered to mice *per os* using a disposable feeding needle (Fuchigami Kikai, Japan) at Zeitgeber time (ZT) 12 or ZT0.

SLEEP RECORDINGS
Mice were anesthetized with sodium pentobarbital, and an electrode was implanted for EEG/EMG recording. Four holes were drilled in the skull, and the arms of the electrode for EEG were implanted at sites approximately 2 mm anterior, ± 2 mm lateral, and 2 mm posterior to the bregma. EMG recording wires made of stainless steel were inserted into the neck muscles bilaterally. Each electrode was fixed rigidly to the skull with dental cement (ESPE Ketac-Cem). After the recovery period (5–6 days after surgery), mice were moved to a recording cage placed in an electrically shielded and sound-attenuated room. The implanted electrode of each mouse was connected to a cable for signal output. They were allowed to move freely with access to food and water *ad libitum*. Signals were amplified through an amplifier (AB-611J, Nihon Koden, Tokyo) and digitally recorded on a computer using EEG/EMG recording software (Vital recorder, Kissei Comtec). Mice were put in recording cages for at least 7 days to allow them to adapt to the recording conditions prior to any EEG/EMG recording session. Following the acclimatization period, 1% methylcellulose as control, C1m and suvorexant were orally administered to mice on separate experimental days with an interval of at least 3 days. Each dose of drugs was explored in different groups of mice ($n = 5$–9/group). We did not use mice repeatedly, in order to avoid the influences of repeated administration procedures and residual effects of drugs. EEG/EMG data for 24 h following drug administration were evaluated as previously described (Hara et al., 2001).

STATISTICAL ANALYSIS
Data were expressed as mean ± s.e.m. Two-Way analysis of variance (ANOVA) followed by Bonfferoni correction as a *post-hoc* test or Student's *t*-test using GraphPad Prism 6.01 was used for comparison among the various treatment groups. Differences were considered significant at $p < 0.05$.

IMMUNOHISTOCHEMISTRY
Mice were anesthetized deeply and perfused with 60 ml ice-cold phosphate buffer saline (PBS) and 40 ml ice-cold 4% paraformaldehyde (PFA) in 0.1 M phosphate buffer 2 h after drug administration at ZT12. The brain was removed and immersed in 4% PFA for 24 h at 4°C, and then in 30% sucrose in 0.1 M PBS for 2 days. The brain was then frozen quickly in embedding solution (Sakura Finetek Co., Ltd., Tokyo, Japan) and cut into coronal sections (30-μm thick) using a cryostat (HM 505E, Micron, Walldorf, Germany). Coronal brain sections were washed three times for 10 min in 0.1 M PBS containing 1% bovine serum albumin and 0.25% Triton-X-100 (PBS-BX). To detect Fos-like immunoreactivity (IR) in orexin-expressing neurons, the sections were incubated overnight at 4°C with guinea pig anti-orexin antibody (1:500) and rabbit anti-cFos antibody Ab-5 (Calbiochem, 1:10,000). After washing three times with PBS-BX, tissue was incubated for 1 h with Alexa Fluor 594-goat anti-guinea pig IgG (Molecular Probes, 1:800) and Alexa

Fluor 488-goat anti-rabbit IgG (Molecular Probes, 1:800) and then washed three times again. The sections were mounted on glass slides and cover-slipped, and the slides were examined by laser-confocal microscopy (Olympus FV10i).

To detect Fos-IR in serotonergic, histaminergic, and noradrenergic neurons, coronal brain sections were incubated with mouse anti-tryptophan hydroxylase (TPH) antibody (Santa Cruz Biotech, 1:200), guinea pig anti-histidine decarboxylase (HDC) antibody (PROGEN Biotechnik Gmbh, 1:4000), or mouse anti-tyrosine hydroxylase (TH) antibody (Santa Cruz Biotech, 1:2000), respectively, with rabbit anti-Fos antibody Ab-5 (Calbiochem, 1:10,000). As a second antibody, Alexa Fluor 594-goat anti-mouse IgG (Molecular Probes, 1:800), Alexa Fluor 594-goat anti-guinea pig IgG (Molecular Probes, 1:800), or Alexa Fluor 488-goat anti-rabbit IgG (Molecular Probes, 1:800) was used.

RESULTS

C1m INCREASED NREM SLEEP TIME WITHOUT AFFECTING REM SLEEP TIME

To examine the effect of C1m on sleep/wakefulness states, we administered it orally to mice at the start of the dark period. Mice administered C1m (30 and 90 mg/kg) showed significantly shorter wakefulness time as compared with vehicle-administered mice for 6 h after administration (**Figure 1A**, **Figure S1A**). Wakefulness time for 6 h post-administration was 17.2 and 22.6% shorter in the 30 and 90 mg/kg C1m groups, respectively, as compared to that in the control group [$F_{(3, 26)} = 9.55$, $p < 0.001$] (**Figure 1A**). Hourly analysis suggested that the effect lasted for 5 h (**Figure S1A**). The decrease of wakefulnes was accompanied by a dose-dependent increase of NREM sleep time (**Figure 1B**, **Figure S1B**), which was significant during the 6 h after administration [$F_{(3, 26)} = 8.54$, $p < 0.01$ for 30 mg/kg, $p < 0.001$ for 90 mg/kg] (**Figure 1B**). Importantly, no significant difference in total REM sleep time was observed between the C1m and vehicle groups, although there was a weak tendency for C1m to increase total REM sleep tine (**Figure 1C**, **Figure S1C**). The C1m-administered group showed shorter wakefulness episode durations as compared with the vehicle-treated group [$F_{(3, 26)} = 5.39$, $p < 0.05$ for 30 mg/kg, $p < 0.01$ for 90 mg/kg] (**Figure 1D**). NREM and REM sleep episode durations were not affected by C1m (**Figures 1E,F**, **Figures S1E,F**).

Latency to NREM sleep onset after administration of C1m show a tendency to be shorter than that in the control group, but the difference was not statistically significant (**Figure 1G**). Latency to the onset of REM sleep after administration was not significantly different between the C1m- and vehicle-administered groups (**Figure 1H**). The power density of EEG in the C1m-administered group (30 and 90 mg/kg) showed no difference from that in the vehicle-administered group, specifically in regard to NREM delta power (0.5–4 Hz) (**Figure 1I**). However, we observed decrease in slow wave power in the low dose (10 mg/kg) group [$F_{(40, 246)} = 2.547$, $p < 0.01$ for 1 Hz, $p < 0.001$ for 2.5 Hz] (**Figure 1I**).

We next administered C1m just prior to the start of the light period (ZT0). The total wakefulness and NREM sleep times were not significantly different between the C1m and vehicle groups during the light period (**Figures 2A,B**, **Figures S2A,B**). REM sleep time for 6 h after the administration in the low dose

C1m group (10 mg/kg) was shorter as compared with the control group, suggesting that low dose of C1m rather shortens REM sleep time (**Figure 2C**, **Figure S2C**). Wakefulness episode duration was also not affected by C1m (**Figure 2D**). However, NREM and REM sleep episode durations were significantly shorter in the C1m groups (30 and 10 mg/kg) than in the control group (**Figures 2E,F**, **Figures S2E,F**). Latencies to NREM and REM sleep onset after administration of C1m were not significantly different from that in the control group (**Figures 2G,H**). The power density of EEG in the C1m-administered groups showed no difference from that in the vehicle-administered group in NREM sleep (**Figure 2I**).

SUVOREXANT DECREASED WAKEFULNESS TIME AND INCREASED BOTH NREM AND REM SLEEP TIMES

To compare the effect of C1m with that of a DORA, we also examined the effect of suvorexant, a DORA, on sleep/wakefulness states of mice under the same recording condition. Mice administered suvorexant (30 mg/kg) at the start of the dark period showed a significantly shorter wakefulness time as compared with vehicle-administered mice for 6 h after administration (**Figure 3A**, **Figure S3A**). The wakefulness time for 6 h post-administration of suvorexant (30 mg/kg) was shortened by 17.8% [$F_{(2, 20)} = 3.74$, $p < 0.05$] (**Figure 3A**). This effect was accompanied by increases of both NREM and REM sleep time (**Figure 3C**, **Figures S3B,C**). Significant differences were also observed in the latter half of the dark period; wakefulness time was rather longer and NREM and REM sleep times were shorter in the suvorexant group than in the control group in this time window (**Figures 3A–C**, **Figures S3A–C**). These effects are likely to be the rebound of wakefulness due to homeostatic mechanisms controlling the amount of sleep.

Episode durations of wakefulness and NREM sleep in the suvorexant group for 6 h after administration were not different from those in the control group (**Figures 3D,E**, **Figures S3D,E**). However, there were significant differences in these parameters in the latter half of the dark period between the suvorexant and control groups [Wakefulness episodes: $F_{(2, 20)} = 10.58$, $p < 0.01$ for 10 mg/kg, $p < 0.001$ for 30 mg/kg, **Figure 3D**] [NREM sleep episodes: $F_{(2, 20)} = 4.86$, $p < 0.05$ for 10 mg/kg, $p < 0.05$ for 90 mg/kg, **Figure 3E**]. The longer episode duration of NREM sleep in the suvorexant group continued in the subsequent light period. These observations suggest that suvorexant consolidates both wakefulness and NREM sleep episodes. REM sleep episode duration was not significantly affected by suvorexant for 12 h after administration (**Figure 3F**). However, hourly analysis showed that high dose (30 mg/kg) suvorexant increased REM sleep duration for several hours (**Figure S3F**). Latency to NREM sleep onset after administration of C1m showed a tendency to be shorter than that in the control group, although the difference was not statistically significant (**Figure 3G**). REM sleep latency after administration was shorter in the 30 mg/kg group than in the vehicle group during the dark period [$F_{(2, 20)} = 4.92$, $p < 0.05$] (**Figure 3H**).

The power density of EEG in the suvorexant-administered group (30 mg/kg) showed slightly, but significantly larger percent of 0.5 and 2.5 Hz component [$F_{(40, 246)} = 2.539$, $p < 0.0001$ for 0.5 Hz, $p < 0.05$ for 2.5 Hz] (**Figure 3I**).

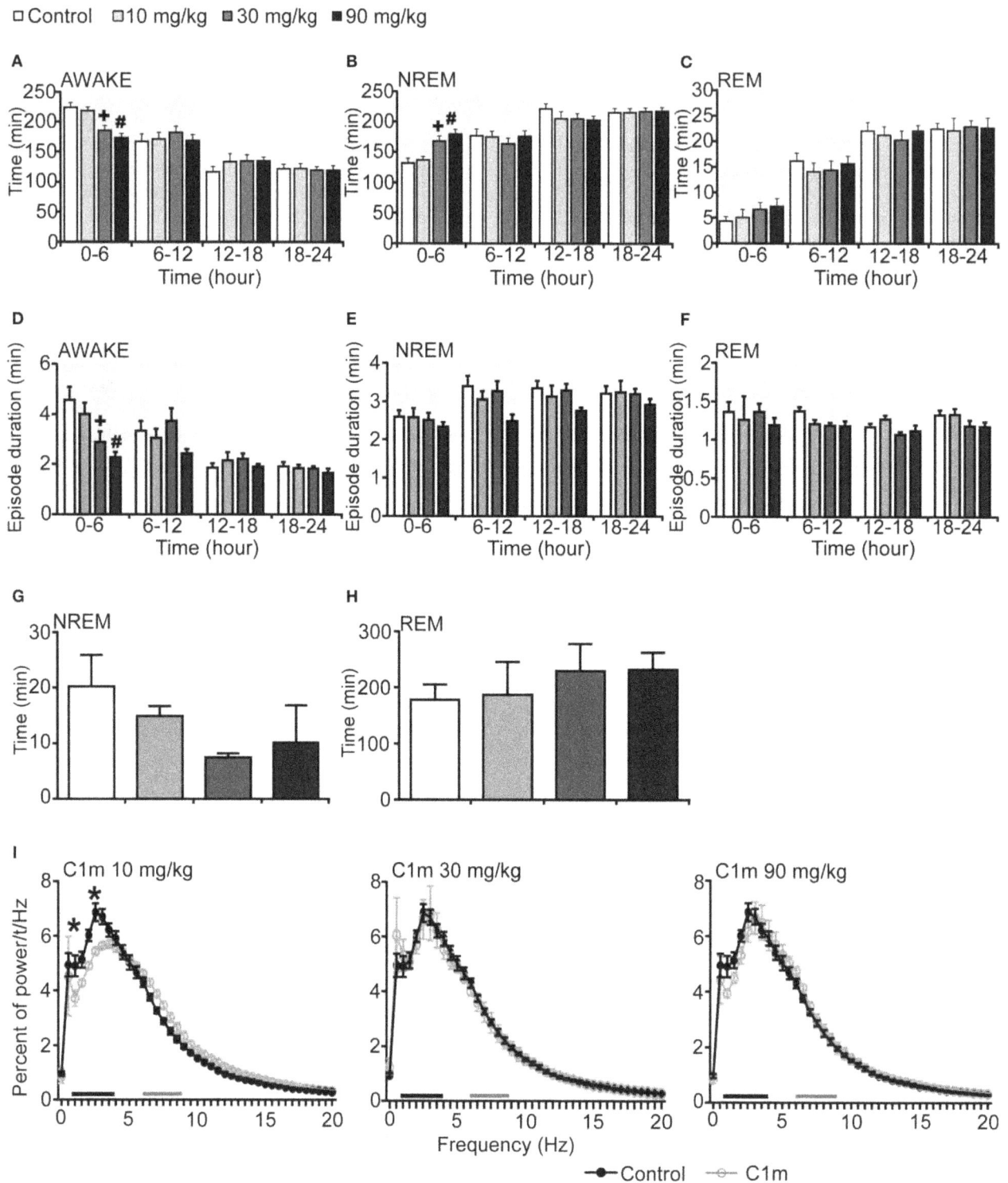

FIGURE 1 | Effects of C1m on basal sleep/wakefulness states in C57BL/6 mice (*n* = 6–9/group) after administration at start of dark period. C1m (10, 30, 90 mg/kg) and methylcellulose as control were administered *per os* at the start of the light period (*t* = 0, *ZT* = 12). (A–C) Total time spent in wakefulness (A), NREM sleep (B), and REM sleep (C) in 6 h time windows over 24 h. (D–F) Mean duration of wakefulness (D), NREM sleep (E) and REM sleep (F) in 6 h time windows over 24 h. Data for the dark and light periods are displayed with light gray and white backgrounds, respectively.

(G,H) Latency to NREM sleep (time to appearance of first NREM sleep after administration) (G) and REM sleep latency (time to appearance of first REM sleep after administration) (H) during dark period. Results are expressed in minutes and presented as mean ± s.e.m. (I) EEG power density during NREM sleep for 3 h after administration shown as mean percentage of total EEG power. The delta range (0.75–4 Hz) is indicated by the black bar and the theta range (6–9 Hz) by the gray bar. *$p < 0.05$ for 10 mg/kg C1m, +$p < 0.05$ for 30 mg/kg C1m, #$p < 0.05$ for 90 mg/kg C1m vs. control.

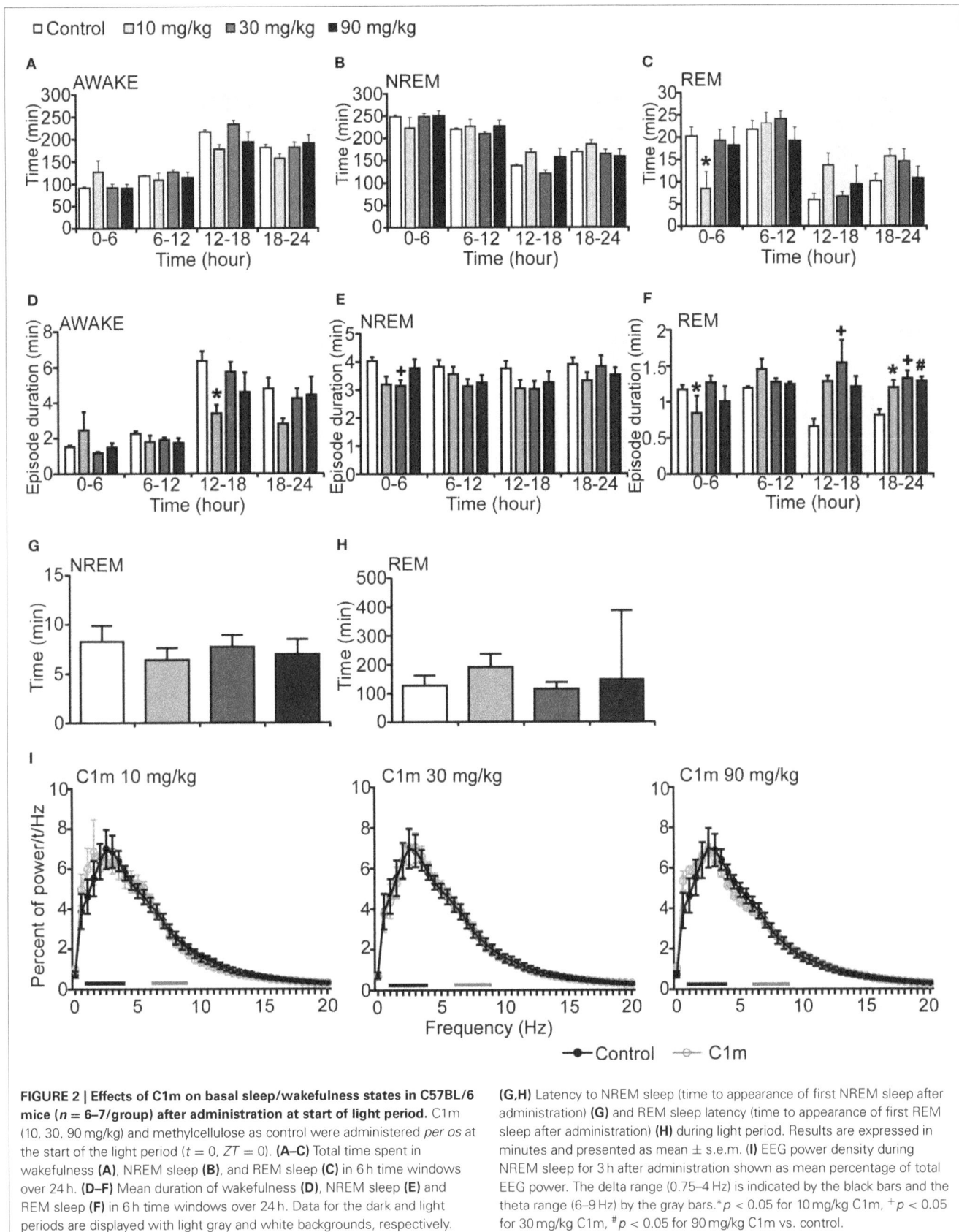

FIGURE 2 | Effects of C1m on basal sleep/wakefulness states in C57BL/6 mice (n = 6–7/group) after administration at start of light period. C1m (10, 30, 90 mg/kg) and methylcellulose as control were administered *per os* at the start of the light period (t = 0, ZT = 0). **(A–C)** Total time spent in wakefulness **(A)**, NREM sleep **(B)**, and REM sleep **(C)** in 6 h time windows over 24 h. **(D–F)** Mean duration of wakefulness **(D)**, NREM sleep **(E)** and REM sleep **(F)** in 6 h time windows over 24 h. Data for the dark and light periods are displayed with light gray and white backgrounds, respectively.

(G,H) Latency to NREM sleep (time to appearance of first NREM sleep after administration) **(G)** and REM sleep latency (time to appearance of first REM sleep after administration) **(H)** during light period. Results are expressed in minutes and presented as mean ± s.e.m. **(I)** EEG power density during NREM sleep for 3 h after administration shown as mean percentage of total EEG power. The delta range (0.75–4 Hz) is indicated by the black bars and the theta range (6–9 Hz) by the gray bars. $*p < 0.05$ for 10 mg/kg C1m, $+p < 0.05$ for 30 mg/kg C1m, $\#p < 0.05$ for 90 mg/kg C1m vs. control.

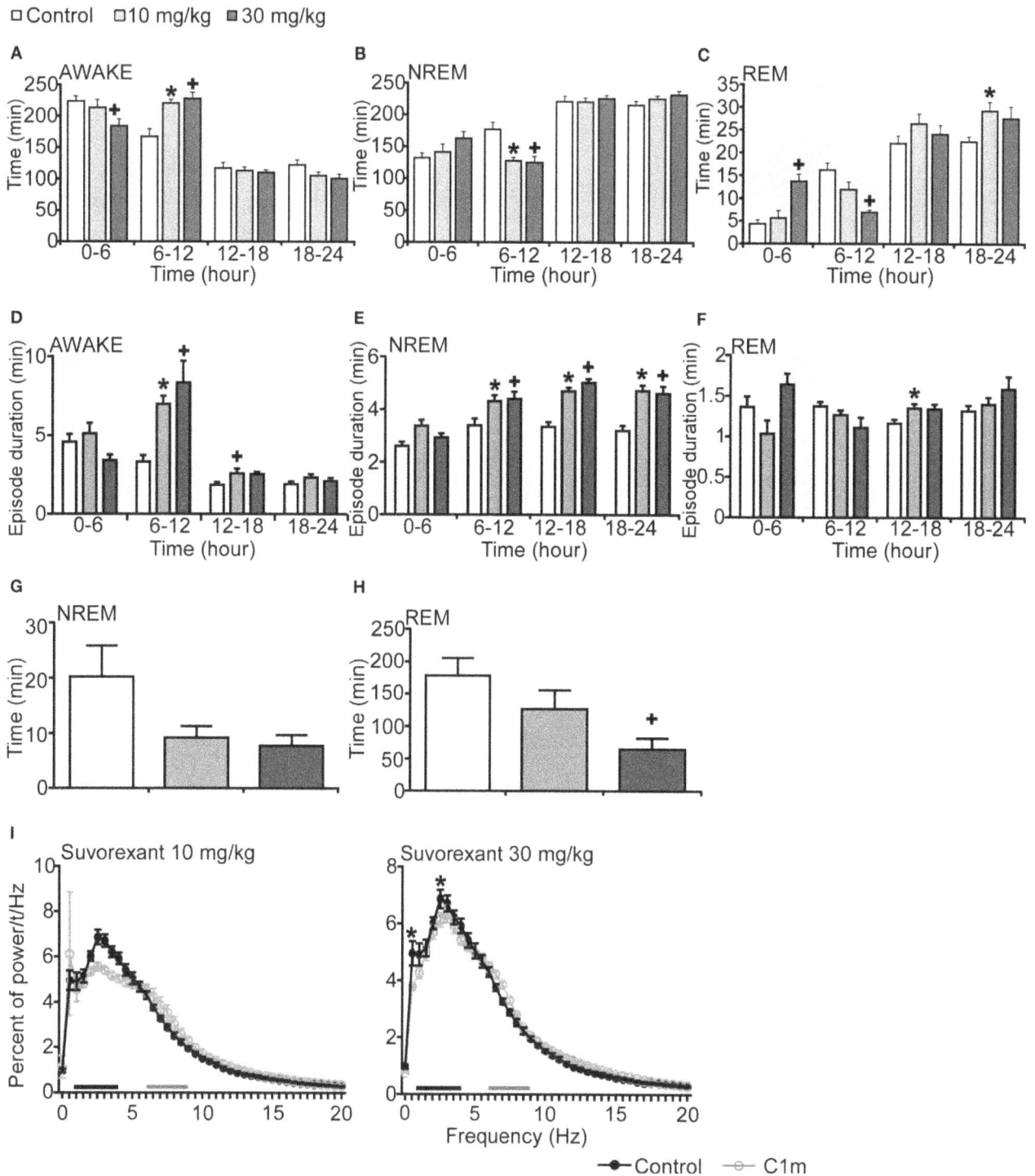

FIGURE 3 | Effects of DORA, suvorexant, on basal sleep/wakefulness states in C57BL/6 mice ($n = 7–9$/group) after administration at ZT12. Suvorexant (10 and 30 mg/kg) and methylcellulose as control were administered *per os* at the start of the dark period ($t = 0$, ZT12). (A–C) Total time spent in wakefulness (A), NREM sleep (B) and REM sleep (C) in 6 h time windows over 24 h. (D–F) Mean duration of wakefulness (D), NREM sleep (E) and REM sleep (F) in 6 h time windows over 24 h. Data for the dark and light periods are displayed with light gray and white backgrounds, respectively. (G,H). Latency to NREM sleep (time to appearance of first NREM sleep after administration) (G) and REM sleep latency (time to appearance of first REM sleep after administration) (H) during dark period. Results are expressed in minutes and presented as mean ± s.e.m. (I) EEG power density during NREM sleep for 3 h after administration shown as mean percentage of total EEG power. The delta range (0.75–4 Hz) is indicated by the black bars and the theta range (6–9 Hz) by the gray bars. *$p < 0.05$ for 10 mg/kg suvorexant, +$p < 0.05$ for 30 mg/kg suvorexant vs. control.

Mice administered suvorexant (30 mg/kg) at the start of light period showed a shorter wakefulness time and longer REM sleep time after administration as compared with vehicle-administered mice (**Figures 4A–C, Figures S4A–C**). During the light phase, suvorexant showed an effect on wakefulness for 1 h and on REM sleep for 3 h (**Figures S4A–C**). Wakefulness and NREM sleep episode durations were not affected by suvorexant administration (**Figures 4D,E**). However, REM sleep episode duration was longer in the suvorexant group. This effect lasted for 24 h (**Figure 4F**). NREM and REM sleep latencies were not different statistically between the suvorexant and vehicle groups (**Figure 4H**). The power density of EEG in the suvorexant-administered group showed no difference from that in the vehicle-administered group (**Figure 4I**).

COMPARISON OF EFFECTS OF C1m vs. SUVOREXANT

Considering the differences in the effective time periods of action of both compounds, we also compared the effects of these drugs in the time window of 2 or 3 h after administration (**Figure 5, Table 1**).

For 2 h after administration at ZT12, both C1m and suvorexant increased NREM sleep time [$F_{(5, 38)} = 5.33$, $p < 0.05$ for C1m 30 mg/kg, $p < 0.05$ for C1m 90 mg/kg, $p < 0.01$ for suvorexant 30 mg/kg] (**Figure 5B**). There was a major difference in the effect on REM sleep time: C1m showed little effect on REM sleep time even at a high dose (90 mg/kg), while suvorexant (30 mg/kg) markedly increased REM sleep time [$F_{(5, 38)} = 14.06$, $p < 0.0001$] (**Figure 5C**). There was also a difference in the effects of both compounds on each episode duration. Both C1m and suvorexant shortened the wakefulness episode duration in a dose-dependent manner [$F_{(5, 38)} = 4.08$, $p < 0.05$ for C1m 30 mg/kg, $p < 0.01$ for C1m 90 mg/kg, $p < 0.05$ for suvorexant 30 mg/kg] (**Figure 5D**). C1m did not change the NREM sleep or REM sleep episode durations (**Figures 1E,F**), whereas suvorexant (30 mg/kg) increased both the REM [$F_{(5, 38)} = 3.76$, $p < 0.05$] and NREM sleep [$F_{(5, 38)} = 5.74$, $p < 0.01$] episode durations (**Figures 5E,F**).

While C1m increased the transition numbers of both wakefulness to NREM sleep and NREM sleep to wakefulness, suvorexant did not show any effects on these parameters (**Table 1**). On the other hand, suvorexant increased NREM to REM sleep and REM to wakefulness transitions, while C1m did not influence them (**Table 1**).

EFFECTS OF C1m AND SUVOREXANT ON ACTIVITY OF OREXINERGIC, NORADRENERGIC, SEROTONERGIC, AND HISTAMINERGIC NEURONS

To define the effects of C1m and suvorexant on activity of arousal-related neurons, we examined Fos-like immunoreactivity (Fos-IR) in orexin neurons, noradrenergic neurons in the locus coeruleus (LC), serotonergic neurons in the dorsal raphe (DR) nucleus, and histaminergic neurons in the tuberomammillary nucleus (TMN). Since Fos-IR generally reflects the activity of neurons for 60–90 min before the time of fixation, we killed mice 2 h after drug administration. Mice were administered drugs at ZT12, and killed at ZT14.

Whereas the numbers of Fos-positive orexin neurons and noradrenergic neurons were not affected by C1m, suvorexant significantly increased the number of Fos-positive orexin

neurons (Control, $67.0 \pm 2.5\%$; suvorexant, $88.0 \pm 1.3\%$, [$F_{(2, 15)} = 8.90$, $p < 0.01$] and decreased the number of Fos-positive noradrenergic neurons [Control, $74.9 \pm 2.8\%$; suvorexant, $57.5 \pm 3.6\%$, $F_{(2, 15)} = 17.65$, $p < 0.01$)] (**Figures 6A,B**). C1m (30 mg/kg) administration significantly decreased the numbers of Fos-positive serotonergic neurons [Control, $44.1 \pm 3.9\%$; C1m, $20.3 \pm 5.0\%$, $F_{(2, 15)} = 13.21$, $p < 0.01$] and histaminergic neurons [Control, $48.7 \pm 6.9\%$; C1m, $24.3 \pm 7.4\%$, $F_{(2, 15)} = 7.57$, $p < 0.05$] (**Figures 6C,D**). Similarly, suvorexant (30 mg/kg) significantly decreased the numbers of Fos-positive serotonergic neurons [Control, $44.1 \pm 3.9\%$; suvorexant, $19.1 \pm 2.2\%$, $F_{(2, 15)} = 13.21$, $p < 0.01$] and histaminergic neurons [Control, $48.7 \pm 6.9\%$; suvorexant, $15.8 \pm 3.5\%$, $F_{(2, 15)} = 7.57$, $p < 0.01$] (**Figures 6C,D**).

DISCUSSION

Orexin receptor antagonists, especially DORAs, are under development as next generation drugs for treating insomnia. Precise knowledge about differential roles of the two orexin receptors would be beneficial for application of orexin agonists/antagonists as treatment for various diseases. It has been thought that OX_2R plays a pivotal role in the maintenance of wakefulness, based on the phenotype of receptor-deficient mice and pharmacological studies using these mice (Sakurai and Mieda, 2011). OX_2R knockout mice show characteristics of narcolepsy (Willie et al., 2003), while OX_1R knockout mice show an almost normal sleep-wake cycle (Willie et al., 2001). However, the phenotype of OX_2R knockout mice is less severe than that found in *prepro-orexin* knockout mice and double receptor knockout mice. Especially, OX_2R knockout mice are almost 33 times less affected by cataplexy and direct transitions to REM sleep from an awake state as compared with orexin ligand knockout mice (Willie et al., 2003). Furthermore, the effects of orexin A on wakefulness and NREM sleep were significantly attenuated in $OX_2R^{-/-}$ mice as compared with wild-type mice and $OX_1R^{-/-}$ mice, although $OX_1R^{-/-}$ mice showed a slightly impaired response (Mieda et al., 2011). Notably, suppression of REM sleep by orexin-A administration was similarly attenuated in both $OX_1R^{-/-}$ and $OX_2R^{-/-}$ mice, suggesting a comparable contribution of the two receptors to REM suppression. These observations suggest that although the OX_2R-mediated pathway has a pivotal role in the promotion of wakefulness, OX_1R also has additional effects on sleep/wakefulness regulation, especially in the inhibitory regulation of REM sleep.

In this study, we examined the effect of a novel 2-SORA, C1m, in mice. We found that C1m (30 and 90 mg/kg) significantly reduced wakefulness time along with an increase in NREM sleep time for 5 h after administration at the start of the dark period (**Figures 1A,B**). The efficacy of C1m in increasing NREM sleep time was comparable (**Figure 5B**) or even stronger (**Figures 1B, 3B**) than that of suvorexant, depending on the observation time. This indicates that the sole blockade of OX_2R is sufficient to increase NREM sleep time. This is consistent with a previous pharmacological study suggesting that wakefulness/NREM sleep transition depends primarily on OX_2R (Mieda et al., 2011). However, while suvorexant increased the NREM sleep episode duration, C1m did not (**Figure 5E**). Likewise, C1m increased the

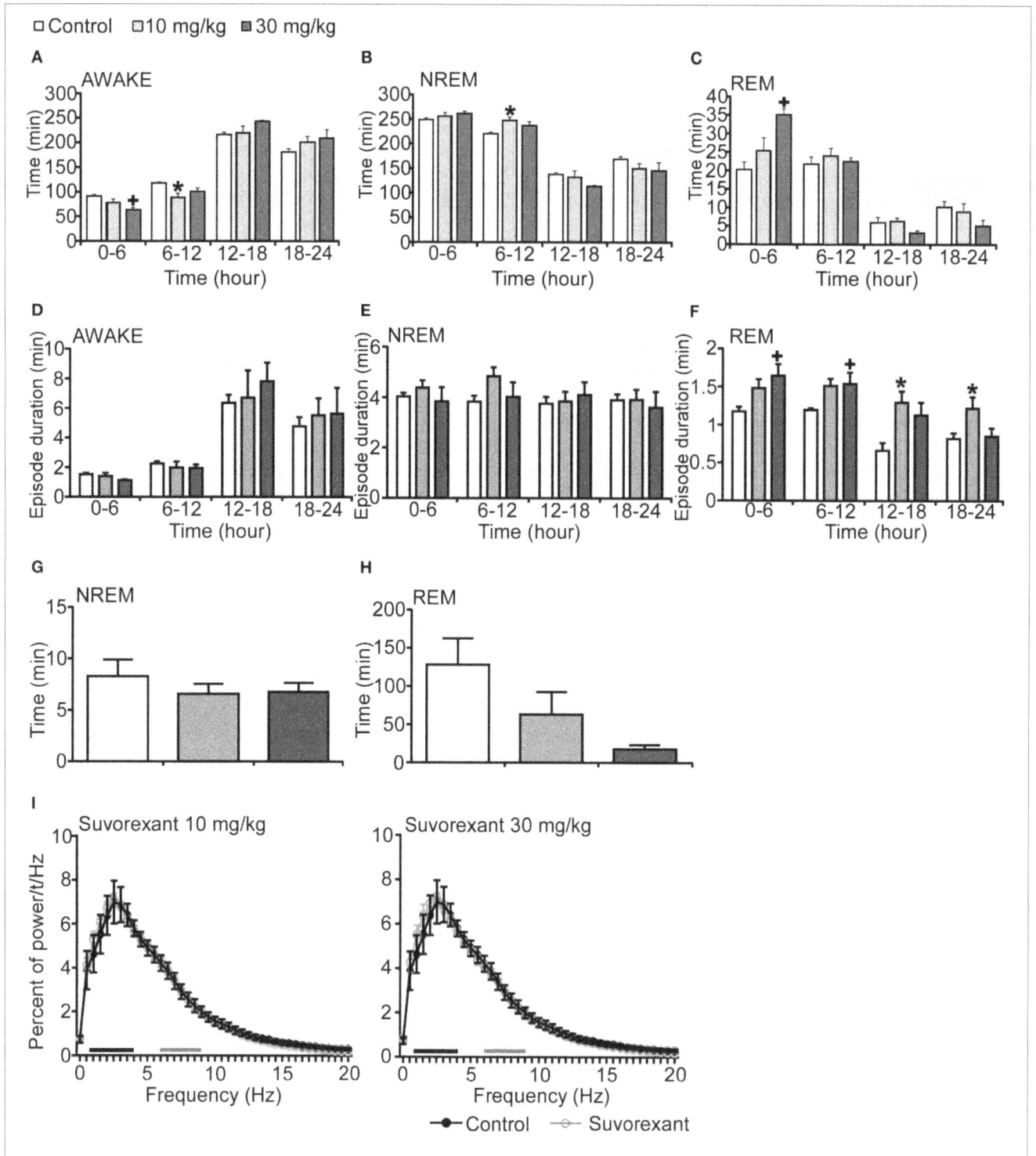

FIGURE 4 | Effects of suvorexant on basal sleep/wakefulness states in C57BL/6 mice (n = 5–7/group) after administration at start of light period. Suvorexant (10 and 30 mg/kg) and methylcellulose as control were administered *per os* at the start of the recording (t = 0, ZT0). **(A–C)** Total time spent in waking **(A)**, NREM sleep **(B)** and REM sleep **(C)** in 6 h time windows over 24 h. **(D–F)** Mean duration of wakefulness **(D)**, NREM sleep **(E)**, and REM **(F)** sleep in 6 h time windows over 24 h. Data for the dark and light periods are displayed with light gray and white backgrounds, respectively.

(G,H) Latency to NREM sleep (time to appearance of first NREM sleep after administration) **(G)** and REM sleep latency (time to appearance of first REM sleep after administration) **(H)** during light period. Results are expressed in minutes and presented as mean ± s.e.m. **(I)** EEG power density during NREM sleep for 3 h after administration shown as mean percentage of total EEG power. The delta range (0.75–4 Hz) is indicated by the black bars and the theta range (6–9 Hz) by the gray bars. *$p < 0.05$ for 10 mg/kg suvorexant, $^+p < 0.05$ for 30 mg/kg suvorexant vs. control.

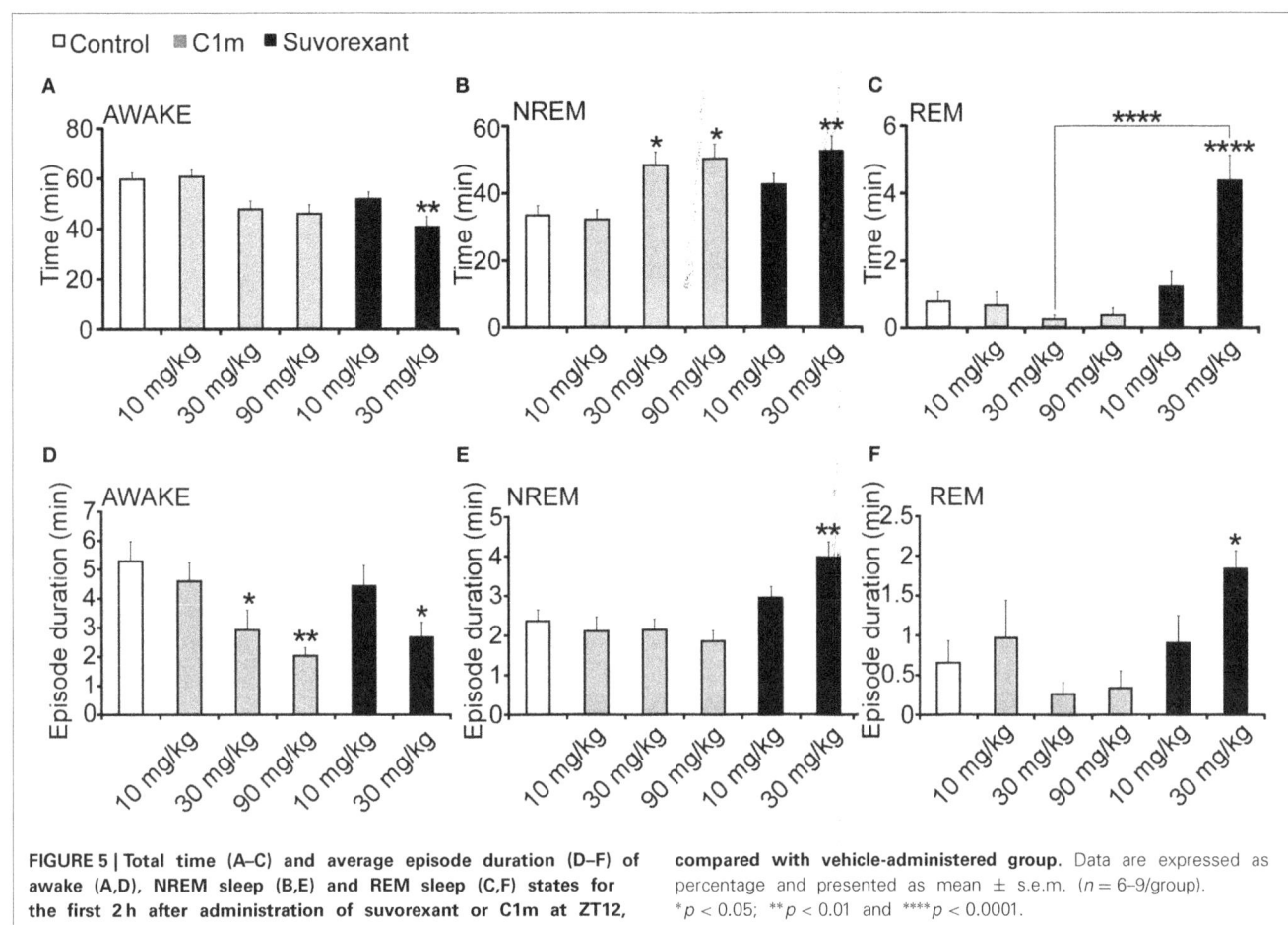

FIGURE 5 | Total time (A–C) and average episode duration (D–F) of awake (A,D), NREM sleep (B,E) and REM sleep (C,F) states for the first 2 h after administration of suvorexant or C1m at ZT12, compared with vehicle-administered group. Data are expressed as percentage and presented as mean ± s.e.m. (n = 6–9/group). *p < 0.05; **p < 0.01 and ****p < 0.0001.

Table 1 | Total number of state transitions after administration of Compound 1 m (10, 30, and 90 mg/kg) and Suvorexant (10 and 30 mg/kg) in wild-type mice at ZT 12.

	Vehicle	Compound 1 m			Suvorexant	
	(n = 6)	10 mg/kg (n = 6)	30 mg/kg (n = 9)	90 mg/kg (n = 6)	10 mg/kg (n = 7)	30 mg/kg (n = 7)
W → NR	25.2 (2.8)	28.0 (5.0)	41.8 (6.8)*	44.7 (5.3)*	22.7 (2.4)	30.4 (1.7)
W → R	0	0	0	0	0	0
NR → W	23.9 (2.9)	26.8 (5.3)	40.7 (7.0)	43.6 (5.5)*	20.4 (2.8)	25.3 (2.1)
NR → R	1.2 (0.4)	0.8 (0.3)	1.0 (0.3)	0.9 (0.5)	2.1 (0.9)	4.4 (0.8)**
R → W	1.2 (0.4)	0.8 (0.3)	1.0 (0.3)	0.9 (0.5)	2.1 (0.9)	4.3 (0.8)**
R → NR	0	0	0	0	0	0

Values (means ± s.e.m.) are calculated for 3 h after administratrion at ZT 12. W, NR, and R represents wake, NREM sleep, and REM sleep, respectively.
*P<0.05 and **P<0.01 for each dose vs. control, one-way ANVA followed by Bonfferoni correction as post-hoc test.*

number of transitions between wakefulness and NREM sleep, while suvorexant did not (**Table 1**). These findings suggest that OX$_1$R might have additional effects of increasing wakefulness, and blocking of OX$_1$R along with OX$_2$R blockade further consolidates NREM sleep. This is again consistent with our previous study showing that ICV orexin-A still increased wakefulness in OX$_2$R$^{-/-}$ mice (Mieda et al., 2011).

Both C1m and suvorexant showed greater sleep-promoting effects in mice during the dark period, in which orexin neurons fire rapidly (Lee et al., 2005), than during the light period.

Still, whereas the administration of C1m just prior to onset of the light phase had only minimal effects on wakefulness, suvorexant (30 mg/kg) was able to significantly decreased wakefulness time (**Figure 4A**) and increase REM sleep time also in the light period (**Figure 4C**, **Figure S4C**). These observations suggest that DORAs might have a more powerful impact on sleep/wakefulness states especially during the light period as compared with 2-SORA. This could suggest a role of OX$_1$R in gating of the transition from NREM sleep to wakefulness during the resting period. The impact of 1 h of suvorexant on wakefulness

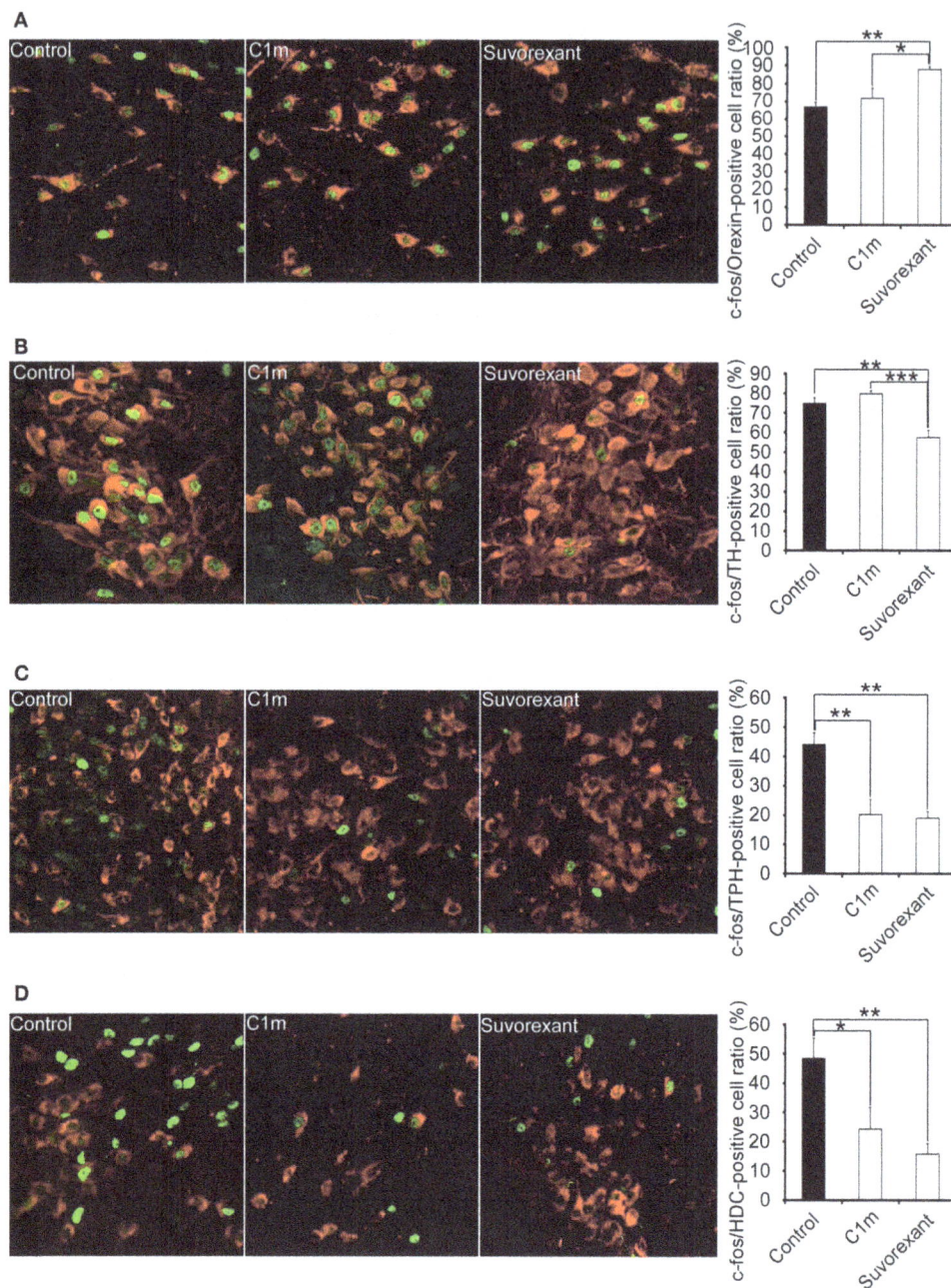

FIGURE 6 | Number of Fos-positive neurons at 2 h after administration of vehicle and drugs (30 mg/kg C1m and suvorexant) at ZT12 in C57BL/6 mice (n = 6/group). Typical images of Fos expression in orexin-IR cells in lateral hypothalamic area **(A)**, TH-IR cells in LC **(B)**, TPH-IR cells in DR **(C)**, and HDC-IR cells in TMN **(D)**. Fos-IR nucleus-positive cells are calculated as the percentage of orexin-IR cells (red) with a Fos-IR nucleus (green) in all orexin neurons, TH-IR cells (red) with a Fos-IR nucleus (green) in all TH-IR cells, TPH-IR cells (red) with a Fos-IR nucleus (green) in all TPH-IR cells, and HDC-IR cells (red) with a Fos-IR nucleus (green) in all HDC-IR cells. Data are expressed as percentage and presented as mean ± s.e.m. $*p < 0.05$, $**p < 0.01$ and $***p < 0.001$. TH, tryptophane hydroxylase; LC, locus coeruleus; TPH, tryptophan hydroxylase; HDC, histidine decarboxylase; TMN, tuberomammillary nucleus.

time when administered during the day (**Figure S3A**) could be due to more rapid onset of action of suvorexant, because administration *per se* has a stimulant effect, and only a compound with a rapid onset of action could show efficacy at that moment.

We observed an increase of wakefulness in the 6–12 h time window after the administration of suvorexant at ZT12

(**Figure 3A**). However, we did not find a rebound increase of wakefulness in the C1m-administered group (**Figure 1A**). This difference is likely the result of the different time periods where both compounds exert biological activity. Alternatively, blocking OX_1R might lead to more profound wakefulness rebound after the time of sleep-induction. This mechanism should be addressed in future studies.

$Orexin^{-/-}$ and $OX_2R^{-/-}$ mice show sleep fragmentation during the dark period, which is accompanied by a shorter NREM episode duration during the dark period (Chemelli et al., 1999; Willie et al., 2003). Although C1m increased the frequency of transitions between wakefulness and NREM sleep states (**Table 1**), it did not significantly shorten NREM sleep episode duration. Suvorexant increased the NREM sleep duration and decreased the frequency of transitions between NREM and REM sleep when it was administered in the dark period (**Figure 5E**). The increase in duration of NREM and REM sleep by DORAs is consistent with the results of previous studies (Winrow et al., 2012). These observations suggest that acute pharmacological blockade of OX_2R or both receptors increases sleep time, but does not induce sleep/wakefulness fragmentation, one of the important characteristics of narcolepsy. These observations suggest that the sleep/wakefulness fragmentation in narcolepsy might be due to chronic compensatory processes in narcoleptic animals resulting from chronic deficiency of orexin signaling (Tsujino et al., 2013).

OX_1R and OX_2R are distributed differently in the brain. Histaminergic neurons in the TMN, which strongly express OX_2R, are thought to play an important role in the arousal-promoting effect of orexin, because the effect of ICV orexin-A administration is markedly attenuated by the histamine H_1 receptor antagonist pyrilamine and is absent in H_1 histamine receptor knockout mice (Huang et al., 2001; Yamanaka et al., 2002). Mochizuki et al. produced a mouse model in which a loxP-flanked gene cassette disrupts production of OX_2R, but normal OX_2R expression can be restored by Cre recombinase (Mochizuki et al., 2011). They showed that targeted Cre expression, i.e., focal restoration of OX_2R expression, in the TMN and adjacent regions abrogated fragmentation of wakefulness in this mouse model, suggesting that the orexin signaling mediated by OX_2R in the TMN and/or its surrounding area in the posterior hypothalamus is sufficient to prevent sleepiness caused by systemic OX_2R deficiency. However, orexins probably promote arousal through many redundant systems because optogenetic activation of orexin neurons still promotes wakefulness in mice lacking histamine (Carter et al., 2009), and mice lacking both OX_1R and histamine H_1 receptors demonstrate no abnormality of sleep/wakefulness (Hondo et al., 2010). Our present study further suggests an additional role of OX_1R in promoting and maintaining wakefulness, and a relatively large impact on REM sleep amount.

To gain an insight into the mechanisms by which both compounds affect sleep/wakefulness states, we examined the effects of the compounds on the number of Fos-IR neurons in orexin-target areas (**Figure 6**). Compounds were administered at the start of the dark period. We found that the number of Fos-IR noradrenergic neurons in the LC was lower in the suvorexant group as compared with the control and C1m-treated groups (**Figure 6B**). This is consistent with the fact that noradrenergic neurons in the LC exclusively express OX_1R (Mieda et al., 2011). The number of Fos-IR serotonergic neurons in the DR was similarly lower in the suvorexant and C1m groups than in the control group (**Figure 6C**). This suggests that orexin mainly excites serotonergic neurons through activation of OX_2R, although these cells also express OX_1R (Mieda et al., 2011). We observed that

the number of Fos-IR neurons in histaminergic neurons in the TMN was lower in both the C1m and suvorexant groups as compared with the control group (**Figure 6D**), consistent with the previous observation that these cells only express OX_2R (Mieda et al., 2011). Unexpectedly, we observed that the suvorexant group showed a larger number of Fos-IR orexin neurons in the LHA as compared with the control and C1m-treated groups (**Figure 6A**), although a previous study suggested that orexin neurons express OX_2R (Yamanaka et al., 2010). The increased number of Fos-IR orexin neurons in the suvorexant group compared with the control group might have resulted from decreased activity of monoaminergic neurons, which were shown to send inhibitory feedback projections to orexin neurons (Sakurai and Mieda, 2011). Inhibitory feedback mechanisms mediated by noradrenergic neurons might play a major role in regulation of orexinergic activity, because C1m did not affect the number of Fos-IR neurons (**Figure 6A**). Alternatively, blockade by suvorexant of OX_1R-mediated activation of GABAergic interneurons that send inhibitory projections to orexin neurons might increase the activity of orexin neurons (Matsuki et al., 2009). The suvorexant-mediated increase in orexin neuronal activity might be one of the possible reasons for the rebound wakefulness seen in suvorexant-administered mice in the latter half of the dark period after administration at ZT12 (**Figure 2A**).

To precisely compare the effects of DORA vs. 2-SORA on sleep/wakefulness states, it would be necessary to compare the effects at equal free brain concentrations and also to have data of brain receptor occupancy. Although we do not have such data, our present results would be useful for further understanding the characteristics of the effects of DORA and 2-SORA and the roles of the two orexin receptors in sleep/wakefulness regulation.

CONCLUSION

Given the comparable values of % reduction of wakefulness time for 6 h after administration of C1m (30 mg/kg) and suvorexant (30 mg/kg), -17.2% [$F_{(3, 26)} = 9.55$, $p < 0.01$] and -17.8% [$F_{(2, 20)} = 3.74$, $p < 0.05$] (**Figures 1A, 3A**), respectively, C1m, a newly developed 2-SORA, sufficiently suppressed wakefulness and promoted sleep with comparable efficacy to that of suvorexant, a potent DORA. However, suvorexant induced more stable sleep with longer NREM sleep episode duration and fewer NREM to wakefulness transitions, suggesting that additional OX_1R blockade confers more stable sleep. On the other hand, C1m showed little effect on REM sleep time while suvorexant significantly increased REM sleep time. These results suggest that the different effects of DORA vs. 2-SORA on orexin-target neurons might reflect differences in the effects of these two drugs on sleep/wake behavior in mice.

AUTHOR CONTRIBUTIONS

Keishi Etori performed all experiments, and wrote the paper. Yuki Saito and Natsuko Tsujino performed the experiments. Takeshi Sakurai designed and supervised the experiments, and wrote the paper.

ACKNOWLEDGMENTS

This study was supported by the Cabinet Office, the Government of Japan, through its "Funding Program for Next Generation

World-Leading Researchers." The authors thank Takeda Pharmaceutical Company for providing C1m. We also thank Dr. Tatsuhiko Fujimoto for valuable discussion.

SUPPLEMENTARY MATERIAL

The Supplementary Material for this article can be found online at: http://www.frontiersin.org/journal/10.3389/fnins.2014.00008/abstract

Figure S1 | Hourly analysis of effects of C1m on basal sleep/wakefulness states in C57BL/6 mice ($n = 6–9$/group) after administration at ZT12. C1m (10, 30, 90 mg/kg) and methylcellulose as control were administered *per os* at the start of the dark period ($t = 0$, ZT12). Total time spent in each state **(A–C)** and average episode duration of each state **(D–F)** over 24 h. Data for the dark and light periods are displayed with light gray and white backgrounds, respectively. $*p < 0.05$ for 10 mg/kg C1m, $^+p < 0.05$ for 30 mg/kg C1m, $^\#p < 0.05$ for 90 mg/kg C1m vs. control, two-way ANOVA followed by Bonfferoni correction as a *post-hoc* test. Results are expressed in minutes and presented as mean $\pm$ s.e.m ($n = 9$ for control, $n = 6$ for 10 mg/kg C1m, $n = 9$ for 30 mg/kg C1m, $n = 6$ for 90 mg/kg C1m).

Figure S2 | Hourly analysis of effects of C1m on basal sleep/wakefulness states in C57BL/6 mice ($n = 6–7$/group) after administration at ZT0. C1m (10, 30, 90 mg/kg) and methylcellulose as control were administered *per os* at the start of the dark period ($t = 0$, ZT0). Total time spent in each state **(A–C)** and average episode duration of each state **(D–F)** over 24 h. Data for the dark and light periods are displayed with light gray and white backgrounds, respectively. $*p < 0.05$ for 10 mg/kg C1m, $^+p < 0.05$ for 30 mg/kg C1m, $^\#p < 0.05$ for 90 mg/kg C1m vs. control, two-way ANOVA followed by Bonfferoni correction as a *post-hoc* test. Results are expressed in minutes and presented as mean $\pm$ s.e.m ($n = 7$ for control, $n = 7$ for 10 mg/kg C1m, $n = 7$ for 30 mg/kg C1m, $n = 6$ for 90 mg/kg C1m).

Figure S3 | Hourly analysis of effects of suvorexant on basal sleep/wakefulness states in C57BL/6 mice ($n = 7–9$/group) after administration at ZT12. Suvorexant (10, 30 mg/kg) and methylcellulose as control were administered *per os* at the start of the dark period ($t = 0$, ZT12). Total time spent in each state **(A–C)** and average episode duration of each state **(D–F)** over 24 h. Data for the dark and light periods are displayed with light gray and white backgrounds, respectively. $*p < 0.05$ for 10 mg/kg suvorexant, $^+p < 0.05$ for 30 mg/kg suvorexant vs. control, two-way ANOVA followed by Bonfferoni correction as a *post-hoc* test. Results are expressed in minutes and presented as mean $\pm$ s.e.m ($n = 9$ for control, $n = 7$ for 10 mg/kg suvorexant, $n = 7$ for 30 mg/kg suvorexant).

Figure S4 | Hourly analysis of effects of suvorexant on basal sleep/wakefulness states in C57BL/6 mice ($n = 5–7$/group) after administration at ZT0. Suvorexant (10, 30 mg/kg) and methylcellulose as control were administered *per os* at the start of the dark period ($t = 0$, ZT0). Time spent in each state **(A–C)** and average episode duration of each state **(D–F)** over 24 h. Data for the dark and light periods are displayed with light gray and white backgrounds, respectively. $*p < 0.05$ for 10 mg/kg suvorexant, $^+p < 0.05$ for 30 mg/kg suvorexant vs. control, two-way ANOVA followed by Bonfferoni correction as a *post-hoc* test. Results are expressed in minutes and presented as mean $\pm$s.e.m. ($n = 7$ for control, $n = 7$ for 10 mg/kg suvorexant, $n = 5$ for 30 mg/kg suvorexant).

REFERENCES

Brisbare-Roch, C., Dingemanse, J., Koberstein, R., Hoever, P., Aissaoui, H., Flores, S., et al. (2007). Promotion of sleep by targeting the orexin system in rats, dogs and humans. *Nat. Med.* 13, 150–155. doi: 10.1038/nm1544

Carter, M. E., Adamantidis, A., Ohtsu, H., Deisseroth, K., and De Lecea, L. (2009). Sleep homeostasis modulates hypocretin-mediated sleep-to-wake transitions. *J. Neurosci.* 29, 10939–10949. doi: 10.1523/JNEUROSCI.1205-09.2009

Chemelli, R. M., Willie, J. T., Sinton, C. M., Elmquist, J. K., Scammell, T., Lee, C., et al. (1999). Narcolepsy in orexin knockout mice: molecular genetics of sleep regulation. *Cell* 98, 437–451. doi: 10.1016/S0092-8674(00)81973-X

Cox, C. D., Breslin, M. J., Whitman, D. B., Schreier, J. D., Mcgaughey, G. B., Bogusky, M. J., et al. (2010). Discovery of the dual orexin receptor antagonist [(7R)-4-(5-chloro-1,3-benzoxazol-2-yl)-7-methyl-1,4-diazepan-1-yl][5-methyl-2-(2H -1,2,3-triazol-2-yl)phenyl]methanone (MK-4305) for the treatment of insomnia. *J. Med. Chem.* 53, 5320–5332. doi: 10.1021/jm100541c

Dietrich, H., and Jenck, F. (2010). Intact learning and memory in rats following treatment with the dual orexin receptor antagonist almorexant. *Psychopharmacology (Berl)* 212, 145–154. doi: 10.1007/s00213-010-1933-5

Dugovic, C., Shelton, J. E., Aluisio, L. E., Fraser, I. C., Jiang, X., Sutton, S. W., et al. (2009). Blockade of orexin-1 receptors attenuates orexin-2 receptor antagonism-induced sleep promotion in the rat. *J. Pharmacol. Exp. Ther.* 330, 142–151. doi: 10.1124/jpet.109.152009

Fujimoto, T., Kunitomo, J., Tomata, Y., Nishiyama, K., Nakashima, M., Hirozane, M., et al. (2011). Discovery of potent, selective, orally active benzoxazepine-based Orexin-2 receptor antagonists. *Bioorg. Med. Chem. Lett.* 21, 6414–6416. doi: 10.1016/j.bmcl.2011.08.093

Hara, J., Beuckmann, C. T., Nambu, T., Willie, J. T., Chemelli, R. M., Sinton, C. M., et al. (2001). Genetic ablation of orexin neurons in mice results in narcolepsy, hypophagia, and obesity. *Neuron* 30, 345–354. doi: 10.1016/S0896-6273(01)00293-8

Hoever, P., De Haas, S., Winkler, J., Schoemaker, R. C., Chiossi, E., Van Gerven, J., et al. (2010). Orexin receptor antagonism, a new sleep-promoting paradigm: an ascending single-dose study with almorexant. *Clin. Pharmacol. Ther.* 87, 593–600. doi: 10.1038/clpt.2010.19

Hondo, M., Nagai, K., Ohno, K., Kisanuki, Y., Willie, J. T., Watanabe, T., et al. (2010). Histamine-1 receptor is not required as a downstream effector of orexin-2 receptor in maintenance of basal sleep/wake states. *Acta physiol.* 198, 287–294. doi: 10.1111/j.1748-1716.2009.02032.x

Hopkins, C. R. (2012). ACS chemical neuroscience molecule spotlight on Suvorexant. *ACS Chem. Neurosci.* 3, 647–648. doi: 10.1021/cn300086a

Huang, Z. L., Qu, W. M., Li, W. D., Mochizuki, T., Eguchi, N., Watanabe, T., et al. (2001). Arousal effect of orexin A depends on activation of the histaminergic system. *Proc. Natl. Acad. Sci. U.S.A.* 98, 9965–9970. doi: 10.1073/pnas.181330998

Lee, M. G., Hassani, O. K., and Jones, B. E. (2005). Discharge of identified orexin/hypocretin neurons across the sleep-waking cycle. *J. Neurosci.* 25, 6716–6720. doi: 10.1523/JNEUROSCI.1887-05.2005

Matsuki, T., Nomiyama, M., Takahira, H., Hirashima, N., Kunita, S., Takahashi, S., et al. (2009). Selective loss of GABA(B) receptors in orexin-producing neurons results in disrupted sleep/wakefulness architecture. *Proc. Natl. Acad. Sci. U.S.A.* 106, 4459–4464. doi: 10.1073/pnas.0811126106

Mieda, M., Hasegawa, E., Kisanuki, Y. Y., Sinton, C. M., Yanagisawa, M., and Sakurai, T. (2011). Differential roles of orexin receptor-1 and -2 in the regulation of non-REM and REM sleep. *J. Neurosci.* 31, 6518–6526. doi: 10.1523/JNEUROSCI.6506-10.2011

Mieda, M., and Sakurai, T. (2013). Orexin (hypocretin) receptor agonists and antagonists for treatment of sleep disorders. Rationale for development and current status. *CNS Drugs* 27, 83–90. doi: 10.1007/s40263-012-0036-8

Mochizuki, T., Arrigoni, E., Marcus, J. N., Clark, E. L., Yamamoto, M., Honer, M., et al. (2011). Orexin receptor 2 expression in the posterior hypothalamus rescues sleepiness in narcoleptic mice. *Proc. Natl. Acad. Sci. U.S.A.* 108, 4471–4476. doi: 10.1073/pnas.1012456108

Morairty, S. R., Revel, F. G., Malherbe, P., Moreau, J. L., Valladao, D., Wettstein, J. G., et al. (2012). Dual hypocretin receptor antagonism is more effective for sleep promotion than antagonism of either receptor alone. *PloS ONE* 7:e39131. doi: 10.1371/journal.pone.0039131

Neubauer, D. N. (2010). Almorexant, a dual orexin receptor antagonist for the treatment of insomnia. *Curr. Opin. Investig. Drugs* 11, 101–110.

Sakurai, T., and Mieda, M. (2011). Connectomics of orexin-producing neurons: interface of systems of emotion, energy homeostasis and arousal. *Trends Pharmacol. Sci.* 32, 451–462. doi: 10.1016/j.tips.2011.03.007

Tsujino, N., Tsunematsu, T., Uchigashima, M., Konno, K., Yamanaka, A., Kobayashi, K., et al. (2013). Chronic alterations in monoaminergic cells in the locus coeruleus in orexin neuron-ablated narcoleptic mice. *PLoS ONE* 8:e70012. doi: 10.1371/journal.pone.0070012

Willie, J. T., Chemelli, R. M., Sinton, C. M., Tokita, S., Williams, S. C., Kisanuki, Y. Y., et al. (2003). Distinct narcolepsy syndromes in Orexin receptor-2 and Orexin null mice: molecular genetic dissection of Non-REM and REM sleep regulatory processes. *Neuron* 38, 715–730. doi: 10.1016/S0896-6273(03)00330-1

Willie, J. T., Chemelli, R. M., Sinton, C. M., and Yanagisawa, M. (2001). To eat or to sleep? Orexin in the regulation of feeding and wakefulness. *Annu. Rev. Neurosci.* 24, 429–458. doi: 10.1146/annurev.neuro.24.1.429

Winrow, C. J., Gotter, A. L., Cox, C. D., Tannenbaum, P. L., Garson, S. L., Doran, S. M., et al. (2012). Pharmacological characterization of MK-6096 - a dual orexin receptor antagonist for insomnia. *Neuropharmacology* 62, 978–987. doi: 10.1016/j.neuropharm.2011.10.003

Winrow, C. J., and Renger, J. J. (2013). Discovery and development of orexin receptor antagonists as therapeutics for insomnia. *Br. J. Pharmacol.* 171, 283–293. doi: 10.1111/bph.12261

Yamanaka, A., Tabuchi, S., Tsunematsu, T., Fukazawa, Y., and Tominaga, M. (2010). Orexin directly excites orexin neurons through orexin 2 receptor. *J. Neurosci.* 30, 12642–12652. doi: 10.1523/JNEUROSCI.2120-10.2010

Yamanaka, A., Tsujino, N., Funahashi, H., Honda, K., Guan, J. L., Wang, Q. P., et al. (2002). Orexins activate histaminergic neurons via the orexin 2 receptor. *Biochem. Biophys. Res. Commun.* 290, 1237–1245. doi: 10.1006/bbrc.2001.6318

Conflict of Interest Statement: The authors declare that the research was conducted in the absence of any commercial or financial relationships that could be construed as a potential conflict of interest.

19

Orexin, cardio-respiratory function, and hypertension

Aihua Li and Eugene Nattie*

Department of Physiology and Neurobiology, Geisel School of Medicine at Dartmouth, Lebanon, NH, USA

Edited by:
Michel A. Steiner, Actelion Pharmaceuticals Ltd., Switzerland

Reviewed by:
Renato Corradetti, University of Florence, Italy
Vincenzo Donadio, IRCCS Istituo delle Scienze Neurologiche di Bologna, Italy
Ling-Ling Hwang, Taipei Medical University, Taiwan

*Correspondence:
Aihua Li, Department of Physiology and Neurobiology, Geisel School of Medicine at Dartmouth 1 Medical Center Drive, Lebanon, NH 03756, USA
e-mail: aihua.li@dartmouth.edu

In this review we focus on the role of orexin in cardio-respiratory functions and its potential link to hypertension. (1) *Orexin, cardiovascular function, and hypertension.* In normal rats, central administration of orexin can induce significant increases in arterial blood pressure (ABP) and sympathetic nerve activity (SNA), which can be blocked by orexin receptor antagonists. In spontaneously hypertensive rats (SHRs), antagonizing orexin receptors can significantly lower blood pressure under anesthetized or conscious conditions. (2) *Orexin, respiratory function, and central chemoreception.* The prepro-orexin knockout mouse has a significantly attenuated ventilatory CO_2 chemoreflex, and in normal rats, central application of orexin stimulates breathing while blocking orexin receptors decreases the ventilatory CO_2 chemoreflex. Interestingly, SHRs have a significantly increased ventilatory CO_2 chemoreflex relative to normotensive WKY rats and blocking both orexin receptors can normalize this exaggerated response. (3) *Orexin, central chemoreception, and hypertension.* SHRs have higher ABP and SNA along with an enhanced ventilatory CO_2 chemoreflex. Treating SHRs by blocking both orexin receptors with oral administration of an antagonist, almorexant (Almxt), can normalize the CO_2 chemoreflex and significantly lower ABP and SNA. We interpret these results to suggest that the orexin system participates in the pathogenesis and maintenance of high blood pressure in SHRs, and the central chemoreflex may be a causal link to the increased SNA and ABP in SHRs. Modulation of the orexin system could be a potential target in treating some forms of hypertension.

Keywords: orexin and orexin receptors, cardiorespiratory function, hypertension, CO2 chemoreflex, blood pressure regulation

INTRODUCTION

Orexins, also known as hypocretins (Hcrt), are two excitatory neuropeptides, orexin A and orexin B (OX-A and OX-B) or hypocretin 1 and hypocretin 2 (Hcrt1 and Hcrt 2), produced by neurons primarily located in the lateral hypothalamic area (LHA) (De Lecea et al., 1998; Sakurai et al., 1998). Both OX-A and OX-B are derived from the same neuropeptide precursor, prepro-orexin (pp-OX or Hcrt gene). The actions of OX-A and OX-B are mediated by two G-protein coupled receptors, orexin receptor-1 (OX$_1$R/HcrtR1) and orexin receptor-2 (OX$_2$R/HcrtR2). Mounting evidence suggests that orexin is not only important to sleep-wake cycle and feeding regulation but also to respiratory and cardiovascular regulation. Furthermore, orexin may play role in some types of hypertension.

OREXIN AND OREXIN RECEPTORS

The anatomical and physiological properties of the orexin system have been reviewed extensively by many recent publications (Sakurai, 2007; Tsujino and Sakurai, 2009; De Lecea, 2012). In this review we focus only on orexin functions of most relevance to cardio-respiratory regulation.

OREXIN NEURONS

In the central nervous system (CNS), the cell bodies of orexin neurons are strictly located in the perifornical area and lateral and dorsal hypothalamic areas (Peyron et al., 1998; Date

et al., 1999; Nambu et al., 1999). Orexin neurons receive afferents from GABA, serotonin and catecholamine neurons, and interact in the LHA with neurons that produce melanin concentrating hormone (MCH) and with neurons that express the leptin receptor (LepR) (Bayer et al., 2005; Leinninger and Myers, 2008; Schone et al., 2011, 2012; Burdakov et al., 2013; Karnani et al., 2013). Serotonin (5-HT) hyperpolarizes orexin neurons through 5-HT$_1$A receptor mediated G-protein-coupled inward rectifier potassium channels (GIRK) in hypothalamic slices prepared from orexin neuron/enhanced green fluorescent protein (EGFP) transgenic mice (Muraki et al., 2004). The majority of orexin-immunoreactive (OX-ir) neurons in LHA are surrounded by dense tyrosine hydroxylase-immunoreactive (TH-ir) axons (Yamanaka et al., 2006), but results of studies on the role of catecholamines in orexin neurons are inconsistent. Bayer et al. showed that noradrenaline depolarized and excited orexin neurons (Bayer et al., 2005), while Yamanaka et al. reported that catecholamines directly and indirectly inhibited orexin neurons via α2-adrenoceptor mediated activation of GIRK channels (Yamanaka et al., 2006).

In the LHA, three major types of neurons OX, MCH, and LepRb expressing neurons are tightly intermingled and have a complex interactive relationship. An emerging hypothesis is that OX-MCH-LepR micro-circuits may act to regulate both autonomic function and energy balance (Leinninger and Myers, 2008; Hall et al., 2010; Leinninger, 2011; Burdakov et al., 2013). OX neurons are most active during wakefulness (Hassani et al., 2009), and activation of orexin receptors promotes wakefulness (De Lecea, 2010, 2012; Sakurai et al., 2010), feeding, and energy metabolism (Tsujino and Sakurai, 2009; Teske et al., 2010; Girault et al., 2012; Nixon et al., 2012), excites breathing, and stimulates sympathetic nerve activity (SNA) leading to an increase in blood pressure (Matsumura et al., 2001; Shirasaka et al., 2002; Zhang et al., 2005; Huang et al., 2010; Shahid et al., 2011, 2012; Nattie and Li, 2012). In contrast, MCH neurons are most active during sleep (Hassani et al., 2009), and MCH promotes sleep or physical inactivity (Nahon, 2006; Peyron et al., 2009; Konadhode et al., 2013; Monti et al., 2013), and regulates the autonomic nervous system. Central administration of MCH via chronic intracerebroventricular infusion (Messina and Overton, 2007) or acute injection into the nucleus of the solitary tract (NTS) (Brown et al., 2007) induces bradycardia and decreases blood pressure. Using a fluorescent-tag to identify LepRb positive neurons, Leinninger and Myers (2008); Leinninger (2011) demonstrated that in the LHA LepRb neurons do not co-express OX or MCH, but rather are co-distributed among the OX neurons (**Figure 1**). Both LepRb and OX neurons are surrounded by the MCH-containing neurons in the LHA (Leinninger and Myers, 2008; Leinninger, 2011). In addition, LHA LepRb neurons have direct synapses with OX neurons suggesting an important modulatory relationship between LepRb and OX neurons in LHA (Louis et al., 2010).

OREXIN PROJECTIONS AND OREXIN RECEPTORS

In contract to the very localized property of the OX neurons, OX axons are widely distributed throughout the CNS, with the exception of the cerebellum (Peyron et al., 1998; Date et al., 1999; Nambu et al., 1999). Based on *in situ* hybridization both OX_1R and OX_2R mRNAs are distributed extensively in the same regions that contain dense OX innervation (Trivedi et al., 1998; Marcus et al., 2001), e.g., the forebrain, the hypothalamus, the brainstem and the spinal cord. Both OX receptors and efferent projections are found in many sites involved in cardiovascular, respiratory and thermo regulation, e.g., the paraventricular nucleus (PVN), NTS, retrotrapezoid nucleus (RTN), locus coeruleus (LC), Kölliker-Fuse nucleus, rostral ventrolateral medulla (RVLM), medullary raphe,

lateral paragigantocellular nucleus, midbrain periaqueductal gray, A5 noradrenergic cell group, parabrachial region, area postrema, intermediolateral cell column of the spinal cord and sympathetic pre-ganglionic neurons (Peyron et al., 1998; Trivedi et al., 1998; Date et al., 1999; Nambu et al., 1999; Marcus et al., 2001). In the brainstem, networks of OX-ir fibers and terminals are expressed on the neurons of all major catecholamine cell groups [adrenaline (Adr): C1, C2, and C3 and noradrenaline (NA): locus coeruleus, A1, A2, A4, A5 and A7] (Puskas et al., 2010). Intracerebroventricular (icv) injection of orexin induces *c-fos* expression in the locus ceruleus, arcuate nucleus, central gray, raphe nuclei, NTS, supraoptic nucleus (SON), and PVN in Wistar rats (Date et al., 1999). The widespread nature and specific connections of the orexin system suggests that orexin may be involved not only in the regulation of the sleep-wake cycle and appetite but also autonomic functions, particularly cardiorespiratory functions. Orexin may act to link the regulation of cardiorespiratory functions to wakefulness and sleep.

SUMMARY OF OREXIN NEURONS AND RECEPTORS

Both orexin projections and orexin receptors are enriched in the neuronal sites that are importantly involved in cardio-respiratory regulation, and they are well positioned to participate in the regulation of cardio-respiratory functions.

THE ROLE OF OREXIN IN CARDIOVASCULAR FUNCTION
OREXIN, BLOOD PRESSURE, AND SYMPATHETIC NERVOUS SYSTEM

The sympathetic nervous system (SNS) plays a crucial role in the regulation of circulation and blood pressure (Guyenet, 2006; Fisher and Paton, 2011; Zubcevic et al., 2011), and many neuronal groups in the lateral hypothaluamus and brainstem are critically involved in such regulation. It is known, that *in vivo*, electrical or chemical stimulation of the perifornical nucleus of the hypothalamus increases blood pressure and heart rate (HR) and activates neurons of the lateral paragigantocellular area (Sun and Guyenet, 1986; Allen and Cechetto, 1992). Soon after orexin and orexin receptors were discovered in 1998, many studies started to examine if orexin in the LHA participation in the regulation of cardiovascular and sympathetic functions (Samson et al., 1999;

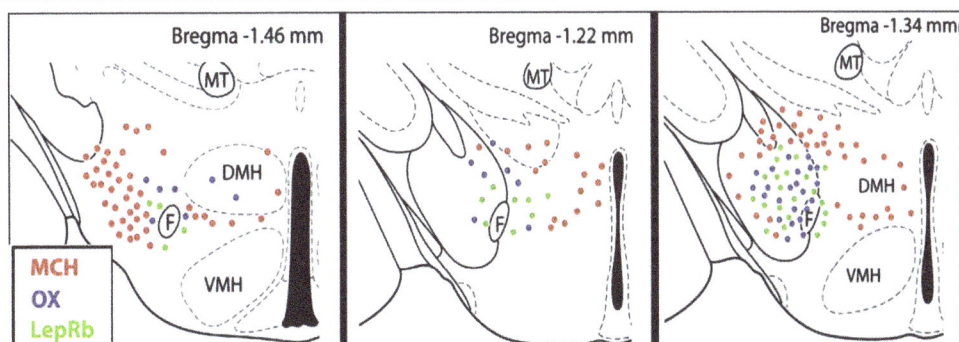

FIGURE 1 | Distribution of orexin (OX), melanin concentrating hormone (MCH) and leptin receptor (LepRb) -expressing neurons in the lateral hypothalamus (LHA). OX, MCH and LepRb-expressing neurons are intermingled in the LHA, but there is no co-expression. Red dots, MCH neurons; blue dots, OX neurons; green dots, LepRb neurons. F, Fornix; VMH, ventromedial hypothalamus; DMH, dorsomedial hypothalamus; MT, mammillothalamic tract (figure adapted with permission from Leinninger, 2011).

Shirasaka et al., 1999; Matsumura et al., 2001). *In vitro*, orexin in a dose-dependent manner, depolarizes neurons that are involved in the regulation of blood pressure and sympathetic nerve activity (SNA), e.g., neurons in the hypothalamic PVN and the RVLM (Shirasaka et al., 2001; Follwell and Ferguson, 2002; Huang et al., 2010), as well as spinal cord sympathetic preganglionic neurons (Antunes et al., 2001). In the RVLM both OX-A and OX-B depolarize neurons in a dose dependent manner, and at 100 nM, orexin excited ~42% of neurons in the area. Application of an OX_2R antagonist (TCS-OX2-29) significantly reduced the number of neurons activated by OX-A, while co-application of OX_1R and OX_2R antagonists completely eliminated orexin A-induced depolarization (**Figure 2**) (Huang et al., 2010). Furthermore, about 88% of adrenergic, 43% of noradrenergic, and 36–41% of rhythmically firing RVLM neurons can be excited by orexin in the RVLM (Huang et al., 2010).

Functional studies *in vivo* have demonstrated that orexin participates in blood pressure regulation. Transgenic orexin deficient animals, both prepro-orexin knockout (pp-OX KO) mice (**Figure 3**) and rats with orexin neurons-genetically ablated (orexin/ataxin-3), have lower resting blood pressure (Kayaba et al., 2003; Schwimmer et al., 2010) relative to their wild type controls. In both anesthetized and unanesthetized normotensive animals, central administration of OX-A or OX-B activates sympathetic activity and increases both arterial blood pressure (ABP) and HR (Samson et al., 1999; Shirasaka et al., 1999, 2002; Chen et al., 2000; Antunes et al., 2001; Matsumura et al., 2001; Machado et al., 2002; Shahid et al., 2011, 2012). In conscious rats and rabbits (Shirasaka et al., 1999; Matsumura et al., 2001; Samson et al., 2007) central administration (icv) of orexin increases ABP (Samson et al., 1999; Shirasaka et al., 1999; Matsumura et al., 2001), and SNA (Shirasaka et al., 1999; Matsumura et al.,

2001) in a dose dependent manner, and the increased ABP, HR and SNA induced by orexin is accompanied by an increase in plasma catecholamines (**Figure 4**) (Shirasaka et al., 1999; Matsumura et al., 2001). Intravenous injection of a ganglionic-blocking agent, pentolinium, can abolish OX-A induced increases in ABP and plasma epinephrine concentrations, which suggests that the pressor response induced by the icv injection of orexin-A can be attributed primarily to enhanced sympathetic outflow (Matsumura et al., 2001). Focal injection of OX-A into the RVLM can also induce a significant increase in ABP and HR in both anesthetized (Chen et al., 2000; Shahid et al., 2012) and conscious (Machado et al., 2002) rats. In anesthetized rats, the increased ABP is accompanied by increased splanchnic SNA(sSNA) and ventilation (phrenic nerve activity) that can be attenuated by blocking OX_1R (Shahid et al., 2012). The peak effects following OX-A injection into the RVLM were observed at a dose of 50 pmol with ~42 mmHg increase in ABP and 45% increase in SNA (Shahid et al., 2012).

Other studies also directly and indirectly support orexin's role in the regulation of blood pressure and SNA, e.g., intrathecal injection of OX-A elicits a dose-dependent increase in ABP, HR (Antunes et al., 2001; Shahid et al., 2011), and sSNA (Shahid et al., 2011), and the effects can be partially attenuated by either beta-adrenergic or alpha-adrenergic receptor antagonists (Antunes et al., 2001) or OX_1R antagonist (Shahid et al., 2011) in anesthetized rats. Microinjection of OX-A into the medullary raphe significantly increases ABP, HR, and body temperature in unanesthetized rats, (Luong and Carrive, 2012). It is well known that orexins are excitatory neuropeptides that also promote locomotion such as chewing and grooming (Shirasaka et al., 1999; Takakusaki et al., 2005; Thorpe and Kotz, 2005). To exclude the possible effects of increased locomotion on the changes in ABP,

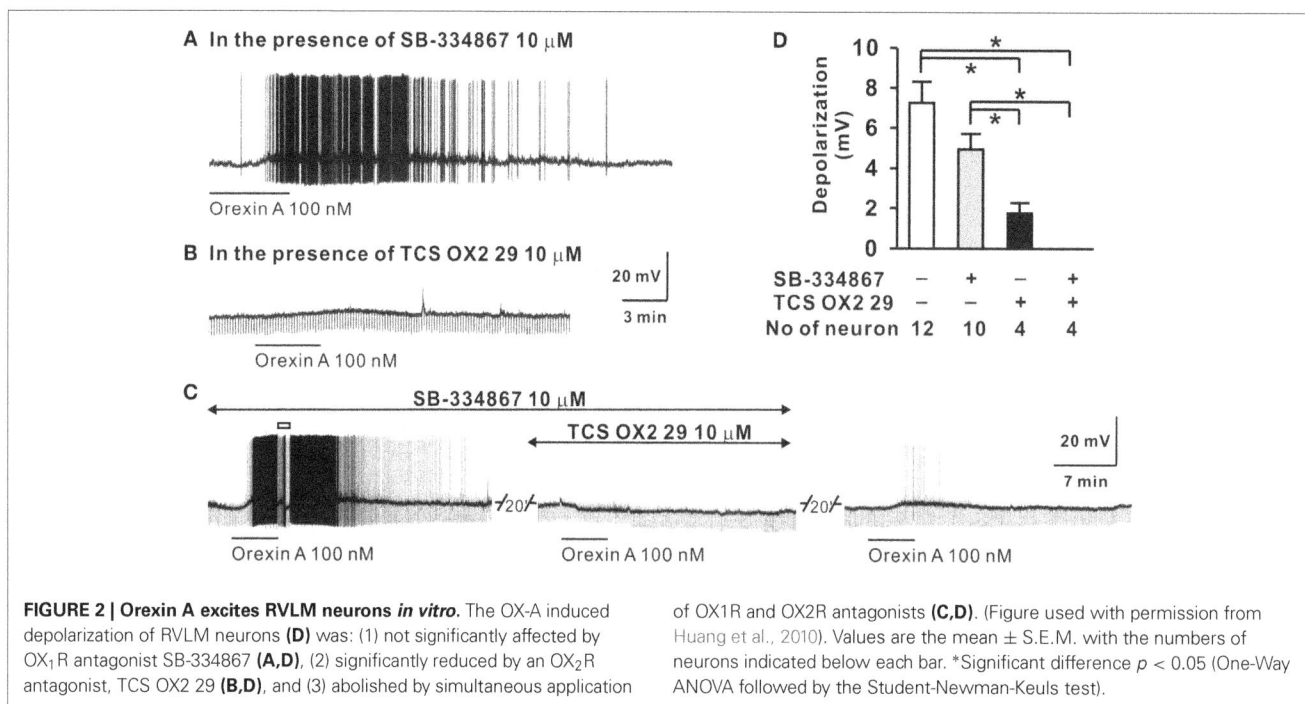

FIGURE 2 | Orexin A excites RVLM neurons *in vitro*. The OX-A induced depolarization of RVLM neurons **(D)** was: (1) not significantly affected by OX_1R antagonist SB-334867 **(A,D)**, (2) significantly reduced by an OX_2R antagonist, TCS OX2 29 **(B,D)**, and (3) abolished by simultaneous application of OX1R and OX2R antagonists **(C,D)**. (Figure used with permission from Huang et al., 2010). Values are the mean ± S.E.M. with the numbers of neurons indicated below each bar. *Significant difference $p < 0.05$ (One-Way ANOVA followed by the Student-Newman-Keuls test).

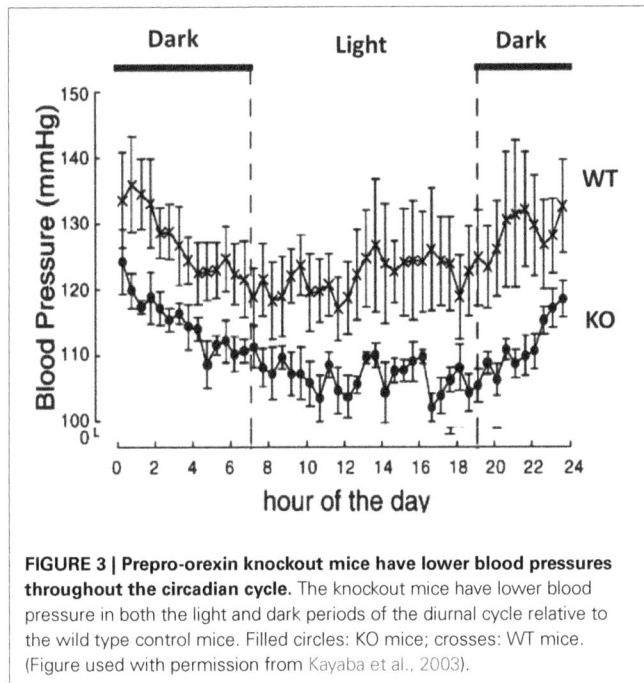

FIGURE 3 | Prepro-orexin knockout mice have lower blood pressures throughout the circadian cycle. The knockout mice have lower blood pressure in both the light and dark periods of the diurnal cycle relative to the wild type control mice. Filled circles: KO mice; crosses: WT mice. (Figure used with permission from Kayaba et al., 2003).

HR and SNA induced by the exogenous orexin in conscious rats, Shirasaka et al. injected OX-A icv in both anesthetized and conscious rats and tested them under the same experimental conditions. They found that OX-A induced a similar significant increase in ABP, HR and SNA in both anesthetized and conscious conditions in these rats (Shirasaka et al., 1999), which suggests that the sympathoexcitatory effects induced by exogenous orexin in the CSN are not due to the activation of locomotion.

Orexin is involved in the cardio-respiratory responses to acute stress, e.g., panic and fear (Kuwaki et al., 2008; Furlong et al., 2009; Iigaya et al., 2012; Johnson et al., 2012; Xiao et al., 2013). For example, in rats, silencing the hypothalamic pp-OX (Hcrt gene) with RNAi or antagonizing OX_1Rs can block blood pressure and HR responses to acute panic stress (Johnson et al., 2010). And antagonizing both orexin receptors can: (1) significantly reduce the "bicuculline" induced stress responses, e.g., hypertension, tachycardia, and renal sympathoexcitation (Iigaya et al., 2012); (2) decrease the fear induced pressor, tachycardic, and locomotor responses (Furlong et al., 2009); and (3) decrease the hypercapnic-induced respiratory chemoreflex without affecting resting breathing (Li and Nattie, 2010).

In summary, studies in normal animals have shown that the central orexin system participates in regulation of blood pressure, HR, and SNA. Activation of OXRs in the CNS, or only the area of RVLM, by exogenous orexin causes sympathetically mediated hypertension and tachycardia, which can be attenuated by OXR antagonists. Orexin is necessary for blood pressure, HR and SNA responses to certain stresses, e.g., panic and fear.

OREXIN AND HYPERTENSION

The observations that: (a) orexin participates in the regulation of cardiovascular homeostasis, (b) exogenous orexins can increase SNA and blood pressure in normal animals, and (c) transgenic orexin deficient animals have lower resting blood pressure, have led two independent groups to test the hypothesis that orexin may participate in the development of neurogenic hypertension in spontaneously hypertensive rats (SHRs) (Lee et al., 2013; Li et al., 2013a). The SHR is one of the most studied animal models of neurogenic hypertension. As in human essential hypertension, the blood pressure of the SHR rises with age, starting at about 6 weeks, accompanied by an overactive sympathetic nervous system (Smith and Hutchins, 1979; Zicha and Kunes, 1999; Simms et al., 2009). We found (Li et al., 2013a,b) in unanesthetized freely moving adult SHRs that: (1) there is a strong trend toward a significant increase in orexin-A mRNA expression in the RVLM (**Figure 5A**), a projection site for orexinergic LHA neurons; (2) blocking both orexin receptors by oral administration of an antagonist, Almxt: (a) significantly lowers blood pressure in wakefulness and sleep during both the dark and light periods of the diurnal cycle, (b) the largest average decrease of ABP after blocking orexin receptors was in wakefulness during the dark period (-37 mmHg) and the smallest average change in NREM sleep during the light period (-25 mmHg) relative to the pretreatment baseline, (c) one dose of Almxt produced a remarkable and long-lasting ($\sim$8 h) reduction of ABP in SHRs (**Figure 6**); (3) the anti-hypertensive effect was accompanied by: (a) a significantly decreased SNA assessed by power spectral analysis of systolic ABP, and (b) decreased noradrenaline levels in cerebrospinal fluid and plasma (**Figures 5B,C**); (4) antagonizing orexin receptors had no effect on resting blood pressure in normotensive WKY rats (**Figure 6B**). Our findings are supported by a recent publication (Lee et al., 2013), which showed that blocking OX_2R centrally by microinjection of an OX_2R antagonist, TCS-OX2-29, into either the cerebral ventricle (icv) or the RVLM in anesthetized SHRs significantly decreased blood pressure (**Figure 7**) (Lee et al., 2013). The significant decrease in ABP following TCS-OX2-29 was observed at 3, 10, and 30 nmol doses, and the maximum reduction of ABP was $\sim$21 or $\sim$30 mmHg at 30 nmol with icv or RVLM injection respectively. It is important to note that in both studies antagonism of orexin receptor(s) with either Almxt or TCS-OX2-29 had no significant effect on ABP in conscious or anesthetized normotensive Wistar- Kyoto (WKY) control rats.

There are data on cardiovascular effects of the orexin system obtained from transgenic animals and hypertensive animal models that directly and indirectly support an orexin link to hypertension. Two recent genetic analysis studies showed that orexin related genes are altered in both SHRs and mice (Schlager BPH/2J) (Marques et al., 2011a,b; Yamamoto et al., 2013). Like SHRs, the Schlager high blood pressure mouse (BPH/2J) is a genetic model of neurogenic hypertension. Using affymetrix GeneChip mouse gene arrays Marques et al. (2011b) identified many genes that are differentially expressed in the hypothalamus of the hypertensive mouse relative to the normotensive BPN/3J control mice. Among these altered genes, the pp-OX (Hcrt) gene, which encodes orexin/hypocretin, is significantly increased or upregulated in the hypothalamus in the hypertensive mice. BPH/2J hypertensive mice also exhibit a larger variation in ABP between the active and inactive periods of the day relative to the normotensive BPN/3J mice, and GeneChip mouse gene arrays showed

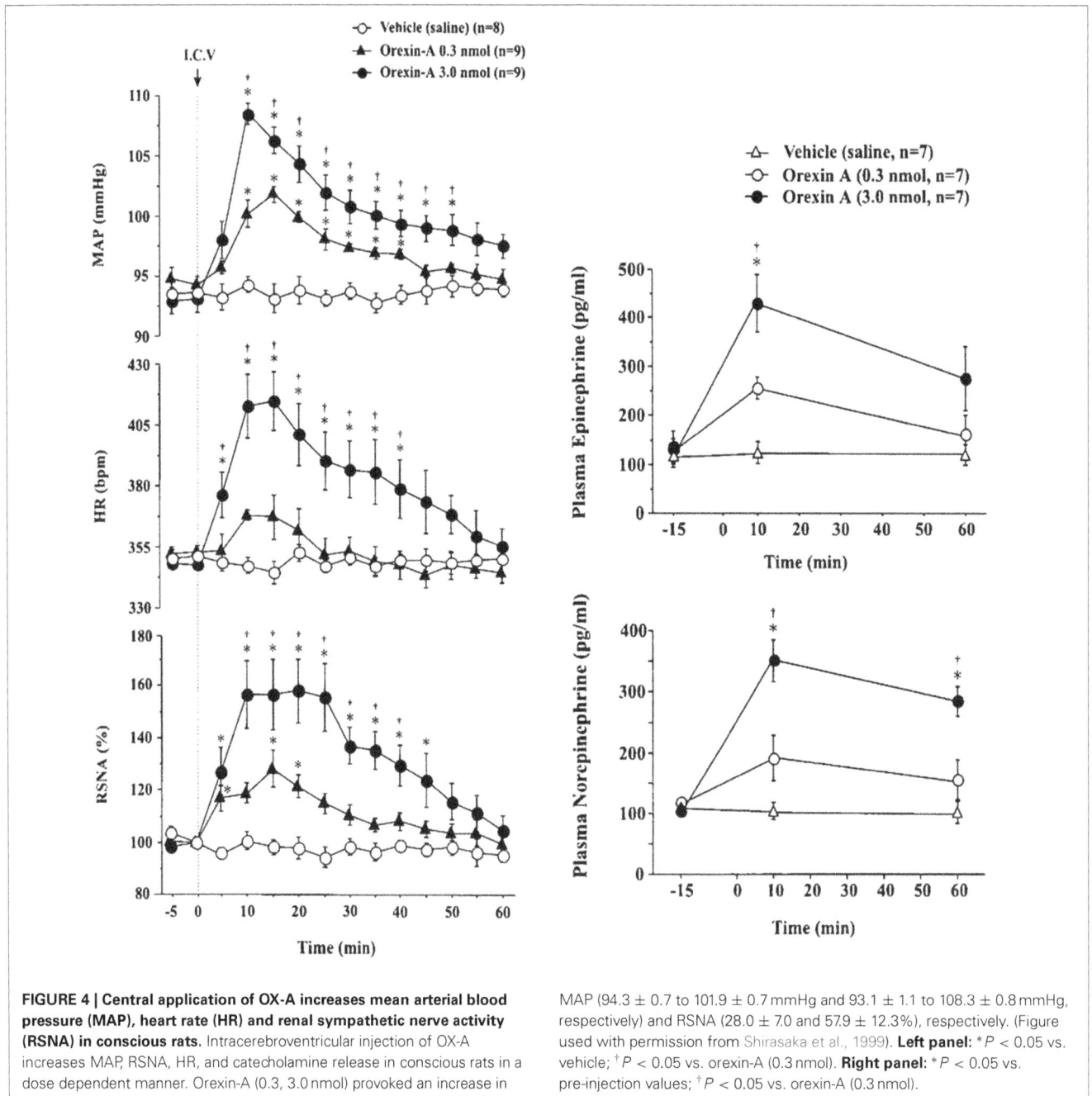

FIGURE 4 | Central application of OX-A increases mean arterial blood pressure (MAP), heart rate (HR) and renal sympathetic nerve activity (RSNA) in conscious rats. Intracerebroventricular injection of OX-A increases MAP, RSNA, HR, and catecholamine release in conscious rats in a dose dependent manner. Orexin-A (0.3, 3.0 nmol) provoked an increase in MAP (94.3 ± 0.7 to 101.9 ± 0.7 mmHg and 93.1 ± 1.1 to 108.3 ± 0.8 mmHg, respectively) and RSNA (28.0 ± 7.0 and 57.9 ± 12.3%), respectively. (Figure used with permission from Shirasaka et al., 1999). **Left panel:** *$P < 0.05$ vs. vehicle; †$P < 0.05$ vs. orexin-A (0.3 nmol). **Right panel:** *$P < 0.05$ vs. pre-injection values; †$P < 0.05$ vs. orexin-A (0.3 nmol).

that the pp-OX/Hcrt gene expression is higher during the active period when ABP is highest than in the inactive period when ABP is lowest in BPH/2J hypertensive mice, and is higher than that of in the normotensive control mice during the same period (Marques et al., 2011a). These genetic and functional studies in the neurogenic hypertensive animal models suggest that an up-regulated or overactive central orexin system may play an important role in developing and maintaining high blood pressure in neurogenic hypertension. It is also interesting to note that Yamamoto et al (Yamamoto et al., 2013) reported that the OX_1R (Hcrtr1) gene is down-regulated in the adrenal gland in SHR and stroke-prone SHR (SHRSP) relative to normotensive WKY

rats. This raises an interesting question of the role of peripheral orexin on cardiovascular function. As mentioned above, orexin neurons are exclusive located in the lateral hypothalamus and send projections to many brain locations. However orexins are found in many peripheral tissues, and the peripheral orexin distributions and functions have been discussed by recent reviews (Kukkonen et al., 2002; Spinazzi et al., 2006; Heinonen et al., 2008; Leonard and Kukkonen, 2013). Orexin receptors have been detected in various peripheral tissues, e.g., the gastrointestinal tract, pancreas, kidney, lung, adrenal gland, and adipose tissue (Kirchgessner and Liu, 1999; Lopez et al., 1999; Johren et al., 2001; Ouedraogo et al., 2003; Heinonen et al., 2008). In rat, both

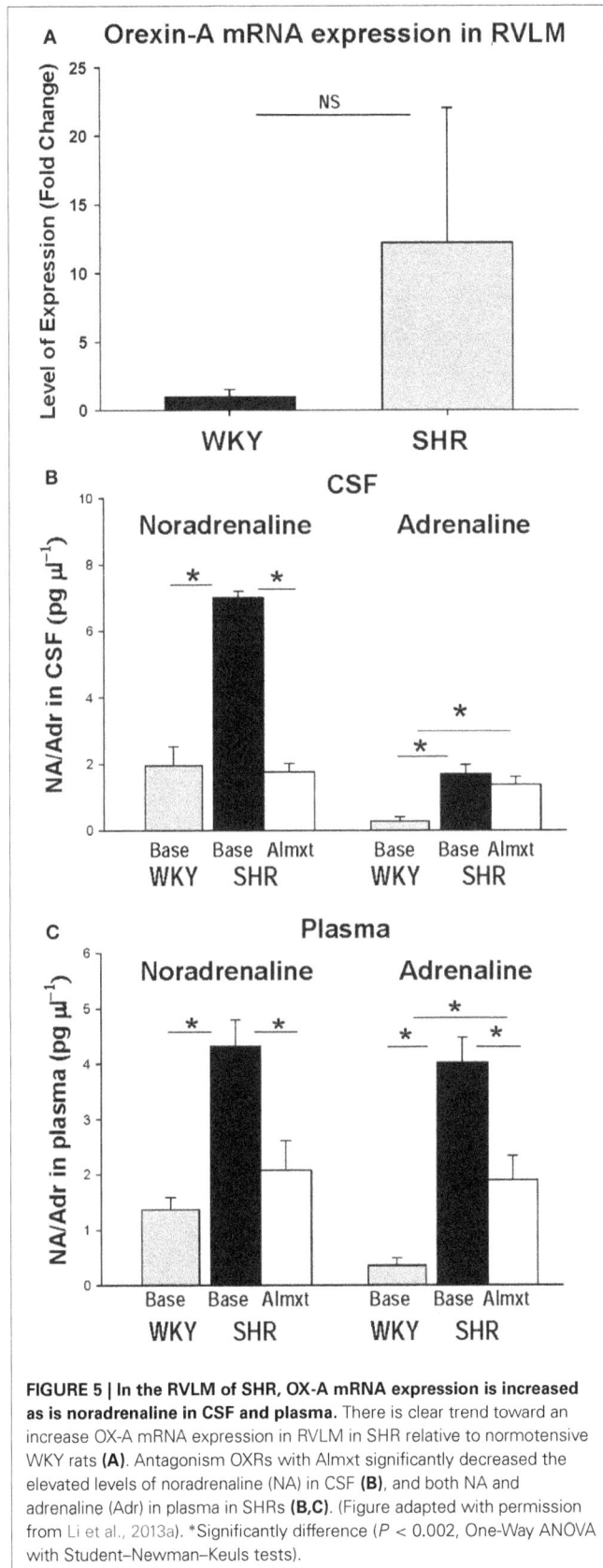

FIGURE 5 | In the RVLM of SHR, OX-A mRNA expression is increased as is noradrenaline in CSF and plasma. There is clear trend toward an increase OX-A mRNA expression in RVLM in SHR relative to normotensive WKY rats **(A)**. Antagonism OXRs with Almxt significantly decreased the elevated levels of noradrenaline (NA) in CSF **(B)**, and both NA and adrenaline (Adr) in plasma in SHRs **(B,C)**. (Figure adapted with permission from Li et al., 2013a). *Significantly difference ($P < 0.002$, One-Way ANOVA with Student–Newman–Keuls tests).

OX_1R and OX_2R mRNA can be detected in adrenal gland (Lopez et al., 1999; Johren et al., 2001), and the expression of OX_2R mRNA in the adrenal is about eight times higher in male than that of female rats (Johren et al., 2001, 2004). The adrenal gland is importantly involved in stress-related cardiovascular function via the hypothalamic-pituitary-adrenal axis, and the significance of a down-regulated Hcrt1R gene in adrenal gland of SHRs needs to be further investigated.

Psychological stresses, e.g., anxiety, prolonged anger, mental stress, have long been considered as a contributing factor in developing hypertension (Zimmerman and Frohlich, 1990; Boone, 1991; Markovitz et al., 1993), and as discussed above orexin is involved in cardiovascular and respiratory responses to the acute stresses, e.g., panic, fear, drug or foot-shock induced, in animal models. Xiao et al. recently investigated possible role of orexin on developing stress related hypertension in adult Sprague-Dawley (SD) rats (Xiao et al., 2013). A stress induced-hypertensive rat (SIHR) was generated by intermittent electric foot-shocks (75–150 V, 0.5 ms duration) every 2–30 s and a buzzer noises (88–98 dB) for 2 h twice daily for 14 consecutive days. Adult normotensive SD rats develop hypertension after day 6 under these conditions. Using tail-cuff method the authors found the systolic blood pressure at 2 h after stress rose from 110 mmHg at baseline to 142 mmHg at day 14 in these SIHRs, and the number of OX-A immunoreactive (OXA-ir) neurons in the LHA and the protein level of OX_1R in RVLM were significantly greater than that of the control rats. Microinjection of a selective OX_1R antagonist (SB-408124), or a selective OX_2R antagonist (TCS OX2 29) into RVLM can partially block the OX-A induced increased SBP and HR in SIHR (Xiao et al., 2013). It is interesting to note that, similar to the neurogenic hypertensive model SHRs, SIHRs also developed an overactive central orexin system. It would be interesting to see if blocking both OXRs by Almxt or a combination of OX_1R and OX_2R antagonists can decrease blood pressure between days 6 and 14 in these SIHRs and prevent the development of hypertension.

The potential peripheral effects of orexins on blood pressure and SNA have been investigated (Chen et al., 2000; Matsumura et al., 2001). Intravenous injection of OX-A or OX-B at a dose as high as 11 nmol/kg had no significant effect on ABP, HR or SNA in anesthetized rats and conscious rabbits, which suggests that the orexin effects on ABP, HR, and SNA are mediated primarily through the CNS (Chen et al., 2000; Matsumura et al., 2001). At the present time there is little evidence to support a role for peripheral orexins in the regulation of cardiovascular function (Heinonen et al., 2008; Kukkonen, 2013).

In summary: (1) Transgenic orexin deficient animals have a lower resting blood pressure. (2) Blocking OXRs significantly lowers blood pressure and SNA in adult SHRs. (3) PP-OX mRNA and gene expression are upregulated in the CNS in hypertensive rats and mice. Based on these findings we suggest that an overactive orexin system in the CNS may participate in the pathogenesis and maintenance of high blood pressure in certain forms of hypertension. Further, modulation of the orexin system could be a potential target in treating some forms of hypertension.

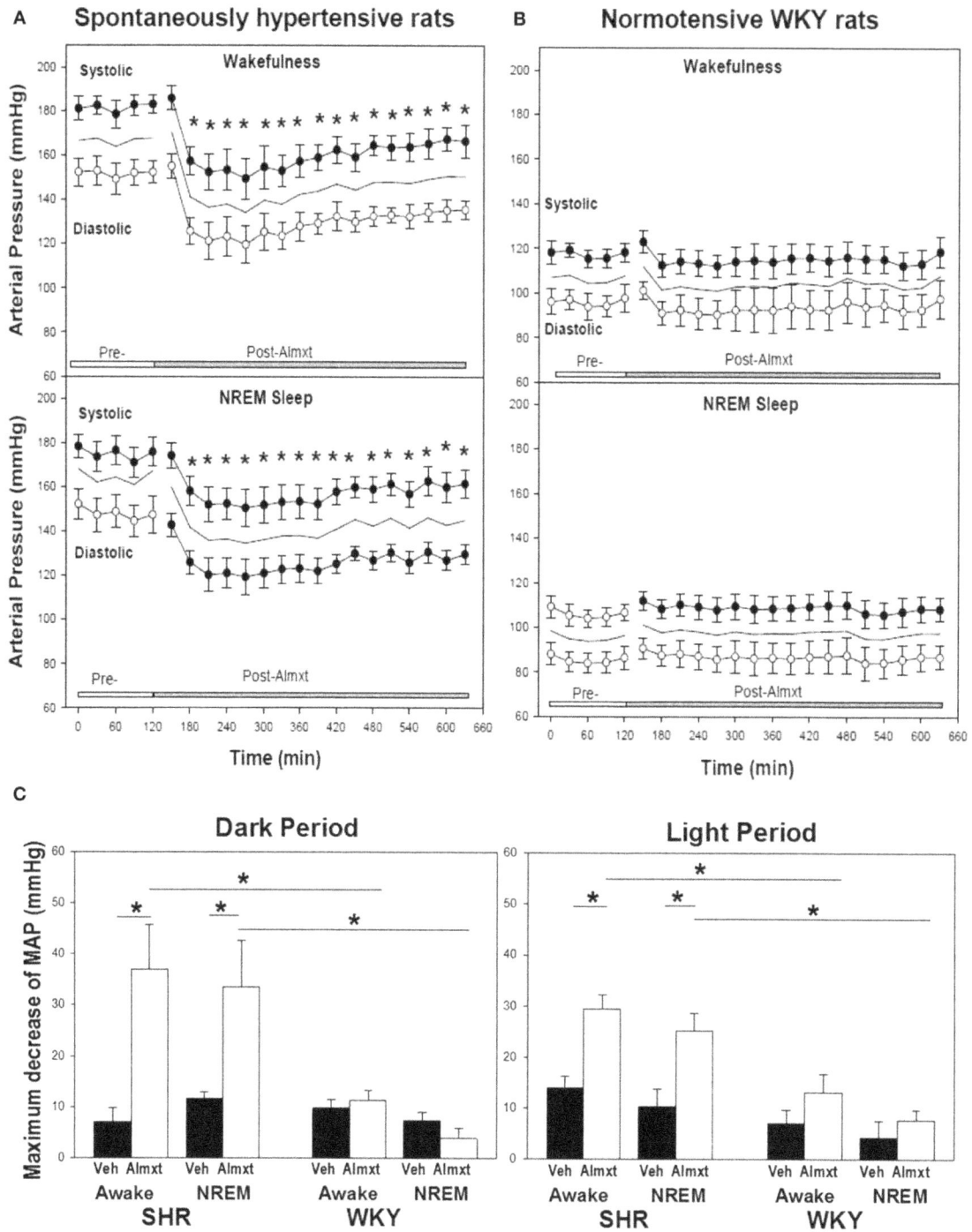

FIGURE 6 | In SHR, antagonism of OXRs with a systemic OXR antagonist, Almxt, decreases arterial pressure. One does of orally administered amlxt significantly decreased arterial pressure in SHR for ~8 h **(A)**, and Almxt had no effect on arterial pressure in normotensive WKY rats **(B)**. The largest decrease of BP after Almxt is in wakefulness during the dark period (−37 mmHg) and smallest change is in NREM sleep during the light period (−25 mmHg) relative to the pretreatment baseline **(C)**. *P < 0.02 (Figure adapted with permission from Li et al., 2013a).

SUMMARY OF THE ROLE OF OREXIN IN CARDIOVASCULAR FUNCTION

In normal animals, activation of OXRs by orexin in the CNS or in areas critically involved in SNA regulation, e.g., the RVLM and spinal cord, induces sympathetically mediated hypertension and tachycardia, which can be attenuated by OXR antagonists. Transgenic orexin deficient animals have a lower resting blood pressure. Spontaneously hypertensive rats and mice may have an overactive orexin system as (1) blocking OXRs produces

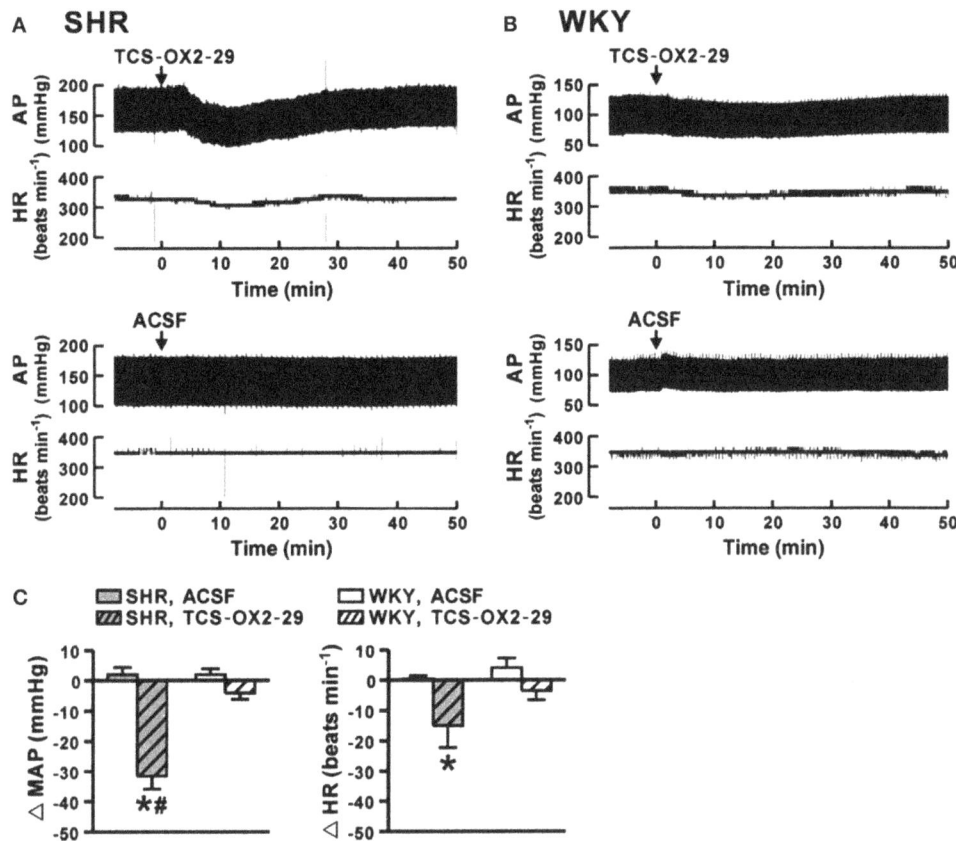

FIGURE 7 | In anesthetized SHR, antagonism of OX$_2$R in RVLM decreases arterial pressure. Microinjection of an OX$_2$R antagonist (TCS-OX2-29) into the RVLM significantly decreased mean AP and HR in anesthetized SHR **(A,C)**, and the maximum change of mean AP and HR being 30 mmHg and 20 bpm respectively (C, gray hatched bars). It is important to note that blocking OX$_2$R in RVLM in normotensive WKY rats had no effect on ABP and HR (B,C, white hatched bars). Control vehicle (ACSF) injection had no effect on AP and HR in SHR and WKY rats **(A,B,C)**. (Figure adapted with permission from Lee et al., 2013). *,#Significant difference ($p < 0.05$).

significant anti-hypertensive effects in SHRs, (2) the expression of OX-A mRNA in increased in RVLM in SHRs and (3) the pp-OX/Hcrt gene is upregulated in hypothalamus in hypertensive BPH/2J mice. Orexin is important in the regulation of SNA and blood pressure and an overactive orexin system may be pathologically linked to the development of neurogenic hypertension.

OREXIN AND RESPIRATION: THE CENTRAL CHEMOREFLEX AND BLOOD PRESSURE REGULATION
OREXIN, RESPIRATION, AND THE HYPERCAPNIC CHEMOREFLEX
Anatomically the orexin system is well positioned to be involved in the regulation of respiration and central chemoreception. Orexin neurons innervate many brainstem respiratory nuclei including the RTN, medullary raphe, LC, NTS, and pre-Bötzinger complex (Peyron et al., 1998; Date et al., 1999; Kukkonen et al., 2002; Young et al., 2005; Puskas et al., 2010; Lazarenko et al., 2011; Tupone et al., 2011; Nixon et al., 2012). Retrograde tracing studies showed that LHA OX-A positive neurons project to the diaphragm (Young et al., 2005; Badami et al., 2010) and raphe pallidus (Tupone et al., 2011). In Phox2b-eGFP transgenic mice, Lazarenko et al. further showed that the orexin-containing axonal varicosities are closely positioned relative to RTN Phox2b expressing neurons (Lazarenko et al., 2011). The expression of OX$_1$R and/or OX$_2$R mRNA is also found abundantly in many respiratory nuclei in the brainstem with a pattern matching that of OX-containing axon terminals (Marcus et al., 2001; Kukkonen et al., 2002).

At the cellular level, using *in vitro* patch-clamp recordings in visualized orexin neurons in brain slices, Williams et al., showed that the orexin neurons are intrinsically CO$_2$ (**Figure 8A**) and pH (**Figure 8B**) sensitive (Williams et al., 2007). The orexin neurons in LHA increase their firing rate during acidification and decrease their firing rate during alkalization (**Figure 8**), while non-orexin neurons are not responsive to such changes (**Figure 8C**) (Williams et al., 2007). These effects are mediated, at least in part, by the TASK-like tandem-pore K$^+$ channels (Williams et al., 2007), and possibly by other acid-sensing channels, e.g., ASICs (Song et al., 2012).

In addition to their intrinsic CO$_2$/pH sensitivity, orexin neurons also modulate the activity of brainstem chemosensitive neurons such as those in medullary raphe nuclei and RTN (Dias et al., 2010; Lazarenko et al., 2011; Tupone et al., 2011; Nattie and Li, 2012). Electrophysiological studies in slices from neonatal (P6-P10) Phox2b-eGFP transgenic mice showed that orexin A excites the acid sensitive eGFP/Phox2b-expressing RTN neurons in a dose dependent manner (ED50 ~250 nM, **Figure 9**), and these

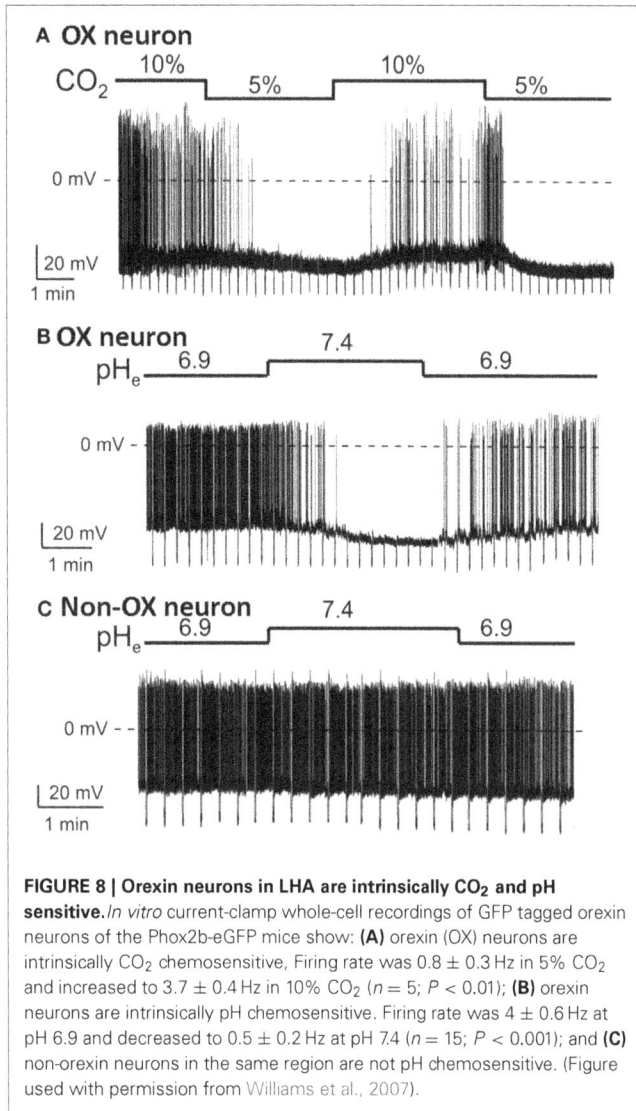

FIGURE 8 | Orexin neurons in LHA are intrinsically CO$_2$ and pH sensitive. *In vitro* current-clamp whole-cell recordings of GFP tagged orexin neurons of the Phox2b-eGFP mice show: **(A)** orexin (OX) neurons are intrinsically CO$_2$ chemosensitive, Firing rate was 0.8 ± 0.3 Hz in 5% CO$_2$ and increased to 3.7 ± 0.4 Hz in 10% CO$_2$ ($n = 5$; $P < 0.01$); **(B)** orexin neurons are intrinsically pH chemosensitive. Firing rate was 4 ± 0.6 Hz at pH 6.9 and decreased to 0.5 ± 0.2 Hz at pH 7.4 ($n = 15$; $P < 0.001$); and **(C)** non-orexin neurons in the same region are not pH chemosensitive. (Figure used with permission from Williams et al., 2007).

neurons increased activity upon bath acidification, decreased firing with alkalization, and exhibited an $\sim$5 Hz dynamic range of response between pH 7.0 and 7.5 (**Figures 9A,B**) (Lazarenko et al., 2011). Functional studies have shown that the orexin system participates in the regulation of respiration and the CO$_2$ central chemoreflex (Dutschmann et al., 2007; Nakamura et al., 2007; Williams et al., 2007; Dias et al., 2009, 2010; Li and Nattie, 2010; Lazarenko et al., 2011). Microinjection of orexin into the RVLM at the level of the pre-Bötzinger complex causes a significant increase in amplitude of integrated phrenic nerve activity (an index of tidal volume) in anesthetized and vagotomized rats (Young et al., 2005; Shahid et al., 2012). Injection of OX-B into the Kölliker–Fuse nucleus significantly increases breathing frequency in P21–42 day rats using the intra-arterially perfused working heart-brainstem preparation (Dutschmann et al., 2007). In the decerebrate cat, OX-A application into the hypoglossal motor nucleus increases genioglossus muscle activity (Peever et al., 2003). The pp-OX knockout mouse with a complete lack of orexin has normal resting breathing but a significantly attenuated respiratory chemoreflex in wakefulness compare to the wide type control mice and supplementation of orexins can partially restore the reflex (Deng et al., 2007; Nakamura et al., 2007). Unilateral administration of an OX$_1$R antagonist (SB334867) in the RTN significantly reduced the respiratory response to hypercapnia (7%CO$_2$) with a substantial effect in wakefulness (-30%; **Figure 10A**) and a much smaller effect in sleep (-9%) (Dias et al., 2009). In the medullary raphe, inhibition of the OX$_1$R produced a significant reduction of the CO$_2$ chemoreflex in wakefulness (-16%; **Figure 10B**) but not in sleep (Dias et al., 2010). Antagonism both OX$_1$R and OX$_2$R by orally administrating a dual OXR antagonist, Almxt, significantly decreased the hypercapnic chemoreflex only in wakefulness during the dark period of diurnal cycle (-31%); the CO$_2$ chemoreflex was not significantly changed in sleep in the dark period and wakefulness and sleep in the light period of the diurnal cycles (**Figure 11**) (Li and Nattie, 2010). Antagonism of orexin receptors had no effect on resting breathing (Dias et al., 2009, 2010; Li and Nattie, 2010).

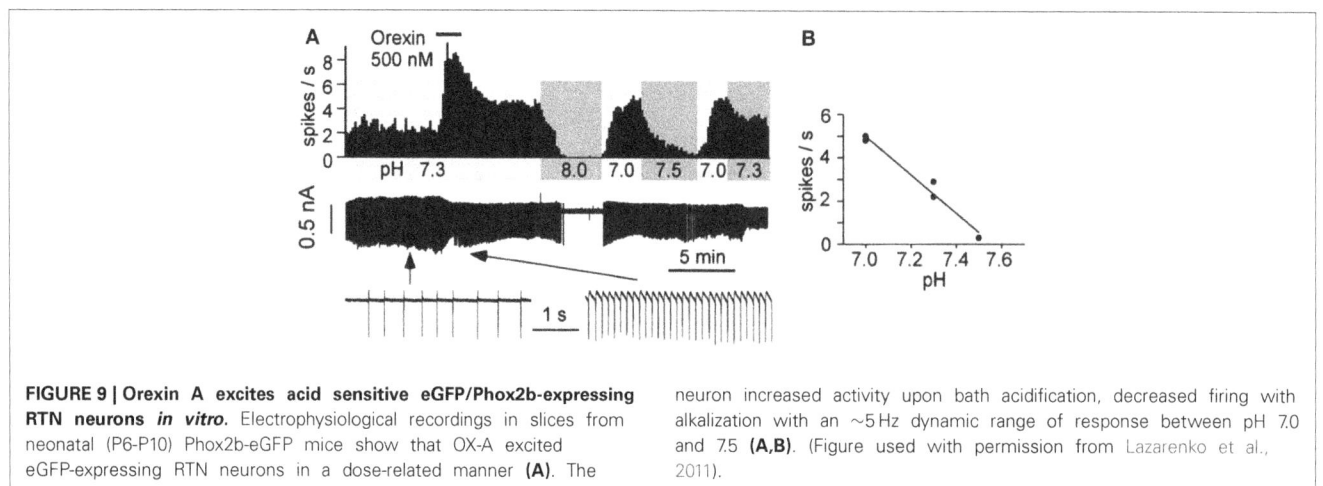

FIGURE 9 | Orexin A excites acid sensitive eGFP/Phox2b-expressing RTN neurons *in vitro*. Electrophysiological recordings in slices from neonatal (P6-P10) Phox2b-eGFP mice show that OX-A excited eGFP-expressing RTN neurons in a dose-related manner **(A)**. The neuron increased activity upon bath acidification, decreased firing with alkalization with an $\sim$5 Hz dynamic range of response between pH 7.0 and 7.5 **(A,B)**. (Figure used with permission from Lazarenko et al., 2011).

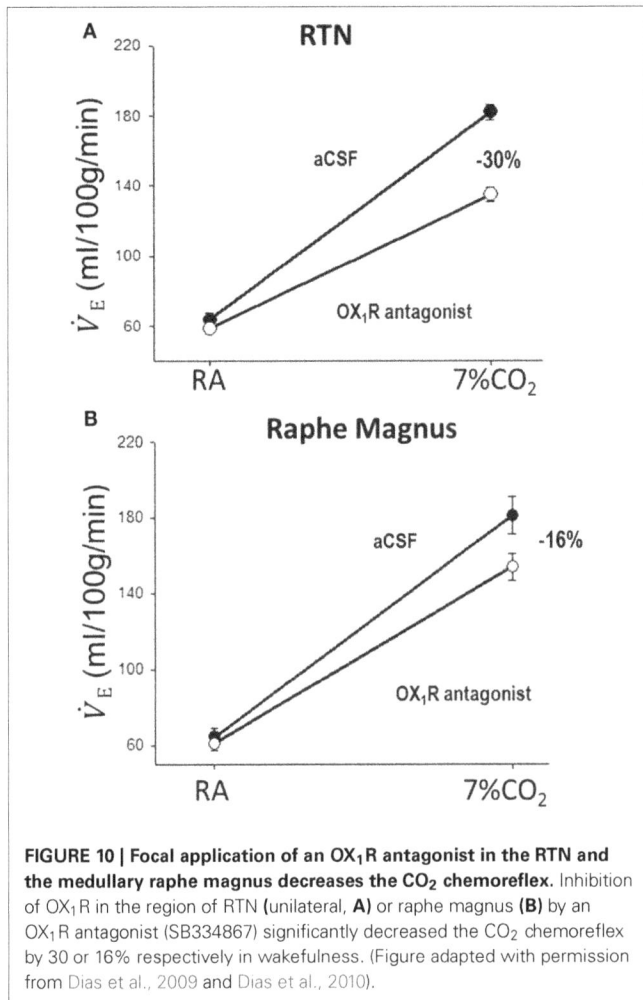

FIGURE 10 | Focal application of an OX_1R antagonist in the RTN and the medullary raphe magnus decreases the CO_2 chemoreflex. Inhibition of OX_1R in the region of RTN (unilateral, A) or raphe magnus (B) by an OX_1R antagonist (SB334867) significantly decreased the CO_2 chemoreflex by 30 or 16% respectively in wakefulness. (Figure adapted with permission from Dias et al., 2009 and Dias et al., 2010).

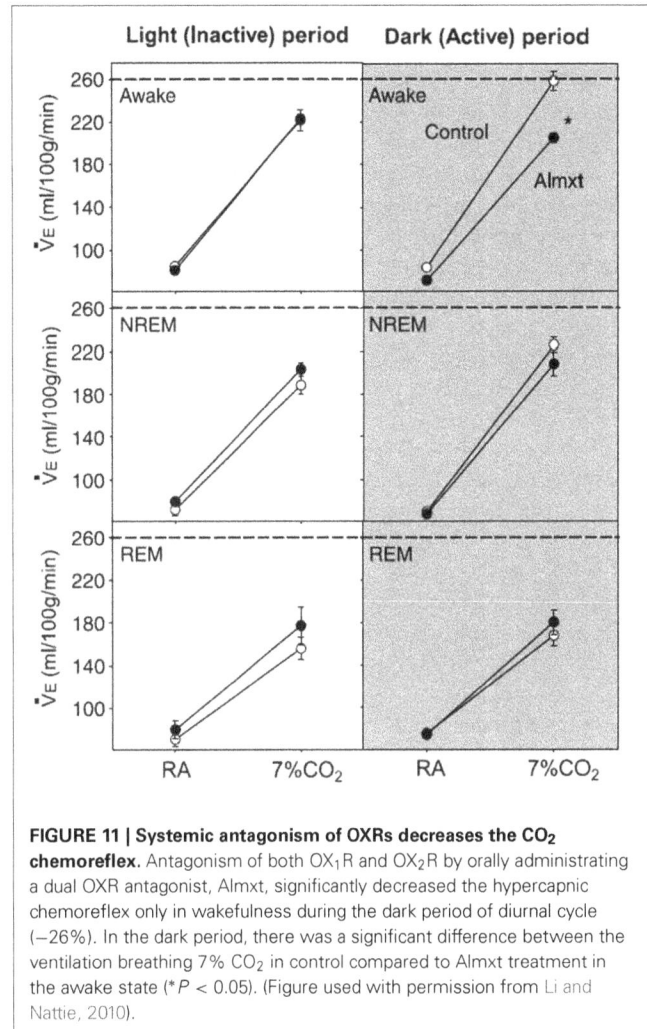

FIGURE 11 | Systemic antagonism of OXRs decreases the CO_2 chemoreflex. Antagonism of both OX_1R and OX_2R by orally administrating a dual OXR antagonist, Almxt, significantly decreased the hypercapnic chemoreflex only in wakefulness during the dark period of diurnal cycle (−26%). In the dark period, there was a significant difference between the ventilation breathing 7% CO_2 in control compared to Almxt treatment in the awake state (*$P < 0.05$). (Figure used with permission from Li and Nattie, 2010).

These *in vitro* and *in vivo* experiments demonstrate that the orexin system is significantly involved in the control of breathing, particularly in the central CO_2 chemoreflex.

In summary: (1) Orexin neurons are intrinsically chemosensitive and send projections to other central chemoreceptor sites, e.g., the RTN and medullary raphe. (2) Orexin may regulate breathing and central chemoreception directly and/or indirectly by recruiting other brainstem chemoreceptor sites, e.g., the RTN and medullary raphe. (3) Orexin modulation of the CO_2 chemoreflex may be vigilance state dependent with the strongest effect being during wakefulness in the dark period. (4) Orexin may be a link between breathing and sleep-wake status.

RESPIRATION AND CENTRAL CHEMORECEPTION IN BLOOD PRESSURE REGULATION

Respiration, sympathetic activity, and blood pressure

Anatomically, many cardiovascular and respiratory related nuclei are closely intertwined within similar regions of the brain, or are even synaptically connected. Many of these nuclei are part of the respiratory-sympathetic network that is critical to the regulation of respiratory and sympathetic activity and blood pressure (Rosin et al., 2006; Zoccal et al., 2009a; Geerling et al., 2010; Guyenet et al., 2010). For example, in the brainstem, both the

RVLM and the caudal ventrolateral medulla (CVLM), sites critically involved in the regulation of sympathetic tone, overlap with the ventral respiratory column including Bötzinger and pre-Bötzinger neurons. The neurons in the RTN, a putative central chemoreceptor site, innervate the entire ventrolateral medulla including the ventral respiratory column (VRC) and areas critically involved in the ABP and SNA regulation, e.g., the RVLM and CVLM (Rosin et al., 2006). The hypothalamic PVN, an important site for autonomic and endocrine homeostasis, is anatomically connected with many putative central chemoreceptors sites, e.g., the RTN, LC, NTS and medullary raphe (Geerling et al., 2010). The sympathetic preganglionic neurons (SPGNs) in the spinal cord receive prominent innervation from spinal interneurons, the RVLM, the midline medulla oblongata including medullary raphe serotonergic neurons, the pontine A5 noradrenergic cell group, the dorsolateral pons, the hypothalamic PVN, and the orexinergic neurons in the LHA (Jansen et al., 1995). The complex anatomical connections between the respiratory sites, central chemoreceptor sites and cardiovascular regulation sites suggest that the central respiratory chemoreflex is positioned to participate in the regulation or modulation of sympathetic activity and blood pressure.

Central chemoreception, SNA and blood pressure

Activation of central chemoreceptors by CO_2/H^+ increases ABP and SNA in both humans and experimental animals (Hanna et al., 1981; Lioy and Trzebski, 1984; Somers et al., 1989; Nattie et al., 1992, 1993; Oikawa et al., 2005; Guyenet et al., 2010). In humans, hyperoxic hypercapnia ($7\%CO_2/93\%O_2$) induced greater increases in ventilation ($\dot{V}_E$), blood pressure and SNA than did hypoxia ($10\%O_2/93\%N_2$) (Somers et al., 1989). In conscious rats (**Figure 12**), Oikawa et al. (2005) showed that hypercapnia induced significant increases in mean ABP, RSNA, and the respiratory rate (**Figure 12B**) in intact animals and in animals with varied peripheral chemoreceptor input, e.g., carotid body destroyed (CBD), aortic nerve denervated (AD), carotid body destroyed plus aortic denervated (CBAD), and sinoaortic denervated (SAD) (**Figure 12C**). There were also no significant differences in the magnitudes of increase in ABP and RSNA during hypercapnia between the intact and the chemo-denervated groups (**Figure 12**). The fact that the increased ABP and rSNA response to hypercapnia was not affected by bilateral carotid chemo-denervation, aortic denervation, or sinoaortic-denervation suggests that the peripheral chemoreceptors do not play a major role in the cardiovascular response to hypercapnia in normal conscious rats (Oikawa et al., 2005). Blockade of glutamate receptors in the RTN or lesion of the rostral part of the RVLM decreased respiratory (phrenic nerve activity, PNA) and SNA responses to hypercapnic stimulation in decerebrate, paralyzed, vagotomized, and servo-ventilated cats (Nattie et al., 1992, 1993).

In summary: (1) Many putative central chemoreceptors sites, e.g., the RTN, NTS and medullary raphe, are involved in the regulation of SNA and blood pressure. (2) Activation of central chemoreceptors by hypercapnia significantly increases blood pressure, SNA and respiration with and without peripheral chemoreceptors. These studies suggest that the hypercapnic induced increase in ABP is due to sympatho-excitation via activation of the central chemoreceptors. The central chemoreceptors directly or indirectly regulate sympathetic vasomotor tone and blood pressure, and can activate the sympathetic outflow in a tonic manner independent of the effects on the central respiratory pattern generator (Moreira et al., 2006; Guyenet et al., 2010).

SUMMARY OF OREXIN AND RESPIRATION: THE CENTRAL CHEMOREFLEX AND BLOOD PRESSURE REGULATION

Orexin neurons are intrinsically chemosensitive and their projections and receptors are found densely in all the major respiratory neuronal groups and central chemoreceptor sites. Activation of central chemoreceptors with and without activation of peripheral chemoreceptors leads to significant sympathoexcitation and hypertension in both human and experimental animals. Respiration and the central chemoreflex are involved in regulation of SNA and blood pressure.

OREXIN, CHEMOREFLEX, AND HYPERTENSION

Overactive vasoconstrictor sympathetic tone, an enhanced peripheral chemoreflex, and an impaired baroreflex have been found in a significant portion of patients with primary hypertensive as well as in SHRs (Izdebska et al., 1982; Simms et al., 2009; Tan et al., 2010). In susceptible individuals, stress or altered physiology initiates increases in sympathetic activity to cardiovascular resistance vessels accompanied by increases in blood pressure. Over time, vascular smooth muscle in resistance vessels hypertrophies resulting in persistent hypertension. The SHR is one of the most used animal models of neurogenic hypertension and SHRs develop hypertension at about 6 weeks of life. Using the working heart–brainstem preparation, Simms et al., showed that the respiratory related sympathetic tone is significantly higher in SHRs relative to normotensive WKY rats starting from postnatal day 9–16, well before the onset of hypertension (Simms et al., 2009). They suggest that this augmented respiratory-sympathetic coupling in SHR and its effect on the vascular tone in early life is a causal factor in developing hypertension (Simms et al., 2009, 2010). However, the mechanisms leading to such changes remain unclear at present time.

PERIPHERAL CHEMOREFLEX AND HYPERTENSION

A link between neurogenic hypertension and an enhanced carotid body chemoreflex has been more extensively studied in patients and in animal models of sleep apnea (Fletcher et al., 1992; Lesske et al., 1997; Fletcher, 2001; Prabhakar et al., 2001, 2005, 2012; Schultz et al., 2007; Simms et al., 2010; Zoccal and Machado, 2011; Costa-Silva et al., 2012; Moraes et al., 2012a,b; Paton et al., 2013). The peripheral chemoreceptor reflex response has been shown to be significantly enhanced in patients with primary hypertension (Trzebski et al., 1982; Tafil-Klawe et al., 1985a,b; Somers et al., 1988a,b; Sinski et al., 2012) and in animal models of systemic hypertension, e.g., SHRs (Fukuda et al., 1987; Simms et al., 2009; Tan et al., 2010). Rats exposed to chronic intermittent hypoxia (CIH) develop hypertension and persistent sympathetic activation, and elimination of the carotid bodies prevents such CIH-induced hypertension (Fletcher et al., 1992; Lesske et al., 1997). Enhanced carotid body activity has been suggested to result in alterations in respiratory–sympathetic coupling (Simms et al., 2009; Zoccal et al., 2009b) and increased muscle vasoconstrictor activity, which may contribute to the development of hypertension (Trzebski et al., 1982; Somers et al., 1988a). The hyperactive carotid chemoreceptors are accompanied by overexpression of ASIC/TASK (acid-sensing ion channel/2-pore domain acid-sensing K^+ channel) channels in young pre-hypertensive SHRs (Tan et al., 2010). Abdala et al., further showed that bilateral denervation of the carotid sinus nerves (CSD) in SHRs can significantly lower the resting blood pressure ($\sim$25 mmHg), respiratory frequency (transiently) and the low frequency component of the frequency analysis of systolic blood pressure, an index of sympathetic vasomotor tone (**Figure 13**), and they suggested that the inputs of carotid sinus nerve from the carotid body are partially responsible for increased SNA and blood pressure in SHR (Abdala et al., 2012).

In summary: an enhanced peripheral chemoreceptor reflex is found in both human hypertension and SHRs, and bilateral denervation of the carotid sinus nerves can partially lower blood pressure in SHRs. It is suggested that this enhanced carotid body activity may contribute to the alterations in respiratory–sympathetic coupling in SHRs.

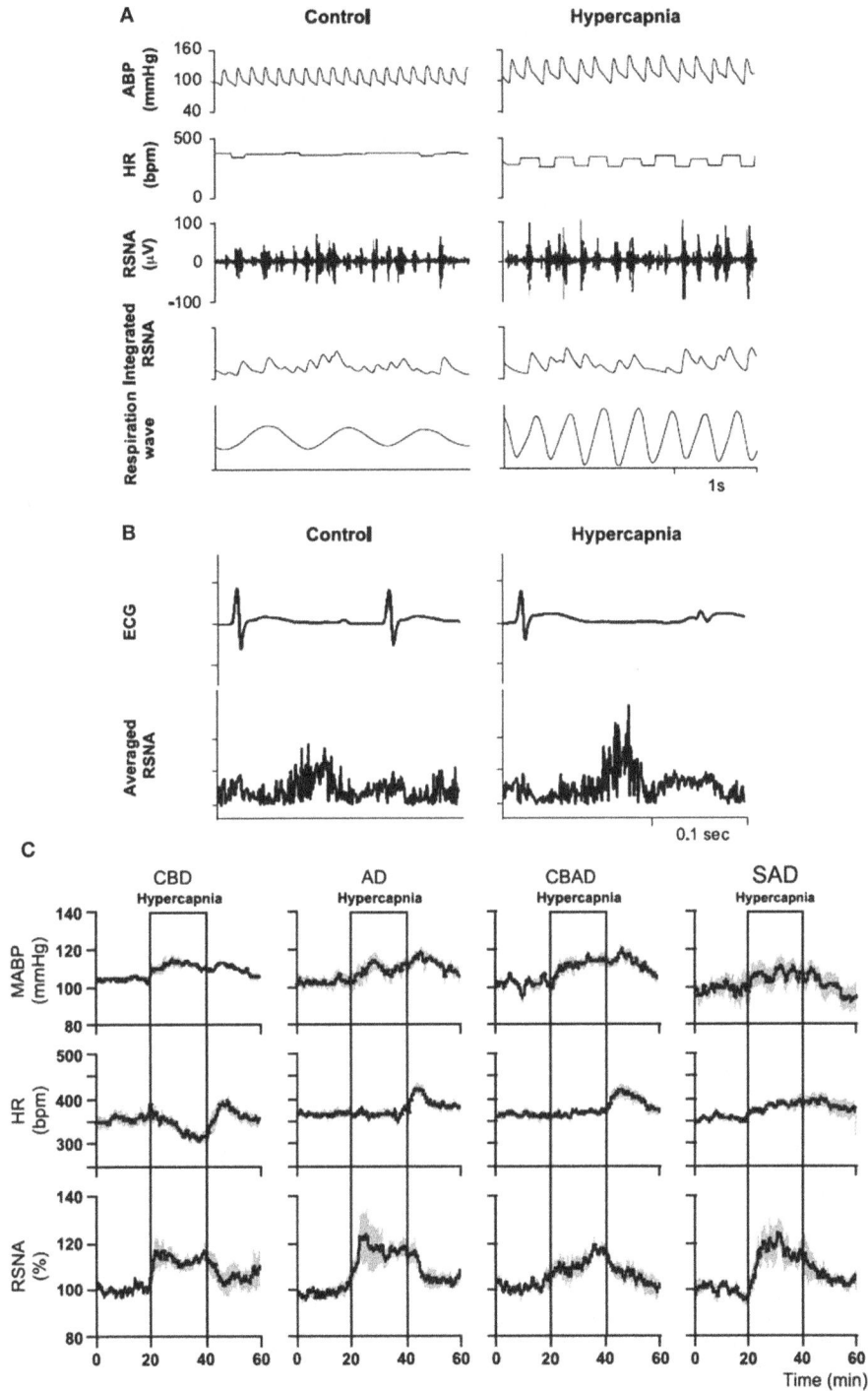

FIGURE 12 | In conscious rats, hypercapnia increases arterial blood pressure (ABP) and renal sympathetic nerve activity (RSNA). Hypercapnia increased mean ABP [from 105 to 117 mm Hg; **(A)**], RSNA [from 100 to 115%, **(A,B)**], and the respiratory rate [from 63 to 151 breaths/min; **(A)**], but decreased HR [from 374 to 302 beats/min; **(A,B)**]. Hypercapnia significantly increased mean ABP and RSNA in intact **(A)**, carotid body destroyed (CBD), aortic nerve denervated (AD), carotid body destroyed and aortic denervated (CBAD), and sinoaortic denervated (SAD) rats **(C)**. There were also no significant differences in the magnitudes of increase in ABP and RSNA during hypercapnia between the intact and the three chemo-denervated groups. (Figure adapted with permission from Oikawa et al., 2005).

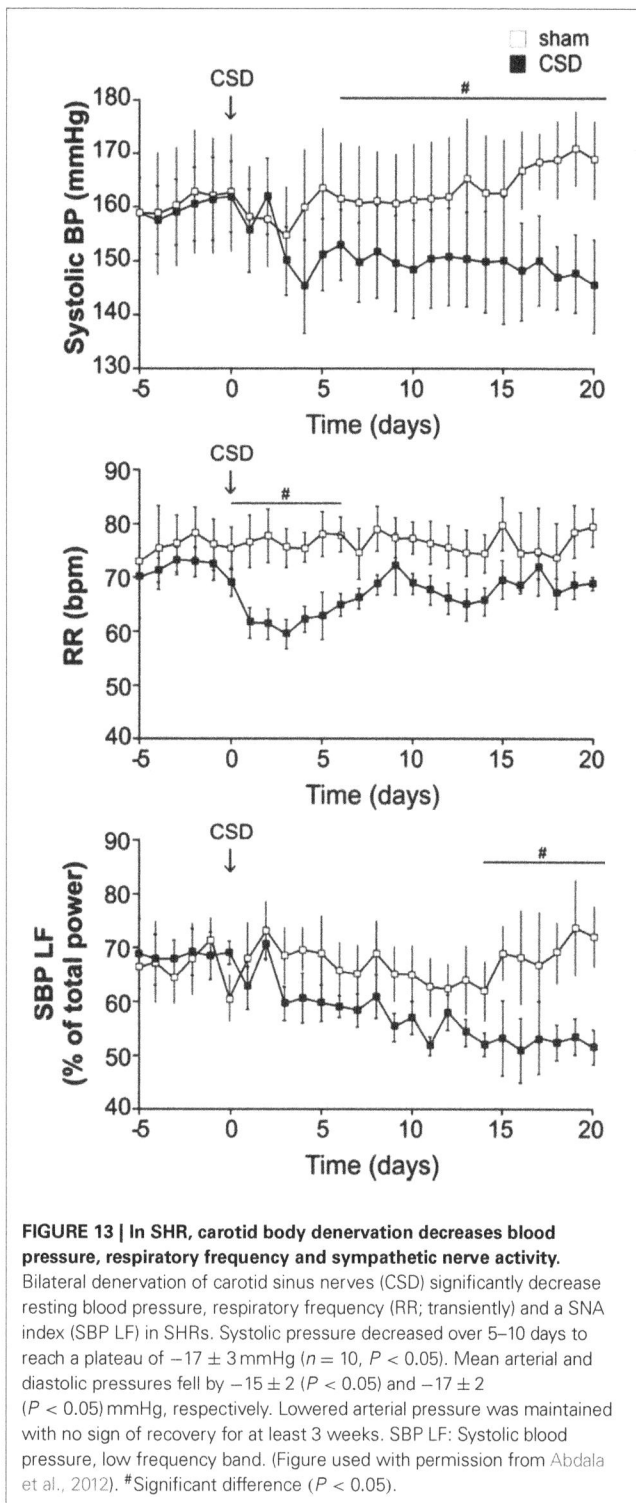

FIGURE 13 | In SHR, carotid body denervation decreases blood pressure, respiratory frequency and sympathetic nerve activity.
Bilateral denervation of carotid sinus nerves (CSD) significantly decrease resting blood pressure, respiratory frequency (RR; transiently) and a SNA index (SBP LF) in SHRs. Systolic pressure decreased over 5–10 days to reach a plateau of -17 ± 3 mmHg ($n = 10$, $P < 0.05$). Mean arterial and diastolic pressures fell by -15 ± 2 ($P < 0.05$) and -17 ± 2 ($P < 0.05$) mmHg, respectively. Lowered arterial pressure was maintained with no sign of recovery for at least 3 weeks. SBP LF: Systolic blood pressure, low frequency band. (Figure used with permission from Abdala et al., 2012). #Significant difference ($P < 0.05$).

CENTRAL CO₂ CHEMORECEPTION, HYPERTENSION

As discussed above it is well established that activation of central chemoreceptors by CO_2 increases breathing, SNA and blood pressure in humans and in anesthetized and conscious animals (Hanna et al., 1981; Lioy and Trzebski, 1984; Somers et al., 1989; Nattie et al., 1992, 1993; Oikawa et al., 2005; Guyenet et al., 2010). In asphyxia, the hypercapnic component is of greater importance than the hypoxic component in causing sympathetically induced increases in ABP and vascular resistance (Morgan et al., 1995; Cooper et al., 2004). However, the links between neurogenic hypertension and the hypercapnic central chemoreflex are not well understood. In human subjects, the hypoxic component of asphyxia reduces the baroreceptor–vascular resistance reflex sensitivity, while the hypercapnic component is responsible for increasing blood pressure (Cooper et al., 2004, 2005). Thus, the effects of both peripheral and central chemoreceptors may contribute to promoting hypertension in patients with obstructive sleep apnea who undergo repeated bouts of asphyxia nightly (Cooper et al., 2005). Combined hypoxia and hypercapnia evoke longer-lasting sympathetic activation in humans than does either hypoxia or hypercapnia alone (Morgan et al., 1995). In patients with heart failure, the central chemoreflex response to hypercapnia is markedly and selectively enhanced (Kara et al., 2003; Yamada et al., 2004), and the enhanced hypercapnic chemosensitivity is correlated significantly with plasma norepinephrine levels suggesting sympathoexcitation (Kara et al., 2003). Administration of 100% oxygen does not lower sympathetic activity in patients with heart failure, providing further evidence against any peripheral chemoreflex potentiation (Kara et al., 2003). In anesthetized SHRs with carotid sinus denervation, systemic hypercapnia increased and hypocapnia decreased the magnitude of both phrenic and sympathetic discharges, and the increased sympathetic discharge during hypercapnia was accompanied by a significant increase in ABP (Czyzyk-Krzeska and Trzebski, 1990).We have recently reported that SHRs have a significantly augmented central hypercapnic chemoreflex relative to the normotensive WKY control rats (Li and Nattie, Neuroscience, 2012). In SHRs, the ventilatory response to normoxic hypercapnia (7% CO_2/21%O_2), or hyperoxic hypercapnia (7%CO_2/93%O_2) when peripheral chemoreceptors are suppressed, is significantly higher in both wakefulness and sleep than that of the normotensive WKY control rats (Li and Nattie, Neuroscience, 2012). It is interesting to note that both peripheral and central chemoreflexes have powerful effects on sympathetic activity (see above), and in SHRs both the peripheral and central chemoreflex are overactive. Asphyxia, a recurring condition in sleep disorders, includes two important components, hypoxia and hypercapnia, which are primarily detected by peripheral and central chemoreceptors, respectively, in normal conditions. Sleep disorders are present in $\sim 40\%$ of obese individuals and both sleep disorders and obesity are closely associated with hypertension (Chau et al., 2012). Many studies have focused on the hypoxic effects of sleep disorders and hypertension with little attention to the role of the central CO_2 chemoreflex in sleep disorders and their link to the development of hypertension. It is also interesting to note that while denervation of the peripheral chemoreceptor in SHRs significantly lower ABP (up to ~ 25 mmHg), ABP remains significantly above the normal even at 21 days post CSD (Abdala et al., 2012) suggesting other possible mechanisms are involved, e.g., an overactive central chemoreflex.

In summary: in SHRs, the respiratory chemoreflex to hypercapnia is exaggerated with and without peripheral carotid chemoreceptor inputs.

OREXIN, CENTRAL CHEMORECEPTORS, AND HYPERTENSION

That activation of orexin receptors evokes increases in breathing, SNA, and ABP, and that SHRs have augmented central and peripheral chemoreflexes suggest that orexin is a key factor that links the cardiovascular and respiratory systems, and that alterations of the orexin system may contribute to some cardio-respiratory diseases. The following observations support this proposed link: (1) The orexin knockout mouse has a decreased respiratory hypercapnic chemoreflex as well as a lower resting ABP (Kayaba et al., 2003; Nakamura et al., 2007). (2) Orexin injections into the CNS increase ABP, HR, SNA, and breathing in both conscious and anesthetized normotensive animals (Shirasaka et al., 1999; Machado et al., 2002; Huang et al., 2010; Shahid et al., 2011, 2012). (3) The SHRs have: (a) an augmented respiratory–sympathetic coupling in reduced preparations (Simms et al., 2009), (b) a hyperactive peripheral chemoreflex (Zoccal et al., 2008; Simms et al., 2009), and (c) a hyperactive central CO_2 chemoreflex (Li and Nattie, Neuroscience, 2012). (4) Blockade of both OXRs can significantly lower ABP, HR, SNA and the hyperactive central CO_2 chemoreflex in conscious SHRs (Li et al., 2013a). Based on these data, we pose the following questions: (1) What is the role of overactive central chemoreceptors in developing hypertension? (2) What is the role of orexin in this augmented CO_2 chemoreflex and hypertension? (3) Can antagonism of OXRs be a target to treat such an augmented CO_2 response and the associated hypertension in SHR? At present, we have found that antagonism of both OXRs using an orally administered dual orexin receptor antagonist, Almxt: (1) significantly reduced the exaggerated CO_2 chemoreflex in SHR to the same level as measured in the control normotensive WKY rats (Li and Nattie, Neuroscience, 2012), and (2) significantly decreased ABP in both resting and hypercapnic condition (Li et al., 2013a) (Li and Nattie, Neuroscience, 2012). We hypothesize that the source of the enhanced SNA and respiratory-sympathetic coupling may involve neurons in the central chemoreceptor sites, and the overactive central orexin system may play an important role in such an alteration. There is no evidence that orexin projections and orexin receptors are located in the peripheral chemoreceptors, e.g., the carotid body, at the present time and the role of peripheral orexins in regulation of cardio-respiratory functions remain unclear (Johren et al., 2001; Nakabayashi et al., 2003; Heinonen et al., 2008).

In summary: transgenic orexin deficient mice and rats have lower resting blood pressure, and a significantly decreased hypercapnic response (pp-OX KO) while SHRs have severe hypertension, a hyperactive central hypercapnic reflex, and possibly an overactive orexin system. Blocking both orexin receptors in SHR can normalize the exaggerated hypercapnic chemoreflex and significantly lower blood pressure, which suggests the overactive central chemoreceptors may be an important link in neurogenic hypertension with orexin as mediator in SHRs.

SUMMARY OF OREXIN, CHEMOREFLEX, AND HYPERTENSION

Orexin knockout mice have both a severely attenuated hypercapnic chemoreflex and lower resting blood pressure, while SHRs have severely increased blood pressure and enhanced peripheral and central chemoreflexes with a possibly upregulated central

orexin system. Antagonism of both orexin receptors can significantly lower SNA and blood pressure and normalize that central hypercapnic chemoreflex in SHRs. We suggest that overactive central chemoreceptors may be an important link to the development and maintenance of high blood pressure in SHRs with orexin as a key mediator.

CONCLUSION

Activation of central CO_2 chemoreceptors is associated with sympatho-excitation, hypertension and tachycardia. In SHRs, the overactive central and peripheral chemoreflex may play an important role in the development of neurogenic hypertension. Orexin links the respiratory and sympathetic nervous systems and an overactive orexin system may be the cause of hyperactive central CO_2 chemoreflex in SHRs and thus the associated hypertension. Antagonism of OXRs can normalize the overactive CO_2 central chemoreflex and significantly lower ABP and SNA in SHRs. Based on the data obtained from SHRs we hypothesize that modulation of the orexin system could be a potential target in treating some forms of hypertension.

REFERENCES

Abdala, A. P., Mcbryde, F. D., Marina, N., Hendy, E. B., Engelman, Z., Fudim, M., et al. (2012). Hypertension is critically dependent on the carotid body input in the spontaneously hypertensive rat. *J. Physiol.* 590, 4269–4277. doi: 10.1113/jphysiol.2012.237800

Allen, G. V., and Cechetto, D. F. (1992). Functional and anatomical organization of cardiovascular pressor and depressor sites in the lateral hypothalamic area: I. Descending projections. *J. Comp. Neurol.* 315, 313–332. doi: 10.1002/cne.903150307

Antunes, V. R., Brailoiu, G. C., Kwok, E. H., Scruggs, P., and Dun, N. J. (2001). Orexins/hypocretins excite rat sympathetic preganglionic neurons *in vivo* and *in vitro*. *Am. J. Physiol. Regul. Integr. Comp. Physiol.* 281, R1801–R1807.

Badami, V. M., Rice, C. D., Lois, J. H., Madrecha, J., and Yates, B. J. (2010). Distribution of hypothalamic neurons with orexin (hypocretin) or melanin concentrating hormone (MCH) immunoreactivity and multisynaptic connections with diaphragm motoneurons. *Brain Res.* 1323, 119–126. doi: 10.1016/j.brainres.2010.02.002

Bayer, L., Eggermann, E., Serafin, M., Grivel, J., Machard, D., Muhlethaler, M., et al. (2005). Opposite effects of noradrenaline and acetylcholine upon hypocretin/orexin versus melanin concentrating hormone neurons in rat hypothalamic slices. *Neuroscience* 130, 807–811. doi: 10.1016/j.neuroscience.2004.10.032

Boone, J. L. (1991). Stress and hypertension. *Prim. Care* 18, 623–649.

Brown, S. N., Chitravanshi, V. C., Kawabe, K., and Sapru, H. N. (2007). Microinjections of melanin concentrating hormone into the nucleus tractus solitarius of the rat elicit depressor and bradycardic responses. *Neuroscience* 150, 796–806. doi: 10.1016/j.neuroscience.2007.10.002

Burdakov, D., Karnani, M. M., and Gonzalez, A. (2013). Lateral hypothalamus as a sensor-regulator in respiratory and metabolic control. *Physiol. Behav.* 121, 117–124. doi: 10.1016/j.physbeh.2013.03.023

Chau, E. H., Lam, D., Wong, J., Mokhlesi, B., and Chung, F. (2012). Obesity hypoventilation syndrome: a review of epidemiology, pathophysiology, and perioperative considerations. *Anesthesiology* 117, 188–205. doi: 10.1097/ALN.0b013e31825add60

Chen, C. T., Hwang, L. L., Chang, J. K., and Dun, N. J. (2000). Pressor effects of orexins injected intracisternally and to rostral ventrolateral medulla of anesthetized rats. *Am. J. Physiol. Regul. Integr. Comp. Physiol.* 278, R692–R697.

Cooper, V. L., Bowker, C. M., Pearson, S. B., Elliott, M. W., and Hainsworth, R. (2004). Effects of simulated obstructive sleep apnoea on the human carotid baroreceptor-vascular resistance reflex. *J. Physiol.* 557, 1055–1065. doi: 10.1113/jphysiol.2004.062513

Cooper, V. L., Pearson, S. B., Bowker, C. M., Elliott, M. W., and Hainsworth, R. (2005). Interaction of chemoreceptor and baroreceptor reflexes by hypoxia and hypercapnia - a mechanism for promoting hypertension in obstructive sleep apnoea. *J. Physiol.* 568, 677–687. doi: 10.1113/jphysiol.2005.094151

Costa-Silva, J. H., Zoccal, D. B., and Machado, B. H. (2012). Chronic intermittent hypoxia alters glutamatergic control of sympathetic and respiratory activities in the commissural NTS of rats. *Am. J. Physiol. Regul. Integr. Comp. Physiol.* 302, R785–R793. doi: 10.1152/ajpregu.00363.2011

Czyzyk-Krzeska, M. F., and Trzebski, A. (1990). Respiratory-related discharge pattern of sympathetic nerve activity in the spontaneously hypertensive rat. *J. Physiol.* 426, 355–368.

Date, Y., Ueta, Y., Yamashita, H., Yamaguchi, H., Matsukura, S., Kangawa, K., et al. (1999). Orexins, orexigenic hypothalamic peptides, interact with autonomic, neuroendocrine and neuroregulatory systems. *Proc. Natl. Acad. Sci. U.S.A.* 96, 748–753.

De Lecea, L. (2010). A decade of hypocretins: past, present and future of the neurobiology of arousal. *Acta Physiol.* 198, 203–208. doi: 10.1111/j.1748-1716.2009.02004.x

De Lecea, L. (2012). Hypocretins and the neurobiology of sleep-wake mechanisms. *Prog. Brain Res.* 198, 15–24. doi: 10.1016/B978-0-444-59489-1.00003-3

De Lecea, L., Kilduff, T. S., Peyron, C., Gao, X., Foye, P. E., Danielson, P. E., et al. (1998). The hypocretins: hypothalamus-specific peptides with neuroexcitatory activity. *Proc. Natl. Acad. Sci. U.S.A.* 95, 322–327. doi: 10.1073/pnas.95.1.322

Deng, B. S., Nakamura, A., Zhang, W., Yanagisawa, M., Fukuda, Y., and Kuwaki, T. (2007). Contribution of orexin in hypercapnic chemoreflex: evidence from genetic and pharmacological disruption and supplementation studies in mice. *J. Appl. Physiol. (1985)* 103, 1772–1779. doi: 10.1152/japplphysiol.00075.2007

Dias, M. B., Li, A., and Nattie, E. (2010). The orexin receptor 1 (OX1R) in the rostral medullary raphe contributes to the hypercapnic chemoreflex in wakefulness, during the active period of the diurnal cycle. *Respir. Physiol. Neurobiol.* 170, 96–102. doi: 10.1016/j.resp.2009.12.002

Dias, M. B., Li, A., and Nattie, E. E. (2009). Antagonism of orexin receptor-1 in the retrotrapezoid nucleus inhibits the ventilatory response to hypercapnia predominantly in wakefulness. *J. Physiol.* 587, 2059–2067. doi: 10.1113/jphysiol.2008.168260

Dutschmann, M., Kron, M., Morschel, M., and Gestreau, C. (2007). Activation of Orexin B receptors in the pontine Kolliker-Fuse nucleus modulates preinspiratory hypoglossal motor activity in rat. *Respir. Physiol. Neurobiol.* 159, 232–235. doi: 10.1016/j.resp.2007.06.004

Fisher, J. P., and Paton, J. F. (2011). The sympathetic nervous system and blood pressure in humans: implications for hypertension. *J. Hum. Hypertens.* 26, 463–475. doi: 10.1038/jhh.2011.66

Fletcher, E. C. (2001). Invited review: physiological consequences of intermittent hypoxia: systemic blood pressure. *J. Appl. Physiol. (1985)* 90, 1600–1605.

Fletcher, E. C., Lesske, J., Behm, R., Miller, C. C. 3rd., Stauss, H., and Unger, T. (1992). Carotid chemoreceptors, systemic blood pressure, and chronic episodic hypoxia mimicking sleep apnea. *J. Appl. Physiol. (1985)* 72, 1978–1984.

Follwell, M. J., and Ferguson, A. V. (2002). Cellular mechanisms of orexin actions on paraventricular nucleus neurones in rat hypothalamus. *J. Physiol.* 545, 855–867. doi: 10.1113/jphysiol.2002.030049

Fukuda, Y., Sato, A., and Trzebski, A. (1987). Carotid chemoreceptor discharge responses to hypoxia and hypercapnia in normotensive and spontaneously hypertensive rats. *J. Auton. Nerv. Syst.* 19, 1–11. doi: 10.1016/0165-1838(87)90139-1

Furlong, T. M., Vianna, D. M., Liu, L., and Carrive, P. (2009). Hypocretin/orexin contributes to the expression of some but not all forms of stress and arousal. *Eur. J. Neurosci.* 30, 1603–1614. doi: 10.1111/j.1460-9568.2009.06952.x

Geerling, J. C., Shin, J. W., Chimenti, P. C., and Loewy, A. D. (2010). Paraventricular hypothalamic nucleus: axonal projections to the brainstem. *J. Comp. Neurol.* 518, 1460–1499. doi: 10.1002/cne.22283

Girault, E. M., Yi, C. X., Fliers, E., and Kalsbeek, A. (2012). Orexins, feeding, and energy balance. *Prog. Brain Res.* 198, 47–64. doi: 10.1016/B978-0-444-59489-1.00005-7

Guyenet, P. G. (2006). The sympathetic control of blood pressure. *Nat. Rev. Neurosci.* 7, 335–346. doi: 10.1038/nrn1902

Guyenet, P. G., Stornetta, R. L., Abbott, S. B., Depuy, S. D., Fortuna, M. G., and Kanbar, R. (2010). Central CO2 chemoreception and integrated neural mechanisms of cardiovascular and respiratory control. *J. Appl. Physiol.* 108, 995–1002. doi: 10.1152/japplphysiol.00712.2009

Hall, J. E., Da Silva, A. A., Do Carmo, J. M., Dubinion, J., Hamza, S., Munusamy, S., et al. (2010). Obesity-induced hypertension: role of sympathetic nervous system, leptin, and melanocortins. *J. Biol. Chem.* 285, 17271–17276. doi: 10.1074/jbc.R110.113175

Hanna, B. D., Lioy, F., and Polosa, C. (1981). Role of carotid and central chemoreceptors in the CO2 response of sympathetic preganglionic neurons. *J. Auton Nerv. Syst.* 3, 421–435.

Hassani, O. K., Lee, M. G., and Jones, B. E. (2009). Melanin-concentrating hormone neurons discharge in a reciprocal manner to orexin neurons across the sleep-wake cycle. *Proc. Natl. Acad. Sci. U.S.A.* 106, 2418–2422. doi: 10.1073/pnas.0811400106

Heinonen, M. V., Purhonen, A. K., Makela, K. A., and Herzig, K. H. (2008). Functions of orexins in peripheral tissues. *Acta Physiol.* 192, 471–485. doi: 10.1111/j.1748-1716.2008.01836.x

Huang, S. C., Dai, Y. W., Lee, Y. H., Chiou, L. C., and Hwang, L. L. (2010). Orexins depolarize rostral ventrolateral medulla neurons and increase arterial pressure and heart rate in rats mainly via orexin 2 receptors. *J. Pharmacol. Exp. Ther.* 334, 522–529. doi: 10.1124/jpet.110.167791

Iigaya, K., Horiuchi, J., Mcdowall, L. M., Lam, A. C., Sediqi, Y., Polson, J. W., et al. (2012). Blockade of orexin receptors with Almorexant reduces cardiorespiratory responses evoked from the hypothalamus but not baro- or chemoreceptor reflex responses. *Am. J. Physiol. Regul. Integr. Comp. Physiol.* 303, R1011–R1022. doi: 10.1152/ajpregu.00263.2012

Izdebska, E., Jodkowski, J., and Trzebski, A. (1982). Central influence of vasopressin on baroreceptor reflex in normotensive rats and its lack in spontaneously hypertensive rats (SHR). *Experientia* 38, 594–595.

Jansen, A. S., Wessendorf, M. W., and Loewy, A. D. (1995). Transneuronal labeling of CNS neuropeptide and monoamine neurons after pseudorabies virus injections into the stellate ganglion. *Brain Res*, 683, 1–24. doi: 10.1016/0006-8993(95)00276-V

Johnson, P. L., Molosh, A., Fitz, S. D., Truitt, W. A., and Shekhar, A. (2012). Orexin, stress, and anxiety/panic states. *Prog. Brain Res.* 198, 133–161. doi: 10.1016/B978-0-444-59489-1.00009-4

Johnson, P. L., Truitt, W., Fitz, S. D., Minick, P. E., Dietrich, A., Sanghani, S., et al. (2010). A key role for orexin in panic anxiety. *Nat. Med.* 16, 111–115. doi: 10.1038/nm.2075

Johren, O., Bruggemann, N., and Dominiak, P. (2004). Orexins (hypocretins) and adrenal function. *Horm. Metab Res.* 36, 370–375. doi: 10.1055/s-2004-814569

Johren, O., Neidert, S. J., Kummer, M., Dendorfer, A., and Dominiak, P. (2001). Prepro-orexin and orexin receptor mRNAs are differentially expressed in peripheral tissues of male and female rats. *Endocrinology* 142, 3324–3331. doi: 10.1210/en.142.8.3324

Kara, T., Narkiewicz, K., and Somers, V. K. (2003). Chemoreflexes–physiology and clinical implications. *Acta Physiol. Scand* 177, 377–384. doi: 10.1046/j.1365-201X.2003.01083.x

Karnani, M. M., Szabo, G., Erdelyi, F., and Burdakov, D. (2013). Lateral hypothalamic GAD65 neurons are spontaneously firing and distinct from orexin- and melanin-concentrating hormone neurons. *J. Physiol.* 591, 933–953. doi: 10.1113/jphysiol.2012.243493

Kayaba, Y., Nakamura, A., Kasuya, Y., Ohuchi, T., Yanagisawa, M., Komuro, I., et al. (2003). Attenuated defense response and low basal blood pressure in orexin knockout mice. *Am. J. Physiol. Regul. Integr. Comp. Physiol.* 285, R581–R593. doi: 10.1152/ajpregu.00671.2002

Kirchgessner, A. L., and Liu, M. (1999). Orexin synthesis and response in the gut. *Neuron* 24, 941–951.

Konadhode, R. R., Pelluru, D., Blanco-Centurion, C., Zayachkivsky, A., Liu, M., Uhde, T., et al. (2013). Optogenetic stimulation of MCH neurons increases sleep. *J. Neurosci.* 33, 10257–10263. doi: 10.1523/JNEUROSCI.1225-13.2013

Kukkonen, J. P. (2013). Physiology of the orexinergic/hypocretinergic system: a revisit in 2012. *Am. J. Physiol. Cell Physiol.* 304, C2–C32. doi: 10.1152/ajpcell.00227.2012

Kukkonen, J. P., Holmqvist, T., Ammoun, S., and Akerman, K. E. (2002). Functions of the orexinergic/hypocretinergic system. *Am. J. Physiol. Cell Physiol.* 283, C1567–C1591. doi: 10.1152/ajpcell.00055.2002

Kuwaki, T., Zhang, W., Nakamura, A., and Deng, B. S. (2008). Emotional and state-dependent modification of cardiorespiratory function: role of orexinergic neurons. *Auton. Neurosci.* 142, 11–16. doi: 10.1016/j.autneu.2008.03.004

Lazarenko, R. M., Stornetta, R. L., Bayliss, D. A., and Guyenet, P. G. (2011). Orexin A activates retrotrapezoid neurons in mice. *Respir Physiol. Neurobiol.* 175, 283–287. doi: 10.1016/j.resp.2010.12.003

Lee, Y. H., Dai, Y. W., Huang, S. C., Li, T. L., and Hwang, L. L. (2013). Blockade of central orexin 2 receptors reduces arterial pressure in spontaneously hypertensive rats. *Exp. Physiol.* 98, 1145–1155. doi: 10.1113/expphysiol.2013.072298

Leinninger, G. M. (2011). Lateral thinking about leptin: a review of leptin action via the lateral hypothalamus. *Physiol. Behav.* 104, 572–581. doi: 10.1016/j.physbeh.2011.04.060

Leinninger, G. M., and Myers, M. G. Jr. (2008). LRb signals act within a distributed network of leptin-responsive neurones to mediate leptin action. *Acta Physiol.* 192, 49–59. doi: 10.1111/j.1748-1716.2007.01784.x

Leonard, C. S., and Kukkonen, J. P. (2013). Orexin/hypocretin receptor signalling: a functional perspective. *Br. J. Pharmacol.* 171, 294–313. doi: 10.1111/bph.12296

Lesske, J., Fletcher, E. C., Bao, G., and Unger, T. (1997). Hypertension caused by chronic intermittent hypoxia–influence of chemoreceptors and sympathetic nervous system. *J. Hypertens* 15, 1593–1603. doi: 10.1097/00004872-199715120-00060

Li, A., Hindmarch, C. C., Nattie, E. E., and Paton, J. F. (2013a). Antagonism of orexin receptors significantly lowers blood pressure in spontaneously hypertensive rats. *J. Physiol.* 591, 4237–4248. doi: 10.1113/jphysiol.2013.256271

Li, A., Hindmarch, C. C., Nattie, E. E., and Paton, J. F. (2013b). Reply from aihua li, charles C. T. Hindmarch, eugene e. Nattie and julian f. R. Paton. *J. Physiol.* 591, 6117. doi: 10.1113/jphysiol.2013.266064

Li, A., and Nattie, E. (2010). Antagonism of rat orexin receptors by almorexant attenuates central chemoreception in wakefulness in the active period of the diurnal cycle. *J. Physiol.* 588, 2935–2944. doi: 10.1113/jphysiol.2010.191288

Li, A., and Nattie, E. E. (2012). "Antagonism of orexin receptors reduces the exaggerated respiratory response to hypercapnia observed in conscious spontaneous hypertensive rats," in *Neuroscience Meeting Planner* (New Orleans, LA: Society for Neuroscience).

Lioy, F., and Trzebski, A. (1984). Pressor effect of CO2 in the rat: different thresholds of the central cardiovascular and respiratory responses to CO2. *J. Auton. Nerv. Syst.* 10, 43–54.

Lopez, M., Senaris, R., Gallego, R., Garcia-Caballero, T., Lago, F., Seoane, L., et al. (1999). Orexin receptors are expressed in the adrenal medulla of the rat. *Endocrinology* 140, 5991–5994.

Louis, G. W., Leinninger, G. M., Rhodes, C. J., and Myers, M. G. Jr. (2010). Direct innervation and modulation of orexin neurons by lateral hypothalamic LepRb neurons. *J. Neurosci.* 30, 11278–11287. doi: 10.1523/JNEUROSCI.1340-10.2010

Luong, L. N., and Carrive, P. (2012). Orexin microinjection in the medullary raphe increases heart rate and arterial pressure but does not reduce tail skin blood flow in the awake rat. *Neuroscience* 202, 209–217. doi: 10.1016/j.neuroscience.2011.11.073

Machado, B. H., Bonagamba, L. G., Dun, S. L., Kwok, E. H., and Dun, N. J. (2002). Pressor response to microinjection of orexin/hypocretin into rostral ventrolateral medulla of awake rats. *Regul. Pept.* 104, 75–81. doi: 10.1016/S0167-0115(01)00351-2

Marcus, J. N., Aschkenasi, C. J., Lee, C. E., Chemelli, R. M., Saper, C. B., Yanagisawa, M., et al. (2001). Differential expression of orexin receptors 1 and 2 in the rat brain. *J. Comp. Neurol.* 435, 6–25. doi: 10.1002/cne.1190

Markovitz, J. H., Matthews, K. A., Kannel, W. B., Cobb, J. L., and D'agostino, R. B. (1993). Psychological predictors of hypertension in the Framingham Study. Is there tension in hypertension? *JAMA* 270, 2439–2443. doi: 10.1001/jama.1993.03510200045030

Marques, F. Z., Campain, A. E., Davern, P. J., Yang, Y. H., Head, G. A., and Morris, B. J. (2011a). Genes influencing circadian differences in blood pressure in hypertensive mice. *PLoS ONE* 6:e19203. doi: 10.1371/journal.pone.0019203

Marques, F. Z., Campain, A. E., Davern, P. J., Yang, Y. H., Head, G. A., and Morris, B. J. (2011b). Global identification of the genes and pathways differentially expressed in hypothalamus in early and established neurogenic hypertension. *Physiol. Genomics* 43, 766–771. doi: 10.1152/physiolgenomics.00009.2011

Matsumura, K., Tsuchihashi, T., and Abe, I. (2001). Central orexin-A augments sympathoadrenal outflow in conscious rabbits. *Hypertension* 37, 1382–1387. doi: 10.1161/01.HYP.37.6.1382

Messina, M. M., and Overton, J. M. (2007). Cardiovascular effects of melanin-concentrating hormone. *Regul. Pept.* 139, 23–30. doi: 10.1016/j.regpep.2006.08.013

Monti, J. M., Torterolo, P., and Lagos, P. (2013). Melanin-concentrating hormone control of sleep-wake behavior. *Sleep Med. Rev.* 17, 293–298. doi: 10.1016/j.smrv.2012.10.002

Moraes, D. J., Zoccal, D. B., and Machado, B. H. (2012a). Medullary respiratory network drives sympathetic overactivity and hypertension in rats

submitted to chronic intermittent hypoxia. *Hypertension* 60, 1374–1380. doi: 10.1161/HYPERTENSIONAHA.111.189332

Moraes, D. J., Zoccal, D. B., and Machado, B. H. (2012b). Sympathoexcitation during chemoreflex active expiration is mediated by L-glutamate in the RVLM/Botzinger complex of rats. *J. Neurophysiol.* 108, 610–623. doi: 10.1152/jn.00057.2012

Moreira, T. S., Takakura, A. C., Colombari, E., and Guyenet, P. G. (2006). Central chemoreceptors and sympathetic vasomotor outflow. *J. Physiol.* 577, 369–386. doi: 10.1113/jphysiol.2006.115600

Morgan, B. J., Crabtree, D. C., Palta, M., and Skatrud, J. B. (1995). Combined hypoxia and hypercapnia evokes long-lasting sympathetic activation in humans. *J. Appl. Physiol. (1985)* 79, 205–213.

Muraki, Y., Yamanaka, A., Tsujino, N., Kilduff, T. S., Goto, K., and Sakurai, T. (2004). Serotonergic regulation of the orexin/hypocretin neurons through the 5-HT1A receptor. *J. Neurosci.* 24, 7159–7166. doi: 10.1523/JNEUROSCI.1027-04.2004

Nahon, J. L. (2006). The melanocortins and melanin-concentrating hormone in the central regulation of feeding behavior and energy homeostasis. *C R Biol.* 329, 623–638; discussion: 653–625. doi: 10.1016/j.crvi.2006.03.021

Nakabayashi, M., Suzuki, T., Takahashi, K., Totsune, K., Muramatsu, Y., Kaneko, C., et al. (2003). Orexin-A expression in human peripheral tissues. *Mol. Cell Endocrinol.* 205, 43–50. doi: 10.1016/S0303-7207(03)00206-5

Nakamura, A., Zhang, W., Yanagisawa, M., Fukuda, Y., and Kuwaki, T. (2007). Vigilance state-dependent attenuation of hypercapnic chemoreflex and exaggerated sleep apnea in orexin knockout mice. *J. Appl. Physiol.* 102, 241–248. doi: 10.1152/japplphysiol.00679.2006

Nambu, T., Sakurai, T., Mizukami, K., Hosoya, Y., Yanagisawa, M., and Goto, K. (1999). Distribution of orexin neurons in the adult rat brain. *Brain Res.* 827, 243–260. doi: 10.1016/S0006-8993(99)01336-0

Nattie, E., and Li, A. (2012). Respiration and autonomic regulation and orexin. *Prog. Brain Res.* 198, 25–46. doi: 10.1016/B978-0-444-59489-1.00004-5

Nattie, E. E., Blanchford, C., and Li, A. (1992). Retrofacial lesions: effects on CO2-sensitive phrenic and sympathetic nerve activity. *J. Appl. Physiol.* 73, 1317–1325.

Nattie, E. E., Gdovin, M., and Li, A. (1993). Retrotrapezoid nucleus glutamate receptors: control of CO2-sensitive phrenic and sympathetic output. *J. Appl. Physiol.* 74, 2958–2968.

Nixon, J. P., Kotz, C. M., Novak, C. M., Billington, C. J., and Teske, J. A. (2012). Neuropeptides controlling energy balance: orexins and neuromedins. *Handb. Exp. Pharmacol.* 209, 77–109. doi: 10.1007/978-3-642-24716-3_4

Oikawa, S., Hirakawa, H., Kusakabe, T., Nakashima, Y., and Hayashida, Y. (2005). Autonomic cardiovascular responses to hypercapnia in conscious rats: the roles of the chemo- and baroreceptors. *Auton. Neurosci.* 117, 105–114. doi: 10.1016/j.autneu.2004.11.009

Ouedraogo, R., Naslund, E., and Kirchgessner, A. L. (2003). Glucose regulates the release of orexin-a from the endocrine pancreas. *Diabetes* 52, 111–117. doi: 10.2337/diabetes.52.1.111

Paton, J. F., Sobotka, P. A., Fudim, M., Engleman, Z. J., Hart, E. C., Mcbryde, F. D., et al. (2013). The carotid body as a therapeutic target for the treatment of sympathetically mediated diseases. *Hypertension* 61, 5–13. doi: 10.1161/HYPERTENSIONAHA.111.00064

Peever, J. H., Lai, Y. Y., and Siegel, J. M. (2003). Excitatory effects of hypocretin-1 (orexin-A) in the trigeminal motor nucleus are reversed by NMDA antagonism. *J. Neurophysiol.* 89, 2591–2600. doi: 10.1152/jn.00968.2002

Peyron, C., Sapin, E., Leger, L., Luppi, P. H., and Fort, P. (2009). Role of the melanin-concentrating hormone neuropeptide in sleep regulation. *Peptides* 30, 2052–2059. doi: 10.1016/j.peptides.2009.07.022

Peyron, C., Tighe, D. K., Van Den Pol, A. N., De Lecea, L., Heller, H. C., Sutcliffe, J. G., et al. (1998). Neurons containing hypocretin (orexin) project to multiple neuronal systems. *J. Neurosci.* 18, 9996–10015.

Prabhakar, N. R., Fields, R. D., Baker, T., and Fletcher, E. C. (2001). Intermittent hypoxia: cell to system. *Am. J. Physiol. Lung. Cell. Mol. Physiol.* 281, L524–L528.

Prabhakar, N. R., Kumar, G. K., and Peng, Y. J. (2012). Sympatho-adrenal activation by chronic intermittent hypoxia. *J. Appl. Physiol. (1985)* 113, 1304–1310. doi: 10.1152/japplphysiol.00444.2012

Prabhakar, N. R., Peng, Y. J., Jacono, F. J., Kumar, G. K., and Dick, T. E. (2005). Cardiovascular alterations by chronic intermittent hypoxia: importance of carotid body chemoreflexes. *Clin. Exp. Pharmacol. Physiol.* 32, 447–449. doi: 10.1111/j.1440-1681.2005.04209.x

Puskas, N., Papp, R. S., Gallatz, K., and Palkovits, M. (2010). Interactions between orexin-immunoreactive fibers and adrenaline or noradrenaline-expressing neurons of the lower brainstem in rats and mice. *Peptides* 31, 1589–1597. doi: 10.1016/j.peptides.2010.04.020

Rosin, D. L., Chang, D. A., and Guyenet, P. G. (2006). Afferent and efferent connections of the rat retrotrapezoid nucleus. *J. Comp. Neurol.* 499, 64–89. doi: 10.1002/cne.21105

Sakurai, T. (2007). The neural circuit of orexin (hypocretin): maintaining sleep and wakefulness. *Nat. Rev. Neurosci.* 8, 171–181. doi: 10.1038/nrn2092

Sakurai, T., Amemiya, A., Ishii, M., Matsuzaki, I., Chemelli, R. M., Tanaka, H., et al. (1998). Orexins and orexin receptors: a family of hypothalamic neuropeptides and G protein-coupled receptors that regulate feeding behavior. *Cell* 92, 573–585. doi: 10.1016/S0092-8674(00)80949-6

Sakurai, T., Mieda, M., and Tsujino, N. (2010). The orexin system: roles in sleep/wake regulation. *Ann. N.Y. Acad. Sci.* 1200, 149–161. doi: 10.1111/j.1749-6632.2010.05513.x

Samson, W. K., Bagley, S. L., Ferguson, A. V., and White, M. M. (2007). Hypocretin/orexin type 1 receptor in brain: role in cardiovascular control and the neuroendocrine response to immobilization stress. *Am. J. Physiol. Regul. Integr. Comp. Physiol.* 292, R382–R387. doi: 10.1152/ajpregu.00496.2006

Samson, W. K., Gosnell, B., Chang, J. K., Resch, Z. T., and Murphy, T. C. (1999). Cardiovascular regulatory actions of the hypocretins in brain. *Brain Res.* 831, 248–253. doi: 10.1016/S0006-8993(99)01457-2

Schone, C., Cao, Z. F., Apergis-Schoute, J., Adamantidis, A., Sakurai, T., and Burdakov, D. (2012). Optogenetic probing of fast glutamatergic transmission from hypocretin/orexin to histamine neurons *in situ*. *J. Neurosci.* 32, 12437–12443. doi: 10.1523/JNEUROSCI.0706-12.2012

Schone, C., Venner, A., Knowles, D., Karnani, M. M., and Burdakov, D. (2011). Dichotomous cellular properties of mouse orexin/hypocretin neurons. *J. Physiol.* 589, 2767–2779. doi: 10.1113/jphysiol.2011.208637

Schultz, H. D., Li, Y. L., and Ding, Y. (2007). Arterial chemoreceptors and sympathetic nerve activity: implications for hypertension and heart failure. *Hypertension* 50, 6–13. doi: 10.1161/HYPERTENSIONAHA.106.076083

Schwimmer, H., Stauss, H. M., Abboud, F., Nishino, S., Mignot, E., and Zeitzer, J. M. (2010). Effects of sleep on the cardiovascular and thermoregulatory systems: a possible role for hypocretins. *J. Appl. Physiol.* 109, 1053–1063. doi: 10.1152/japplphysiol.00516.2010

Shahid, I. Z., Rahman, A. A., and Pilowsky, P. M. (2011). Intrathecal orexin A increases sympathetic outflow and respiratory drive, enhances baroreflex sensitivity and blocks the somato-sympathetic reflex. *Br. J. Pharmacol.* 162, 961–973. doi: 10.1111/j.1476-5381.2010.01102.x

Shahid, I. Z., Rahman, A. A., and Pilowsky, P. M. (2012). Orexin A in rat rostral ventrolateral medulla is pressor, sympatho-excitatory, increases barosensitivity and attenuates the somato-sympathetic reflex. *Br. J. Pharmacol.* 165, 2292–2303. doi: 10.1111/j.1476-5381.2011.01694.x

Shirasaka, T., Kunitake, T., Takasaki, M., and Kannan, H. (2002). Neuronal effects of orexins: relevant to sympathetic and cardiovascular functions. *Regul. Pept.* 104, 91–95. doi: 10.1016/S0167-0115(01)00352-4

Shirasaka, T., Miyahara, S., Kunitake, T., Jin, Q. H., Kato, K., Takasaki, M., et al. (2001). Orexin depolarizes rat hypothalamic paraventricular nucleus neurons. *Am. J. Physiol. Regul. Integr. Comp. Physiol.* 281, R1114–R1118.

Shirasaka, T., Nakazato, M., Matsukura, S., Takasaki, M., and Kannan, H. (1999). Sympathetic and cardiovascular actions of orexins in conscious rats. *Am. J. Physiol.* 277, R1780–R1785.

Simms, A. E., Paton, J. F., Allen, A. M., and Pickering, A. E. (2010). Is augmented central respiratory-sympathetic coupling involved in the generation of hypertension? *Respir Physiol. Neurobiol.* 174, 89–97. doi: 10.1016/j.resp.2010.07.010.

Simms, A. E., Paton, J. F., Pickering, A. E., and Allen, A. M. (2009). Amplified respiratory-sympathetic coupling in the spontaneously hypertensive rat: does it contribute to hypertension? *J. Physiol.* 587, 597–610. doi: 10.1113/jphysiol.2008.165902

Sinski, M., Lewandowski, J., Przybylski, J., Bidiuk, J., Abramczyk, P., Ciarka, A., et al. (2012). Tonic activity of carotid body chemoreceptors contributes to the increased sympathetic drive in essential hypertension. *Hypertens. Res.* 35, 487–491. doi: 10.1038/hr.2011.209

Smith, T. L., and Hutchins, P. M. (1979). Central hemodynamics in the developmental stage of spontaneous hypertension in the unanesthetized rat. *Hypertension* 1, 508–517.

Somers, V. K., Mark, A. L., and Abboud, F. M. (1988a). Potentiation of sympathetic nerve responses to hypoxia in borderline hypertensive subjects. *Hypertension* 11, 608–612.

Somers, V. K., Mark, A. L., and Abboud, F. M. (1988b). Sympathetic activation by hypoxia and hypercapnia–implications for sleep apnea. *Clin. Exp. Hypertens A* 10(Suppl. 1), 413–422.

Somers, V. K., Mark, A. L., Zavala, D. C., and Abboud, F. M. (1989). Contrasting effects of hypoxia and hypercapnia on ventilation and sympathetic activity in humans. *J. Appl. Physiol.* 67, 2101–2106.

Song, N., Zhang, G., Geng, W., Liu, Z., Jin, W., Li, L., et al. (2012). Acid sensing ion channel 1 in lateral hypothalamus contributes to breathing control. *PLoS ONE* 7:e39982. doi: 10.1371/journal.pone.0039982

Spinazzi, R., Andreis, P. G., Rossi, G. P., and Nussdorfer, G. G. (2006). Orexins in the regulation of the hypothalamic-pituitary-adrenal axis. *Pharmacol. Rev.* 58, 46–57. doi: 10.1124/pr.58.1.4.

Sun, M. K., and Guyenet, P. G. (1986). Hypothalamic glutamatergic input to medullary sympathoexcitatory neurons in rats. *Am. J. Physiol.* 251, R798–R810.

Tafil-Klawe, M., Trzebski, A., and Klawe, J. (1985a). Contribution of the carotid chemoreceptor reflex to the mechanism of respiratory sinus arrhythmia in young healthy and hypertensive humans. *Acta Physiol. Pol.* 36, 59–64.

Tafil-Klawe, M., Trzebski, A., Klawe, J., and Palko, T. (1985b). Augmented chemoreceptor reflex tonic drive in early human hypertension and in normotensive subjects with family background of hypertension. *Acta Physiol. Pol.* 36, 51–58.

Takakusaki, K., Takahashi, K., Saitoh, K., Harada, H., Okumura, T., Kayama, Y., et al. (2005). Orexinergic projections to the cat midbrain mediate alternation of emotional behavioural states from locomotion to cataplexy. *J. Physiol.* 568, 1003–1020. doi: 10.1113/jphysiol.2005.085829

Tan, Z. Y., Lu, Y., Whiteis, C. A., Simms, A. E., Paton, J. F., Chapleau, M. W., et al. (2010). Chemoreceptor hypersensitivity, sympathetic excitation, and overexpression of ASIC and TASK channels before the onset of hypertension in SHR. *Circ. Res.* 106, 536–545. doi: 10.1161/CIRCRESAHA.109.206946

Teske, J. A., Billington, C. J., and Kotz, C. M. (2010). Hypocretin/orexin and energy expenditure. *Acta Physiol.* 198, 303–312. doi: 10.1111/j.1748-1716.2010.02075.x

Thorpe, A. J., and Kotz, C. M. (2005). Orexin A in the nucleus accumbens stimulates feeding and locomotor activity. *Brain Res.* 1050, 156–162. doi: 10.1016/j.brainres.2005.05.045

Trivedi, P., Yu, H., Macneil, D. J., Van Der Ploeg, L. H., and Guan, X. M. (1998). Distribution of orexin receptor mRNA in the rat brain. *FEBS Lett.* 438, 71–75.

Trzebski, A., Tafil, M., Zoltowski, M., and Przybylski, J. (1982). Increased sensitivity of the arterial chemoreceptor drive in young men with mild hypertension. *Cardiovasc. Res.* 16, 163–172.

Tsujino, N., and Sakurai, T. (2009). Orexin/hypocretin: a neuropeptide at the interface of sleep, energy homeostasis, and reward system. *Pharmacol Rev.* 61, 162–176. doi: 10.1124/pr.109.001321

Tupone, D., Madden, C. J., Cano, G., and Morrison, S. F. (2011). An orexinergic projection from perifornical hypothalamus to raphe pallidus increases rat brown adipose tissue thermogenesis. *J. Neurosci.* 31, 15944–15955. doi: 10.1523/JNEUROSCI.3909-11.2011

Williams, R. H., Jensen, L. T., Verkhratsky, A., Fugger, L., and Burdakov, D. (2007). Control of hypothalamic orexin neurons by acid and CO2. *Proc. Natl. Acad. Sci. U.S.A.* 104, 10685–10690. doi: 10.1073/pnas.0702676104

Xiao, F., Jiang, M., Du, D., Xia, C., Wang, J., Cao, Y., et al. (2013). Orexin A regulates cardiovascular responses in stress-induced hypertensive rats. *Neuropharmacology* 67, 16–24. doi: 10.1016/j.neuropharm.2012.10.021

Yamada, K., Asanoi, H., Ueno, H., Joho, S., Takagawa, J., Kameyama, T., et al. (2004). Role of central sympathoexcitation in enhanced hypercapnic chemosensitivity in patients with heart failure. *Am. Heart J.* 148, 964–970. doi: 10.1016/j.ahj.2004.05.030

Yamamoto, H., Okuzaki, D., Yamanishi, K., Xu, Y., Watanabe, Y., Yoshida, M., et al. (2013). Genetic analysis of genes causing hypertension and stroke in spontaneously hypertensive rats. *Int. J. Mol. Med.* 31, 1057–1065. doi: 10.3892/ijmm.2013.1304

Yamanaka, A., Muraki, Y., Ichiki, K., Tsujino, N., Kilduff, T. S., Goto, K., et al. (2006). Orexin neurons are directly and indirectly regulated by catecholamines in a complex manner. *J. Neurophysiol.* 96, 284–298. doi: 10.1152/jn.01361.2005

Young, J. K., Wu, M., Manaye, K. F., Kc, P., Allard, J. S., Mack, S. O., et al. (2005). Orexin stimulates breathing via medullary and spinal pathways. *J. Appl. Physiol.* 98, 1387–1395. doi: 10.1152/japplphysiol.00914.2004

Zhang, W., Fukuda, Y., and Kuwaki, T. (2005). Respiratory and cardio-vascular actions of orexin-A in mice. *Neurosci. Lett.* 385, 131–136. doi: 10.1016/j.neulet.2005.05.032

Zicha, J., and Kunes, J. (1999). Ontogenetic aspects of hypertension development: analysis in the rat. *Physiol. Rev.* 79, 1227–1282.

Zimmerman, R. S., and Frohlich, E. D. (1990). Stress and hypertension. *J. Hypertens. Suppl.* 8, S103–S107.

Zoccal, D. B., Bonagamba, L. G., Paton, J. F., and Machado, B. H. (2009a). Sympathetic-mediated hypertension of awake juvenile rats submitted to chronic intermittent hypoxia is not linked to baroreflex dysfunction. *Exp. Physiol.* 94, 972–983. doi: 10.1113/expphysiol.2009. 048306

Zoccal, D. B., Paton, J. F., and Machado, B. H. (2009b). Do changes in the coupling between respiratory and sympathetic activities contribute to neurogenic hypertension? *Clin. Exp. Pharmacol. Physiol.* 36, 1188–1196. doi: 10.1111/j.1440-1681.2009.05202.x

Zoccal, D. B., and Machado, B. H. (2011). Coupling between respiratory and sympathetic activities as a novel mechanism underpinning neurogenic hypertension. *Curr. Hypertens. Rep.* 13, 229–236. doi: 10.1007/s11906-011-0198-7

Zoccal, D. B., Simms, A. E., Bonagamba, L. G., Braga, V. A., Pickering, A. E., Paton, J. F., et al. (2008). Increased sympathetic outflow in juvenile rats submitted to chronic intermittent hypoxia correlates with enhanced expiratory activity. *J. Physiol.* 586, 3253–3265. doi: 10.1113/jphysiol.2008.154187

Zubcevic, J., Waki, H., Raizada, M. K., and Paton, J. F. (2011). Autonomic-immune-vascular interaction: an emerging concept for neurogenic hypertension. *Hypertension* 57, 1026–1033. doi: 10.1161/HYPERTENSIONAHA.111.169748

Conflict of Interest Statement: The authors declare that the research was conducted in the absence of any commercial or financial relationships that could be construed as a potential conflict of interest.

20

Differential actions of orexin receptors in brainstem cholinergic and monoaminergic neurons revealed by receptor knockouts: implications for orexinergic signaling in arousal and narcolepsy

Kristi A. Kohlmeier[1], Christopher J. Tyler[2], Mike Kalogiannis[2], Masaru Ishibashi[2], Morten P. Kristensen[1], Iryna Gumenchuk[2], Richard M. Chemelli[3], Yaz Y. Kisanuki[3†], Masashi Yanagisawa[3] and Christopher S. Leonard[2]*

[1] Department of Drug Design and Pharmacology, Faculty of Health and Medical Sciences, University of Copenhagen, Copenhagen, Denmark
[2] Department of Physiology, New York Medical College, Valhalla, NY, USA
[3] Howard Hughes Medical Institute, University of Texas Southwestern Medical Center, Dallas, TX, USA

Edited by:
Christopher J. Winrow, Merck & Co., Inc., USA

Reviewed by:
Gregg Stanwood, Vanderbilt University, USA
Jafri M. Abdullah, Universiti Sains Malaysia, Malaysia
Christie D. Fowler, The Scripps Research Institute, USA

*Correspondence:
Christopher S. Leonard, Department of Physiology, New York Medical College, 15 Dana Road, Valhalla, NY 10595, USA
e-mail: chris_leonard@nymc.ed
†

Orexin neuropeptides influence multiple homeostatic functions and play an essential role in the expression of normal sleep-wake behavior. While their two known receptors (OX_1 and OX_2) are targets for novel pharmacotherapeutics, the actions mediated by each receptor remain largely unexplored. Using brain slices from mice constitutively lacking either receptor, we used whole-cell and Ca^{2+} imaging methods to delineate the cellular actions of each receptor within cholinergic [laterodorsal tegmental nucleus (LDT)] and monoaminergic [dorsal raphe (DR) and locus coeruleus (LC)] brainstem nuclei—where orexins promote arousal and suppress REM sleep. In slices from $OX_2^{-/-}$ mice, orexin-A (300 nM) elicited wild-type responses in LDT, DR, and LC neurons consisting of a depolarizing current and augmented voltage-dependent Ca^{2+} transients. In slices from $OX_1^{-/-}$ mice, the depolarizing current was absent in LDT and LC neurons and was attenuated in DR neurons, although Ca^{2+}-transients were still augmented. Since orexin-A produced neither of these actions in slices lacking both receptors, our findings suggest that orexin-mediated depolarization is mediated by both receptors in DR, but is exclusively mediated by OX_1 in LDT and LC neurons, even though OX_2 is present and OX_2 mRNA appears elevated in brainstems from $OX_1^{-/-}$ mice. Considering published behavioral data, these findings support a model in which orexin-mediated excitation of mesopontine cholinergic and monoaminergic neurons contributes little to stabilizing spontaneous waking and sleep bouts, but functions in context-dependent arousal and helps restrict muscle atonia to REM sleep. The augmented Ca^{2+} transients produced by both receptors appeared mediated by influx via L-type Ca^{2+} channels, which is often linked to transcriptional signaling. This could provide an adaptive signal to compensate for receptor loss or prolonged antagonism and may contribute to the reduced severity of narcolepsy in single receptor knockout mice.

Keywords: laterodorsal tegmental nucleus, dorsal raphe nucleus, locus coeruleus, whole-cell patch-clamp recording, Ca^{2+} signaling

INTRODUCTION

Orexin-A and Orexin-B, also called hypocretin-1 and -2, are two hypothalamic neuropeptides (De Lecea et al., 1998; Sakurai et al., 1998) that influence feeding, metabolism, arousal, reward, and stress substrates in the CNS (for review, see Tsujino and Sakurai, 2009). The orexin system plays a particularly important role in the normal expression of waking and sleep since its disruption underlies the sleep disorder narcolepsy with cataplexy in humans (Peyron et al., 2000; Thannickal et al., 2000) and produces a narcolepsy phenotype with unstable behavioral states, sleep attacks and cataplexy-like motor arrests in animals (Chemelli et al., 1999; Lin et al., 1999; Hara et al., 2001; Willie et al., 2003; Beuckmann et al., 2004; Mochizuki et al., 2004; Kalogiannis et al., 2011).

Orexin actions are mediated by two G-protein coupled receptors (Sakurai et al., 1998), termed orexin-1 (OX_1) and orexin-2 (OX_2) receptors, which have partly overlapping and widespread expression patterns in the CNS (Trivedi et al., 1998; Hervieu et al., 2001; Marcus et al., 2001). These receptors are attractive targets for the development of a range of novel therapeutic agents with potential for treating sleep disorders, obesity, stress-related disorders, and addiction. The first orexin-related drugs to appear will be the dual orexin receptor antagonists (DORAs) for the treatment of insomnia (Uslaner et al., 2013; Winrow and Renger, 2013), but there is significant interest in developing single orexin receptor-specific antagonists (SORAs). However, much remains unknown about the cellular actions of each receptor and the behavioral consequences of activation or inhibition of each receptor at their many targets.

In this study, we focus on mesopontine cholinergic [laterodorsal tegmental nucleus (LDT)] and monoaminergic [dorsal raphe (DR) and locus coeruleus (LC)] neurons, which participate in a spectrum of functions that include the control of arousal and sleep (Jones, 2005; Brown et al., 2012), the maintenance of motor activity and muscle tone during arousal (Jacobs and Fornal, 1993; Michelsen et al., 2007), the mediation of stress related actions and adaptation (Lowry et al., 2005; Valentino and Van Bockstaele, 2008) and the stimulation of motivated behavior via projections to midbrain dopamine systems (Maskos, 2008; Mena-Segovia et al., 2008). These structures, and especially the LC, receive substantial orexinergic innervation (Peyron et al., 1998; Chemelli et al., 1999; Nambu et al., 1999), and orexin terminals have been shown to synapse upon tyrosine hydroxylase immunoreactive neurons in LC (Horvath et al., 1999), cholinergic neurons in the LDT (Cid-Pellitero and Garzón, 2011) and DR neurons (Del Cid-Pellitero and Garzón, 2011). Evidence from *in-situ* hybridization studies in rat (Marcus et al., 2001) indicate that moderate levels of OX_1 mRNA are expressed in LDT and DR while especially high levels of OX_1 mRNA are expressed in the LC. These studies also found moderate levels of OX_2 mRNA levels in the DR with lower levels in the LDT and LC. Consistent with this innervation pattern and receptor distribution, exogenously applied orexins directly depolarize LDT (Burlet et al., 2002; Kohlmeier et al., 2008) and related PPT (Kim et al., 2009) neurons, along with DR (Brown et al., 2002; Liu et al., 2002; Kohlmeier et al., 2008) and LC neurons (Horvath et al., 1999; Ivanov and Aston-Jones, 2000; Li et al., 2002; Hoang et al., 2003; Murai and Akaike, 2005) partly, by activating a cation current. Orexin-A has also been shown previously to have a distinct modulatory role in the LDT and DR by augmenting the Ca^{2+} influx mediated by L-type Ca^{2+} channels (Kohlmeier et al., 2008). However, the roles played by each receptor in these actions are unknown.

Early studies of orexin receptors using heterologous expression found that both receptors stimulate Ca^{2+}-release from intracellular stores (Sakurai et al., 1998; Smart et al., 1999) and activate phospholipase C (PLC) (Lund et al., 2000; Holmqvist et al., 2002), suggesting they are G_q coupled receptors. More recent studies indicate these receptors can couple to multiple G-proteins and therefore may utilize more diverse signaling cascades, however, much less is known about the signaling targets of native orexin receptors (for review see Kukkonen and Leonard, 2013). Evidence from studies of brain slices or freshly dissociated neurons indicate that native orexin receptors mediate neuronal depolarization from resting membrane potential by activating three classes of effectors (for review see Leonard and Kukkonen, 2013): closure of K^+ channels (Ivanov and Aston-Jones, 2000; Hwang et al., 2001; Bayer et al., 2002; Grabauskas and Moises, 2003; Hoang et al., 2003, 2004; Ishibashi et al., 2005; Bisetti et al., 2006), forward activation of the electrogenic Na^+/Ca^{2+} exchanger (Eriksson et al., 2001; Wu et al., 2002, 2004; Burdakov et al., 2003), activation of a cation current (Brown et al., 2002; Yang and Ferguson, 2002, 2003; Murai and Akaike, 2005; Kohlmeier et al., 2008) and can elevate intracellular $[Ca^{2+}]$ (Van Den Pol et al., 1998; Van Den Pol, 1999; Uramura et al., 2001; Xu et al., 2002; Kohlmeier et al., 2004,

2008; Ishibashi et al., 2005). Only limited information is available about the particular receptors mediating these actions, especially since receptor overlap is common and subtype-specific antagonists are lacking. Conclusions about native receptor function has often relied upon the relative potencies of orexin-A and -B, based on the high potency of orexin-A for both receptors and the ~10-fold lower potency of orexin-B for OX_1 expressed in CHO cells (Sakurai et al., 1998). However, agonist-based receptor determinations have numerous potential confounds (see Leonard and Kukkonen, 2013) including differing stability of agonists, differing receptor levels and the possibility of biased agonism, as has been proposed for expressed orexin receptors (Putula et al., 2011).

To avoid these potential limitations, we sought to determine the actions of each receptor in LDT, DR, and LC neurons using a genetic dissection approach: We examined the actions by each receptor using whole-cell recording and Ca^{2+} imaging methods in brain slices from knockout mice constitutively lacking either receptor thereby allowing us to determine the functional capacity of each receptor in isolation. This revealed that OX_1 and OX_2 have both convergent and unique functions in LDT, DR, and LC neurons. These findings have implications for understanding the cellular functions of orexin receptors, the behavioral consequences of orexin signaling at these loci and some consequences for using receptor specific antagonists as therapeutics.

MATERIALS AND METHODS

All procedures complied with National Institutes of Health (US) and institutional guidelines (New York Medical College) for ethical use of animals and were approved by the New York Medical College Institutional Animal Care and Use Committee (IACUC).

ANIMALS AND GENOTYPING

Brain slices for whole cell recordings were prepared from 14 to 32 day old C57BL6, background control (orexin receptor wild-type; OxrWT), $OX_2^{-/-}$, $OX_1^{-/-}$, and $OX_1^{-/-}/OX_2^{-/-}$ double knockout (DKO) mice. In those cases where calcium imaging was being performed with the cell permeant fura-2AM, mice aged 9–15 days old were utilized. Both male and female mice were used in this study and receptor knockout mice were the offspring of breeders that were both homozygous for the null alleles on mixed C57BL6 and 129SvEv genetic backgrounds. The OxrWT mice were bred from the wild-type progeny of the $OX_2^{+/-}$ parents used to make the $OX_2^{-/-}$ mice. The OxrWT, $OX_2^{-/-}$, $OX_1^{-/-}$, and DKO mice have been described previously (Willie et al., 2003; Kalogiannis et al., 2011; Mieda et al., 2011).

To confirm genotypes, tail biopsies were obtained during slice preparation and subsequently analyzed by PCR. One set of primers were used to determine if the mouse was either a wild-type or knockout for each orexin receptor. The three primers for OX_1 consisted of a common primer (5'-CTCTTTC TCCACAGAGCCCAGGACTC-3'), a knockout primer (5'-TGA GCGAGTAACAACCCGTCGGATTC-3') and a wild-type primer (5'gCAAGAATGGGTATGAAGGGAAGGGC-3'). The expected product sizes were ~320 base pairs for the wild-type allele and ~500 base pairs for the knockout allele. The three primers for OX_2 consisted of a common primer (5'-CTGGTGCAAATCCCC TGCAAA-3'), a knockout primer (5'-GGTTTTCCCAGTCAC

GACGTTGTA-3′) and a wild-type primer (5′-AATCCTTCTAGA GATCCCTCCTAG-3′). The expected product sizes were ~620 base pairs for wild-type allele and ~300 base pairs for the knock-out allele. These two sets of primers for different orexin receptors were processed separately. PCR amplification consisted of denaturation at 95°C for 8 min followed by 35 cycles of 94°C (30 s), 62°C (30 s) and 72°C (1 min), followed by one cycle at 72°C for 10 min. The result of each PCR reaction was then separated using a 2% agarose gel, and the PCR product was visualized with ethidium bromide.

BRAIN SLICES AND ELECTROPHYSIOLOGY

Brain slices (250 μm) were prepared using a Leica vibratome (VT1000S) in ice-cold artificial cerebrospinal fluid (ACSF) which contained (in mM): 121 NaCl, 5 KCl, 1.2 NaH_2PO_4, 2.7 $CaCl_2$, 1.2 $MgSO_4$, 26 $NaHCO_3$, 20 dextrose, 4.2 lactic acid and was oxygenated by bubbling with carbogen (95% O_2 and 5% CO_2). Slices containing the LDT, DR, or LC were incubated at 35°C for 15 min in oxygenated ACSF, and were then stored at room temperature in continuously oxygenated ACSF, until they were utilized for recordings.

For recording, slices were placed in a submersion chamber on a fixed-stage microscope (Olympus BX50WI) and superfused (1–2 ml/min) with ACSF (23 ± 2°C). Regions for recording were chosen from within the boundaries of the LDT, DR, or LC nuclei determined using a 4X objective and brightfield illumination. Neurons were then visualized with a video camera and DIC optics using a 40X water immersion objective (Olympus; NA 0.8). Large to medium sized multipolar neurons were selected for gigaseal recording in voltage clamp or current clamp mode using an Axoclamp 2A or Axopatch 2A or 2B amplifier (Axon Instruments). Borosilicate patch pipettes (2–5 MOhms; cat number 8050, AM systems) containing a solution of (in mM) 144 K-Gluconate, 0.2 EGTA, 3 $MgCl_2$, 10 HEPES, 0.3 NaGTP, 4 Na_2ATP. Biocytin (0.1%) with the Na-GTP added to the pipette solution just before use.

DRUGS AND EXPERIMENTAL SOLUTIONS

Normal ACSF contained (in mM) 124 NaCl, 5 KCl, 1.2 NaH_2PO_4, 2.7 $CaCl_2$, 1.2 $MgSO_4$, 26 $NaHCO_3$ and 10 dextrose (295–305 mOsm). To block voltage-gated sodium channels and fast synaptic potentials, the ACSF (DABST-containing) contained the ionotropic receptor antagonists DNQX (15 μM, Sigma), APV (50 μM, Sigma), bicuculline (10 μM, Sigma), and strychnine (2.5 μM, Sigma) with TTX (500 nM, Alomone). To measure the average orexin-A mediated post-synaptic current and its I-V relation in LDT and DR neurons, CsCl (2 or 3 mM) was added to the DABST to block H-current and a low Ca^{2+} ACSF was used to inhibit voltage-gated Ca^{2+} currents. [Ca^{2+}] was buffered to <20 μM by the addition of 2.7 mM EGTA (calculated with Patcher's Power Tools XOP for Igor Pro). Orexin-A (Sigma, USA; Phoenix Pharmaceuticals, USA; American Peptides, USA; Peptide international, USA) was dissolved in deionized water or physiological saline in 1 mM aliquots and frozen (−80°C). Aliquots were dissolved in ACSF to a final concentration of 300 nM immediately before use. The L-type Ca^{2+} channel antagonist nifedipine and agonist, Bay-K-8644 (Bay-K; Sigma, USA) were dissolved

in DMSO to a stock concentration of 10 mM and delivered at the final concentration of 10 μM in ACSF. Bisindolylmaleimide I, HCl (Calbiochem, EMD Biosciences) was dissolved in DMSO to a stock concentration of 5 mM. On the day of experiments it was diluted in TTX-ACSF to a final concentration of 1 μM and applied for 5 min prior to application of orexin. Final dilutions of these drugs were made immediately before application and light exposure was minimized throughout preparation and application.

Ca^{2+} IMAGING

Fluorescence related to intracellular calcium concentration was measured from neurons in slices that had been either individually filled with bis-fura-2 from patch pipettes or bulk-loaded with fura-2AM. The patch solution for Ca^{2+} imaging contained the potassium salt of bis-fura-2 (50 μM, Molecular Probes) dissolved in a solution containing (in mM) 144 K-gluconate, 3 $MgCl_2$, 10 HEPES, 0.3 NaGTP, and 4 Na_2ATP. Biocytin (0.1%) or biotinylated Alexa-594 (25 μM; Invitrogen) was included in all experiments for cell identification following slice fixation.

For bulk loading neurons with fura-2, slices from young mice (P6-P17) were incubated in ACSF containing 15 μM fura-2AM (Molecular Probes) prepared from a 3.3 mM stock of fura-2AM in DMSO. Slices were incubated for 30 min at 36°C in a small volume equilibrated with Carbogen (5% CO_2/95% O_2). Slices were then transferred to the recording chamber and rinsed for at least 30 min to ensure de-esterification and temperature equilibration. After locating a recording region in the LDT, DR, or LC, individual cells were imaged with the 40× water immersion lens.

Ca^{2+} transients were monitored by measuring the emission at 515 nm resulting from excitation of fura-2 with 380 nm (F_{380}; 71000 Chroma fura-2 filter set) from a shuttered 75W Xenon light source. Optical recordings were made using a back illuminated, frame-transfer, cooled CCD camera system (EEV 57 chip, Micromax System, Roper Scientific) that was controlled with custom software (TI Workbench) running on a Mac OS computer. Images were either acquired discontinuously (every 1–4 s) with the shutter closed between images (600 ms exposure) or continuously (~50 ms/frame), with the shutter open for the entire epoch. Changes in intracellular calcium concentration were inferred from changes in delta F/F (dF/F) where F is the fluorescence at rest within a ROI following subtraction of background fluorescence. dF is the change in fluorescence following subtraction of the average F prior to stimulation. dF/F was usually corrected for photobleaching. Since rises in [Ca^{2+}] produce a decrease in F_{380} with fura-2, all dF/F measures are inverted so positive-going traces indicate elevation of [Ca^{2+}]$_i$.

IMMUNOCYTOCHEMISTRY

Recorded neurons were identified as cholinergic, serotonergic or noradrenergic by using conventional immunocytochemistry following slice fixation in 4% paraformaldehyde, cryoprotection and re-sectioning at 40 μm on a freezing microtome. Filled neurons were visualized with avidin-Texas Red or Alexa-594 biocytin. Cholinergic neurons in the LDT selectively co-localize the enzyme neuronal nitric oxide synthase (nNOS; Vincent et al., 1983) and were identified by immunolabeling for nNOS (1:400 rabbit polyclonal, Sigma, Cat N7280). Serotonergic neurons in the DR were identified by immunolabeling for tryptophan hydroxylase (TpH; 1:400 sheep polyclonal, Abcam, 3907 and Covance, PSH-327P). Catecholamine neurons in the LC were identified by immunolabeling for tyrosine hydroxylase (TH; 1:1000, rabbit polyclonal, Abcam, Cat 112). For immunofluorescence, primary antibodies were visualized with FITC or Alexa 488-labeled secondary antibodies. Following washing and mounting, cleared sections were imaged using appropriate filter sets with a CCD camera (Coolsnap, Roper Scientific or QICam, QImaging) mounted on an epi-fluorescence microscope (BX60; Olympus). For immunohistochemistry primary antibodies were visualized with biotinylated secondary antibodies and the tissue was processed with a Vector ABC kit as per the manufacturer's instructions and reacted with Sigma's FastDAB kit for 5 min (Sigma-Aldrich, St. Louis, MO). The precipitation reaction was stopped with three rises of PBS and the sections were mounted on slides and coverslipped.

RNA ISOLATION FROM WHOLE BRAINSTEM

To isolate RNA from whole brainstems, C57BL6, $OX_1^{-/-}$, $OX_2^{-/-}$, DKO, and 129SvEv mice were anesthetized and decapitated as for brain slices. The brainstems were then rapidly dissected from the whole brain starting ~5 mm anterior to the superior colliculus to the medulla, and the cerebellum was removed. The brainstems were then flash-frozen in liquid nitrogen. Total RNA was isolated from the frozen tissue using the RNeasy Lipid Tissue Mini kit (Qiagen). RNA quality and quantity was determined by the A260/A280 ratio from the spectrophotometer.

Standards were generated from cDNA isolated from the C57BL6 brainstem. The cDNA was loaded with primers of the gene of interest and amplified using a conventional PCR for 35 cycles. The product was then run on a gel to determine the specificity of the amplification. If there was a single band of the predicted size, the concentration of the PCR product was determined through spectrophotometry and serially diluted. This technique was utilized with all the primers to create scales unique for each gene of interest. These scales were used to correlate target mRNA fluorescence to sample starting concentration. Scales were created for OX_1 and for each of the two splice variants of OX_2 identified in mouse: $OX_2\alpha$ and $OX_2\beta$ (Chen and Randeva, 2004; Chen et al., 2006). OX_1 mRNA scales ranged from 1.8×10^{-2} to $1.8 \times 10^{-5}\,\mu g/ml$. $OX_2\alpha$ mRNA scales ranged from 7.7×10^{-2} to $7.7 \times 10^{-5}\,\mu g/ml$. $OX_2\beta$ mRNA scale ranged from 9.0×10^{-3} to $9.0 \times 10^{-6}\,\mu g/ml$.

LIGHT CYCLER REAL TIME PCR

A 20 μl volume of the RNA solution, with ~1 μg of total RNA from each sample was reverse transcribed using random primers and the Improm II Reverse Transcription (RT) kit (Promega). The samples were incubated with random primers for 5 min at 70°C, 5 min at 4°C and 1 h at 37°C followed by 70°C for 15 min. The RT product was then aliquoted and stored at −20°C. Two microliters of the RT product were loaded with SYBR green I reagent, 25 mM MgCl₂ and primers to a final volume of 20 μl. Primers for OX_1, $OX_2\alpha$, and $OX_2\beta$ were loaded at a constant concentration (10 μM) for their respective runs (Invitrogen). The following sequences were used to amplify the genes of interest: OX_1 forward: 5′-TGCCGCCAACCCTATC

ATCT-3′ reverse: 5′-GTGACGGTGGTCAGCACGAC-3′ (which corresponds to pubmed genbank NM_198959, 1364-1547); $OX_2\alpha$ forward: 5′-GAGACAAGCTTGCAGCACTGAG-3′ reverse: 5′-TGAGTCGGGTATCCTCATCATAG-3′; $OX_2\beta$ forward: 5′-GAG ACAAGCTTGCAGCACTGAG-3′ reverse: 5′-GGTCGGTCAATG TCCAATGTTC-3′ (Chen and Randeva, 2004; Chen et al., 2006). Each sample was loaded in duplicate (Roche, Lightcycler RT-PCR). Light cycler protocols for mRNA quantification consisted of denaturation at 95°C (485 s), cycling 40 times at 94°C (5 s), 64°C (10 s), and 76°C (14 s). The same amount of total RNA was loaded into each capillary tube for the lightcycler. The measured starting amount of target mRNA was then normalized by the amount of total RNA loaded. The mRNA/total RNA ratios were subsequently compared between samples obtained from C57BL6, $OX_1^{-/-}$, $OX_2^{-/-}$, DKO, and 129SvEv mice. Lightcycler products were then visualized with ethidium bromide in 2% agarose gels to confirm the presence of the RT-PCR target.

DATA ANALYSIS

Data analysis and figure preparation was done using Igor Pro (Wavemetrics) software. Differences between means were determined by paired or unpaired Student's t-test or a One Way ANOVA using MS excel or DataDesk 6 software (Data Description, Inc). Non-parametric comparisons were conducted utilizing Chi-Square analysis using excel or DataDesk 6 or the Kolmogorov-Smirnov test using Igor Pro. Numerical results are reported as mean ± SEM.

RESULTS

PRINCIPAL NEURONS IN THE LDT, DR, AND LC APPEAR NORMAL IN OREXIN RECEPTOR NULL MICE

To determine if the absence of orexin receptors resulted in gross anomalies in the development of brainstem cholinergic and monoaminergic nuclei, we inspected immunohistochemically stained tissue sections through the LDT, DR, and LC. We examined nNOS, TpH, and TH staining in sections from C57BL6 mice ($n = 2$) and from mice lacking one or both receptors ($n = 2$ for each genotype). **Figure 1** shows comparable tissue sections through the LDT, DR, and LC from a C57BL6 mouse (left column) and a DKO mouse (right column) stained for nNOS (top row), TpH (middle row), and TH (bottom row). Immunoreactivity appeared highly specific and the expected pools of labeled neurons were observed in sections from each genotype. No gross differences were observed in distribution of stained neurons or in the range of cell shapes in any of the receptor knockouts. This suggests that mesopontine cholinergic and monoaminergic neurons will be found in their expected locations and will be encountered at about the same rate in brain slice experiments from normal and receptor knockout mice. Of course, this qualitative observation does not rule out quantitative differences that might be present between knockout and wild type mice (see Kalogiannis et al., 2010; Valko et al., 2013).

OREXIN-A PRODUCES COMPARABLE NOISY INWARD CURRENT IN SLICES FROM C57BL6 AND HYBRID BACKGROUND CONTROL MICE

In our previous studies of orexin actions on LDT and DR neurons, we conducted whole-cell recordings and Ca²⁺ imaging using slices made from C57BL6 mice (Burlet et al., 2002;

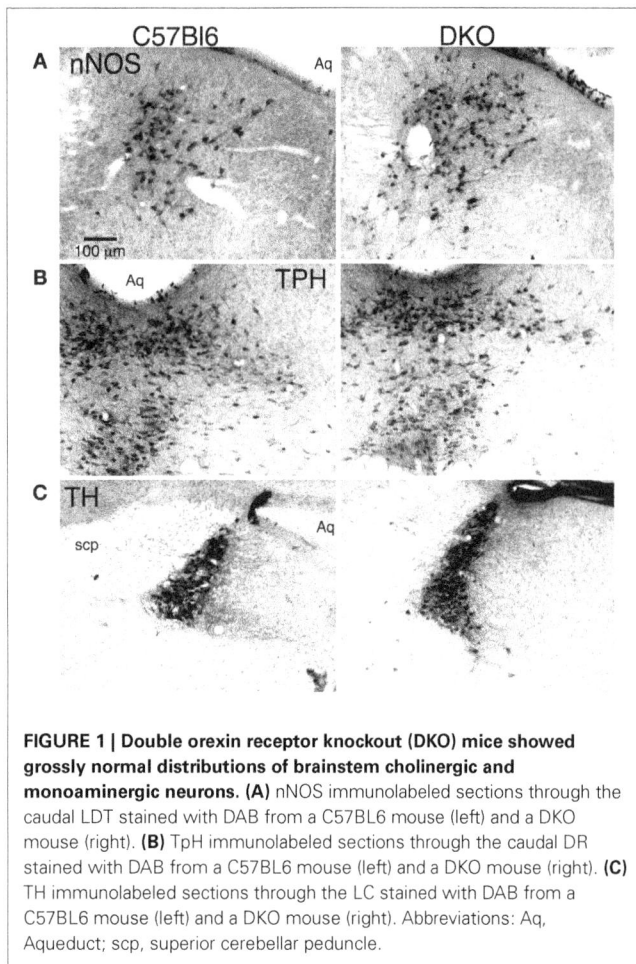

FIGURE 1 | Double orexin receptor knockout (DKO) mice showed grossly normal distributions of brainstem cholinergic and monoaminergic neurons. (A) nNOS immunolabeled sections through the caudal LDT stained with DAB from a C57BL6 mouse (left) and a DKO mouse (right). (B) TpH immunolabeled sections through the caudal DR stained with DAB from a C57BL6 mouse (left) and a DKO mouse (right). (C) TH immunolabeled sections through the LC stained with DAB from a C57BL6 mouse (left) and a DKO mouse (right). Abbreviations: Aq, Aqueduct; scp, superior cerebellar peduncle.

Kohlmeier et al., 2004, 2008). Since receptor null mice were on C57BL6/129SvEv hybrid background, we initially examined the ability of a bath application of orexin-A (300 nM) to evoke an inward current from a holding potential of −60 mV in LDT and DR neurons in slices from C57BL6 and background control mice (OxrWT). As expected, orexin-A activated a noisy inward current in both nuclei and this current appeared identical in both strains. In the LDT, we recorded 16 neurons from 13 C57BL6 mice and 7 neurons from 6 OxrWT mice. There was no difference in the mean current (C57BL6: −19.1 ± 2.4 pA; OxrWT: −15.2 ± 3.1 pA; $P = 0.38$) and there was no difference in the distribution of current amplitudes, including the three C57BL6 and two OxrWT neurons that didn't respond (Kolmogorov-Smirnov test, $P = 0.24$). In the DR, we recorded 31 neurons from 22 C57BL6 mice and 16 neurons from 8 OxrWT mice. There was no difference in the mean current from cells that responded to orexin (C57BL6: −36.3 ± 2.9 pA; OxrWT: −36.9 ± 3.2 pA; $P = 0.89$) and there was no difference in the distributions, including the one C57BL6 and two OxrWT neurons that didn't respond (Kolmogorov-Smirnov test, $P = 1$). This suggests that the differences in genetic background of C57BL6 and hybrid mice has little influence on the expression of orexin currents.

ACTIVATION OF OX$_1$ PRODUCES INWARD CURRENT AND ENHANCED Ca^{2+} TRANSIENTS IN LDT, DR, AND LC NEURONS

To test the ability of OX$_1$ to sustain orexin signaling in the LDT, DR, and LC, we recorded from slices made from OX$_2^{-/-}$ mice and compared the orexin responses obtained in these knockouts with those in slices obtained from C57BL6 mice (Figure 2). In each nucleus, we examined the ability of a bath application of orexin-A (300 nM) to evoke an inward current from a holding potential of −60 mV and to enhance the Ca^{2+} influx produced by a voltage-step from −60 to −30 mV.

In LDT neurons recorded from OX$_2^{-/-}$ mice, orexin-A evoked a slowly developing inward current, often with an increase in frequency and amplitude of sEPSPs (Figure 2A$_1$; normal ACSF) that appeared quite similar to the responses previously described in nNOS+ LDT neurons (Burlet et al., 2002). We did not analyze the increase in sEPSC frequency in detail, but we compared the average magnitude of the slowly developing inward orexin current recorded from a holding potential of −60 mV (low-Ca^{2+} DABST-containing ACSF with Cs). This post-synaptic depolarizing current was −40.7 ± 13.0 pA ($n = 7$) which was not statistically different from the inward current measured from LDT neurons in slices from C57BL6 mice recorded under identical conditions (32.8 ± 10.6 pA; $n = 8$; $P > 0.05$; Figure 2D$_1$). Orexin-A (300 nM) also enhanced the Ca^{2+}-transient evoked by a 5 s voltage-jump from −60 to −30 mV by 30.4 ± 6.4% ($n = 9/12$) in neurons from OX$_2^{-/-}$ mice (Figure 2A$_2$; DABST-containing ACSF). The magnitude of this Ca^{2+} transient enhancement was also not different from that measured in LDT neurons from C57BL6 mice (31.1 ± 7.7%; $n = 9/13$; $P > 0.05$; Figure 2D$_2$).

In DR neurons recorded in slices from OX$_2^{-/-}$ mice, orexin A (300 nM) also evoked a slow inward current (Figure 2B$_1$; normal ACSF) as observed previously (Brown et al., 2002; Liu et al., 2002; Kohlmeier et al., 2008). These inward currents were not accompanied by increases in sEPSCs, as expected from a previous study (Haj-Dahmane and Shen, 2005). The average amplitude of the orexin-evoked slow inward current was −55.2 ± 14.4 pA ($n = 8$; low-Ca^{2+} DABST-containing ACSF with Cs). This was not statistically different from the orexin-evoked current measured from DR neurons in slices from C57BL6 mice under the same conditions (88.0 ± 24.1 pA; $n = 7$; $P > 0.05$; Figure 2D$_1$). In the voltage-step paradigm, orexin-A (300 nM) also enhanced the Ca^{2+}-transient evoked by steps from −60 to −30 mV by 32.3 ± 8.7% ($n = 13/18$) in neurons from OX$_2^{-/-}$ mice (Figure 2A$_2$; DABST-containing ACSF) as reported in wild-type DR neurons (Kohlmeier et al., 2008). This enhancement in neurons from OX$_2^{-/-}$ mice was also not different from that measured in DR neurons from C57BL6 mice (28.6 ± 3.5, $n = 9/14$; $P > 0.05$; Figure 2D$_2$) recorded under the same conditions.

In LC neurons from OX$_2^{-/-}$ mice, orexin-A (300 nM) produced a small, slow inward current (Figure 2C$_1$; normal ACSF). The average current evoked by orexin-A was 11.4 ± 1.2 pA ($n = 28$; DABST-containing ACSF) and was not different from the average current measured from LC neurons in slices from C57BL6 mice under the same conditions (12.4 ± 1.8 pA; $n = 12$; $P > 0.05$; Figure 2D$_1$). Orexin-A (300 nM) also produced a strong enhancement of the Ca^{2+} transient evoked by a voltage step

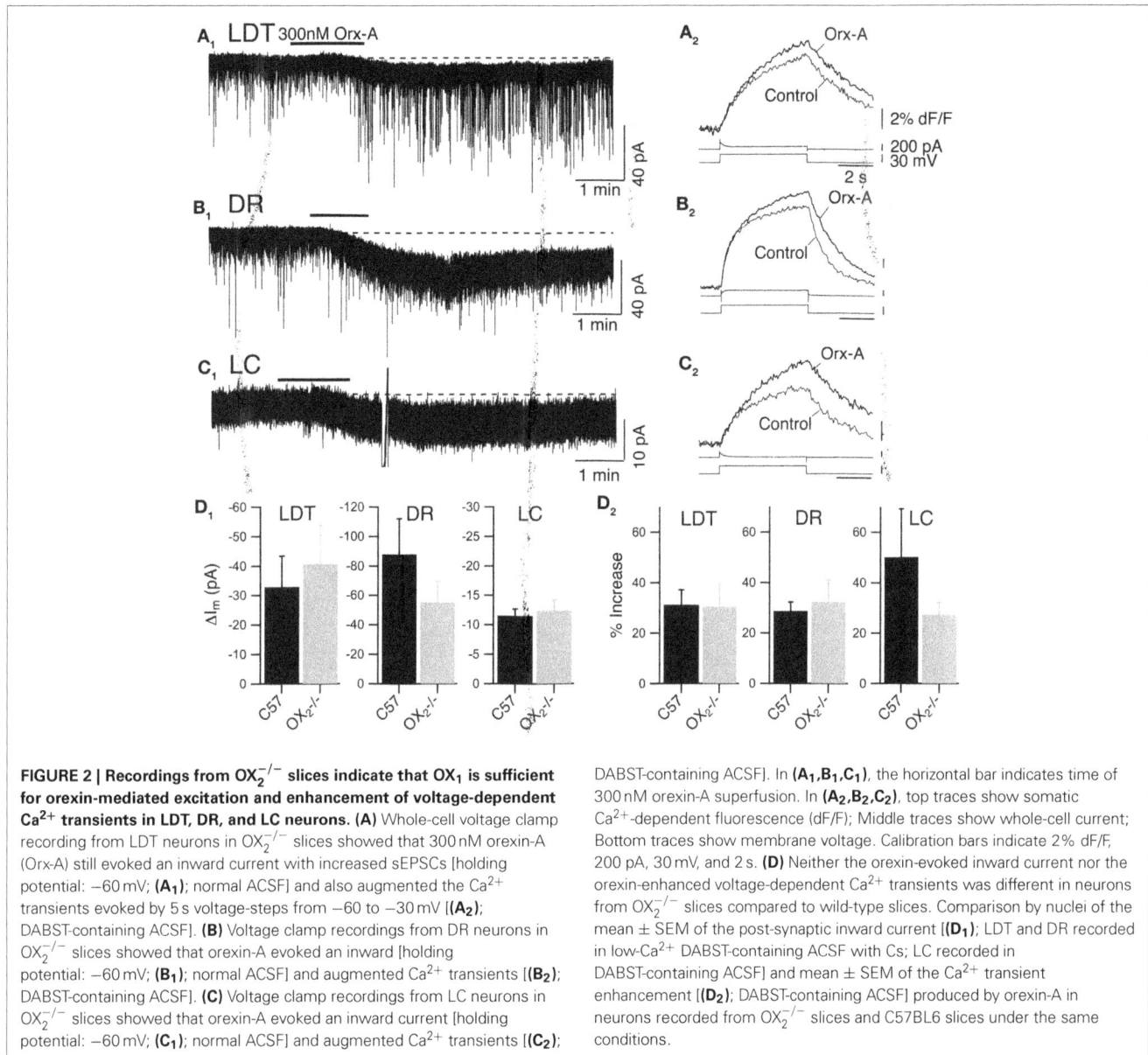

FIGURE 2 | Recordings from $OX_2^{-/-}$ slices indicate that OX_1 is sufficient for orexin-mediated excitation and enhancement of voltage-dependent Ca^{2+} transients in LDT, DR, and LC neurons. (A) Whole-cell voltage clamp recording from LDT neurons in $OX_2^{-/-}$ slices showed that 300 nM orexin-A (Orx-A) still evoked an inward current with increased sEPSCs [holding potential: −60 mV; **(A₁)**; normal ACSF] and also augmented the Ca^{2+} transients evoked by 5 s voltage-steps from −60 to −30 mV [**(A₂)**; DABST-containing ACSF]. **(B)** Voltage clamp recordings from DR neurons in $OX_2^{-/-}$ slices showed that orexin-A evoked an inward [holding potential: −60 mV; **(B₁)**; normal ACSF] and augmented Ca^{2+} transients [**(B₂)**; DABST-containing ACSF]. **(C)** Voltage clamp recordings from LC neurons in $OX_2^{-/-}$ slices showed that orexin-A evoked an inward current [holding potential: −60 mV; **(C₁)**; normal ACSF] and augmented Ca^{2+} transients [**(C₂)**;

DABST-containing ACSF]. In **(A₁,B₁,C₁)**, the horizontal bar indicates time of 300 nM orexin-A superfusion. In **(A₂,B₂,C₂)**, top traces show somatic Ca^{2+}-dependent fluorescence (dF/F); Middle traces show whole-cell current; Bottom traces show membrane voltage. Calibration bars indicate 2% dF/F, 200 pA, 30 mV, and 2 s. **(D)** Neither the orexin-evoked inward current nor the orexin-enhanced voltage-dependent Ca^{2+} transients was different in neurons from $OX_2^{-/-}$ slices compared to wild-type slices. Comparison by nuclei of the mean ± SEM of the post-synaptic inward current [**(D₁)**; LDT and DR recorded in low-Ca^{2+} DABST-containing ACSF with Cs; LC recorded in DABST-containing ACSF] and mean ± SEM of the Ca^{2+} transient enhancement [**(D₂)**; DABST-containing ACSF] produced by orexin-A in neurons recorded from $OX_2^{-/-}$ slices and C57BL6 slices under the same conditions.

from −60 to −30 mV (**Figure 2C₂**; DABST-containing ACSF) in LC neurons. This enhancement was on average 27.2 ± 4.8% ($n = 11/17$) and was not different from that obtained from LC neurons from C57BL6 mice (50.19 ± 19.1%; $n = 6/8$; $P > 0.05$; **Figure 2D₂**) recorded under the same conditions. Collectively, these data indicate that OX_1 is sufficient to mediate two normal actions of orexin on LDT, DR, and LC neurons: (1) post-synaptic activation of a slowly developing inward current and (2) the enhancement of voltage-dependent Ca^{2+} influx.

To determine if OX_1 mediated these actions in principal neurons from each nucleus, we processed brain slices from $OX_2^{-/-}$ mice for immunocytochemistry to identify the transmitter phenotype of recorded neurons. In the LDT, we confirmed that OX_1 activation produced an inward current in six nNOS+ neurons and that OX_1 activation enhanced the voltage-step

evoked Ca^{2+} transient in four nNOS+ neurons. In the DR, we confirmed that OX_1 activation produced an inward current in nine TpH+ neurons and enhanced the voltage-step evoked Ca^{2+} transient in four TpH+ neurons. Similarly, in the LC, we confirmed that OX_1 activation produced an inward current in 24 TH+ neurons and enhanced the voltage-step evoked Ca^{2+} transient in 2/4 TH+ neurons. **Figure 3** illustrates examples of an nNOS+ neuron recorded in the LDT (**Figure 3A**), a TPH+ neuron recorded in the DR (**Figure 3B**) and a TH+ neuron recorded in the LC. Each of these neurons showed an OX_1-mediated inward current and an enhancement of the Ca^{2+} transient evoked by voltage steps from −60 to −30 mV. From these data we conclude that OX_1 is sufficient to mediate major direct orexin actions on principal cells of these nuclei.

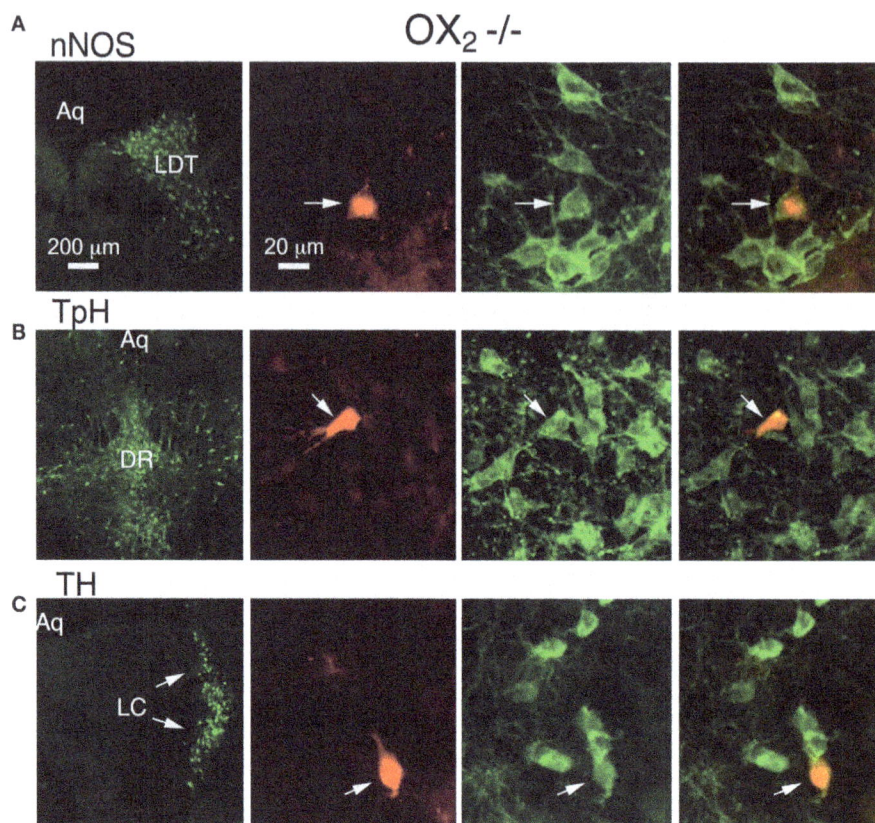

FIGURE 3 | Stimulation of OX$_1$ alone is sufficient to produce inward currents and augmented voltage-dependent Ca^{2+} transients in nNOS+ LDT neurons (A), TpH+ DR neurons (B), and TH+ LC neurons (C). Left column illustrates low-power fluorescent micrographs of the recorded slices immunostained and visualized with an Alexa-488-label (green) for nNOS in LDT **(A)**, TpH in DR **(B)**, and TH in the LC **(C)**. The second column illustrates a higher-power image of the recorded and red fluorescently labeled neuron (arrow; Alexa 594) in each nucleus. The third column shows the same field with Alexa 488 visualized. The right column merges the Alexa 488 and 594 images and indicates that each recorded neuron was immunopositive for nNOS, TpH, and TH, respectively.

OX$_1$ ACTIVATES A NOISY CATION CURRENT IN LDT AND DR NEURONS AND ENHANCES Ca^{2+} TRANSIENTS MEDIATED BY L-TYPE Ca^{2+} CHANNELS IN LDT, DR, AND LC NEURONS

As noted above, previous studies of LDT and DR neurons indicate that a noisy non-selective cation current is an important effector mediating the slow membrane depolarization produced by orexin-A. We therefore examined the change in membrane noise and the current-voltage relation of the current evoked in LDT and DR neurons from OX$_2^{-/-}$ mice to determine if OX$_1$ is competent to activate a similar current. Since current evoked by orexin-A in LC neurons was quite small in our recordings, and since they did not show a similar increase in noise, we did not further characterize their orexin currents. In both LDT (**Figure 4A$_1$**) and DR (**Figure 4B$_1$**) neurons from OX$_2^{-/-}$ mice, orexin-A (300 nM) produced an inward current that was accompanied by a large increase in membrane current noise, similar to that reported in wild-type mice (Kohlmeier et al., 2008). The membrane current noise increased by $118.4 \pm 59.3\%$ in LDT neurons ($n = 8$) and by $307 \pm 87.0\%$ in DR neurons ($n = 7$) which was not different from values in LDT ($86.8 \pm 31.3\%$, $n = 8$; $P > 0.05$) and DR ($380.5 \pm 85.2\%$; $n = 7$; $P >$

0.05) from C57BL6 mice. Similarly, the I-V relation for the orexin mediated current in LDT (**Figure 4A$_2$**) and DR neurons (**Figure 4B$_2$**) from OX$_2^{-/-}$ mice was computed from voltage ramps between -100 and -35 mV. It appeared roughly linear over this range as previously described for C57BL6 neurons in these nuclei (Kohlmeier et al., 2008) suggesting that OX$_1$ activates the same channel or channels that are activated in C57BL6 mice.

In LDT and DR neurons from C57BL6 mice, the orexin mediated enhancement of voltage-dependent Ca^{2+} transients produced by voltage-steps from -60 to -30 mV is produced almost entirely by the enhancement of Ca^{2+} transients generated by L-type Ca^{2+} channels (Kohlmeier et al., 2008). We therefore tested whether the L-channel antagonist nifedipine (10 μM), also occludes this enhancement in LDT, DR, and LC neurons in slices from OX$_2$ mice. Nifedipine alone, attenuated the Ca^{2+} transient produced by a voltage-step from -30 to -60 mV in LDT (**Figure 4C**), DR (**Figure 4D**), and LC (**Figure 4E**) neurons indicating that activation of L-type channels contribute to these transients. In the presence of nifedipine, orexin failed to significantly enhance the calcium transient in all cells examined

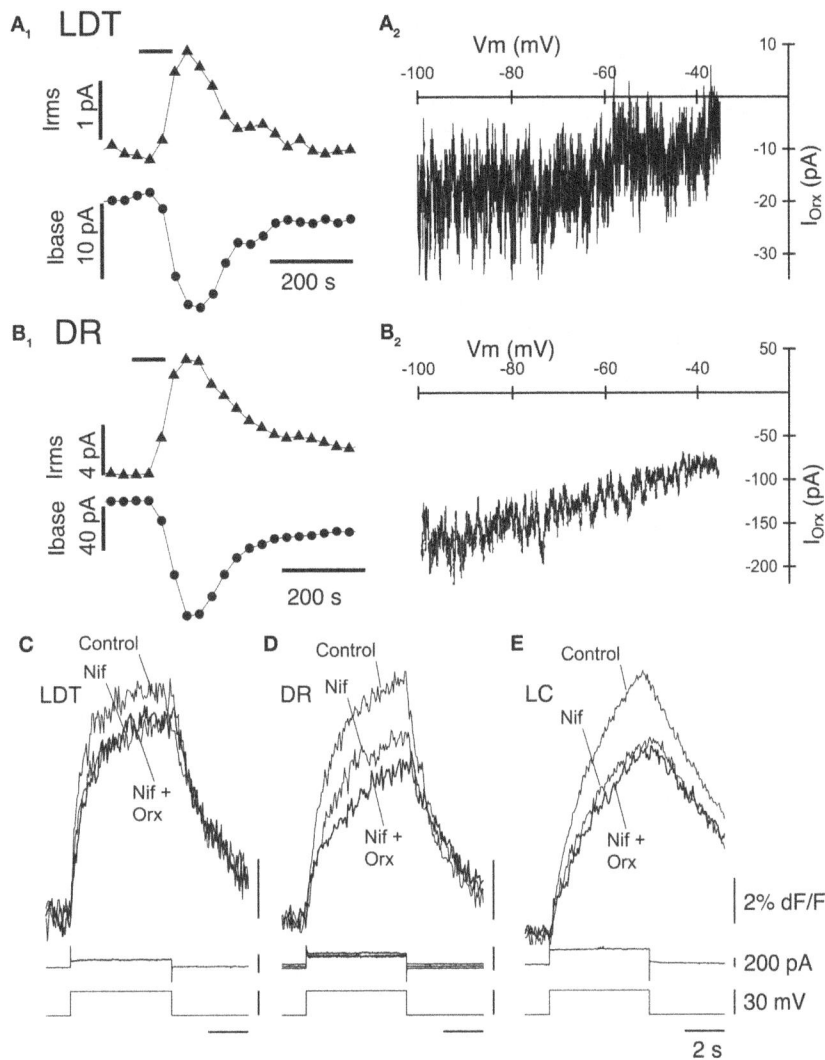

FIGURE 4 | Stimulation of OX$_1$ alone activates a noisy cation current in LDT and DR neurons and enhance voltage-dependent Ca^{2+} transients mediated by L-type Ca^{2+} channels in LDT, DR, and LC neurons. (A$_1$) Holding current (at −60 mV; Ibase; bottom trace) and membrane current noise (Irms; top trace) were measured every 30 s starting before bath application of 300 nM orexin-A (horizontal bar) from LDT neurons in OX$_2^{-/-}$ slices. Orexin produced an inward shift in holding current that was accompanied by an increase in current noise. **(A$_2$)** The I-V curve of the orexin-evoked inward current (I$_{Orx}$) was obtained by subtracting the membrane current produced by a voltage ramp between −100 and −35 mV prior to orexin-A application from that obtained during the peak of the orexin-A-evoked inward current. These currents were similar to those obtained from LDT neurons in C57BL6 slices. **(B$_1$)** Orexin-A (300 nM) has a similar, but larger effect on the holding current (Ibase, bottom) and membrane current noise (Irms, top) in DR neurons recorded in OX$_2^{-/-}$ slices. **(B$_2$)** The I-V relation for the orexin-evoked inward current (I$_{Orx}$) in a DR neuron from an OX$_2^{-/-}$ slice was similar that that observed in DR neurons from C57BL6 slices. **(C,D,E)**. The L-channel antagonist, nifedipine (Nif, 10 μM) attenuated the Ca^{2+}-transients evoked by voltage-steps from −60 to −30 mV in LDT **(C)**, DR **(D)**, and LC **(E)** neurons from OX$_2^{-/-}$ slices and completely blocked the enhancement of these transients by orexin-A (300 nM). Top traces show somatic Ca^{2+}-dependent fluorescence (dF/F); Middle traces show whole-cell current; Bottom traces show membrane voltage. Calibration bar labels in **(E)**, also apply to **(C)** and **(D)**.

within the LDT, DR, or LC (LDT: 9% reduction in the transient, $P > 0.05$, $n = 4$; DR: 5.2% reduction in the transient, $P > 0.05$, $n = 4$; LC: 1.8% increase in the transient, $P > 0.05$, $n = 4$). These data suggest that the Ca^{2+} transients augmented by OX$_1$ signaling are mediated by enhanced influx via L-type Ca^{2+} channels. Thus, activation of OX$_1$ alone is sufficient to activate a noisy cation current in LDT and DR neurons and to enhance Ca^{2+} transients which appear generated by L-type Ca^{2+} channels in the LDT, DR, and LC.

ACTIVATION OF OX$_2$ EXCITES DR NEURONS AND ENHANCES Ca^{2+} TRANSIENTS IN LDT, DR, AND LC NEURONS

To determine whether activation of OX$_2$ alone can influence membrane currents and Ca^{2+} transients in LDT, DR, and LC neurons, we examined the action of orexin-A in slices prepared from mice lacking OX$_1$. Whole-cell recordings from LDT ($n = 14$) and LC ($n = 45$) neurons revealed that in that absence of OX$_1$, 300 nM orexin-A failed to induce a detectable inward current at a holding potential of −60 mV (**Figures 5A$_1$,C$_1$**).

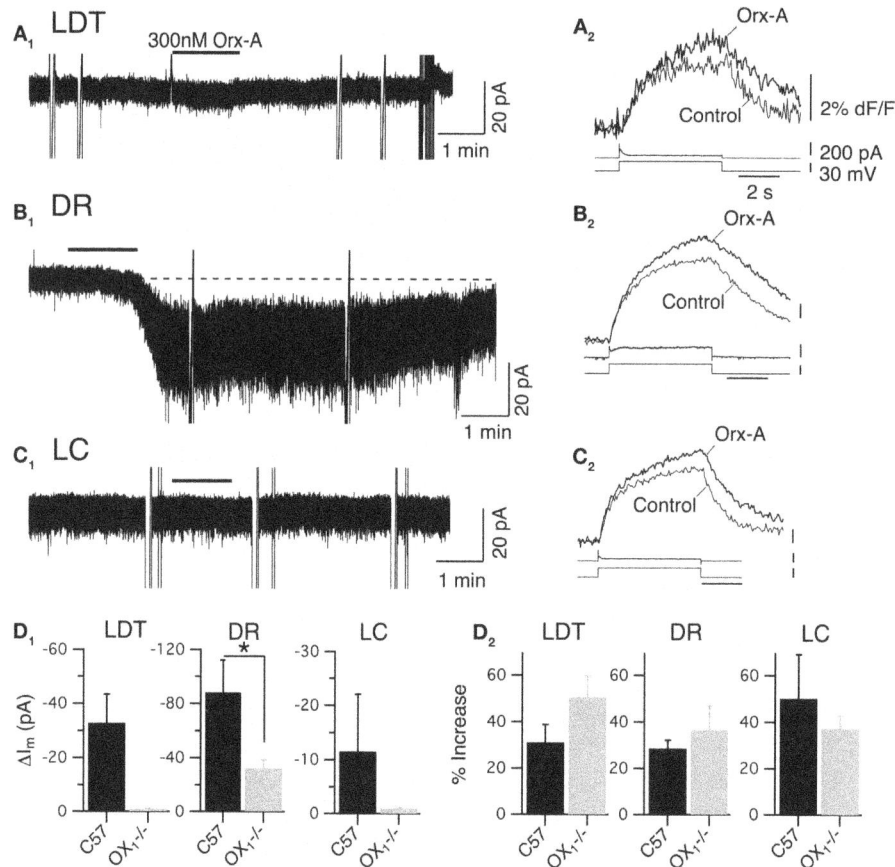

FIGURE 5 | Stimulation of OX$_2$ alone is sufficient to produce an inward current in DR neurons and to enhance voltage-dependent Ca^{2+} transients in LDT, DR, and LC neurons. (A) Whole-cell voltage clamp recordings obtained from LDT neurons in OX$_1^{-/-}$ slices showed that 300 nM orexin-A (Orx-A) failed to evoke a current at −60 mV (A$_1$) but augmented voltage-dependent Ca^{2+} transients evoked by 5 s voltage-steps from −60 to −30 mV (A$_2$). (B) Voltage clamp recordings obtained from DR neurons in OX$_1^{-/-}$ slices showed that orexin-A evoked both a noisy inward current (holding potential: −60 mV; B$_1$) and augmented voltage-dependent Ca^{2+} transients (B$_2$). (C) Voltage clamp recordings obtained from LC neurons in OX$_1^{-/-}$ slices showed that orexin-A failed to evoke an inward current (holding

potential: −60 mV; C$_1$) but augmented voltage-dependent Ca^{2+} transients (C$_2$). In (A$_1$,B$_1$,C$_1$), the horizontal bar indicates time of 300 nM orexin-A superfusion. In (A$_2$,B$_2$,C$_2$), Top traces show somatic Ca^{2+}-dependent fluorescence (dF/F); Middle traces show whole-cell current; Bottom traces show membrane voltage. Calibration bars indicate 2% dF/F, 200 pA, 30 mV and 2 s. (D) The orexin-A evoked inward current was absent in LDT and LC neurons and was significantly smaller in DR neurons from OX$_1^{-/-}$ slices than in DR neurons from C57BL6 slices (D$_1$; *P < 0.05). In contrast, the magnitude of the Ca^{2+} transient enhancement produced by orexin-A was the same in LDT, DR, and LC neurons from OX$_1^{-/-}$ slices compared to those recorded in C57BL6 slices.

In contrast, orexin-A application to DR neurons resulted in significant inward current with a large increase in membrane noise (**Figure 5B$_1$**). Nevertheless, the average peak inward current elicited by orexin-A in DR neurons (32.2 ± 6.3 pA; n = 8) was significantly lower than observed in control recordings from DR neurons in slices from C57BL6 mice (88.0 ± 24.1 pA; n = 7; P < 0.05; **Figure 5D$_1$**).

Despite being unable to stimulate inward currents in LDT and LC neurons from OX$_1^{-/-}$ mice, orexin-A was effective at enhancing Ca^{2+} transients evoked by voltage-jumps from −60 to −30 mV in LDT, DR and LC neurons (**Figures 5A$_2$,B$_2$,C$_2$**). In fact, on average the magnitude of the enhancement in the absence of OX$_1$ (LDT: 50.6 ± 9.0%, n = 7/17; DR: 36.5 ± 10.4, n = 11/18; LC: 37.3 ± 5.5, n = 8/13) was as large as observed in control neurons from C57BL6 mice (**Figure 5D$_2$**; P > 0.05

for each cell type). In a some recordings, we were able to verify that the recorded neurons were nNOS+ in the LDT (n = 6), TpH+ in the DR (n = 9), and TH+ in the LC (n = 13; **Figure 6**). This confirmed that OX$_2$ alone is insufficient to excite neurons in the LDT and LC at subthreshold membrane potentials but is sufficient to do so in TpH+ DR neurons. In spite of this, OX$_2$ activation is able to augment the step-activated Ca^{2+} transients in principal neurons of each of these nuclei. This implies that released orexin would enhance Ca^{2+} influx during persistent activity in each nucleus, even in OX$_1$ null mice.

We also examined the I–V relation between −100 and −30 mV in LDT and DR neurons. This confirmed that no observable subthreshold currents were activated by orexin-A in LDT neurons (**Figures 7A$_1$,A$_2$**) and that the noisy inward current activated in

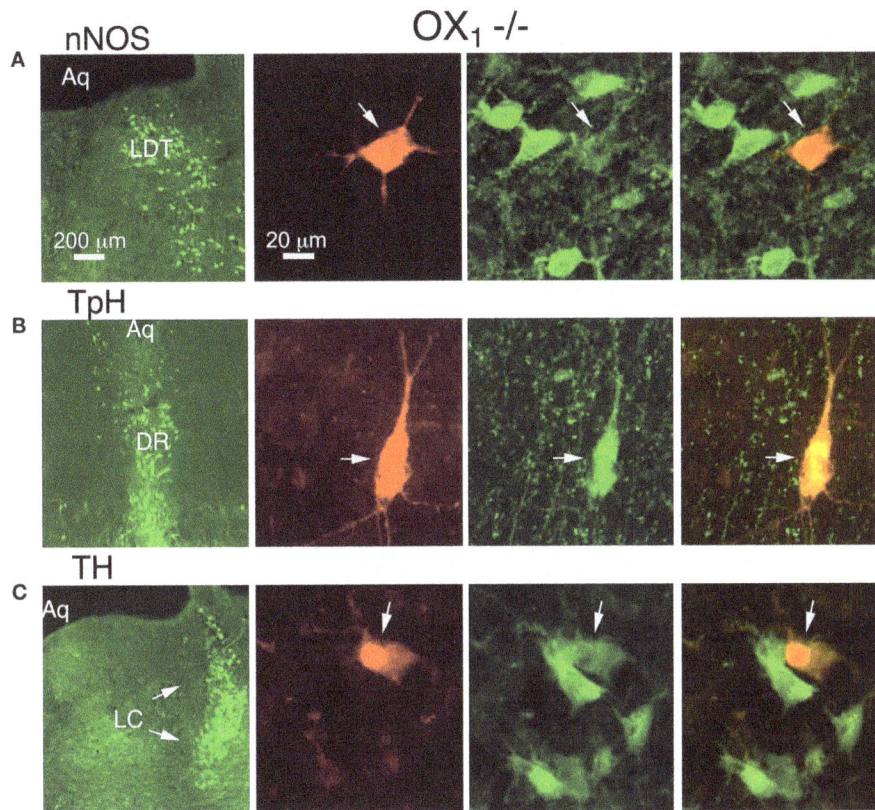

FIGURE 6 | Orexin augments voltage-dependent Ca²⁺ transients in nNOS+ LDT neurons, TpH+ DR neurons, and TH+ LC neurons in slices from OX₁⁻/⁻ mice. Orexin-A augmented the voltage-dependent Ca²⁺ transient in identified neurons. Left column illustrates low-power fluorescent micrographs of the recorded slices immunostained with Alexa-488 (green) for nNOS in LDT **(A)**, TpH in DR **(B)**, and TH in the LC **(C** arrows). The second column illustrates a higher-power image of the recorded and fluorescently labeled neurons (Alexa-594) from each nucleus. The third column shows the same field with Alexa-488 visualized. The right column shows the images merged, revealing that each recorded neuron was immunopositive for nNOS, TpH, and TH, respectively.

DR neurons was approximately linear over this voltage range, having similar characteristics to the non-selective cation current observed in C57BL6 DR neurons (**Figures 7B₁,B₂**). Similarly, we determined whether L-type Ca²⁺ channels are a target of OX₂ by testing whether nifedipine occluded the orexin-A enhancement of Ca²⁺ transients (**Figures 7C,D,E**). In LDT, DR, and LC neurons obtained from mice lacking OX₁, nifedipine blocked the enhancement produced by orexin-A (300 nM) application. In the presence of nifedipine, orexin-A application produced a 0.6 ± 0.4% increase in LDT ($n = 4$), a 4.0 ± 2.1% increase in DR ($n = 5$) and a 3.6 ± 3.3% increase in LC neurons ($n = 6$). These changes were not significantly different from zero ($P > 0.05$) and all of these differences were significantly less than changes produced in neurons from C57BL6 mice ($P < 0.05$). Thus, activation of OX₂ alone is sufficient to activate a noisy cation current in DR neurons but not in LDT or LC neurons. Despite this, OX₂ activation is sufficient to enhance Ca²⁺ transients in the LDT, DR, and LC. Moreover, the magnitude of this enhancement was comparable to the enhancement measured in LDT, DR, and LC neurons from C57BL6 mice and also appear mediated by L-type Ca²⁺ channels.

OX₁ SIGNALING IS DOMINANT IN THE LDT AND LC BUT IS MORE EVENLY SHARED BY BOTH RECEPTORS IN THE DR

To obtain a better estimate of the fraction of neurons activated by each orexin receptor, we utilized fura-2AM loading of slices obtained from mice lacking each receptor (**Figure 8**). Under these conditions, orexin-A (300 nM) evokes Ca²⁺ transients by both depolarization and subsequent activation of a voltage-dependent Ca²⁺ influx and by specific enhancement of the Ca²⁺ transient evoked by L-type Ca²⁺ channel activation (Kohlmeier et al., 2004, 2008). As expected from whole-cell Ca²⁺ transient measurements, 300 nM orexin-A evoked Ca²⁺ transients in slices obtained from mice lacking OX₂ (**Figure 8A**) and mice lacking OX₁ (**Figure 8B**). We found that in each genotype and nucleus, these transients recapitulated the range of temporal profiles we observed in DR and LDT slices from C57BL6 mice (Kohlmeier et al., 2004). Moreover, when the magnitude of the "plateau" type Ca²⁺ responses, which we could confidently measure, were compared, the transients from knockout slices were not smaller than the transients from C57BL6 slices. In OX₂ null tissue, the average plateau responses were 11.9 ± 1.8% in LDT ($n = 13$); 9.9 ± 1.9% in DR ($n = 18$); and 12.1 ± 2.4% in LC

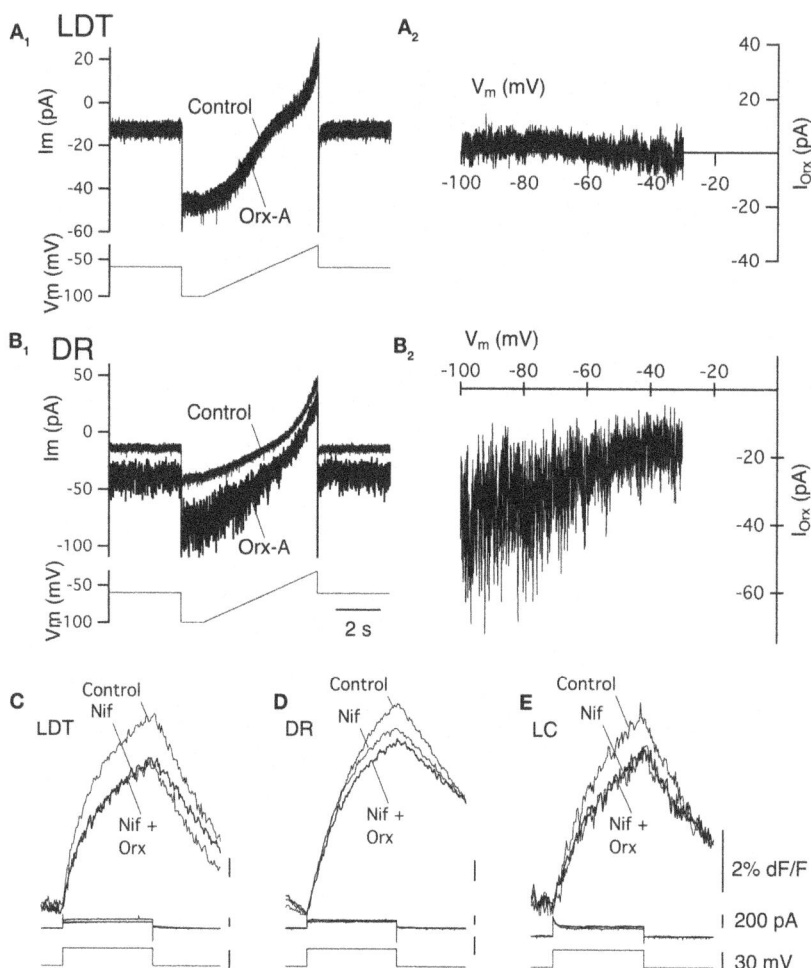

FIGURE 7 | Stimulation of OX_2 alone activate a noisy cation current in DR neurons and enhance Ca^{2+} transients mediated by L-type Ca^{2+} channels in LDT, DR, and LC neurons. (A_1) Whole-cell voltage clamp currents (upper traces) from an LDT neuron in an $OX_1^{-/-}$ slice recorded before and after bath superfusion with orexin-A (Orx-A, 300 nM). These currents were produced by the voltage-ramp in the bottom trace (−100 to −35 mV). Orexin failed to produce an inward shift in holding current in LDT neurons from $OX_1^{-/-}$ mice. **(A_2)** The difference between the currents in **(A_1)** plotted as a function of membrane voltage (Vm) shows the I-V relation. No orexin current was detectable throughout the voltage range studied. **(B_1)** Orexin-A (300 nM) produced an inward shift in holding current and a large increase in membrane current noise in DR neurons recorded in $OX_1^{-/-}$ slices. **(B_2)** The I-V relation for the difference current from **(B_1)** appeared nearly linear and was characteristic of the cation current observed in DR neurons from C57BL6 slices. **(C,D,E)** The L-channel antagonist, nifedipine (Nif, 10 μM) attenuated the Ca^{2+}-transients evoked by voltage-steps from −60 to −30 mV in LDT **(C)**, DR **(D)**, and LC **(E)** neurons from $OX_1^{-/-}$ slices and prevented the enhancement of these transients by orexin-A (300 nM). Top traces show somatic Ca^{2+}-dependent fluorescence (dF/F); Middle traces show whole-cell current; Bottom traces show membrane voltage. Calibration bar labels in **(E)**, also apply to **(C,D)**.

($n = 12$), which were not different ($P > 0.05$) from responses measured in slices from C57BL6 mice ($11.0 \pm 2.2\%$ in LDT, $n = 29$; $13.8 \pm 2.6\%$ in DR, $n = 49$; and $12.7 \pm 2.3\%$ in LC, $n = 24$). Similarly, in OX_1 null slices, the average plateau response were not different ($P > 0.05$) from those in C57BL6 slices (OX_1 null responses: $12.0 \pm 4.3\%$ in LDT, $n = 12$; $16.1 \pm 2.5\%$ in DR, $n = 15$; and $15.1 \pm 5.1\%$ in LC, $n = 5$). However, the likelihood of encountering orexin-A responsive cells (**Figure 8C**) was much lower in slices from OX_1 null mice in both the LDT and LC. The proportion of fura-2AM labeled cells responding to orexin was only 20% in LDT ($n = 113$) and 10% in LC ($n = 82$) compared to estimates of 60–70% responding in

slices from C57BL6 mice. Interestingly, in the DR from OX_1 null mice, the fraction of responders was only reduced to 47.1% from about 70% in the C57BL6 mice. Presumably this high percent responding in the DR reflects the ability of OX_2 to drive depolarizations in DR neurons unlike in LDT and LC neurons.

OX_1 AND OX_2 SIGNALING IS ATTENUATED BY PKC INHIBITION

In the next series of experiments we examined whether the PKC inhibitor Bis I attenuates the Ca^{2+} transients evoked by activity of one or both receptors. In these experiments, we first obtained control responses with bath application of orexin-A

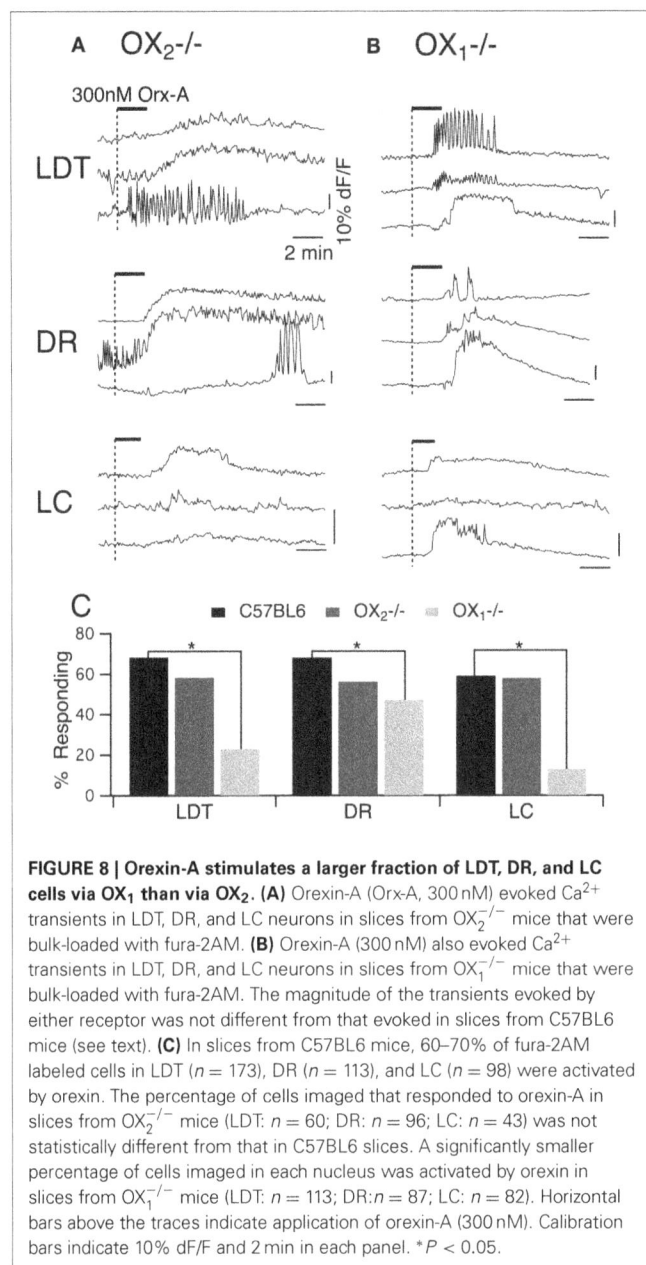

FIGURE 8 | Orexin-A stimulates a larger fraction of LDT, DR, and LC cells via OX$_1$ than via OX$_2$. (A) Orexin-A (Orx-A, 300 nM) evoked Ca^{2+} transients in LDT, DR, and LC neurons in slices from OX$_2^{-/-}$ mice that were bulk-loaded with fura-2AM. **(B)** Orexin-A (300 nM) also evoked Ca^{2+} transients in LDT, DR, and LC neurons in slices from OX$_1^{-/-}$ mice that were bulk-loaded with fura-2AM. The magnitude of the transients evoked by either receptor was not different from that evoked in slices from C57BL6 mice (see text). **(C)** In slices from C57BL6 mice, 60–70% of fura-2AM labeled cells in LDT ($n = 173$), DR ($n = 113$), and LC ($n = 98$) were activated by orexin. The percentage of cells imaged that responded to orexin-A in slices from OX$_2^{-/-}$ mice (LDT: $n = 60$; DR: $n = 96$; LC: $n = 43$) was not statistically different from that in C57BL6 slices. A significantly smaller percentage of cells imaged in each nucleus was activated by orexin in slices from OX$_1^{-/-}$ mice (LDT: $n = 113$; DR: $n = 87$; LC: $n = 82$). Horizontal bars above the traces indicate application of orexin-A (300 nM). Calibration bars indicate 10% dF/F and 2 min in each panel. *$P < 0.05$.

(300 nM) from OX$_2^{-/-}$ or OX$_1^{-/-}$ slices containing LDT, DR, or LC (**Figures 9**, left column in **A,B**). The slices were then superfused with ACSF containing bis I (1 μM; Bis) for 20 min, to inhibit PKC. This completely attenuated the orexin-mediated enhancement of L-type Ca^{2+} transients but did not block the orexin mediated depolarization in all LDT and DR neurons (Kohlmeier et al., 2008). Here, we found that the Ca^{2+} transients evoked in each nucleus were strongly attenuated by Bis in slices from both OX$_2$ and OX$_1$ null mice (**Figures 9**, right column in **A,B**). The average amplitude of plateau responses was reduced by 62.0 ± 7.7% in slices from OX$_2$ null mice ($n = 34$) and by 59.3 ± 8.3 in slices from OX$_1^{-/-}$ mice ($n = 25$). Thus, Ca^{2+} transients evoked by activation of either orexin receptor involves PKC signaling.

OREXIN ACTIONS IN THE LDT, DR, AND LC REQUIRE THE TWO KNOWN OREXIN RECEPTORS

Interpretation of our data from single receptor knockouts presupposes that there are only two orexin receptors responsible for orexin actions and that our test concentration of orexin-A is specific for these receptors. We directly tested this by examining the action of orexin-A on slices made from mice lacking both orexin receptors. As can be seen in **Figure 10A**, orexin-A (300 nM) did not evoke Ca^{2+} transients in slices from DKO mice. To verify that each of the cells recorded under these conditions remained viable, we followed orexin application with a bolus application of glutamate (5 mM), which rapidly and effectively evoked Ca^{2+} transients in these same cells (**Figure 10B**). We also examined extracellular recordings using cell-attached patch recordings, whole-cell currents and the ability of orexin to augment the Ca^{2+} transients produced by step depolarizations to −30 mV. In each of these tests, orexin-A failed to produce a response. Collectively these data strongly indicate that 300 nM orexin-A is specific for native orexin receptors and that OX$_1$ and OX$_2$ are the only functional orexin receptors expressed in the LDT, DR and LC.

WHOLE BRAINSTEM OX$_2$ mRNA LEVELS ARE HIGHER IN MICE LACKING OX$_1$

A potential complication to the interpretation of data from constitutive knockouts is the possibility that the loss of one receptor alters the expression of the other. Indeed, like any lesion study, knockouts can't reveal the function of the missing component but can only reveal the capacity remaining in the absence of that component. We therefore compared OX$_1$ and OX$_2$ mRNA levels isolated from whole brainstems of C57BL6 and receptor knockout mice using quantitative RT-PCR to (**Figure 11**). Since two splice variants of the OX$_2$ were identified in mice (Chen and Randeva, 2004; Chen et al., 2006), we designed primers for OX$_1$ and both OX$_2$ receptors. The primers used for each receptor were specific since PCR produced single amplicons of the predicted sizes. These amplicons were undetectable in samples from the corresponding single receptor knockout or double receptor knockouts (**Figure 11**, see gel insets). Results from ANOVAs comparing target mRNA levels by genotype were highly significant for each transcript ($P < 0.001$). *Post-hoc* testing revealed that the fraction of OX$_1$ mRNA per total mRNA in brainstems from C57BL6 mice (9.75E-6 ± 2.00E-6, $n = 28$ samples from 14 mice) was not different from that measured from OX$_2^{-/-}$ brainstems (1.07E-5 ± 1.39E-6, $n = 28$ samples from 14 mice; $P = 0.62$; **Figure 11A**). In contrast, we found that in OX$_1^{-/-}$ mice, levels of both the OX$_2$α (9.48E-5 ± 2.52E-5, $n = 20$ samples from 10 mice) and OX$_2$β (1.88E-4 ± 3.97E-5, $n = 26$ samples from 13 mice) splice variants were significantly higher compared to those from C57BL6 mice (OX$_2$α: 7.16E-6 ± 2.27E-6, $n = 14$ samples from 7 mice, $P < 0.0001$; OX$_2$β: 1.94E-5 ±3.78E-6, $n = 14$ samples from 7 mice, $P < 0.0005$; **Figures 11B,C**).

Since these differences could indicate upregulation of OX$_2$ expression resulting from the absence of OX$_1$ and since the single receptor knockouts were on a mixed C57BL6 and 129SvEv background, we also measured receptor levels in 129SvEv mice. This comparison indicated that levels of OX$_1$ are higher in

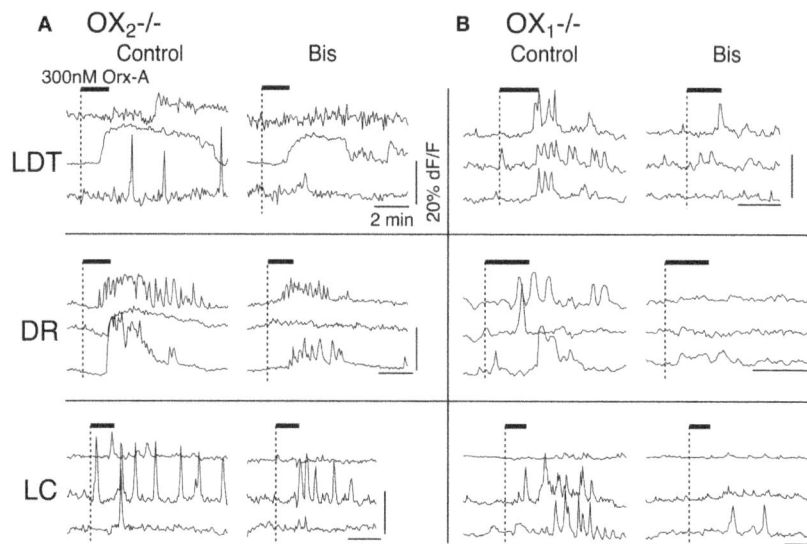

FIGURE 9 | Inhibition of PKC by Bis I attenuated Ca²⁺-transients evoked by activation OX₁ or OX₂. (A) Ca²⁺ transients in LDT, DR, and LC neurons in slices from OX₂⁻/⁻ mice were attenuated by prior application of Bis I. **(B)** Similarly, Ca²⁺ transients in LDT, DR, and LC neurons in slices from OX₁⁻/⁻ mice were attenuated by prior application of Bis I. Horizontal bars above the traces indicate application of orexin-A (300 nM). Calibration bars indicate 20% dF/F and 2 min in each panel.

129SvEv brainstems than in either C57BL6 or OX₂⁻/⁻ brainstems (2.89E-5 ± 2.04-06, $n = 16$ samples from 8 mice, $P < 0.0001$ for both; **Figure 9A**). Interestingly, levels of OX₂α (4.08E-5 ± 1.46E-5, $n = 16$ samples from 8 mice) and OX₂β (7.21E-5 ± 3.22E-5, $n = 15$ samples from 8 mice) from 129SvEv brainstems were not statistically different from those in C57BL6 brainstems (OX₂α: $P = 0.18$; OX₂β: $P = 0.17$) but were significantly lower than those from OX₁⁻/⁻ brainstems (OX₂α : $P < 0.02$; OX₂β: $P < 0.02$; **Figures 11B,C**). These findings suggest that background alone is not the reason that OX₂ mRNA levels are higher in brainstems from OX₁⁻/⁻ mice and therefore imply some level of compensation.

DISCUSSION

A major finding of this study is that OX₁ exclusively mediates direct depolarization of nNOS+ LDT and TH+ LC neurons, while both receptors mediate direct depolarization of TpH+ DR neurons. In contrast, augmentation of depolarization-induced Ca²⁺ transients was mediated by OX₁ and OX₂ in each nucleus and likely involved L-type Ca²⁺ channels and PKC signaling. Finally, we found whole-brainstem OX₂ mRNA levels were elevated in OX₁⁻/⁻ mice. These findings have implications for understanding the cellular function of native orexin receptors, for understanding the roles played by orexin signaling at these loci in the control of behavioral state and for understanding the consequences of using receptor specific antagonists as therapeutics.

Interpretation of our results are predicated on the idea that the different observed actions of orexin in OX₁ null and OX₂ null slices result from the absence of orexin receptors rather than from differences in genetic background between each mouse. Since genetic drift occurs and there is allelic variation in each parent strain, possibly in modifier genes, there is some uncertainty to this interpretation (Doetschman, 2009). We found that orexin currents had the same variation of responses and mean amplitude in both C57BL6 mice and in OxrWT, which have the same mixed genetic background as our knockout mice. In both strains, slices from each mouse showed responses to orexin and neither strain showed symptoms of narcolepsy (Kalogiannis et al., 2011) indicating that despite genetic drift and the allelic variations present, orexin signaling at our targets was equivalent in both backgrounds. Moreover, in DKO mice there were no response in any of the cells recorded in any mouse tested, and these mice show severe signs of narcolepsy (Kalogiannis et al., 2011). These considerations, and the recent evidence that the distribution of orexin receptor mRNA is not altered in LDT, DR, or LC in orexin receptor knockouts (Mieda et al., 2011) suggest it is unlikely that the absence of orexin responses result from background effects rather than the loss of the receptor. We therefore interpret our data in terms of receptor loss, mindful of the possibility that responses might also be modulated by background effects.

BOTH NATIVE OREXIN RECEPTORS CAN COUPLE TO A NOISY CATION CURRENT AND L-TYPE Ca²⁺ CHANNELS

Recordings from DR neurons in slices from mice lacking either OX₂ or OX₁ revealed that activation of either receptor evoked a noisy inward current appearing identical to the cation current evoked in wild-type slices (Brown et al., 2002; Liu et al., 2002; Kohlmeier et al., 2008). Since orexin-A did not activate this current in slices lacking both receptors, we conclude that signaling by either receptor converges onto this current and that there are no additional orexin-binding receptors sufficient to mediate this action. The ability of both receptors to augment depolarization-induced Ca²⁺ transients mediated by L-type Ca²⁺ channels via a PKC-sensitive pathway further supports

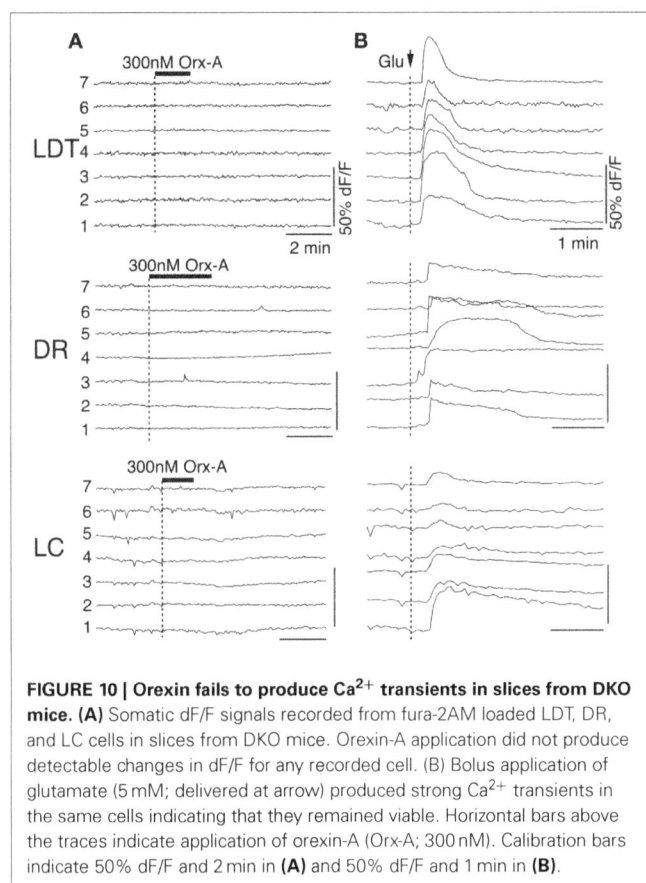

FIGURE 10 | Orexin fails to produce Ca^{2+} transients in slices from DKO mice. (A) Somatic dF/F signals recorded from fura-2AM loaded LDT, DR, and LC cells in slices from DKO mice. Orexin-A application did not produce detectable changes in dF/F for any recorded cell. (B) Bolus application of glutamate (5 mM; delivered at arrow) produced strong Ca^{2+} transients in the same cells indicating that they remained viable. Horizontal bars above the traces indicate application of orexin-A (Orx-A; 300 nM). Calibration bars indicate 50% dF/F and 2 min in **(A)** and 50% dF/F and 1 min in **(B)**.

convergent or redundant functions of native OX_1 and OX_2 in DR neurons. Immunofluorescence identification demonstrated that this convergence includes serotonergic DR neurons (TpH+). These findings fit well with double *in-situ* hybridization evidence indicating both receptors are co-localized within a large fraction of TpH-expressing neurons in mouse DR (Mieda et al., 2011), and with single-cell RT-PCR evidence indicating both OX_1 and OX_2 mRNA is typically recovered from TpH neurons in rat (Brown et al., 2002). Together, these data suggest that both orexin receptors normally excite TpH neurons and augment their intracellular Ca^{2+}-levels during periods of prolonged depolarization.

Since the average OX_1–evoked inward current was somewhat larger than the OX_2–evoked current, and since OX_1 activation produced Ca^{2+} transients in a greater fraction of DR neurons than did OX_2 activation, it is plausible that OX_1 normally mediates the larger part of the orexin-mediated depolarization of DR neurons. A previous pharmacological study of rat DR slices concluded that OX_2 is primarily responsible for orexin-evoked spiking (Soffin et al., 2004). However, that conclusion was based on data that was acknowledged to be difficult to interpret and suffered from limitations related to the use of selective agonists for receptor subtype identification (see also Leonard and Kukkonen, 2013). Co-expression and convergent action of these receptors also likely contributed to interpretive difficulties (e.g., the relatively weak effect of the OX_1-selective antagonist SB 334867). Use of conditional receptor knockouts and development

of subtype-specific receptor antagonists should help to further clarify the natural role of each receptor.

In contrast to the DR, OX_1 was necessary for orexin to elicit depolarizing currents in principal LDT and LC neurons, which fits well with the high levels of OX_1 mRNA in these structures from adult rodents (Marcus et al., 2001; Mieda et al., 2011). Since OX_2 is competent to activate a similar depolarizing current in DR neurons, it is possible that OX_2 is either not expressed, or is incapable of activating available depolarizing channels in LDT and LC neurons. Isotopic *in-situ* hybridization indicates OX_2 message is much less abundant than OX_1 but is above background in both the LDT and LC (Marcus et al., 2001), suggesting that low levels of OX_2 are present. Recent double, non-isotopic, *in-situ* hybridization studies detected OX_2 only in non-cholinergic LDT neurons and non-TH+ LC neurons (Mieda et al., 2011). Nevertheless, we found clear examples of LDT and LC neurons where orexin-A enhanced depolarization-induced Ca^{2+} transients in OX_1 null slices, albeit fewer LDT and LC neurons were activated compared to slices from wild-type or OX_2 null mice (**Figure 8**). Moreover, we recovered nNOS+ and TH+ neurons showing orexin-augmented Ca^{2+}-transients, indicating that OX_2 signaling influences at least a sub-population of these neurons (**Figure 6**). These latter findings are consistent with the possibility that OX_2 expression in LDT and LC neurons might be developmentally regulated and could be lower in adult mice compared to the 2–4 week-old-mice used here, or simply that functional OX_2 receptors are present, but that mRNA levels are too low to be detected with double *in-situ* hybridization methods, which are generally less sensitive than isotopic methods. If this is the case, how then does OX_2 augment the depolarization-induced Ca^{2+} influx without also producing a depolarization? One possibility is that there is spatial segregation of OX_1 and OX_2 and their respective effectors such that OX_2 signaling can't activate the depolarization channels. Another possibility is that each receptor activates different second messenger cascades and the depolarizing channels in LDT and LC are only activated by the cascade(s) from OX_1. Neither scenario has been demonstrated for native orexin receptors and both deserve further investigation. In general, the messenger cascades underlying native orexin receptor actions are poorly understood, although they appear more diverse that originally thought (for review see Kukkonen and Leonard, 2013). Moreover, the cascades mediating depolarization in these neurons have not been identified, although since PKC is involved with augmenting Ca^{2+}-transients, both receptors may activate PLC, as has been often found elsewhere (for review see Kukkonen and Leonard, 2013). While the cation currents activated in LDT and DR appear quite similar, we did find previously that low-Ca^{2+} ACSF augments the DR current, but not the LDT current (Kohlmeier et al., 2008), suggesting the possibility that different channels may mediate the orexin-activated cation current in these neurons. Future experiments are needed to clarify the signaling pathways and effectors utilized by each receptor in these neurons.

Finally, it is also possible that the orexin-enhanced Ca^{2+} transients were produced indirectly by an unknown mediator released from OX_2-expressing nNOS- and TH- neurons in response to orexin-A. This seems unlikely since blocking action potentials with TTX, did not attenuate the orexin effects. However, this is

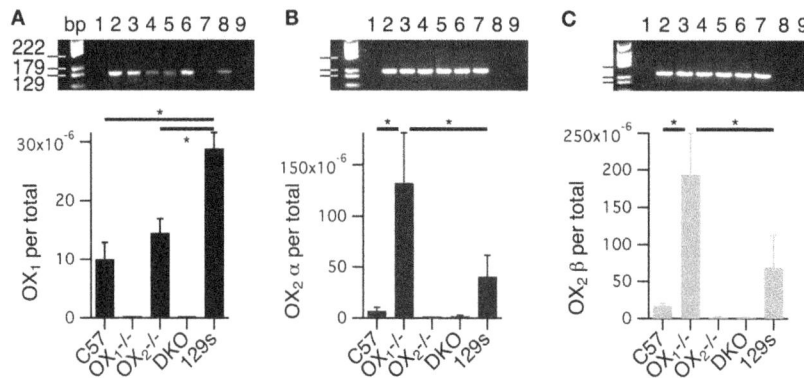

FIGURE 11 | Levels of whole brainstem OX$_2$ mRNA are higher in OX$_1^{-/-}$ mice compared to wild-type mice. (A–C) Top Gel images of the amplicons resulting from probes for OX$_1$ **(A)**, OX$_2\alpha$ **(B)**, and OX$_2\beta$ **(C)**. Samples for each lane were 1: blank, 2–5: scales for corresponding receptor, 6: C57 sample, 7: OX$_1^{-/-}$ sample, 8: OX$_2^{-/-}$ sample, 9: DKO sample. **(A)** Bottom RNA for OX$_1$ (OX$_1$ per total) was quantified from whole brainstems of C57BL6(C57; 28 samples from 14 mice), OX$_1^{-/-}$ (9 samples from 5 mice), OX$_2^{-/-}$ (28 samples from 14 mice), double orexin receptor knockouts (DKO; 8 samples from 4 mice) and 129SvEv (129s; 16 samples from 8 mice) mice by RT-PCR. OX$_1$ mRNA was undetectable in tissue from OX$_{1-/-}$ and DKO mice. Despite significantly higher levels of OX$_1$ mRNA in brainstems from 129s mice compared to C57 and OX$_2^{-/-}$ brainstems (*$P < 0.0001$), there was no significant difference between mRNA levels measured in brainstems from C57 and OX$_2^{-/-}$ mice. **(B)** Bottom mRNA levels for OX$_2\alpha$ (OX$_2\alpha$ per total) were measured from isolates obtained from the same mice used in **(A)**. OX$_2\alpha$ mRNA was undetectable in tissue from OX$_2^{-/-}$ (7 samples from 4 mice) and DKOs (20 samples from 10 mice). OX$_2\alpha$ mRNA levels were higher in OX$_1^{-/-}$ samples (20 samples from 10 mice) than in either C57 (14 samples from 7 mice) or 129s (16 samples from 8 mice) samples (*$P < 0.02$). **(C)** Bottom Similarly, mRNA levels for OX$_2\beta$ (OX$_2\beta$ per total) were measured from mRNA isolates from the same mice in A. OX$_2\beta$ mRNA was undetectable in tissue from OX$_2^{-/-}$ (14 samples from 7 mice) and DKOs (20 samples from 10 mice). OX$_2\beta$ mRNA levels were higher in tissue from OX$_1^{-/-}$ mice (26 samples from 13 mice) than in tissue from either C57 (14 samples from 7 mice) or 129s mice (15 samples from 8 mice, *$P < 0.02$).

difficult to rule out since conventional procedures to block Ca^{2+}-dependent release, like lowering extracellular Ca^{2+} or adding Co^{2+} or Cd^{2+}, also block the Ca^{2+} influx we monitored. Future studies using acutely isolated neurons could help address this issue.

ROLES OF OREXIN SIGNALING IN RETICULAR ACTIVATING SYSTEM NEURONS

Our main finding demonstrates that OX$_1$ is required for orexin-mediated excitation of LC and LDT neurons but that either receptor is sufficient to mediate excitation of DR neurons. While subtle developmental changes in orexin receptor distribution cannot be ruled out, this main finding, obtained from young mice, agrees very well with orexin receptor mRNA levels in these neurons from adult mice (Mieda et al., 2011). It is therefore possible to compare the impairment of excitation observed here to the degree of behavioral impairment reported for each knockout, in order to gain insight into the functional consequences of orexin receptor signaling at these loci. Deletion of both receptors produces a narcolepsy phenotype (Hondo et al., 2010; Kalogiannis et al., 2011) similar to that seen in the prepro-orexin knockouts (Chemelli et al., 1999; Mochizuki et al., 2004), with fragmented waking states, spontaneous sleep attacks and frequent cataplexy. Since orexin-A normally stimulates a large fraction of LDT, DR, and LC neurons, the loss of orexin action at these sites in the DKOs is consistent with a role for orexin signaling at these loci in promoting wake and sleep consolidation, suppressing REM sleep, preventing sleep attacks and suppressing cataplexy. Indeed, optogenetic excitation of orexin neurons promotes sleep-to-wake

transitions (Adamantidis et al., 2007) and optogenetic inhibition of orexin neurons promotes slow-wave sleep and reduced firing of DR neurons (Tsunematsu et al., 2011), while focal orexin injection into the LDT (Xi et al., 2001) or LC (Bourgin et al., 2000) prolongs waking bouts and suppresses REM sleep. Moreover, optogenetic inhibition of TH+ LC neurons blocks the ability of orexin neuron stimulation to promote sleep-to-wake transitions (Carter et al., 2012), while ontogenetic stimulation of TH+ LC neurons both prolongs waking (Carter et al., 2010) and enhances the wake-promoting effect of orexin neuron stimulation (Carter et al., 2012). This indicates orexin–excitation of TH+ LC neurons is necessary for orexin neuron activity to promote sleep-to-wake transitions. Nevertheless, it is the OX$_2$ knockouts that show fragmented spontaneous waking and sleep states and have sleep attacks at the same frequency as prepro-orexin knockouts (Willie et al., 2003), even though orexin-mediated excitation of LDT, DR, and LC neurons is preserved (**Figure 2**). This might indicate that orexin neuron firing and orexin release is impaired through the loss of OX$_2$-mediated positive feedback (Yamanaka et al., 2010) and/or that residual OX$_1$-excitation of LDT, DR, and LC neurons is insufficient to maintain normal duration bouts of spontaneous waking and sleep in the absence of OX$_2$, even though ICV orexin still prolongs waking and suppresses REM sleep in OX$_2^{-/-}$ mice (Mieda et al., 2011). Conversely, OX$_1^{-/-}$ mice appear to have normal sleep-wake states without fragmentation or sleep attacks (Hondo et al., 2010; Mieda et al., 2011), even though orexin excitation is abolished in LDT and LC neurons and is reduced in DR neurons (**Figure 5**), in spite of possible upregulation of OX$_2$ (**Figure 11**). Thus, it appears intact orexin excitation in the LDT, DR, and LC is neither necessary nor sufficient for the expression of normally consolidated bouts of spontaneous sleep and waking. Since, OX_1 signaling in LDT, DR, and LC promotes arousal, but is not necessary for consolidated spontaneous waking, orexin signaling at these loci may promote context-dependent arousal associated with, for example, stress, anxiety, panic, and/or food and drug seeking behavior (Winskey-Sommerer et al., 2004; Boutrel et al., 2005; Harris et al., 2005; Nair et al., 2008; Johnson et al., 2012; Piccoli et al., 2012; Steiner et al., 2012; Heydendael et al., 2013). Orexin signaling at these loci may also support other functions. For example, $OX_1^{-/-}$ mice show impaired acquisition and expression of cued and contextual fear conditioning and the re-expression of OX_1 in TH+ LC neurons rescues the expression of cued fear (Soya et al., 2013). Future studies using receptor rescue approaches (Mochizuki et al., 2011) or the local application of OX_1-specific antagonists will be needed to further explore OX_1 functions at these loci.

Our findings are also consistent with a cataplexy-suppressing role for orexin excitation in the LDT, DR and LC. $OX_2^{-/-}$ mice have cataplexy but it occurs rarely compared with prepro-orexin null mice (Willie et al., 2003). Since DKO mice show frequent cataplexy-like arrests (Kalogiannis et al., 2011), the less severe cataplexy in $OX_2^{-/-}$ mice is likely related to residual OX_1 signaling. Since orexin injections into the LDT and LC suppress REM sleep, and knockdown of OX_1 in LC increases REM during the dark phase (Chen et al., 2010) it is plausible that remaining OX_1-excitation in LDT, LC, and perhaps DR, reduces cataplexy in $OX_2^{-/-}$ mice. Nevertheless, $OX_1^{-/-}$ mice do not have cataplexy, indicating that the loss of orexin-excitation in LDT and LC and reduced orexin excitation in the DR is not sufficient to produce cataplexy, at least in these knockouts, where OX_2 may also be up regulated.

IMPLICATIONS FOR SINGLE OREXIN RECEPTOR PHARMACOTHERAPEUTICS

DORAs show significant promise for improved treatment of insomnia (Uslaner et al., 2013; Winrow and Renger, 2013) and are currently being considered for FDA approval. Given that orexins regulate numerous functions beyond normal waking and sleep and that their receptors are differentially distributed, it seems likely that subtype-specific orexin receptor antagonists (SORAs) will have even greater therapeutic potential. The development of sub-type specific drugs will accelerate preclinical investigations of receptor function and, may allow better targeting of different orexin-dependent behaviors and a fine-tuning of their sleep-promoting effects. For example, OX_2 antagonists appear more effective at sleep promotion than DORAs (Dugovic et al., 2009), perhaps by targeting hypothalamic circuits promoting histamine release and consolidated waking (Dugovic et al., 2009; Mochizuki et al., 2011). Conversely, OX_1 antagonists may provide better relief for hyperarousal and other maladaptive behaviors associated with stress, as noted above, perhaps by dampening OX_1 excitation of noradrenergic, serotonergic and cholinergic reticular neurons and midbrain dopamine systems. Nevertheless, much more needs to be learned about how each orexin receptor impacts

their cellular targets and how these targets influence behavior. These interactions are likely to be complex: as demonstrated here for key elements of the reticular activating system, each receptor can have common effectors (i.e., both receptors activating depolarizing channels and enhancing voltage-dependent Ca^{2+} transients in TpH DR neurons) or act differentially with respect to one effector while having a common action on another effector (i.e., OX_1 is necessary for depolarization while both receptors enhance voltage-dependent Ca^{2+} transients in LDT and LC neurons). It will also be important in future experiments to evaluate the degree to which persistent alteration of signaling by either orexin receptor impacts synaptic plasticity (Borgland et al., 2006; Selbach et al., 2010), neurotransmitter phenotypes (Kalogiannis et al., 2010; Valko et al., 2013) and orexin receptor expression (i.e., elevated brainstem OX_2 message levels in OX_1 null mice), as each of these could lead to deleterious side-effects and diminished therapeutic potential.

ACKNOWLEDGMENTS
Research was supported by NIH grants NS27881 and HL64150

REFERENCES
Adamantidis, A. R., Zhang, F., Aravanis, A. M., Deisseroth, K., and De Lecea, L. (2007). Neural substrates of awakening probed with optogenetic control of hypocretin neurons. *Nature* 450, 420–424. doi: 10.1038/nature06310

Bayer, L., Eggermann, E., Saint-Mleux, B., Machard, D., Jones, B. E., Muhlethaler, M., et al. (2002). Selective action of orexin (hypocretin) on nonspecific thalamocortical projection neurons. *J. Neurosci.* 22, 7835–7839.

Beuckmann, C. T., Sinton, C. M., Williams, S. C., Richardson, J. A., Hammer, R. E., Sakurai, T., et al. (2004). Expression of a poly-glutamine-ataxin-3 transgene in orexin neurons induces narcolepsy-cataplexy in the rat. *J. Neurosci.* 24, 4469–4477. doi: 10.1523/JNEUROSCI.5560-03.2004

Bisetti, A., Cvetkovic, V., Serafin, M., Bayer, L., Machard, D., Jones, B. E., et al. (2006). Excitatory action of hypocretin/orexin on neurons of the central medial amygdala. *Neuroscience* 142, 999–1004. doi: 10.1016/j.neuroscience.2006.07.018

Borgland, S. L., Taha, S. A., Sarti, F., Fields, H. L., and Bonci, A. (2006). Orexin A in the VTA is critical for the induction of synaptic plasticity and behavioral sensitization to cocaine. *Neuron* 49, 589–601. doi: 10.1016/j.neuron.2006.01.016

Bourgin, P., Huitron-Resendiz, S., Spier, A. D., Fabre, V., Morte, B., Criado, J. R., et al. (2000). Hypocretin-1 modulates rapid eye movement sleep through activation of locus coeruleus neurons. *J. Neurosci.* 20, 7760–7765.

Boutrel, B., Kenny, P. J., Specio, S. E., Martin-Fardon, R., Markou, A., Koob, G. F., et al. (2005). Role for hypocretin in mediating stress-induced reinstatement of cocaine-seeking behavior. *Proc. Natl. Acad. Sci. U.S.A.* 102, 19168–19173. doi: 10.1073/pnas.0507480102

Brown, R. E., Basheer, R., McKenna, J. T., Strecker, R. E., and McCarley, R. W. (2012). Control of sleep and wakefulness. *Physiol. Rev.* 92, 1087–1187. doi: 10.1152/physrev.00032.2011

Brown, R. E., Sergeeva, O. A., Eriksson, K. S., and Haas, H. L. (2002). Convergent excitation of dorsal raphe serotonin neurons by multiple arousal systems (orexin/hypocretin, histamine and noradrenaline). *J. Neurosci.* 22, 8850–8859.

Burdakov, D., Liss, B., and Ashcroft, F. M. (2003). Orexin excites GABAergic neurons of the arcuate nucleus by activating the sodium–calcium exchanger. *J. Neurosci.* 23, 4951–4957.

Burlet, S., Tyler, C. J., and Leonard, C. S. (2002). Direct and indirect excitation of laterodorsal tegmental neurons by hypocretin/orexin peptides: implications for wakefulness and narcolepsy. *J. Neurosci.* 22, 2862–2872.

Carter, M. E., Brill, J., Bonnavion, P., Huguenard, J. R., Huerta, R., and De Lecea, L. (2012). Mechanism for Hypocretin-mediated sleep-to-wake transitions. *Proc. Natl. Acad. Sci. U.S.A.* 109, E2635–E2644. doi: 10.1073/pnas.1202526109

Carter, M. E., Yizhar, O., Chikahisa, S., Nguyen, H., Adamantidis, A., Nishino, S., et al. (2010). Tuning arousal with optogenetic modulation of locus coeruleus neurons. *Nat. Neurosci.* 13, 1526–1533. doi: 10.1038/nn.2682

Chemelli, R. M., Willie, J. T., Sinton, C. M., Elmquist, J. K., Scammell, T., Lee, C., et al. (1999). Narcolepsy in orexin knockout mice: molecular genetics of sleep regulation. *Cell* 98, 437–451. doi: 10.1016/S0092-8674(00)81973-X

Chen, J., Karteris, E., Collins, D., and Randeva, H. S. (2006). Differential expression of mouse orexin receptor type-2 (OX2R) variants in the mouse brain. *Brain Res.* 1103, 20–24. doi: 10.1016/j.brainres.2006.05.054

Chen, J., and Randeva, H. S. (2004). Genomic organization of mouse orexin receptors: characterization of two novel tissue-specific splice variants. *Mol. Endocrinol.* 18, 2790–2804. doi: 10.1210/me.2004-0167

Chen, L., McKenna, J. T., Bolortuya, Y., Winston, S., Thakkar, M. M., Basheer, R., et al. (2010). Knockdown of orexin type 1 receptor in rat locus coeruleus increases REM sleep during the dark period. *Eur. J. Neurosci.* 32, 1528–1536. doi: 10.1111/j.1460-9568.2010.07401.x

Cid-Pellitero, E. D., and Garzón, M. (2011). Hypocretin1/orexinA axon targeting of laterodorsal tegmental nucleus neurons projecting to the rat medial prefrontal cortex. *Cereb. Cortex* 21, 2762–2773. doi: 10.1093/cercor/bhr070

Del Cid-Pellitero, E., and Garzón, M. (2011). Medial prefrontal cortex receives input from dorsal raphe nucleus neurons targeted by hypocretin1/orexinA-containing axons. *Neuroscience* 172, 30–43. doi: 10.1016/j.neuroscience.2010.10.058

De Lecea, L., Kilduff, T. S., Peyron, C., Gao, X., Foye, P. E., Danielson, P. E., et al. (1998). The hypocretins: hypothalamus-specific peptides with neuroexcitatory activity. *Proc. Natl. Acad. Sci. U.S.A.* 95, 322–327. doi: 10.1073/pnas.95.1.322

Doetschman, T. (2009). Influence of genetic background on genetically engineered mouse phenotypes. *Methods Mol. Biol.* 530, 423–433. doi: 10.1007/978-1-59745-471-1_23

Dugovic, C., Shelton, J. E., Aluisio, L. E., Fraser, I. C., Jiang, X., Sutton, S. W., et al. (2009). Blockade of orexin-1 receptors attenuates orexin-2 receptor antagonism-induced sleep promotion in the rat. *J. Pharmacol. Exp. Ther.* 330, 142–151. doi: 10.1124/jpet.109.152009

Eriksson, K. S., Sergeeva, O., Brown, R. E., and Haas, H. L. (2001). Orexin/hypocretin excites the histaminergic neurons of the tuberomammillary nucleus. *J. Neurosci.* 21, 9273–9279.

Grabauskas, G., and Moises, H. C. (2003). Gastrointestinal-projecting neurones in the dorsal motor nucleus of the vagus exhibit direct and viscerotopically organized sensitivity to orexin. *J. Physiol.* 549, 37–56. doi: 10.1113/jphysiol.2002.029546

Haj-Dahmane, S., and Shen, R. Y. (2005). The wake-promoting peptide orexin-B inhibits glutamatergic transmission to dorsal raphe nucleus serotonin neurons through retrograde endocannabinoid signaling. *J. Neurosci.* 25, 896–905. doi: 10.1523/JNEUROSCI.3258-04.2005

Hara, J., Beuckmann, C. T., Nambu, T., Willie, J. T., Chemelli, R. M., Sinton, C. M., et al. (2001). Genetic ablation of orexin neurons in mice results in narcolepsy, hypophagia, and obesity. *Neuron* 30, 345–354. doi: 10.1016/S0896-6273(01)00293-8

Harris, G. C., Wimmer, M., and Aston-Jones, G. (2005). A role for lateral hypothalamic orexin neurons in reward seeking. *Nature* 437, 556–559. doi: 10.1038/nature04071

Hervieu, G. J., Cluderay, J. E., Harrison, D. C., Roberts, J. C., and Leslie, R. A. (2001). Gene expression and protein distribution of the orexin-1 receptor in the rat brain and spinal cord. *Neuroscience* 103, 777–797. doi: 10.1016/S0306-4522(01)00033-1

Heydendael, W., Sengupta, A., Beck, S., and Bhatnagar, S. (2013). Optogenetic examination identifies a context-specific role for orexins/hypocretins in anxiety-related behavior. *Physiol. Behav.* doi: 10.1016/j.physbeh.2013.10.005. [Epub ahead of print].

Hoang, Q. V., Bajic, D., Yanagisawa, M., Nakajima, S., and Nakajima, Y. (2003). Effects of orexin (hypocretin) on GIRK channels. *J. Neurophysiol.* 90, 693–702. doi: 10.1152/jn.00001.2003

Hoang, Q. V., Zhao, P., Nakajima, S., and Nakajima, Y. (2004). Orexin (hypocretin) effects on constitutively active inward rectifier K+ channels in cultured nucleus basalis neurons. *J. Neurophysiol.* 92, 3183–3191. doi: 10.1152/jn.01222.2003

Holmqvist, T., Åkerman, K. E. O., and Kukkonen, J. P. (2002). Orexin signaling in recombinant neuron-like cells. *FEBS Lett.* 526, 11–14. doi: 10.1016/S0014-5793(02)03101-0

Hondo, M., Nagai, K., Ohno, K., Kisanuki, Y., Willie, J. T., Watanabe, T., et al. (2010). Histamine-1 receptor is not required as a downstream effector of orexin-2 receptor in maintenance of basal sleep/wake states. *Acta Physiol. (Oxf.)* 198, 287–294. doi: 10.1111/j.1748-1716.2009.02032.x

Horvath, T. L., Peyron, C., Diano, S., Ivanov, A., Aston-Jones, G., Kilduff, T. S., et al. (1999). Hypocretin (orexin) activation and synaptic innervation of the locus coeruleus noradrenergic system. *J. Comp. Neurol.* 415, 145–159. doi: 10.1002/(SICI)1096-9861(19991213)415:2<145::AID-CNE1>3.0.CO;2-2

Hwang, L. L., Chen, C. T., and Dun, N. J. (2001). Mechanisms of orexin-induced depolarizations in rat dorsal motor nucleus of vagus neurones *in vitro. J. Physiol.* 537, 511–520. doi: 10.1111/j.1469-7793.2001.00511.x

Ishibashi, M., Takano, S., Yanagida, H., Takatsuna, M., Nakajima, K., Oomura, Y., et al. (2005). Effects of orexins/hypocretins on neuronal activity in the paraventricular nucleus of the thalamus in rats *in vitro. Peptides* 26, 471–481. doi: 10.1016/j.peptides.2004.10.014

Ivanov, A., and Aston-Jones, G. (2000). Hypocretin/orexin depolarizes and decreases potassium conductance in locus coeruleus neurons. *Neuroreport* 11, 1755–1758. doi: 10.1097/00001756-200006050-00031

Jacobs, B. L., and Fornal, C. A. (1993). 5-HT and motor control: a hypothesis. *Trends Neurosci.* 16, 346–352. doi: 10.1016/0166-2236(93)90090-9

Johnson, P. L., Samuels, B. C., Fitz, S. D., Lightman, S. L., Lowry, C. A., and Shekhar, A. (2012). Activation of the orexin 1 receptor is a critical component of CO2-mediated anxiety and hypertension but not bradycardia. *Neuropsychopharmacology* 37, 1911–1922. doi: 10.1038/npp.2012.38

Jones, B. E. (2005). From waking to sleeping: neuronal and chemical substrates. *Trends Pharmacol. Sci.* 26, 578–586. doi: 10.1016/j.tips.2005.09.009

Kalogiannis, M., Grupke, S. L., Potter, P. E., Edwards, J. G., Chemelli, R. M., Kisanuki, Y. Y., et al. (2010). Narcoleptic orexin receptor knockout mice express enhanced cholinergic properties in laterodorsal tegmental neurons. *Eur. J. Neurosci.* 32, 130–142. doi: 10.1111/j.1460-9568.2010.07259.x

Kalogiannis, M., Hsu, E., Willie, J. T., Chemelli, R. M., Kisanuki, Y. Y., Yanagisawa, M., et al. (2011). Cholinergic modulation of narcoleptic attacks in double orexin receptor knockout mice. *PLoS ONE* 6:e18697. doi: 10.1371/journal.pone.0018697

Kim, J., Nakajima, K., Oomura, Y., Wayner, M. J., and Sasaki, K. (2009). Electrophysiological effects of orexins/hypocretins on pedunculopontine tegmental neurons in rats: an *in vitro* study. *Peptides* 30, 191–209. doi: 10.1016/j.peptides.2008.09.023

Kohlmeier, K. A., Inoue, T., and Leonard, C. S. (2004). Hypocretin/orexin peptide signaling in the ascending arousal system: elevation of intracellular calcium in the mouse dorsal raphe and laterodorsal tegmentum. *J. Neurophysiol.* 92, 221–235. doi: 10.1152/jn.00076.2004

Kohlmeier, K. A., Watanabe, S., Tyler, C. J., Burlet, S., and Leonard, C. S. (2008). Dual orexin actions on dorsal raphe and laterodorsal tegmentum neurons: noisy cation current activation and selective enhancement of Ca transients mediated by L-type calcium channels. *J. Neurophysiol.* 100, 2265–2281. doi: 10.1152/jn.01388.2007

Kukkonen, J. P., and Leonard, C. S. (2013). Orexin/hypocretin receptor signalling cascades. *Br. J. Pharmacol.* doi: 10.1111/bph.12324. [Epub ahead of print].

Leonard, C. S., and Kukkonen, J. P. (2013). Orexin/hypocretin receptor signalling: a functional perspective. *Br. J. Pharmacol.* doi: 10.1111/bph.12296. [Epub ahead of print].

Li, Y., Gao, X. B., Sakurai, T., and Van Den Pol, A. N. (2002). Hypocretin/Orexin excites hypocretin neurons via a local glutamate neuron-A potential mechanism for orchestrating the hypothalamic arousal system. *Neuron* 36, 1169–1181. doi: 10.1016/S0896-6273(02)01132-7

Lin, L., Faraco, J., Li, R., Kadotani, H., Rogers, W., Lin, X., et al. (1999). The sleep disorder canine narcolepsy is caused by a mutation in the hypocretin (orexin) receptor 2 gene. *Cell* 98, 365–376. doi: 10.1016/S0092-8674(00)81965-0

Liu, R. J., Van Den Pol, A. N., and Aghajanian, G. K. (2002). Hypocretins (orexins) regulate serotonin neurons in the dorsal raphe nucleus by excitatory direct and inhibitory indirect actions. *J. Neurosci.* 22, 9453–9464.

Lowry, C. A., Johnson, P. L., Hay-Schmidt, A., Mikkelsen, J., and Shekhar, A. (2005). Modulation of anxiety circuits by serotonergic systems. *Stress* 8, 233–246. doi: 10.1080/10253890500492787

Lund, P. E., Shariatmadari, R., Uustare, A., Detheux, M., Parmentier, M., Kukkonen, J. P., and Åkerman, K. E. O. (2000). The orexin OX1 receptor activates a novel Ca2+ influx pathway necessary for coupling to phospholipase C. *J. Biol. Chem.* 275, 30806–30812. doi: 10.1074/jbc.M002603200

Marcus, J. N., Aschkenasi, C. J., Lee, C. E., Chemelli, R. M., Saper, C. B., Yanagisawa, M., et al. (2001). Differential expression of orexin receptors 1 and 2 in the rat brain. *J. Comp. Neurol.* 435, 6–25. doi: 10.1002/cne.1190

Maskos, U. (2008). The cholinergic mesopontine tegmentum is a relatively neglected nicotinic master modulator of the dopaminergic system: relevance to drugs of abuse and pathology. *Br. J. Pharmacol.* 153(Suppl. 1), S438–S445. doi: 10.1038/bjp.2008.5

Mena-Segovia, J., Winn, P., and Bolam, J. P. (2008). Cholinergic modulation of midbrain dopaminergic systems. *Brain Res. Rev.* 58, 265–271. doi: 10.1016/j.brainresrev.2008.02.003

Michelsen, K. A., Schmitz, C., and Steinbusch, H. W. (2007). The dorsal raphe nucleus–from silver stainings to a role in depression. *Brain Res. Rev.* 55, 329–342. doi: 10.1016/j.brainresrev.2007.01.002

Mieda, M., Hasegawa, E., Kisanuki, Y. Y., Sinton, C. M., Yanagisawa, M., and Sakurai, T. (2011). Differential roles of orexin receptor-1 and -2 in the regulation of non-REM and REM sleep. *J. Neurosci.* 31, 6518–6526. doi: 10.1523/JNEUROSCI.6506-10.2011

Mochizuki, T., Arrigoni, E., Marcus, J. N., Clark, E. L., Yamamoto, M., Honer, M., et al. (2011). Orexin receptor 2 expression in the posterior hypothalamus rescues sleepiness in narcoleptic mice. *Proc. Natl. Acad. Sci. U.S.A.* 108, 4471–4476. doi: 10.1073/pnas.1012456108

Mochizuki, T., Crocker, A., McCormack, S., Yanagisawa, M., Sakurai, T., and Scammell, T. (2004). Behavioral State Instability in Orexin Knockout Mice. *J. Neurosci.* 24, 6291–6300. doi: 10.1523/JNEUROSCI.0586-04.2004

Murai, Y., and Akaike, T. (2005). Orexins cause depolarization via nonselective cationic and K+ channels in isolated locus coeruleus neurons. *Neurosci. Res.* 51, 55–65. doi: 10.1016/j.neures.2004.09.005

Nair, S. G., Golden, S. A., and Shaham, Y. (2008). Differential effects of the hypocretin 1 receptor antagonist SB 334867 on high-fat food self-administration and reinstatement of food seeking in rats. *Br. J. Pharmacol.* 154, 406–416. doi: 10.1038/bjp.2008.3

Nambu, T., Sakurai, T., Mizukami, K., Hosoya, Y., Yanagisawa, M., and Goto, K. (1999). Distribution of orexin neurons in the adult rat brain. *Brain Res.* 827, 243–260. doi: 10.1016/S0006-8993(99)01336-0

Peyron, C., Faraco, J., Rogers, W., Ripley, B., Overeem, S., Charnay, Y., et al. (2000). A mutation in a case of early onset narcolepsy and a generalized absence of hypocretin peptides in human narcoleptic brains. *Nat. Med.* 6, 991–997. doi: 10.1038/79690

Peyron, C., Tighe, D. K., Van Den Pol, A. N., De Lecea, L., Heller, H. C., Sutcliffe, J. G., et al. (1998). Neurons containing hypocretin (orexin) project to multiple neuronal systems. *J. Neurosci.* 18, 9996–10015.

Piccoli, L., Micioni Di Bonaventura, M. V., Cifani, C., Costantini, V. J., Massagrande, M., Montanari, D., et al. (2012). Role of orexin-1 receptor mechanisms on compulsive food consumption in a model of binge eating in female rats. *Neuropsychopharmacology* 37, 1999–2011. doi: 10.1038/npp.2012.48

Putula, J., Turunen, P. M., Jäntti, M. H., Ekholm, M. E., and Kukkonen, J. P. (2011). Agonist ligand discrimination by the two orexin receptors depends on the expression system. *Neurosci. Lett.* 494, 57–60. doi: 10.1016/j.neulet.2011.02.055

Sakurai, T., Amemiya, A., Ishii, M., Matsuzaki, I., Chemelli, R. M., Tanaka, H., et al. (1998). Orexins and orexin receptors: a family of hypothalamic neuropeptides and G protein-coupled receptors that regulate feeding behavior. *Cell* 92, 573–585. doi: 10.1016/S0092-8674(00)80949-6

Selbach, O., Bohla, C., Barbara, A., Doreulee, N., Eriksson, K. S., Sergeeva, O. A., et al. (2010). Orexins/hypocretins control bistability of hippocampal long-term synaptic plasticity through co-activation of multiple kinases. *Acta Physiol. (Oxf.)* 198, 277–285. doi: 10.1111/j.1748-1716.2009.02021.x

Smart, D., Jerman, J. C., Brough, S. J., Rushton, S. L., Murdock, P. R., Jewitt, F., et al. (1999). Characterization of recombinant human orexin receptor pharmacology in a Chinese hamster ovary cell-line using FLIPR. *Br. J. Pharmacol.* 128, 1–3. doi: 10.1038/sj.bjp.0702780

Soffin, E. M., Gill, C. H., Brough, S. J., Jerman, J. C., and Davies, C. H. (2004). Pharmacological characterisation of the orexin receptor subtype mediating postsynaptic excitation in the rat dorsal raphe nucleus. *Neuropharmacology* 46, 1168–1176. doi: 10.1016/j.neuropharm.2004.02.014

Soya, S., Shoji, H., Hasegawa, E., Hondo, M., Miyakawa, T., Yanagisawa, M., et al. (2013). Orexin receptor-1 in the locus coeruleus plays an important role in cue-dependent fear memory consolidation. *J. Neurosci.* 33, 14549–14557. doi: 10.1523/JNEUROSCI.1130-13.2013

Steiner, M. A., Lecourt, H., and Jenck, F. (2012). The brain orexin system and almorexant in fear-conditioned startle reactions in the rat. *Psychopharmacology (Berl.)* 223, 465–475. doi: 10.1007/s00213-012-2736-7

Thannickal, T. C., Moore, R. Y., Nienhuis, R., Ramanathan, L., Gulyani, S., Aldrich, M., et al. (2000). Reduced number of hypocretin neurons in human narcolepsy. *Neuron* 27, 469–474. doi: 10.1016/S0896-6273(00)00058-1

Trivedi, P., Yu, H., Macneil, D. J., Van Der Ploeg, L. H., and Guan, X. M. (1998). Distribution of orexin receptor mRNA in the rat brain. *FEBS Lett.* 438, 71–75. doi: 10.1016/S0014-5793(98)01266-6

Tsujino, N., and Sakurai, T. (2009). Orexin/hypocretin: a neuropeptide at the interface of sleep, energy homeostasis, and reward system. *Pharmacol. Rev.* 61, 162–176. doi: 10.1124/pr.109.001321

Tsunematsu, T., Kilduff, T. S., Boyden, E. S., Takahashi, S., Tominaga, M., and Yamanaka, A. (2011). Acute optogenetic silencing of orexin/hypocretin neurons induces slow-wave sleep in mice. *J. Neurosci.* 31, 10529–10539. doi: 10.1523/JNEUROSCI.0784-11.2011

Uramura, K., Funahashi, H., Muroya, S., Shioda, S., Takigawa, M., and Yada, T. (2001). Orexin-a activates phospholipase C- and protein kinase C-mediated Ca2+ signaling in dopamine neurons of the ventral tegmental area. *Neuroreport* 12, 1885–1889. doi: 10.1097/00001756-200107030-00024

Uslaner, J. M., Tye, S. J., Eddins, D. M., Wang, X., Fox, S. V., Savitz, A. T., et al. (2013). Orexin receptor antagonists differ from standard sleep drugs by promoting sleep at doses that do not disrupt cognition. *Sci. Transl. Med.* 5, 179ra144. doi: 10.1126/scitranslmed.3005213

Valentino, R. J., and Van Bockstaele, E. (2008). Convergent regulation of locus coeruleus activity as an adaptive response to stress. *Eur. J. Pharmacol.* 583, 194–203. doi: 10.1016/j.ejphar.2007.11.062

Valko, P. O., Gavrilov, Y. V., Yamamoto, M., Reddy, H., Haybaeck, J., Mignot, E., et al. (2013). Increase of histaminergic tuberomammillary neurons in narcolepsy. *Ann. Neurol.* doi: 10.1002/ana.24019. [Epub ahead of print].

Van Den Pol, A. N. (1999). Hypothalamic hypocretin (orexin): robust innervation of the spinal cord. *J. Neurosci.* 19, 3171–3182.

Van Den Pol, A. N., Gao, X. B., Obrietan, K., Kilduff, T. S., and Belousov, A. B. (1998). Presynaptic and postsynaptic actions and modulation of neuroendocrine neurons by a new hypothalamic peptide, hypocretin/orexin. *J. Neurosci.* 18, 7962–7971.

Vincent, S. R., Satoh, K., Armstrong, D. M., and Fibiger, H. C. (1983). NADPH-Diaphorase: A selective histochemical marker for the cholinergic neurons of the pontine reticular formation. *Neurosci. Lett.* 43, 31–36. doi: 10.1016/0304-3940(83)90124-6

Willie, J. T., Chemelli, R. M., Sinton, C. M., Tokita, S., Williams, S. C., Kisanuki, Y. Y., et al. (2003). Distinct narcolepsy syndromes in orexin receptor-2 and orexin null mice. molecular genetic dissection of non-REM and REM sleep regulatory processes. *Neuron* 38, 715–730. doi: 10.1016/S0896-6273(03)00330-1

Winrow, C. J., and Renger, J. J. (2013). Discovery and development of orexin receptor antagonists as therapeutics for insomnia. *Br. J. Pharmacol.* doi: 10.1111/bph.12261. [Epub ahead of print].

Winskey-Sommerer, R., Yamanaka, A., Diano, S., Borok, E., Roberts, A. J., Sakurai, T., et al. (2004). Interaction between corticotropin-releasing factor system and hypocretins (Orexins): a novel circuit mediating stress response. *J. Neurosci.* 24, 11439–11448. doi: 10.1523/JNEUROSCI.3459-04.2004

Wu, M., Zaborszky, L., Hajszan, T., Van Den Pol, A. N., and Alreja, M. (2004). Hypocretin/orexin innervation and excitation of identified septohippocampal cholinergic neurons. *J. Neurosci.* 24, 3527–3536. doi: 10.1523/JNEUROSCI.5364-03.2004

Wu, M., Zhang, Z., Leranth, C., Xu, C., Van Den Pol, A. N., and Alreja, M. (2002). Hypocretin increases impulse flow in the septohippocampal GABAergic pathway: implications for arousal via a mechanism of hippocampal disinhibition. *J. Neurosci.* 22, 7754–7765.

Xi, M., Morales, F. R., and Chase, M. H. (2001). Effects on sleep and wakefulness of the injection of hypocretin-1 (orexin-A) into the laterodorsal tegmental nucleus of the cat. *Brain Res.* 901, 259–264. doi: 10.1016/S0006-8993(01)02317-4

Xu, R., Wang, Q., Yan, M., Hernandez, M., Gong, C., Boon, W. C., et al. (2002). Orexin-A augments voltage-gated Ca2+ currents and synergistically increases growth hormone (GH) secretion with GH-releasing hormone in primary cultured ovine somatotropes. *Endocrinology* 143, 4609–4619. doi: 10.1210/en.2002-220506

Yamanaka, A., Tabuchi, S., Tsunematsu, T., Fukazawa, Y., and Tominaga, M. (2010). Orexin directly excites orexin neurons through orexin 2 receptor. *J. Neurosci.* 30, 12642–12652. doi: 10.1523/JNEUROSCI.2120-10.2010

Yang, B., and Ferguson, A. V. (2002). Orexin-A depolarizes dissociated rat area postrema neurons through activation of a nonselective cationic conductance. *J. Neurosci.* 22, 6303–6308.

Yang, B., and Ferguson, A. V. (2003). Orexin-A depolarizes nucleus tractus solitarius neurons through effects on nonselective cationic and K+ conductances. *J. Neurophysiol.* 89, 2167–2175. doi: 10.1152/jn.01088.2002

Conflict of Interest Statement: The authors declare that the research was conducted in the absence of any commercial or financial relationships that could be construed as a potential conflict of interest.

Permissions

All chapters in this book were first published in IBETPORA, by Frontiers Media SA; hereby published with permission under the Creative Commons Attribution License or equivalent. Every chapter published in this book has been scrutinized by our experts. Their significance has been extensively debated. The topics covered herein carry significant findings which will fuel the growth of the discipline. They may even be implemented as practical applications or may be referred to as a beginning point for another development.

The contributors of this book come from diverse backgrounds, making this book a truly international effort. This book will bring forth new frontiers with its revolutionizing research information and detailed analysis of the nascent developments around the world.

We would like to thank all the contributing authors for lending their expertise to make the book truly unique. They have played a crucial role in the development of this book. Without their invaluable contributions this book wouldn't have been possible. They have made vital efforts to compile up to date information on the varied aspects of this subject to make this book a valuable addition to the collection of many professionals and students.

This book was conceptualized with the vision of imparting up-to-date information and advanced data in this field. To ensure the same, a matchless editorial board was set up. Every individual on the board went through rigorous rounds of assessment to prove their worth. After which they invested a large part of their time researching and compiling the most relevant data for our readers.

The editorial board has been involved in producing this book since its inception. They have spent rigorous hours researching and exploring the diverse topics which have resulted in the successful publishing of this book. They have passed on their knowledge of decades through this book. To expedite this challenging task, the publisher supported the team at every step. A small team of assistant editors was also appointed to further simplify the editing procedure and attain best results for the readers.

Apart from the editorial board, the designing team has also invested a significant amount of their time in understanding the subject and creating the most relevant covers. They scrutinized every image to scout for the most suitable representation of the subject and create an appropriate cover for the book.

The publishing team has been an ardent support to the editorial, designing and production team. Their endless efforts to recruit the best for this project, has resulted in the accomplishment of this book. They are a veteran in the field of academics and their pool of knowledge is as vast as their experience in printing. Their expertise and guidance has proved useful at every step. Their uncompromising quality standards have made this book an exceptional effort. Their encouragement from time to time has been an inspiration for everyone.

The publisher and the editorial board hope that this book will prove to be a valuable piece of knowledge for researchers, students, practitioners and scholars across the globe.

List of Contributors

Pascal Carrive
Blood Pressure, Brain and Behavior Laboratory, School of Medical Sciences, University of New South Wales, Sydney, NSW, Australia

Thomas Dürst
Neuroscience, Novartis Institutes for BioMedical Research, Basel, Switzerland

Markus Fendt
Neuroscience, Novartis Institutes for BioMedical Research, Basel, Switzerland
Center of Behavioral Brain Sciences, Institute for Pharmacology and Toxicology, Otto-von-Guericke University Magdeburg, Magdeburg, Germany

Laura H. Jacobson
Neuroscience, Novartis Institutes for BioMedical Research, Basel, Switzerland
The Florey Institute of Neuroscience and Mental Health, The University of Melbourne, Parkville, VIC, Australia

Claudia Betschart, Samuel Hintermann, Dirk Behnke, Simona Cotesta and Silvio Ofner
Global Discovery Chemistry, Novartis Institutes for BioMedical Research, Basel, Switzerland

Grit Laue
Metabolism and Pharmacokinetics, Novartis Institutes for BioMedical Research, Basel, Switzerland

Eric Legangneux
Translational Medicine, Novartis Institutes for BioMedical Research, Basel, Switzerland

Christine E. Gee
Neuroscience, Novartis Institutes for BioMedical Research, Basel, Switzerland
Center for Molecular Neuroscience Hamburg, Institute for Synaptic Physiology, Hamburg, Germany

Andres D. Ramirez, Anthony L. Gotter, Terrence McDonald, Joseph Brunner, Susan L. Garson, Duane R. Reiss, John J. Renger and Christopher J. Winrow
Merck Research Laboratories, Department of Neuroscience, Merck & Co., Inc., West Point, PA, USA

Steven V.Fox, Pamela L. Tannenbaum, Lihang Yao, Spencer J. Tye, Jason M. Uslaner, Robert Hodgson and Susan E. Browne
Merck Research Laboratories, Department of In Vivo Pharmacology, Merck & Co., Inc., West Point, PA, USA

Scott D. Kuduk and Paul J.Coleman
Merck Research Laboratories, Department of Medicinal Chemistry, Merck & Co., Inc., West Point, PA, USA

Ana C. Equihua and Rene Drucker-Colin
Neuropatología Molecular, Instituto de Fisiología Celular, Universidad Nacional Autónoma de México, Mexico City, México

Alberto K. De La Herrán-Arita
Center for Sleep Sciences and Medicine, Stanford University, Palo Alto, CA, USA

Emilio Merlo Pich
Neuroscience DTA, F. Hoffman – La Roche, Basel, Switzerland

Sergio Melotto
Legnago, Italy

Luis de Lecea
Department of Psychiatry and Behavioral Sciences, Stanford University School of Medicine, Stanford, CA, USA

Ramón Huerta
BioCircuits Institute, University of California, San Diego, La Jolla, CA, USA

Silvia Tortorella, Margarita L. Rodrigo-Angulo, Angel Núñez and Miguel Garzón
Departamento de Anatomía, Histología y Neurociencia, Facultad de Medicina, Research Institute, Universidad Autonoma de Madrid, La Paz University Hospital (IDIPAZ), Madrid, Spain

Rachel I. Anderson
Medical University of South Carolina, Charleston, SC, USA
Charleston Alcohol Research Center, Charleston, SC, USA

Howard C. Becker
Medical University of South Carolina, Charleston, SC, USA
Charleston Alcohol Research Center, Charleston, SC, USA
Ralph H. Johnson VA Medical Center, USA

Benjamin L. Adams, Cynthia D. Jesudason and Linda M. Rorick-Kehn
Lilly Research Laboratories, Eli Lilly and Company, Indianapolis, IN, USA

Jiann Wei Yeoh, Erin J. Campbell, Morgan H. James, Brett A. Graham and Christopher V. Dayas
Neurobiology of Addiction Laboratory, The Centre for Translational Neuroscience and Mental Health Research, School of Biomedical Sciences and Pharmacy, University of Newcastle and the Hunter Medical Research Institute, Newcastle, NSW, Australia

Christine Dugovic, Jonathan E. Shelton, Sujin Yun, Pascal Bonaventure, Brock T. Shireman and Timothy W. Lovenberg
Neuroscience, Janssen Research & Development, L.L.C., San Diego, CA, USA

Stephen R. Morairty, Alan J. Wilk, Webster U. Lincoln and Thomas S. Kilduff
SRI International, Center for Neuroscience, Biosciences Division, Menlo Park, CA, USA

Thomas C. Neylan
Department of Psychiatry, SF VA Medical Center/ NCIRE/University of California, San Francisco, CA, USA

Michel A. Steiner and Francois Jenck
CNS Pharmacology Neurobiology, Actelion Pharmaceuticals Ltd., Allschwil, Switzerland

Carla Sciarretta
Immunology, Actelion Pharmaceuticals Ltd., Allschwil, Switzerland

Anne Pasquali
Cardiology, Actelion Pharmaceuticals Ltd., Allschwil, Switzerland

Gabrielle E. Callander
Department of Pharmacology and Therapeutics, Faculty of Medicine, Dentistry and Health Sciences, School of Medicine, The University of Melbourne, Parkville, VIC, Australia
The Florey Institute of Neuroscience and Mental Health, The University of Melbourne, Parkville, VIC, Australia

Morenike Olorunda, Dominique Monna, Edi Schuepbach and Daniel Langenegger
Department of Neuroscience, Novartis Institutes for Biomedical Research, Basel, Switzerland

Emmanuelle Briard
Global Discovery Chemistry, Novartis Institutes for Biomedical Research, Basel, Switzerland

Christine E. Gee
Department of Neuroscience, Novartis Institutes for Biomedical Research, Basel, Switzerland
Centre for Neurobiology Hamburg, Institute for Synaptic Physiology, Hamburg, Germany

Daniel Hoyer
Department of Pharmacology and Therapeutics, Faculty of Medicine, Dentistry and Health Sciences, School of Medicine, The University of Melbourne, Parkville, VIC, Australia
The Florey Institute of Neuroscience and Mental Health, The University of Melbourne, Parkville, VIC, Australia
Department of Neuroscience, Novartis Institutes for Biomedical Research, Basel, Switzerland

África Flores, Rafael Maldonado and Fernando Berrendero
Laboratory of Neuropharmacology, Department of Experimental and Health Sciences, Universitat Pompeu Fabra, Barcelona, Spain

Thomas E. Fitch, Mark J. Benvenga, Charity Zink, Amy B. Vandergriff, Michelle M. Menezes and Douglas A. Schober
Lilly Research Laboratories, Department of Neuroscience, Eli Lilly and Company, Indianapolis, IN, USA

Miles D. Thompson
University of Toronto Epilepsy Research Program, Department of Pharmacology, University of Toronto, Toronto, ON, Canada

Henri Xhaard
Faculty of Pharmacy, Centre for Drug Research, University of Helsinki, Helsinki, Finland

Innocenzo Rainero
Department of Neuroscience, University of Turin, Torino, Italy

Jyrki P. Kukkonen
Biochemistry and Cell Biology, Department of Veterinary Biosciences, University of Helsinki, Helsinki, Finland

Damien Colas
Department of Biology, Stanford University, Stanford, CA, USA
Laboratory of Neurodegeneration and Axon Dynamics, European Brain Research Institute, Rome, Italy

Annalisa Manca and Jean-Dominique Delcroix
Laboratory of Neurodegeneration and Axon Dynamics, European Brain Research Institute, Rome, Italy

Philippe Mourrain
Department of Psychiatry and Behavioral Sciences, Center for Sleep Sciences, Beckman Center, Stanford University, Stanford, CA, USA
INSERM 1024, Ecole Normale Supérieure, Paris, France

Keishi Etori, Yuki C. Saito, Natsuko Tsujino and Takeshi Sakurai
Department of Molecular Neuroscience and Integrative Physiology, Faculty of Medicine, Institute of Medical, Pharmaceutical and Health Sciences, Kanazawa University, Kanazawa, Japan

Aihua Li and Eugene Nattie
Department of Physiology and Neurobiology, Geisel School of Medicine at Dartmouth, Lebanon, NH, USA

Kristi A. Kohlmeier and Morten P. Kristensen
Department of Drug Design and Pharmacology, Faculty of Health and Medical Sciences, University of Copenhagen, Copenhagen, Denmark

Christopher J. Tyler, Mike Kalogiannis, Masaru Ishibashi, Iryna Gumenchuk and Christopher S. Leonard
Department of Physiology, New York Medical College, Valhalla, NY, USA

Richard M. Chemelli, Yaz Y. Kisanuki and Masashi Yanagisawa
Howard Hughes Medical Institute, University of Texas Southwestern Medical Center, Dallas, TX, USA

Index

A

Acetylcholine, 41-42, 44, 54, 124, 189

Analgesia, 116, 125, 131, 145, 160, 162

Antinociception, 116, 121, 125, 128-130, 154, 162

Arousal Stability, 41

Arousal Threshold, 41, 46, 76, 157

C

Cannabinoid Receptor, 116-117, 127-131

Cannabinoid-hypocretin, 116

Cataplexy, 5-6, 8-9, 12, 29, 31, 38-42, 55, 78-79, 83-84, 107, 112-113, 144, 160-161, 163, 169, 192, 194, 208-209

Catecholaminergic Receptors, 48, 54

Cerebrospinal Fluid, 44, 46, 49, 70, 73, 75-76, 142-144, 153, 155, 179, 196

Chinese Hamster Ovary, 16, 106, 108, 126, 211

Cluster Headache, 13, 144-145, 150-155

Cognitive Impairment, 86, 104-105

D

Dopaminergic, 38, 42, 44, 95, 117, 123-124, 129, 141, 211

Double Orexin Receptor Knockout, 12, 32, 114, 198, 210

Drug Development, 31, 110, 148, 160

E

Electrophysiology, 121-122, 196

Endocannabinoids, 116-117, 119-120, 122-123, 125-128, 130-131

Energy Homeostasis, 46, 56, 94-95, 105, 107, 117, 131, 141, 155, 175, 191-192, 211

F

Functional Magnetic Resonance Imaging, 32, 39, 42, 74, 84

G

Gabaergic Receptors, 48, 51, 53

Gene Variants, 145, 152

Genetic Variation, 145-146, 148, 150

H

Haplotype Analysis, 13, 152, 155

Hcrt Neurons, 41-44, 156-158, 160

Heteromerization, 116, 119, 122, 128

Hypervigilance, 35, 41

Hypocretin, 5-8, 22-25, 28, 32-41, 44-49, 73-77, 84, 86, 92-93, 104-105, 114, 116-131, 133, 158, 174, 176, 179, 189-192, 194, 209-211

Hypocretin Receptors, 117-118, 126, 153

Hypocretinergic System, 25, 116, 124-125, 129, 146-147, 154, 190

Hypocretins, 5-6, 25, 32, 34-35, 39-41, 44-46, 48, 55, 57, 65, 74-76, 84, 86, 92, 104, 113, 116-117, 119-120, 122-129, 131, 142, 153-155, 161, 163, 176, 189-190, 192, 210-211

Hypothalamic Cells, 141, 151

Hypothalamic Regulators, 120

I

Immunocytochemistry, 121, 161, 196, 199

In-situ Hybridization, 195, 207

Intracellular Calcium Concentration, 196

Intracerebroventricular Administration, 132, 144, 151

L

Laterodorsal Tegmental Nucleus, 28, 34, 42, 46, 56, 194-195, 210-211

Locomotor Performance, 14-15, 17, 19-21

Locus Coeruleus, 3, 12, 15, 28, 32, 38, 40, 42, 44-45, 48, 54-56, 68, 76, 78, 83-84, 107, 117-118, 130, 142, 150-151, 153, 163, 169, 172, 175, 177, 194-195, 209-211

M

Mesopontine Cholinergic, 194-195, 197

Microiontophoresis, 49

Monoaminergic Neurons, 42-43, 164, 173, 194, 197-198

Monoamines, 41-42, 151

Mutagenesis, 145-147, 153

N

Narcolepsy, 5-9, 12-14, 22-23, 31-35, 37-39, 41, 49, 66, 74, 76, 78-79, 83-85, 107, 125-126, 129, 131, 142, 144, 148, 151-154, 156, 160-163, 169, 173-175, 194, 206, 208-211

Narcoleptic Patients, 5, 41, 83

Nasopharyngitis, 26-27, 31

Neurobiotin, 49-50, 52, 67

Neuromodulators, 41, 44, 116-117

Noradrenergic, 42, 53-55, 68, 74, 141, 150, 153, 163, 165, 169, 173, 177-178, 185, 196, 209-210

Norepinephrine, 26-29, 41, 44, 54, 82, 84, 134, 141, 151, 188

O

Opioid Receptors, 147

Optogenetics, 28, 41

Orexin Neurons, 1-7, 12, 21, 24, 28, 45-47, 55-57, 66-68, 70-71, 73-76, 83, 105, 107, 126, 129, 132-134, 142, 151, 157, 162-163, 169, 180, 183-186, 190-192, 208-212

Orexin Receptor Antagonists, 1, 3-4, 8, 12-17, 19-23, 25-26, 29, 31, 33, 38-39, 41, 66, 72-73, 92-93, 106-107, 141, 148, 150, 152, 155, 163, 169, 175-176, 194, 209, 211

Orexin Receptors, 1-3, 23, 28-30, 33, 38-40, 46, 55, 58, 65, 70, 72, 78, 104-109, 126, 128-130, 143-148, 151-153, 160, 169, 173, 184, 189-192, 194-197, 210-211

Orexin Signaling, 8-9, 14, 19, 40, 64, 67, 70-73, 75, 78, 105, 131, 133, 139, 141-142, 152-153, 173, 195, 198, 206, 208-210

Orexin-mediated Excitation, 194, 199, 208

Orx Receptors, 49

P
Perifornical Area, 1, 4, 48, 66, 139, 176

Pharmacogenetics, 144, 148, 152, 155

Pharmacokinetics, 8, 12, 22, 84, 96, 106, 110-113, 141

Pharmacotherapeutics, 194, 209

Phosphorylation, 35, 117-118, 147

Polydipsia-hyponatremia, 144, 153

Protein Kinases, 127, 145

Proteolytic Processing, 145, 148

R
Rebound Insomnia, 26-27, 31

Receptor Sequence Variation, 150, 152

S
Sleep Fragmentation, 93, 173

Sleep Latencies, 26, 30, 169

Slice Fixation, 196

Spatial Reference Memory, 86-88, 90

Spatial Working Memory, 86-89, 91

Suvorexant Competition Curves, 109, 111

Synaptic Interactions, 48, 54

www.ingramcontent.com/pod-product-compliance
Lightning Source LLC
Chambersburg PA
CBHW080627200326
41458CB00013B/4535

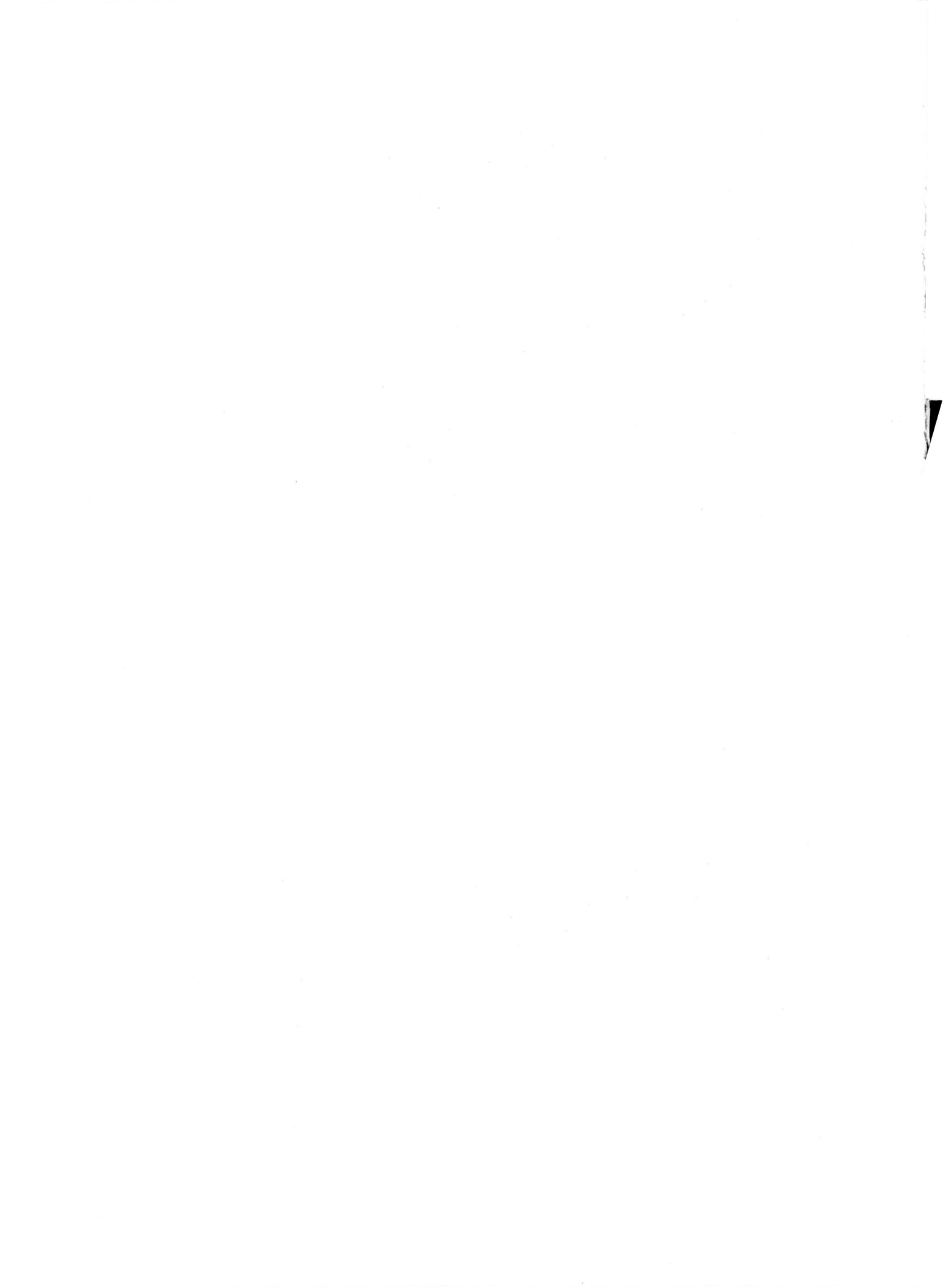